John Brittenden • Damian J.M. Tolan
Editors

Radiology of the Post Surgical Abdomen

Springer

Editors
John Brittenden, MBChB, MRCP, FRCR
Department of Radiology
Mid Yorkshire Hospitals NHS Trust
Wakefield
UK

Damian J.M. Tolan, MBChB, MRCP, FRCR
Department of Clinical Radiology
Leeds Teaching Hospitals NHS Trust
Lincoln Wing
St James's University Hospital
Leeds
UK

ISBN 978-1-4471-2774-1 e-ISBN 978-1-4471-2775-8
DOI 10.1007/978-1-4471-2775-8
Springer London Heidelberg New York Dordrecht

Library of Congress Control Number: 2012933966

Printed on acid-free paper

Springer is part of Springer Science+Business Media (www.springer.com)

To our teachers and patients.
To our wives, our children and our parents.

John and Damian

Foreword

I am very grateful to have been asked to write the Foreword for *Radiology of the Post Surgical Abdomen*, edited by John Brittenden and Damian Tolan.

Generally, I refuse when asked to do this sort of thing – writing a decent Foreword means (to me at least) that you have to read the book. That takes time so the topic just has to be interesting; it often isn't. I also think that anyone taking on the task of assembling a medical textbook in this day and age is either very brave, very foolish, or a bit of both: Books are dwindling in importance as the Internet assumes prominence for those seeking rapid answers. Books are not indexed in medical databases (so why not write a research article instead?), and – most importantly – they are a phenomenal amount of work for relatively little reward (if any).

However, when I saw the topic, I agreed immediately. For many years I worked at a hospital dedicated solely to small bowel and lower-gastrointestinal surgery. I rapidly found out (to my cost) that the cornerstone of sensible radiological diagnosis was a deep understanding of the surgical procedures undertaken, their post operative appearances, and their potential complications. Believe me, declaring the blind loop of an end-to-side anastomosis a "leak" wins you few friends and simultaneously makes you look an idiot. A few years ago I moved to a hospital that does a lot of upper gastrointestinal surgery. I will admit that I have never really taken this head on, preferring to stay within my colorectal comfort zone. Furthermore, the surgeons are rather "remote", so the opportunity for face-to-face interaction is uncommon, especially since there is no upper GI surgery MDT on our site. So, Chapters 2 and 3 of this book were the perfect opportunity to put this straight, as it was increasingly embarrassing for the Professor of Gastrointestinal Radiology to be ignorant of such matters.

And when I read them, I was struck immediately by how informative they are. I found myself straying into the other chapters very easily – everything is here, both gastrointestinal tube and solid organs. Even those retroperitoneal things that GI radiologists (and gynaecologists!) cannot avoid no matter how hard they try are included. I said above that books are a phenomenal amount of work and it really shows here: There are loads of medical images and, even better, tons of informative line diagrams of the sort you wished the surgeon had penned on the back of the request form (but never does). Some of these are really quite exquisite and a huge amount of work in themselves. The Chapter Authors are well known and can write with credibility and authority.

So, was this a phenomenal amount of work? Yes, clearly! Quite frankly, I am gob smacked at the volume of effort here. Were the Editors and their co-Authors mad to take this on? No, I think not because, for once, I do genuinely believe that this book covers a very important gap in the market. A very wise mentor of mine once described abdomino-pelvic radiology as the last bastion of "general radiology". None of us can avoid the "abdo/pelvis CT scan please", especially in the postoperative patient who is "going off" Crackerjack style (...it's Friday, it's 5 o'clock…). For those situations and others, this book is immediately useful and immensely practical. It is destined to be one of the most useful "bench books" in any department.

March 2012

Steve Halligan
Professor of Gastrointestinal Radiology
University College London

Preface

When we first commenced this project, our intention was to create a comprehensive bench book for practicing radiologists to address one of the most difficult areas of practice – 'the post surgical abdomen'. This is an area that most radiologists lack confidence in, due to the multiplicity and complexity of modern surgical procedures. However, all radiologists are expected to be able to provide imaging interpretation on such cases as part of an emergency out-of-hours imaging service.

As we developed our ideas we realized the size of the task ahead. We were extremely fortunate to be able to enlist the support and expertise of radiology and surgical colleagues in the North of England to create this volume. In it we have tried to provide a practical guide covering all abdominal procedures including detailed line drawings of post operative anatomy, which is often only properly understood by surgeons and highly specialized gastrointestinal radiologists. In addition there are tips for interpretation and techniques, both for understanding post surgical anatomy and associated complications as well as advice on how to avoid common pitfalls.

We have tried to be as thorough as possible in providing examples of normal and abnormal imaging, using all radiological modalities. These are all cases from our institutions, gathered over the last 5 years and we must thank our surgeons, radiologists and most importantly our patients for the great enjoyment and satisfaction that this work gives us.

In our day to day practice, close cooperation between surgeons and radiologists enormously benefits patients and improves their outcome from surgery. We hope that this textbook will also provide general surgeons with a better understanding of what assistance imaging and radiologists can offer to augment their clinical assessment of post operative patients: indeed this is an area that is increasingly assessed in post graduate surgery examinations.

We ourselves have learned a great deal. We would particularly like to thank our wives (Geraldine and Emma) and our children who have shown great perseverance and forbearance for the many hours we have been immersed in writing this. We hope that you find it useful and that it serves your patients well.

March 2012

John Brittenden
Damian Tolan

Contents

1 **Introduction to the Post Surgical Abdomen** 1
Alan G. Chalmers, David Macafee, Damian J.M. Tolan, and John Brittenden

2 **The Esophagus** 41
Damian J.M. Tolan, Keith M. Harris, Deepak Prasad, and Samir P. Mehta

3 **The Stomach and Duodenum** 71
Damian J.M. Tolan, Keith M. Harris, Deepak Prasad, and Samir P. Mehta

4 **The Pancreas** 127
Krishna Menon, John Brittenden, Simon McPherson, Nikhil M. Bhuskute, and Andrew Smith

5 **The Biliary Tree** 153
Vamshi P. Jagadesham, Maria Sheridan, J. Peter A. Lodge, and John Brittenden

6 **The Liver** 187
J. Ashley Guthrie, Hajamohideen M. Salahudeen, and J. Peter A. Lodge

7 **The Small Bowel** 227
James C. Lenton, Adeshina S. Fawole, John Brittenden, and Damian J.M. Tolan

8 **The Colon** 255
Chris Macklin, John Brittenden, David Jayne, and Damian J.M. Tolan

9 **Genitourinary System** 295
Christopher Wilkinson

Index 317

Contributors

Nikhil M. Bhuskute, MBBS, MS, MRCS, FRCR Department of Radiology, Calderdale and Huddersfield NHS Foundation Trust, Huddersfield, UK

John Brittenden, MBChB, MRCP, FRCR Department of Radiology, Mid Yorkshire Hospitals NHS Trust, Wakefield, UK

Alan G. Chalmers, MBChB, MRCP, FRCR Department of Radiology, Leeds General Infirmary, Leeds Teaching Hospitals NHS Trust, Leeds, UK

Adeshina S. Fawole, MBBS, MD, FRCS Department of Surgery, Mid Yorkshire Hospitals NHS Trust, Wakefield, UK

J. Ashley Guthrie, BA, MB, BChir, MRCP, FRCR Department of Radiology, Leeds Teaching Hospitals NHS Trust, Leeds, UK

Keith M. Harris, FRCSEd, FRCR Department of Clinical Radiology, Leeds Teaching Hospitals NHS Trust, Bexley Wing, St James's University Hospital, Leeds, UK

Vamshi P. Jagadesham, BSc (Hons), MBChB (Hons), MRCS, M.D. Department of Surgery, Yorkshire and Humber Deanery, Leeds, UK

David Jayne, BSc, MB, BCh, MD, FRCS Department of Surgery, St James's University Hospital, Leeds Teaching Hospitals NHS Trust, Leeds, UK

James C. Lenton, MBChB, MRCS(Ed), FRCR Department of Radiology, Mid Yorkshire Hospitals NHS Trust, Wakefield, UK

J. Peter A. Lodge, MD, FRCS Department of Surgery, Leeds Teaching Hospitals NHS Trust, Leeds, UK

David Macafee, MA, DM, FRCS Department of Surgery, James Cook University Hospital, Teesside, Middlesbrough, UK

Chris Macklin, BMedSci, BM, BS, FRCS (Gen Surg), D.M. Department of Surgery, Mid Yorkshire Hospitals NHS Trust, Wakefield, UK

Simon McPherson, MRCP, FRCR, BSc Department of Radiology, Leeds General Infirmary, Leeds Teaching Hospitals NHS Trust, Leeds, UK

Samir P. Mehta, MA, DM (Oxon), FRCS Department of Upper Gastrointestinal Surgery, Leeds Teaching Hospitals NHS Trust, Bexley Wing, St James's University Hospital, Leeds, UK

Krishna Menon, MS, FRCS Department of Surgery, Leeds Teaching Hospitals NHS Trust, Bexley Wing, St James's University Hospital, Leeds, UK

Deepak Prasad, MBBS, MRCP, FRCR Department of Radiology, Bradford Teaching Hospitals NHS Trust, Bradford Royal Infirmary, Bradford, UK

Hajamohideen M. Salahudeen, MBBS, MD, MRCP, FRCR Department of Radiology, Calderdale and Huddersfield NHS Foundation Trust, Huddersfield, UK

Maria Sheridan, MBChB, MRCP, FRCR Department of Radiology, Leeds Teaching Hospitals NHS Trust, Leeds, UK

Andrew Smith, MBBS, DM, FRCS, BSc Department of Surgery, Leeds Teaching Hospitals NHS Trust, Bexley Wing, St James's University Hospital, Leeds, UK

Damian J.M. Tolan, MBChB, MRCP, FRCR Department of Clinical Radiology, Leeds Teaching Hospitals NHS Trust, Bexley Wing, St James's University Hospital, Leeds, UK

Christopher Wilkinson, BSc, MBChB, FRCR Department of Radiology, York NHS Trust, York, UK

List of Abbreviations

APER	Abdominoperineal excision of rectum
AR	Anterior resection
BFFE	Balanced fast field echo
ERCP	Endoscopic retrograde cholangiopancreatography
EUS	Endoscopic ultrasound
FDG	Fluorine 18 flurodeoxyglucose
FIESTA	Fast imaging employing steady state acquisition
FSE	Fast spin echo
HASTE	Half-Fourier acquisition single-shot turbo spin echo
HIDA	Hepatobiliary imino diacetic acid
HCC	Hepatocellular carcinoma
IOC	Intra operative cholangiogram
IRA	Ileorectal anastomosis
LHC	Left hemicolectomy
MIP	Maximum intensity projection
MRCP	Magnetic resonance cholangiopancreatography
PC	Proctocolectomy
PET	Positron emission tomography
RFA	Radiofrequency ablation
RHC	Right hemicolectomy
RIG	Radiological insertion of gastrostomy
STC	Subtotal colectomy
TACE	Trans catheter arterial chemoembolisation
TC	Total colectomy
True FISP	Fast imaging with steady state precession

Introduction to the Post Surgical Abdomen

1

Alan G. Chalmers, David Macafee, Damian J.M. Tolan, and John Brittenden

Contents

1.1 **Introduction** ... 2

1.2 **CT Protocol/Technique Optimization for Postoperative Imaging** ... 2
1.2.1 Luminal Contrast ... 2
1.2.2 Intravenous Contrast ... 3
1.2.3 Slice Thickness/Collimation ... 5
1.2.4 Anatomical Coverage ... 5
1.2.5 Single-Phase Versus Multiphase Acquisition ... 5

1.3 **The Normal Postoperative Abdomen** ... 6
1.3.1 "Smoke of Battle" ... 6
1.3.2 Postoperative Free Gas ... 6
1.3.3 The "Wet" Patient ... 7
1.3.4 Basal Pulmonary Atelectasis ... 7

1.4 **Postoperative Findings That Serve to Confuse** ... 8
1.4.1 Preexisting Pathology ... 8
1.4.2 Surgical Material Left Behind Deliberately ... 9

1.5 **The Abnormal Postoperative Abdomen** ... 11
1.5.1 Generalized Peritonitis ... 11
1.5.2 Fluid Collections and Abscesses ... 11
1.5.3 Spontaneous Bacterial Peritonitis ... 13
1.5.4 Postoperative Leaks ... 13
1.5.5 Bowel Obstruction Versus Ileus and Pseudoobstruction ... 14

1.6 **Iatrogenic Postoperative Problems** ... 16
1.6.1 Drain-Related Events ... 16
1.6.2 Intraoperative Injury ... 18
1.6.3 Hemorrhage ... 19
1.6.4 Omental Infarction ... 19
1.6.5 Specific Patterns of Postoperative Complications ... 20
1.6.6 Surgical Material Left in Error ... 21
1.6.7 Retained Foreign Material ... 21

1.7 **Complications Related to Laparoscopic Surgery** ... 22
1.7.1 General Surgical Principles of Laparoscopic Surgery ... 22
1.7.2 Patterns of Complications ... 25
1.7.3 Specific Complications ... 27

1.8 **Wound Complications** ... 28

1.9 **Assorted Problems in the Postoperative Abdomen** ... 29
1.9.1 Acute Colitis ... 29
1.9.2 Small Bowel Ischemia ... 30
1.9.3 Portal Vein Thrombosis (PVT) ... 32
1.9.4 Neutropenic Enterocolitis ... 32
1.9.5 The Other Postoperative "-itis's" ... 32

1.10 **Image-Guided Drainage** ... 34
1.10.1 Route of Access ... 34

A.G. Chalmers, MBChB, MRCP, FRCR
Department of Radiology, Leeds General Infirmary, Leeds Teaching Hospitals NHS Trust, Leeds, UK

D. Macafee, MA, DM, FRCS
Department of Surgery, James Cook University Hospital, Teesside, Middlesbrough, UK

D.J.M. Tolan, MBChB, MRCP, FRCR (✉)
Department of Clinical Radiology, Leeds Teaching Hospitals NHS Trust, Lincoln Wing, St James's University Hospital, LS9 7JT, Leeds, UK
e-mail: damian.tolan@leedsth.nhs.uk

J. Brittenden, MBChB, MRCP, FRCR
Department of Radiology, Mid Yorkshire Hospitals NHS Trust, Wakefield, UK
e-mail: john.brittenden@midyorks.nhs.uk

J. Brittenden, D.J.M. Tolan (eds.), *Radiology of the Post Surgical Abdomen*,
DOI 10.1007/978-1-4471-2775-8_1,

1.10.2 Choice of Modality ... 34
1.10.3 Consent ... 35
1.10.4 Assessment of Coagulation Status ... 35
1.10.5 Drainage Technique ... 36

1.11 Principles of Fluoroscopy and Ultrasound in the Postoperative Patient ... 37
1.11.1 Fluoroscopy: General Considerations ... 37
1.11.2 Ultrasound: General Considerations ... 38

References ... 39

1.1 Introduction

In any hospital with a busy acute and elective surgical service, complications associated with a patient's postoperative recovery account for a significant number of requests for acute imaging. These requests also account for an increasing proportion of the workload for radiologists providing an on-call service, who have varying degrees of expertise in gastrointestinal imaging. It is therefore important for radiologists who are asked to report these studies to be familiar with the postoperative anatomy of the more commonly encountered surgical procedures and their potential complications. This chapter aims to address the basics of postoperative imaging, with an emphasis on CT, and give an overview of what might be encountered in the post surgical abdomen. Specific surgical techniques and the radiological changes they produce will be addressed in subsequent dedicated chapters.

In general terms, reporting a postoperative study is usually a straightforward exercise, assuming the radiologist is aware of the post surgical anatomy and the specific clinical concerns that led to the request. The most common queries are:

- Is ileus or obstruction present?
- Is there any support for ischemic compromise?
- Has the anastomosis leaked, and are there any drainable collections?

These and similar issues will be addressed in the sections that follow along with an assortment of more chance findings that can have important management implications.

This chapter will focus on CT appearances, but it should be remembered that ultrasound has a complementary role to play especially in children and younger females. However, drain sites, abdominal wall dressings, and problems associated with gas-filled bowel loops may conspire to make ultrasound a technically difficult procedure with limited exclusion value in this group of patients.

As with most radiological interpretation, the difficulty often lies in differentiating between what are acceptable and expected postoperative/post surgical changes ("the smoke of battle") from significant pathologies that might require an alteration in patient management. Close clinical and radiological dialogue is paramount when reporting studies of the postoperative abdomen, as often the clinical detail on the radiology request card may not tell the whole story.

1.2 CT Protocol/Technique Optimization for Postoperative Imaging

CT is the modality of choice for imaging the postoperative abdomen in most complex cases (Bader et al. 2009), and a brief review of the various protocols follows. Multidetector CT (MDCT) has had a major impact. This technology allows rapid image acquisition and multiplanar reconstruction, which has advantages when imaging the sick patient and interpreting complex appearances of the post surgical abdomen. For the radiologist supervising the study, the following factors require consideration:

- Choice of bowel contrast
- Choice of slice thickness reconstruction
- Whether intravenous contrast is indicated or necessary
- Choice of single or multiphase study

1.2.1 Luminal Contrast

The use of oral bowel contrast varies from department to department, and what follows is very much a personal view based on the author's current departmental practice. Positive or neutral contrast options are available. For a general postoperative survey, which accounts for the majority of studies, positive contrast should be considered the norm. Whether dilute barium or dilute water-soluble contrast is chosen depends on local preference. Iodinated water-soluble agents such as Gastrografin (sodium diatrizoate and meglumine diatrizoate, Bayer Schering Pharma, Newbury, UK) occasionally cause diarrhea. This is an added complication when managing a sick postoperative patient. Neutral contrast, such as water, offers a more benign alternative but is infrequently used in routine practice. Contrast agents that provide a degree of small bowel distension such as Volumen (Bracco, Princeton, USA) which is not licensed in Europe or mannitol are unlikely to be required for this patient group.

The use of oral contrast can be considered in four general situations:

1.2.1.1 Oral Contrast Advisable

For most general postoperative survey examinations and especially when the question posed is whether a collection is present or not (assuming the patient can drink or contrast can be delivered via a nasogastric tube) positive oral contrast has clear benefits for distinguishing between what lies within and what lies outside the gastrointestinal tract. In terms of the volume of oral contrast given, a pragmatic approach should be adopted to achieve a balance between an optimal diagnostic study and what the sick patient can reasonably tolerate. Volumes between 500 and 1,000 ml are typically used.

1.2.1.2 Oral Contrast Unnecessary

For most cases of small and large bowel obstruction, particularly when plain film evidence supports obstruction as the likely diagnosis, oral contrast is best avoided. The fluid content of the obstructed small and large bowel provides excellent natural contrast that makes the use of oral contrast agents both unnecessary and less than kind for a patient who is often vomiting.

1.2.1.3 Oral Contrast Optional

There is an argument for using oral contrast if subacute obstruction is the likely diagnosis. If contrast has reached the colon, after a delay of up to 3–4 h, then complete mechanical small bowel obstruction is effectively excluded. Identifying leaked oral contrast at the site of gastrointestinal perforation can be very helpful, but bowel contrast is not a prerequisite to establishing this diagnosis. Where perforation leads to a contrast leak, water-soluble agents have no adverse effect. If small bowel ischemia is the primary concern, some radiologists choose to avoid positive oral contrast, preferring neutral agents or no oral contrast at all so that any change to the enhancement characteristics of the bowel wall can be better appreciated. The down side of withholding oral contrast is that the assessment of mural enhancement in collapsed segments of bowel can be difficult.

1.2.1.4 Positive Oral Contrast Contraindicated

If the detection of acute GI tract bleeding is the primary clinical concern, positive oral contrast must be avoided in order to optimize the chances of detecting extravasated intravenous contrast within the bowel lumen. Highly concentrated positive oral contrast agents can cause scatter artifact and degrade reconstructed CT angiographic images. They should therefore be avoided particularly where specific endovascular treatments may be required such as embolization.

1.2.1.5 Rectal Contrast

This is potentially underutilized when investigating the postoperative abdomen but on occasion can be very useful to differentiate between leaks and fistulae of small or large bowel origin (Fig. 1.1), as well as aiding the detection of iatrogenic colonic injury. Again, any leaked water-soluble contrast used for colonic opacification will result in no adverse effect.

1.2.2 Intravenous Contrast

Unless contraindicated because of prior contrast allergy or current renal impairment, intravenous contrast is a standard component of most CT

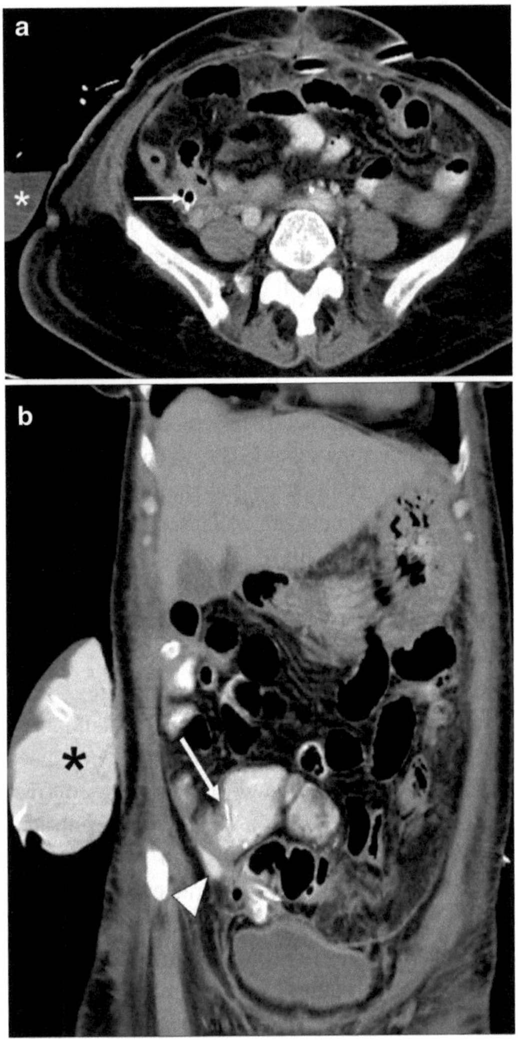

Fig. 1.1 Subtotal colectomy with a suspected leak from the ileorectal anastomosis. Relaparotomy failed to find a source of perforation. (**a**) CT with oral contrast did not identify the source of the leak. The right iliac fossa drain (*white arrow*) contains water density enteric fluid (*asterisk*). (**b**) Repeat CT a few minutes later after infusion of rectal contrast confirms a leak with contrast collecting in the drainage bag (*asterisk*) and right paracolic gutter (*arrowhead*) adjacent to anastomosis (*white arrow*)

protocols for the postoperative abdomen. Typically, a single portal venous phase study works best. Contrast is delivered by a power injector with total injected volumes of 100 ml at a rate of 2.5–3 ml/s. The portal venous phase may be acquired between 60 and 75 s following contrast injection.

In certain clinical situations, adding in additional vascular phases to the CT examination can augment a single-phase study. Examples include investigation of suspected intra-abdominal bleeding or obscure GI tract bleeding when combinations of noncontrast, arterial, portal venous and delayed phases are required to establish the diagnosis. Bolus tracking is mandatory to optimize timing for arterial phase imaging, to mitigate for variations in cardiac output. If iatrogenic renal tract injury is suspected, additional delayed excretory phase can be used to detect collecting system or ureteric abnormalities (Sects. 9.3 and 9.4).

In general, the volume of intravenous contrast used should be as low as possible to minimize the risk of contrast-induced nephropathy, while being enough to allow an accurate diagnosis to be made. Patients at risk of contrast-induced nephropathy are a group including those with the following conditions:

- Preexisting chronic kidney disease (CKD stage 3 or more – eGFR <60 ml/min)
- Dehydration/hypovolemia
- Sepsis or hypotension
- Cardiovascular disease
- Age over 60
- Concomitant use of nephrotoxic drugs (e.g., NSAIDs, ACE inhibitors)

It is obvious that a number of postoperative patients will have one or more of the risk factors on this list. In this setting, it is essential to ensure adequate intravascular volume replacement prior to scanning and that the eGFR is known before the scan in order to stratify risk from contrast injection. Where eGFR is less than 30 ml/min (CKD stage 4 or 5) in a critical care setting, it is appropriate to discuss with a renal specialist regarding contrast administration as predialysis patients may lose a small but important degree of residual renal function that would precipitate introduction of renal support (such as hemofiltration or dialysis).

Although assessment of serum creatinine is a method of charting changes in renal function for an individual, it does not give an accurate measure of renal function alone as other factors such as sex, weight, ethnicity, and age should also be taken into account (e.g., a serum creatinine of

120 μmol/l in a young adult male may be normal but in a small elderly female indicate significant renal dysfunction). The eGFR calculation takes these factors into account along with the creatinine concentration to provide a more accurate estimation of renal function than serum creatinine alone.

It is also important to consider whether there is another imaging modality that could answer the question (e.g., MRI or ultrasound) or whether contrast-enhanced CT is required rather than a noncontrast-enhanced study. If the noncontrast study reveals an obvious abnormality (e.g., bowel obstruction or abscess) as a cause for deterioration, then any risk of nephrotoxicity has been avoided. Where the diagnosis remains unclear (e.g., where there is concern for ischemia or bleeding), then at this stage, contrast injection can be considered in balance with the risks from giving contrast against those from withholding it (and a nondiagnostic study for that specific indication). In these cases, a multidisciplinary approach is required canvassing opinions from the surgical team, critical care specialists, and radiologists.

1.2.3 Slice Thickness/Collimation

In the majority of departments with access to MDCT (eight slice or greater), scans are acquired with a detector collimation of 1 mm or less and reconstructed to 2.5–5 mm slice thickness. This offers a balance between the numbers of images acquired and diagnostic image quality, as noise is more noticeable with a slice thickness of less than 2.5 mm. In most instances, standard reconstruction protocols provide coronal images to allow the supervising radiologist to use a PACS workstation for reporting. However, there are specific instances where additional reconstructions are required for interpretation, such as for mesenteric angiography where thinner slices are required for vessel analysis (typically 1 mm). Specific postprocessing may be necessary for these cases on either a dedicated workstation or integrated reconstruction package within PACS. It is important for the reporting radiologist to recognize situations where returning to the source data and manipulating the reconstructed images can assist in improving the accuracy of diagnosis.

1.2.4 Anatomical Coverage

Images should be acquired from just above the diaphragm to just below the symphysis pubis, assuming there is no concern for thoracic pathology (e.g., pulmonary embolus). Limiting coverage to only the abdomen and excluding the pelvis makes no sense when examining the postoperative abdomen since both compartments are interconnected, and complications do not respect this arbitrary boundary. For the remainder of this chapter, it is assumed that full coverage is obtained. The only potential exception may be where follow-up of a localized collection is required, inaccessible to ultrasound evaluation (e.g., deep pelvic abscess or pancreatic collection).

Generally, the thorax is not scanned unless there are clear clinical indications, usually based on the surgical procedure (e.g., esophagogastric surgery) or any specific clinical concerns at the time (e.g., respiratory compromise).

1.2.5 Single-Phase Versus Multiphase Acquisition

Although MDCT can provide rapid whole body coverage with multiple-phase acquisitions, a balance must be struck between the protocol chosen and the likely benefit to the patient taking account the resulting radiation dose. This will be proportional to the area of coverage and number of phases acquired. Modern CT scanners employ dose reduction, such as real-time dose modulation, iterative reconstruction and collimation modification to help reduce radiation dose, but a postoperative patient can receive a significant cumulative radiation dose when frequent repeat studies are requested in a patient with a prolonged postoperative complication. It is the responsibility of the radiologist to ensure that studies using ionizing radiation are kept to the minimum necessary for safe patient management while at the same time considering alternative options such as ultrasound and MRI where appropriate.

1.3 The Normal Postoperative Abdomen

The most commonly encountered findings can be broadly grouped into the following categories:

- Post surgical changes ("smoke of battle")
- Postoperative free gas
- The "wet" patient
- Basal pulmonary atelectasis
- Postoperative findings that serve to confuse (i.e., preexisting pathology and surgical material left behind deliberately)

1.3.1 "Smoke of Battle"

Images of the postoperative abdomen are rarely free of post surgical change, even when the procedure has been straightforward and free from complications. Patchy increased peritoneal or retroperitoneal fat density will usually be found in the immediate perioperative bed and in the abdominal wall around the incision site. These findings are largely of no clinical consequence and their description (e.g., edematous change, "dirty fat", or other terms should reflect that). Such changes are frequently reported as "inflammatory." They may or may not be, but it is important when reporting not to give the impression of significant "corruption" heralding a serious complication.

Some surgical operations are more complex than others, and the imaging findings can raise alarm (Fig. 1.2). Following upper GI surgery, small fluid collections are seen anterior to the pancreatic bed that can be mistaken for intraoperative pancreatic injury or acute pancreatitis. Being aware that these findings may be encountered after an uncomplicated upper GI surgical procedure can be helpful in preventing a diagnostic overcall, but as always, clinicoradiological correlation is required before any firm conclusions are drawn.

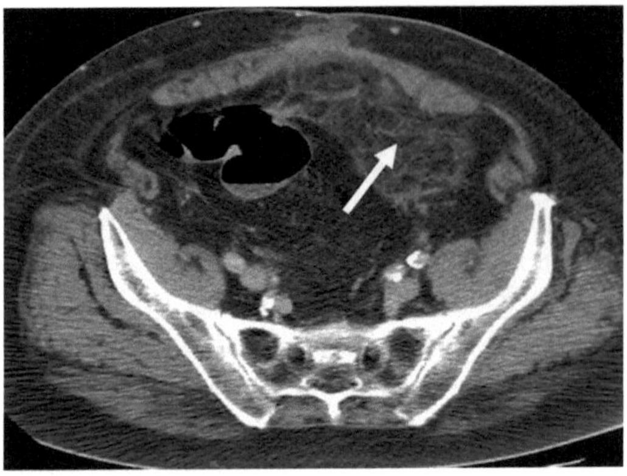

Fig. 1.2 "Smoke of battle." One week post subtotal colectomy. Increased fat density involving the infracolic omentum with mass-like elements supporting omental infarction (*arrow*). Follow-up imaging (*not shown*) several months later showed complete resolution

Where there has been significant and prolonged bowel handling (e.g., following extensive adhesiolysis), the small bowel may appear very abnormal. Mural thickening, variable bowel caliber and interloop edema can produce an alarming appearance and closely mimic the findings of ischemic change. Again, correlation with the patient's clinical status and biochemistry is necessary.

1.3.2 Postoperative Free Gas

Free intraperitoneal gas on a postoperative CT can be problematic for the radiologist when trying to decide whether all can be attributed to retained post surgical air alone or whether the gas is a consequence of perforation, anastomotic leak, or infection. The traditional radiological literature on postoperative intraperitoneal gas is based on plain abdominal radiograph findings (Earls et al. 1993). CT is significantly more sensitive in detecting postoperative gas than conventional radiographs especially in the obese patient or in the presence of a postoperative ileus, with CT demonstrating free gas in 87% on day 3 and 50% on day 6 compared with 53% and 8% with plain films taken at the same time (Earls et al. 1993). The reported average prevalence of persisting free gas on a CT is approximately 44% on postoperative day 3 and 30% between days 4 and 18

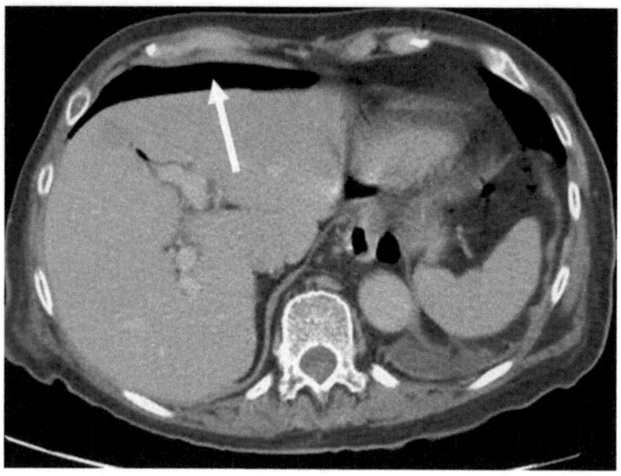

Fig. 1.3 Excess intraperitoneal air 10 days post laparoscopic sigmoid colectomy. Gas is noted in the right anterior perihepatic space (*arrow*) along with multiple smaller foci in the left upper quadrant anterior to the spleen and adjacent to the gastroesophageal junction

(Gayer et al. 2000). However, small traces of free gas can be demonstrated for up to 24 days following surgery, indicating a potential extended time line for this finding.

The advent of laparoscopic surgery has complicated interpretation by introducing an alternative time line due to carbon dioxide dissipating at a significantly faster rate than air. Animal studies have suggested that gas should be expected to resolve by day 2, with any persisting gas after this time likely to reflect a pathological process. Nevertheless, interpretation is often a matter of judgment as to whether an excess of free gas remains. As a rule of thumb, gas from an open procedure should have largely resolved by 7–10 days and for a laparoscopic procedure by day 2 (Fig. 1.3). When doubt remains, the option of a follow-up CT study may help. Uncomplicated postoperative gas should always diminish with time. Any increasing free gas volume should alert the radiologist to consider infection or an anastomotic leak as a likely explanation.

Distinction should be made between intraperitoneal and retroperitoneal gas. Unless drainage catheters are located in the retroperitoneal spaces, gas here generally indicates pathology. Examples would include perforation from the duodenum and rectosigmoid, retroperitoneal infection, and trauma either resulting from iatrogenic injury (e.g., ERCP or endoscopy) or another cause.

1.3.2.1 Iatrogenic Causes of Free Intraperitoneal Air

Surgical drains, radiologically placed catheters and peritoneal dialysis catheters can all lead to free intraperitoneal gas and should be factored in to any discussion regarding the significance of free gas, particularly when present in only a small volume.

1.3.3 The "Wet" Patient

Fluid retention, fluid overload, and hypoproteinemia are common findings in the postoperative patient with comorbidities such as cardiac or renal failure. This typically results in a picture of generalized fluid retention that may produce combinations of the following:

- Bilateral pleural effusions (not always of equal volume)
- Low-volume ascites
- Generalized subcutaneous fat edema
- Edematous mesenteric fat
- A small increase in the expected volume of pericardial fluid

The above should be differentiated from excessive localized fluid or edematous change resulting from inflammation, postoperative leaks, or collections. Some conditions, such as acute pancreatitis, result in fairly predictable distributions of fluid involving the retroperitoneal and peritoneal spaces. Similarly localized and loculated fluid alone (e.g., in one paracolic gutter or between leaves of the mesenteries) should not be readily dismissed as simply related to edema without other explanations being excluded such as ischemia. Always check the appearance of the pleural surfaces when pleural fluid is noted. Pleural enhancement may indicate an empyema that offers an alternative explanation for the patient's pyrexia and elevated white cell count.

1.3.4 Basal Pulmonary Atelectasis

Some atelectasis is almost the norm for a postoperative patient, and varying degrees of collapsed enhancing lung will be present at both lung bases. Enhancement is characteristic, and with an

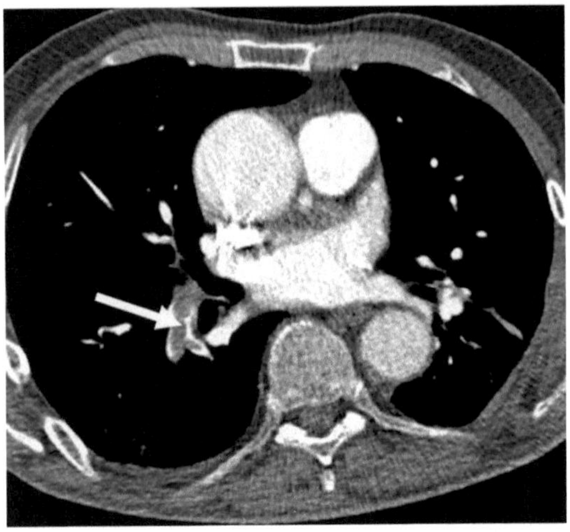

Fig. 1.4 Occult pulmonary embolic disease. Postoperative abdominal CT demonstrated a possible filling defect in a right lower lobe segmental artery at the level of the lung bases (*not shown*). The patient was recalled for a CT pulmonary angiogram which confirmed extensive pulmonary embolic disease (*arrow*)

absence of a recognizable air bronchogram, the often used description "consolidation" is best avoided. This is generally not infection but represents passive atelectasis occurring with or without an associated pleural effusion and of limited or no clinical consequence. For intensive care patients, these changes can be particularly prominent. Although the whole chest is not routinely covered as part of a standard postoperative abdominal examination, a few sections through the lung bases will be provided in most patients. Careful review of the basal pulmonary arterial branches may reveal occult pulmonary embolic disease. This can be a difficult diagnosis if reconstructed slice thickness is wide, but if there is sufficient suspicion and no firm diagnosis is possible, a recall for a dedicated CT pulmonary angiogram is appropriate (Fig. 1.4).

1.4 Postoperative Findings That Serve to Confuse

- Preexisting pathology
- Surgical material left on purpose

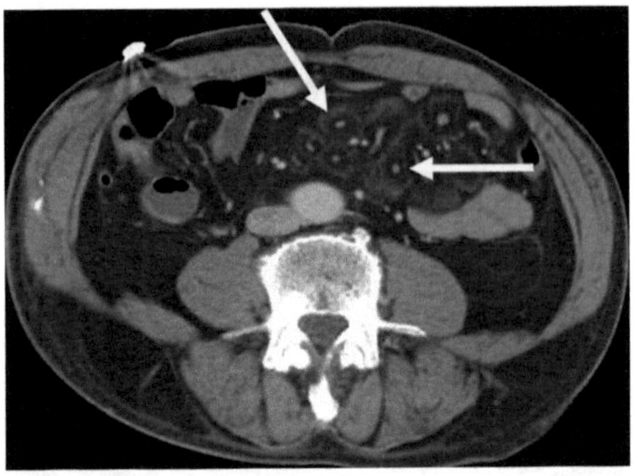

Fig. 1.5 Mesenteric panniculitis. Classic example of increased mesenteric fat density, with normal fat density retained around the mesenteric vessels. This appearance is described as the *fat halo sign* (*arrows*)

1.4.1 Preexisting Pathology

It is probable that any preexisting pathology will have already been documented on a preoperative imaging study. Nevertheless, emergency surgery may have been performed without any prior imaging and referral to earlier examinations on PACS, or reports in the clinical record may help. In some cases, liaison with outside hospitals is required to obtain relevant imaging, particularly where a patient has been referred for very specialist surgery.

Incidental "pathology" such as mesenteric panniculitis, a usually asymptomatic benign inflammatory condition of the mesentery, can lead to confusion. Here, the CT abnormalities range from subtle increased mesenteric fat density, the "misty mesentery," to the more mass-mimicking desmoid disease. The characteristic central mesenteric location, an encapsulated periphery, a perivascular fat halo (Fig. 1.5), and low-volume mesenteric lymphadenopathy should help differentiate from a more acute postoperative inflammatory process.

Similarly, the presence of hydronephrosis or ureteric dilatation may be long standing or acute. While cortical atrophy may indicate chronicity along with small renal size, reduced renal enhancement and perinephric fat stranding may indicate acute pathology; comparison with prior imaging is important to help prioritize the need and appropriateness of urgent intervention such as nephrostomy or ureteric stent placement.

1.4.2 Surgical Material Left Behind Deliberately

1.4.2.1 Hemostatic Compounds

Any material deliberately left behind can create diagnostic difficulty, and especially problematic are the changes related to the use of hemostatic agents of which Surgicel (Ethicon, Livingston, UK) is one of the more widely encountered. This is a bioabsorbable hemostatic agent made of oxidized regenerated cellulose that may be removed from the abdomen following control of bleeding or left behind after abdominal closure. When left behind, Surgicel is gradually reabsorbed over 7–14 days, but there are reports of significantly longer retention.

There are two fundamental points to remember regarding the use of Surgicel or other hemostatic agents:

- Surgeons rarely tell you when they have used this product (!).
- The imaging appearance of Surgicel can closely mimic an intra-abdominal abscess.

Surgicel appears as a low attenuation mass on CT that characteristically contains punctate, linear, and often peripheral gas foci (Young et al. 1993). If unenhanced and postcontrast images are available, Surgicel will show no contrast enhancement. Surgicel is hypointense on T2W MR imaging compared to a true abscess that would typically be hyperintense. Unexpected gas containing collections at sites away from where the clinical concerns lie should be viewed with suspicion and referred to the surgeon for clarification. Specifically, whether hemostatic agents have been used or not should be established before any diagnosis of unexpected abscess is made. Common sites for the use of Surgicel include around the pancreatic tail and spleen, both of which can be injured during mobilization of the left colon (Sect. 8.2.4.7); in the gallbladder fossa following cholecystectomy; and in the pelvis after rectal or gynecological surgery (Figs. 1.6 and 1.7).

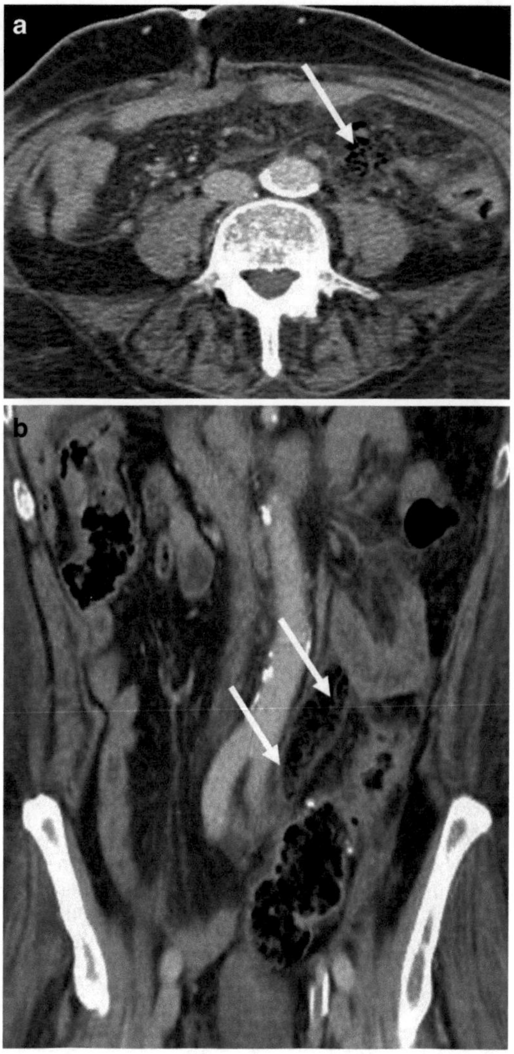

Fig. 1.6 Surgicel. (**a**) Axial and (**b**) coronal CT images from a patient who recently underwent a sigmoid colectomy complicated intraoperatively by bleeding below the pancreatic tail at the time of splenic flexure mobilization. Hemostasis was achieved by application of Surgicel (*arrows*) which can mimic focal abscess formation. Information regarding the use of hemostatic agents is rarely shared with the radiologist prior to CT

1.4.2.2 Meshes

The majority of meshes in current use for abdominal surgery are made of polypropylene or polyfluoroethylene and are sometimes identified by the coil like metallic studs or rivets anchoring it along the anterior abdominal wall (Fig. 1.8). When mesh studs detach, hernia recurrence is likely. Occasionally, a detached mesh can lead to an acute abdomen, for example, small bowel obstruction (Fig. 1.9). There are concerns regarding the use of mesh products for the repair of

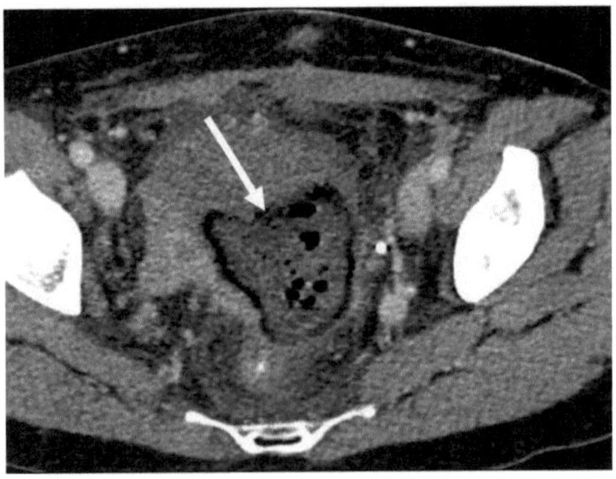

Fig. 1.7 Surgicel. Post-hysterectomy patient in whom pelvic and retroperitoneal bleeding required control with Surgicel packing (*arrow*). Note the predominantly peripheral location of the gas foci, which is a common finding with hemostatic agents

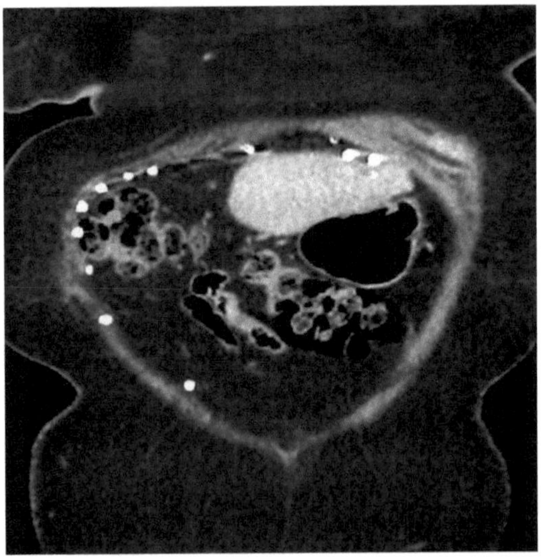

Fig. 1.8 Coronal CT showing peripheral metallic stud alignment following an uncomplicated anterior abdominal wall mesh

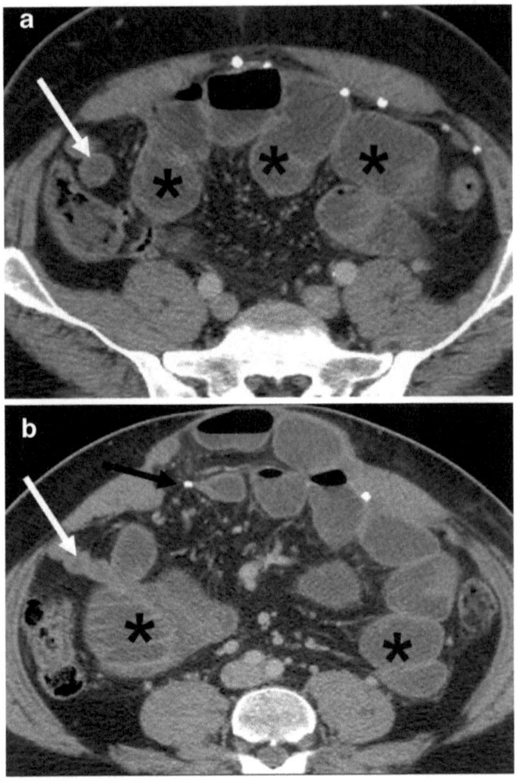

Fig. 1.9 Detached mesh. (**a**) CT shows normal mesh attachments but a combination of fluid-filled dilated small bowel loops (*asterisks*), and segments of nondistended small bowel (*white arrows*) indicate established small bowel obstruction. (**b**) Several centimeters cephalad, there is a detached segment of mesh with recurrence of the anterior hernia. A mesh stud lies at the point of small bowel transition (*black arrow*). This was confirmed at laparotomy where a section of mesh had become detached, allowing herniation of a small bowel loop anteriorly through the defect and leading to small bowel obstruction

parastomal and other hernias due to risk of small bowel erosion, leading to perforation and abscess formation (Fig. 1.10) (Ott et al. 2005).

Rarely, meshes made from pigskin are encountered that can lead to diagnostic and interventional difficulties. On a postcontrast study, a pigskin mesh can closely mimic the abnormal peritoneal enhancement seen in patients with peritonitis (Fig. 1.11). The other signs of peritonitis will usually be absent which will help with diagnosis. Another problem with any meshes is that they act as a very effective barrier to needle puncture, therefore limiting any interventional approach to an underlying collection.

Special consideration should be made when performing image-guided intervention in patients with abdominal meshes in two specific instances. First, in patients with a clearly infected mesh, this acts as a foreign body and conservative treatment with antibiotics, and drainage of collections is

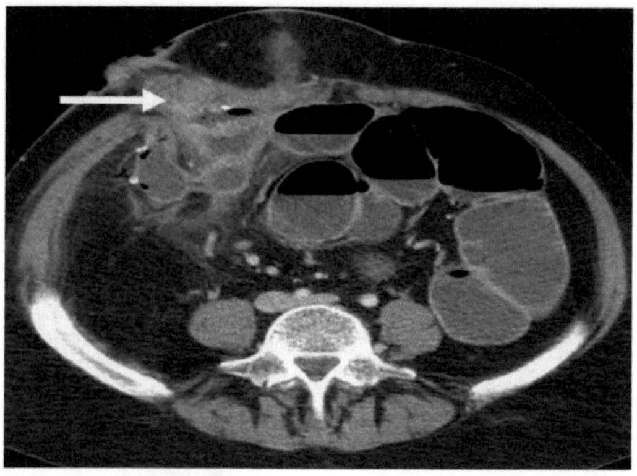

Fig. 1.10 Mesh-related erosion. Patient with an ileostomy and parastomal hernia who underwent mesh repair. Axial CT shows dilated loops of small bowel, and an inflammatory phlegmon in the right anterior abdominal wall (*arrow*) tethered to the adjacent small bowel. At operation, mesh had eroded into the adjacent small bowel, leading to perforation, abscess formation, and small bowel obstruction

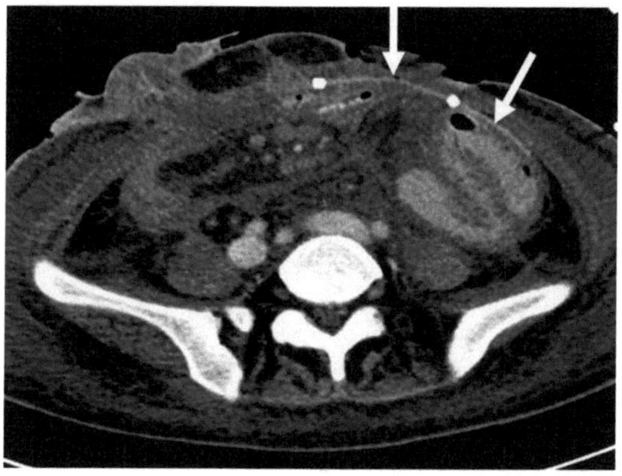

Fig. 1.11 Pigskin mesh. Postoperative study in an edematous patient showing the apparent "enhancement" of high-density pigskin mesh (*arrows*). These are rarely used but can be easily misinterpreted as increased peritoneal enhancement found with peritonitis

seldom successful and usually requires removal of the mesh that is the nidus of infection. Second, radiologists should exercise particular care in traversing a mesh to treat intra-abdominal collections for two reasons: the mesh may itself become infected, and inserting a drain through a mesh is virtually impossible.

1.5 The Abnormal Postoperative Abdomen

1.5.1 Generalized Peritonitis

This is usually a straightforward clinical diagnosis, but CT has an important role and is highly accurate (Bader et al. 2009). Radiology in this scenario may also indicate unexpected peritonitis in patients that are difficult to assess clinically such as those who are immunosuppressed, the obese, and unconscious patients in intensive care units.

Signs to look for include:

- Patchy increased attenuation of the mesenteric fat
- Variable amounts of ascites (typically low-volume) and pockets of interloop fluid
- Thickening and enhancement of peritoneal reflections (Fig. 1.12)

1.5.2 Fluid Collections and Abscesses

Uncomplicated intraperitoneal fluid tends to configure to the space it finds itself in, as well as accumulating in the more dependent peritoneal recesses such as in the pelvis. It is important to assess the density of fluid, and an "eyeball" comparison with known simple fluid density structures such as the urinary bladder should help differentiate transudate from a postoperative hemoperitoneum (Fig. 1.13).

Abscesses are fluid collections that can have an impact and influence on neighboring anatomy, with a tendency to displace and distort adjacent structures. They typically show an enhancing margin of variable thickness with gas only in the minority of cases (Fig. 1.14).When an abscess or cavity contains semisolid feculent material rather than simple fluid content, and an anastomosis has clearly dehisced, percutaneous drainage is less likely to succeed, and surgical intervention is often required (Fig. 1.15). However, clinical discussion is required in this circumstance as some patients can be effectively temporized by initial

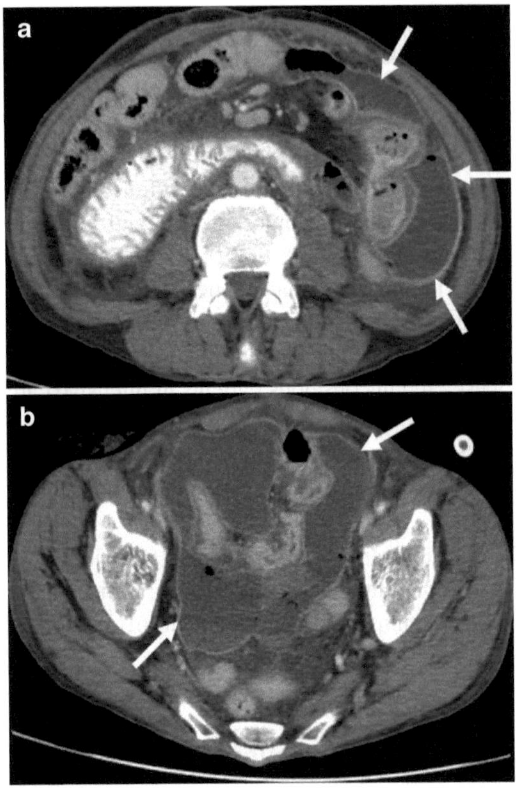

Fig. 1.12 (**a**, **b**) An example of increased peritoneal enhancement in a patient with peritonitis and multiple abdominal collections following a leak from an ileoanal pouch (*arrows*). Note similarity to the pigskin mesh appearances in Fig. 1.11

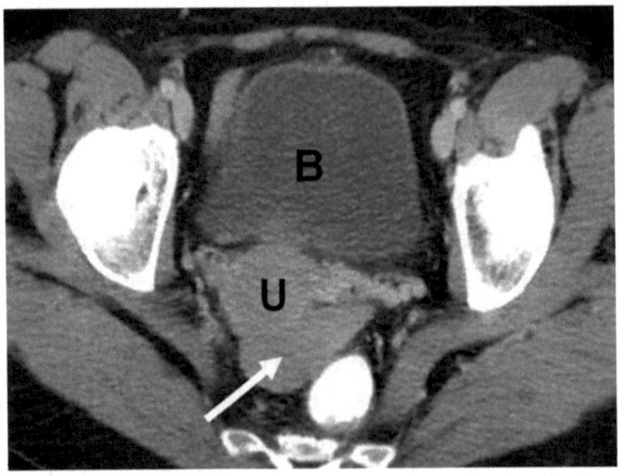

Fig. 1.13 Hemoperitoneum. Axial CT from a female patient showing high-density fluid (*arrow*) located between contrast-filled rectum posteriorly and uterus (*U*) and bladder (*B*) anteriorly. Water density of the urinary bladder serves as useful point of reference when evaluating the density of pelvic fluid

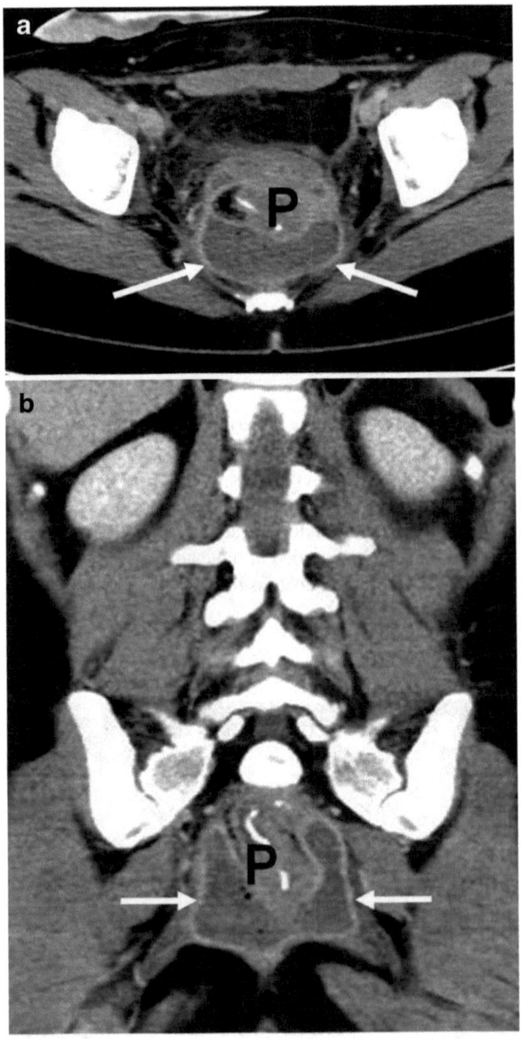

Fig. 1.14 Pelvic abscess 2 weeks post proctectomy. (**a**) Axial and (**b**) coronal CT images show a peripouch abscess that adopts a horseshoe configuration around the posterior margin of the pouch (*P*). The collection has an enhancing margin (*arrows*) and contains several tiny foci of gas

percutaneous drainage, particularly where they are unfit to return to theater immediately.

It must be remembered that CT is a poor technique for characterizing the internal characteristics of fluid collections. What can appear as simple fluid density on CT can in practice be predominantly solid or multiloculated, a situation not uncommonly encountered when assessing

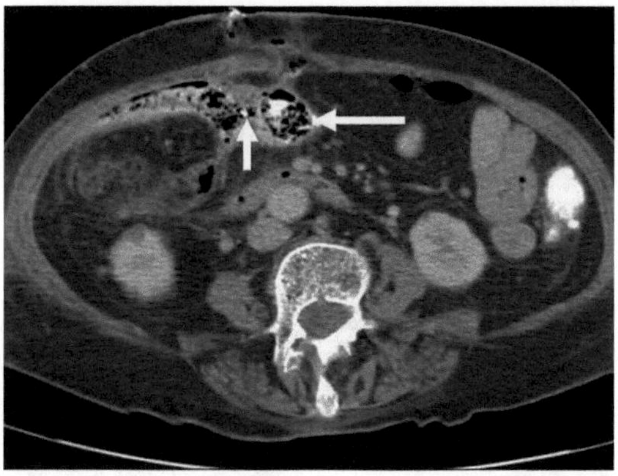

Fig. 1.15 Anastomotic leak 1 week post right hemicolectomy. Disruption of the anastomosis (*small arrow*) associated with a leak of contrast and feculent material (*long arrow*). This was not amenable to percutaneous drainage

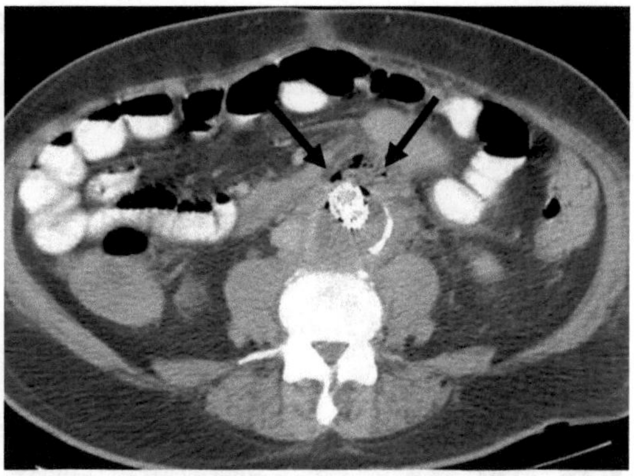

Fig. 1.16 Patient after endovascular abdominal aortic aneurysm repair developed an aortoenteric fistula as a postprocedure complication. During surgical fistula repair, a piece of omentum was interposed between small bowel and the aorta that subsequently became infected. The poorly demarcated soft tissue and gas densities anterior to the aortic stent graft represent the infected interposed omentum (*black arrows*)

pancreatitis-related collections. Ultrasound and MR are superior for characterizing the content of potentially drainable collections (Sects. 1.10.2 and 1.11.2).

Unusual patterns of sepsis may be encountered as a consequence of the surgical procedure. Omental interposition may be used during vascular surgery with enteric complications. This can become infected, leading to confusing appearances on CT (Fig. 1.16). Again, the usual rule applies; discussion with the referring clinician or reference to the surgical record often explains peculiarities found on postoperative imaging.

Any mention of a collection in a CT report invariably triggers a surgical "knee jerk" response with an instant request for percutaneous drainage. It is therefore helpful when a collection is found that the size, location, confidence that it represents an abscess (e.g. rim enhancement), and the potential for safe image-guided drainage should be recorded. Direct clinical discussion following the study is often best to correlate with the patient clinical status.

1.5.3 Spontaneous Bacterial Peritonitis

This is an acute bacterial infection of ascitic fluid with typically no causative source of sepsis identified. Adults with cirrhosis are at particular risk, but the condition can be encountered in noncirrhotics who are undergoing peritoneal dialysis (Ergün and Lakadamyal 2012). When established, the prognosis is poor. Imaging has little role to play other than excluding other causes of peritonitis (e.g., presence of free gas or colonic wall thickening). If suspected in a postoperative patient, peritoneal fluid aspiration and culture are required to confirm the diagnosis.

1.5.4 Postoperative Leaks

Spiking temperatures, a rising white cell count, raised inflammatory markers, and a failure of the patient to progress as clinically expected are often the hallmarks of a postoperative leak. On CT, specific features to evaluate are:

- An excess of fluid in the surgical bed adjacent to an anastomosis (Fig. 1.17)
- An excess of extraluminal gas
- A disrupted anastomotic staple line (Fig. 1.18)

Postoperative leaks are discussed in greater detail in later chapters.

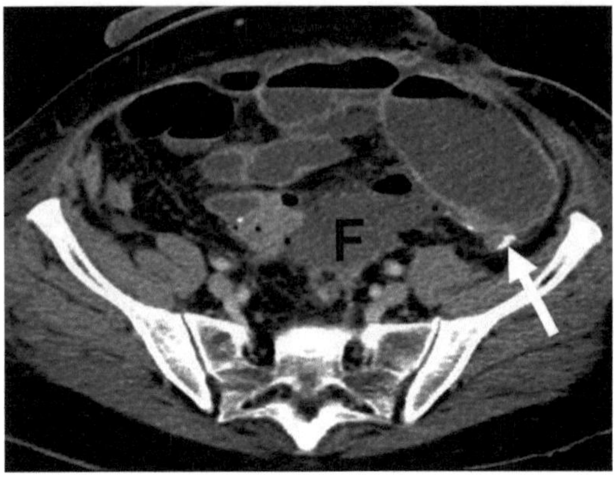

Fig. 1.17 Postoperative leak. A prolonged surgical procedure that included a small bowel resection, extensive adhesiolysis, and multiple enterotomies. Poorly marginated pelvic fluid collection (*F*) lying in the midline just above the urinary bladder with an air fluid level. Anastomosis (*arrow*). There is no route for image guided drainage

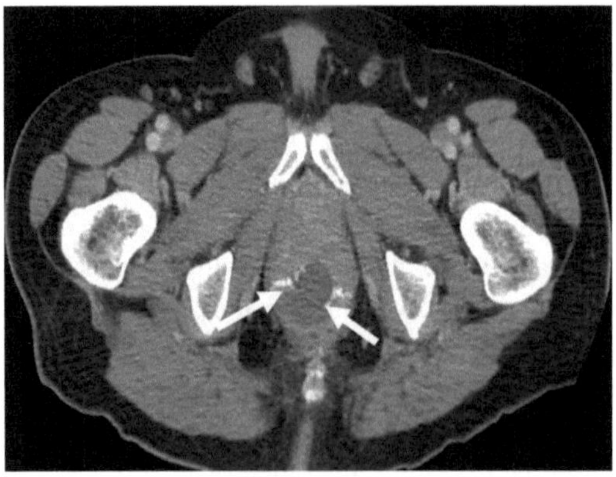

Fig. 1.18 Anastomotic breakdown post low anterior resection. Axial section showing an open surgical suture line (*arrows*)

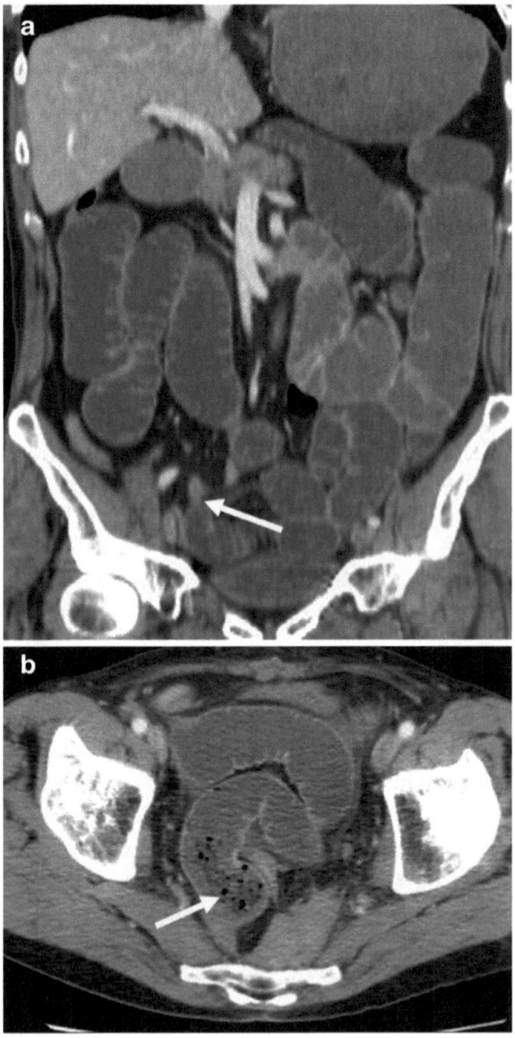

Fig. 1.19 Small bowel obstruction 1 week post anterior resection secondary to adhesions. (**a**) The coronal CT image shows segments of dilated and collapsed small bowel indicating small bowel obstruction along with a point of transition (*arrow*), indicating the point of obstruction. (**b**) Axial section shows the small bowel feces sign (*arrow*) in a segment just proximal to the point of obstruction

1.5.5 Bowel Obstruction Versus Ileus and Pseudoobstruction

In the postoperative patient, a distinction must be made between small bowel obstruction and small bowel ileus, while for the colon, the differential lies between mechanical large bowel obstruction and pseudoobstruction.

1.5.5.1 Small Bowel Obstruction

Specific features to look for include (Frager et al. 1995):

- Dilated proximal small bowel.
- Collapsed distal small bowel.
- A focal transition zone (Fig. 1.19a).
- Small bowel feces sign, stagnant particulate feculent matter lying within a segment of dilated small bowel immediately proximal to the point of obstruction (Fig. 1.19b).
- Exclusion of hernia (e.g., hernial orifices, laparoscopic port sites).
- If no cause is identified, the obstruction is likely to be adhesive.

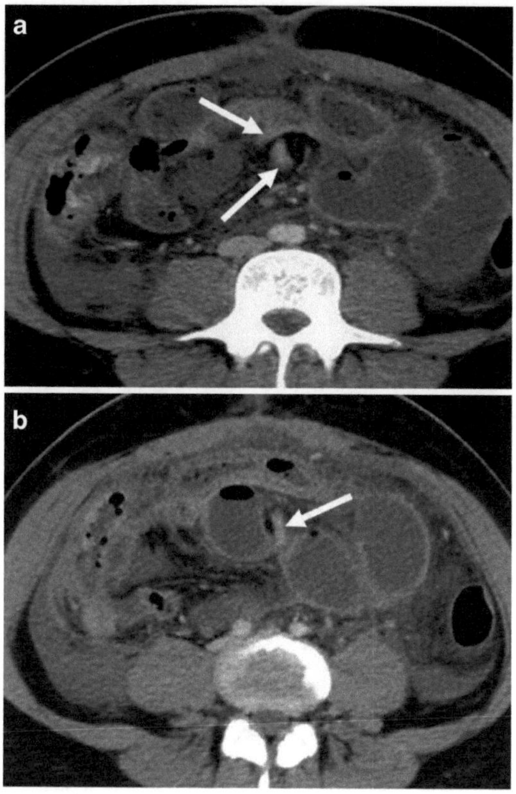

Fig. 1.20 (**a**, **b**) Closed-loop small bowel obstruction due to a strangulated adhesive band following appendicectomy. The *arrows* indicate the transition zone of obstructed small bowel in the central mesentery. The whirling appearance secondary to a small bowel twist or volvulus is always better appreciated on workstation review rather than selected static images

- Look for signs of strangulation/ischemic compromise (Elsayes et al. 2007) (Fig. 1.20). These include:
  - Localized edema within the mesentery that subtends the abnormal small bowel loop.
  - Small bowel mural change; this can lead to hyperenhancement secondary to vasodilatation, hyperattenuation due to intramural bleeding, or alternatively hypoenhancement reflecting reduced perfusion. Changes are usually related to venous ischemia, and findings may be minimal in the early stages. A high index of suspicion is required when there is any clinical possibility of ischemia.
  - Pneumatosis.
  - Portal vein gas.

Predictors for failure of conservative management include intraperitoneal fluid, mesenteric edema, vascular engorgement, pneumatosis, and small bowel thickening as well as elevated serum lactate (Zielinski et al. 2010). There is a proposed role for a therapeutic small bowel oral contrast study in this setting (Catena et al. 2011) (Sect. 1.11.1).

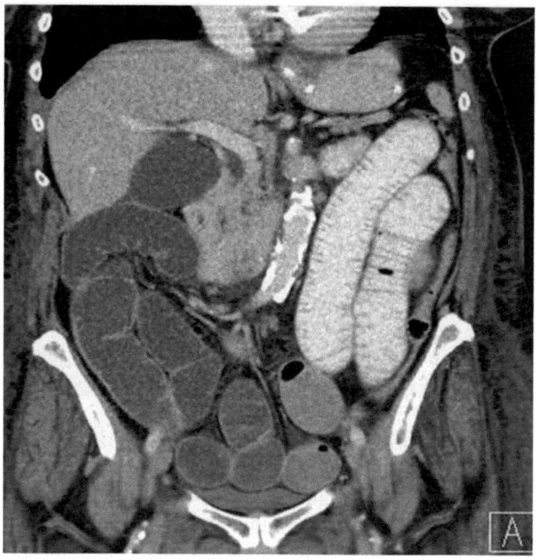

Fig. 1.21 Patient 4 days post right hemicolectomy with persistent vomiting. Coronal CT shows globally dilated small bowel with no transition zone, consistent with ileus

1.5.5.2 Small Bowel Ileus

With ileus, the typical finding is a generalized, often modest, small bowel dilatation with no recognizable zone of transition or distal bowel collapse (Fig. 1.21). The small bowel changes are often accompanied by colonic dilatation usually extending to just beyond the splenic flexure, with the distal colon collapsed – this is probably a function of raised intra-abdominal pressure and dependency of the descending colon, which lies posteriorly.

1.5.5.3 Colonic Pseudoobstruction

Acute colonic pseudoobstruction, sometimes referred to as Ogilvie syndrome, leads to marked colonic dilatation with all the clinical signs and symptoms of true obstruction but with no mechanical cause. The condition usually occurs in hospitalized patients who have significant comorbidity, and if not corrected, there is a risk of colonic perforation. The cecum, being the most distensible section of large bowel, is the most likely to perforate. Increasing unrelieved

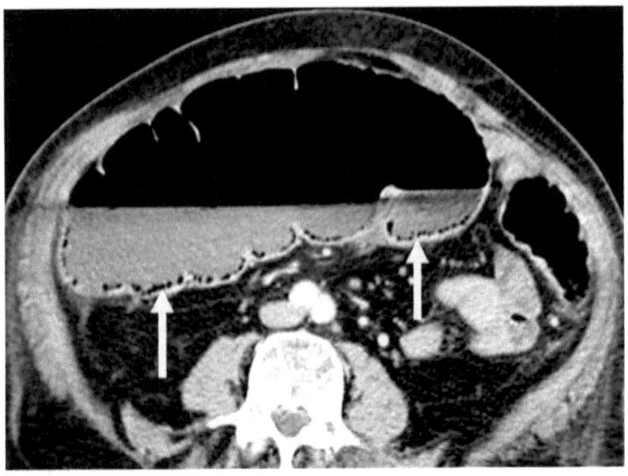

Fig. 1.22 Air trapping in the cecum mimicking pneumatosis. Axial CT section showing multiple foci of gas along the posterior cecal wall behind fluid content (*arrows*). Note the absence of comparable findings along the anterior cecal wall away from the fluid and adjacent to the air/wall interface. There is also an absence of mural edema or perimural change, findings that would be expected if cecal ischemia were present

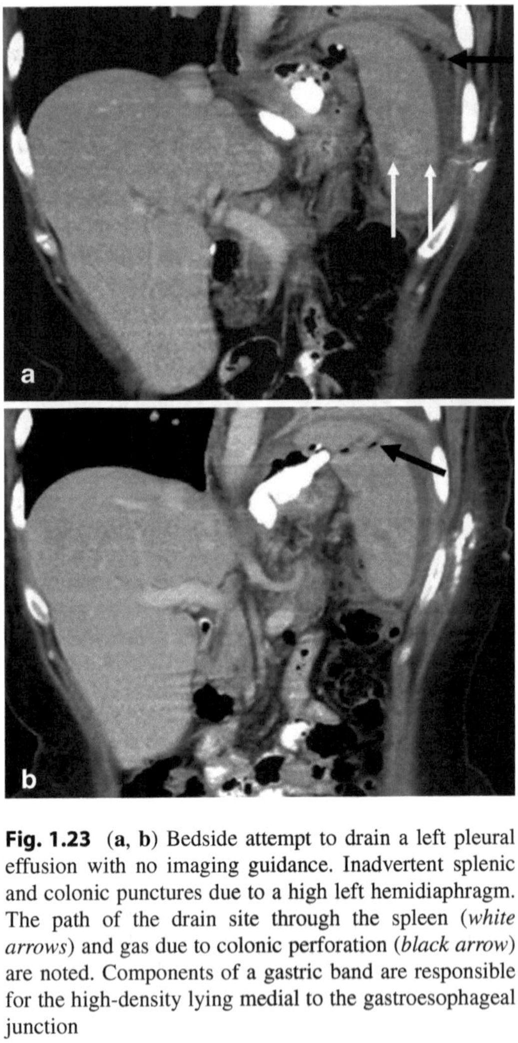

Fig. 1.23 (**a**, **b**) Bedside attempt to drain a left pleural effusion with no imaging guidance. Inadvertent splenic and colonic punctures due to a high left hemidiaphragm. The path of the drain site through the spleen (*white arrows*) and gas due to colonic perforation (*black arrow*) are noted. Components of a gastric band are responsible for the high-density lying medial to the gastroesophageal junction

colonic distension will eventually lead to ischemic changes with serosal splitting and perforation. The risk of perforation is related to both the degree of distension and the duration of distension. The earlier a radiological diagnosis can be made, the earlier therapeutic measures can be taken (e.g., the insertion of a flatus tube, colonoscopic decompression, or cecostomy) (Sect. 8.6.2). Where there is doubt in the differentiation of obstruction from ileus (e.g., collapsed sigmoid segment), CT can be augmented with rectal contrast administration or a supplementary fluoroscopic water-soluble enema study performed.

1.5.5.4 Large Bowel Obstruction

This is a less common event than small bowel obstruction in the postoperative period. As with pseudoobstruction, the cecum is at the greatest risk of perforation, particularly when the diameter reaches 10–12 cm. Cecal wall and pericecal fat edema in the presence of large bowel obstruction are indicators of potential perforation if the obstruction is not treated promptly.

Beware of overcalling cecal ischemia and mural pneumatosis. Air trapping between the bowel wall and semisolid fecal material is especially prevalent in the cecum and can be difficult to differentiate from true mural air. Air trapping will typically involve only the posterior sections of the cecal circumference, with normal wall morphology seen anterior to the air/fluid interface. If in doubt, turning the patient decubitus/prone and rescanning through the cecal pole will usually show a resolution or a change in location of what was thought to be mural gas (Fig. 1.22).

1.6 Iatrogenic Postoperative Problems

1.6.1 Drain-Related Events

As part of surgical "elective enhanced recovery programs," drains are being used less frequently, although some remain essential such as chest and pericardial drains in cardiothoracic surgery,

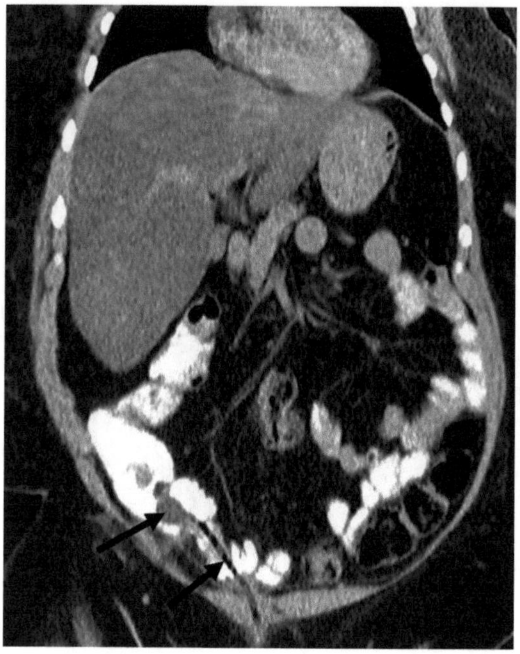

Fig. 1.24 Attempted bedside placement of suprapubic catheter with no imaging guidance. Catheter (*black arrows*) shown to lie in a loop of small bowel

perihepatic drains after bile duct and liver surgery, or abdominal drains following emergency surgery for peritonitis where significant contamination has been found.

The majority of postoperative drain placements are now performed under imaging guidance. Two cases illustrate why image guided drainage should be considered best practice. In the first example (Fig. 1.23), a bedside procedure to drain a left pleural effusion resulted in two separate splenic punctures with the more caudal puncture also producing a colonic injury. In a second example, a bedside suprapubic catheter placement is located in an adjacent small bowel loop (Fig. 1.24).

Caution should be observed when considering draining seromas related to incisional and other mesh-based hernia repairs. The most challenging late postoperative complication is mesh infection, which often necessitates mesh removal. With large hernias, this produces an immediate recurrence of a symptomatic hernia and a major challenge for the next surgery. A conservative approach may resolve some, or alternatively surgical drainage (under local anesthesia) in theater probably carries a lower risk of mesh infection. A detailed request

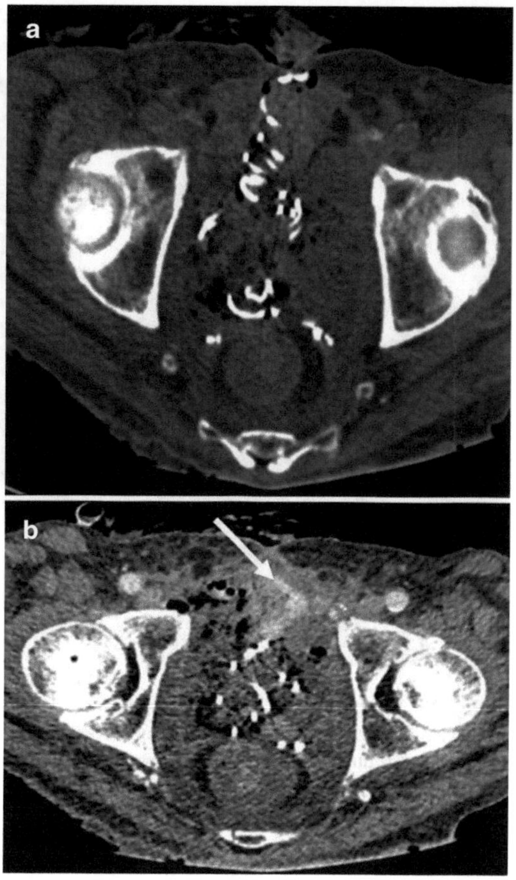

Fig. 1.25 Pre- and postcontrast CT images showing active bleeding into a surgically packed cavity after trauma. (**a**) Serpiginous high-density metallic markers are related to packed gauze on the unenhanced section. (**b**) Active contrast extravasation (*arrow*) shown on the post-contrast series. Subsequent angiography (*not shown*) and therapeutic embolization identified the origin of bleeding from the left inferior epigastric artery

card is essential, as occasionally meshes may also be used to close the perineal defect following major pelvic surgery, a situation which is likely to become more widespread as the cylindrical abdominoperineal excision of rectum (APER) is used to reduce local recurrence rates for low rectal cancers. The mesh can be confused for a collection, and once again inappropriate drainage could convert a sterile seroma into an infected mesh.

Bleeding from drain sites is not common, but CT may be requested when there are clinical concerns of hemorrhage from a drain site, or acute bleeding may be encountered during a CT study for another reason (Fig. 1.25).

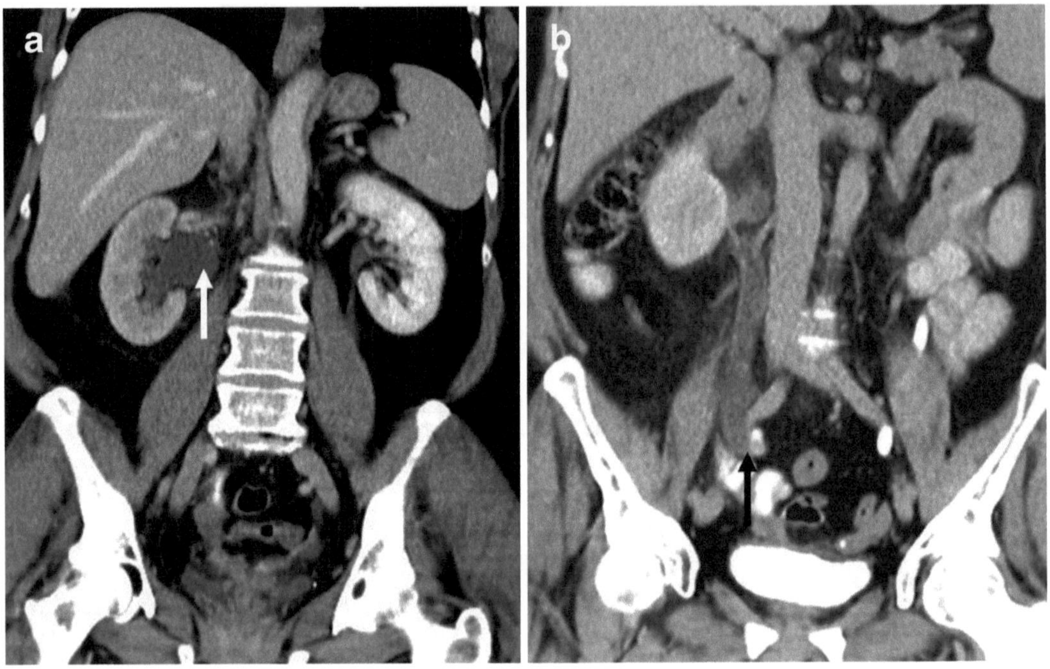

Fig. 1.26 Ureteric injury. CT study performed 4 days post–vaginal hysterectomy. (**a**) Hydronephrosis (*white arrow*) and reduced cortical enhancement of the right kidney compared to normal left kidney. (**b**) Dilated right ureter with the point of compromise located at the point of accidental ligation (*black arrow*)

When bleeding is suspected on clinical grounds, dual-phase imaging with arterial and portal venous phases is recommended, while some radiologists find an initial noncontrast series helpful. As discussed earlier, it is very important not to administer positive oral contrast as this may mask hemorrhage. If active bleeding is confirmed by contrast extravasation, the interventional radiologist should be contacted at the earliest opportunity with view to therapeutic embolization of the bleeding vessel.

Splenic preservation after splenic traumatic injury is now well established although the decision making in such cases requires close collaboration between surgeons and radiologists. The use of embolization for posterior duodenal ulcers and for pelvic bleeding after pelvic fracture potentially offers more rapid and considerably less invasive hemostatic control than emergency laparotomy, which is generally reserved now for salvage when endovascular techniques have failed.

1.6.2 Intraoperative Injury

Some injuries follow fairly predictable patterns such as trauma to the spleen or pancreatic tail during left hemicolectomy, where mobilization of the splenic flexure has been technically difficult. The more common indicators of splenic injury are areas of parenchymal infarction or perisplenic hemorrhage. While splenectomy may be an intended part of the surgical procedure (e.g., distal pancreatectomy), an absent spleen may indicate a more problematic surgical procedure. A knowledge of the most common postoperative problems also helps when informing clinical colleagues; imaging diagnosis of acute gastric distension after splenectomy and resolution with simple nasogastric tube drainage by alerting the clinical team is a simple potentially life-saving intervention.

Injuries to the urinary tract are encountered less commonly in modern practice but do occur in general, gynecological, and urological surgeries. They may be identified on postoperative CT performed

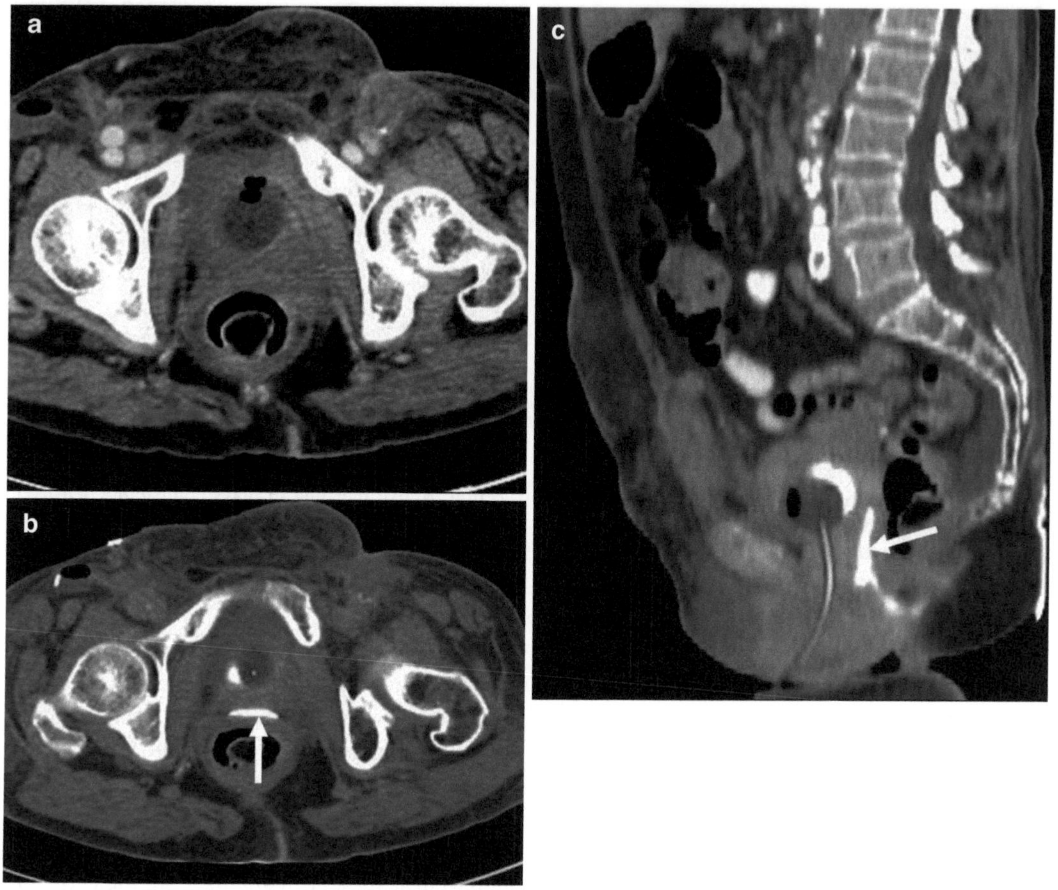

Fig. 1.27 Bladder injury. Femoral-femoral crossover procedure using a left transobturator approach that resulted in bladder trauma. (**a**) Axial CT section from portal venous phase and (**b**) axial and (**c**) sagittal sections from a 10-min delayed series. Contrast leak demonstrated on delayed imaging between the rectum and bladder (*arrow*)

for another suspected complication (Fig. 1.26) Hydronephrosis, hydroureter, and urinoma may occur secondary to ureteric injury, while renal infarction may be seen if there has been injury to the renal vascular pedicle. Direct bladder trauma can occur with both open and laparoscopic procedures (Fig. 1.27). While the distribution of fluid may indicate the site of leak, excretory phase CT imaging may be augmented with CT cystography to define the location of injury.

1.6.3 Hemorrhage

Intraoperative hemorrhage resulting from direct vessel or organ injury is usually recognized at the time of surgery. This bleeding is usually controlled with sutures, surgical clips, tissue glues, and hemostatic agents. Certain hemostatic agents can be seen on postoperative imaging (e.g., oxidized cellulose) and misinterpreted as a collection or abscess (Sect. 1.4.2.1). Some surgical procedures, such as extensive debulking of peritoneal tumor, can cause more delayed or insidious bleeding that may only become apparent in the late postoperative period (Fig. 1.28).

1.6.4 Omental Infarction

Spontaneous segmental omental infarction and epiploic appendagitis are well-recognized causes of an acute abdomen. Perhaps, less well recognized is omental infarction (Kerr et al. 2012,

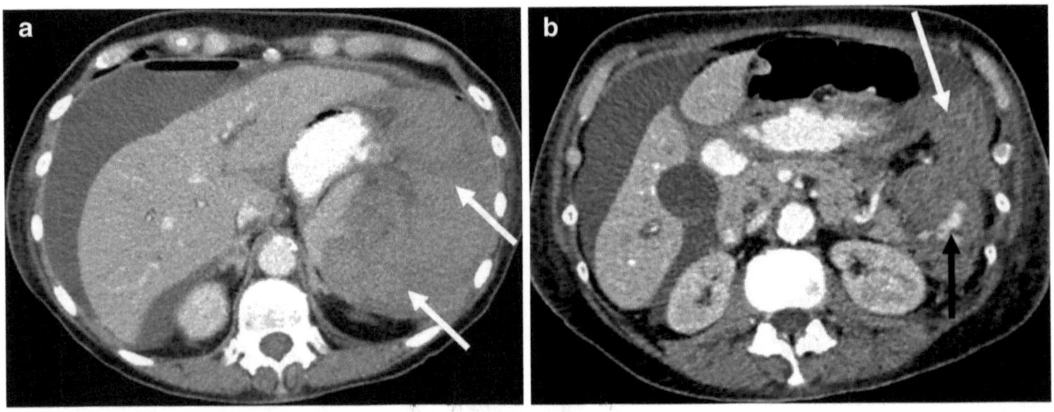

Fig. 1.28 Debulking procedure for intraperitoneal ovarian malignancy complicated by delayed postoperative bleeding. (**a**) Large perisplenic hematoma (*white arrows*). Note the higher density of recently formed hematoma compared with the more fluid density of the right-sided ascites. (**b**) Contrast extravasation (*black arrow*) shown within the hematoma (*white arrow*) on the more caudad section. Active bleeding displays comparable density to the intravascular contrast in adjacent aorta

Singh et al. 2006) developing as a complication of intra-abdominal surgery (Fig. 1.2). The finding of soft tissue masses in the omentum, often accompanied by a more diffuse increase in omental fat density, can be encountered after a variety of intra-abdominal surgical procedures including hemicolectomy, hysterectomy, and gastric surgery. The finding of omental abnormality after an extended hemicolectomy for colonic malignancy can lead to concerns for apparent omental tumor spread. If diagnostic doubt remains, percutaneous biopsy may be required at some stage since the imaging findings may persist for many months and appear to "progress" in the early postoperative period. While omental infarction in the acute abdomen setting is characteristically not associated with an elevated white cell count or a raised CRP, in the postoperative patient, the pattern of inflammatory markers may be more confusing.

1.6.5 Specific Patterns of Postoperative Complications

Table 1.1 provides some common and unusual but serious complications related to particular surgical procedures of the gastrointestinal tract. It serves to highlight the importance of a radiologist's knowledge of the surgical operations and also how important the request card details are in helping delineate any abnormalities on the subsequent CT scan.

To illustrate, gastric bands can slip or erode in bariatric surgery, while the complicated anatomy of a duodenal switch operation can make it challenging to delineate and exclude an anastomotic leak. Heller myotomy on the other hand risks esophageal perforation as does Nissens' fundoplication. The variable anatomy in the biliary tree and hepatic vasculature can lead to a variety of postoperative complications post laparoscopic cholecystectomy, ranging from cystic duct and common bile duct leakage to right hepatic artery ligation and subsequent hepatic infarction. Transplant surgery brings with it the inherent challenges of surgery in immunocompromised and very unwell patients. In acute colitis where a subtotal colectomy has been performed, there is a risk of rectal stump blowout with subsequent pelvic infection. Left colonic and rectal resections risk injury to the left ureter and pelvic side wall structures, while the spleen may also be at risk when splenic flexure mobilization is required.

Table 1.1 Gastrointestinal operations and some of the specific complications identified

Gastrointestinal specialty	Operation	Potential complication
All specialties	Any operation	Bleeding, infection (wound, intra-abdominal, chest, urine, pelvis, adhesions, bowel herniation, obstruction)
Upper GI	Esophagectomy	Anastomotic leak
	Nissens fundoplication	Esophageal injury, wrap migration leading to recurrent symptoms, pneumothorax
HPB and transplant	Cholecystectomy	Bile duct leak or injury
	Hepatic resection	Major bleeding, bile leak
	Transplant surgery	Vascular inflow or outflow occlusion/stenosis
		Early thrombosis, stricture formation requiring vascular stenting (e.g., caval or portal vein), abscess, or collections, anastomotic leak (ureteric in renal, CBD in biliary)
Colorectal	Rectal resection	Ureteric injury, pelvic side wall or sacral venous bleeding, splenic injury
	Right hemicolectomy	Right ureteric injury, duodenal injury, anastomotic leak
	Restorative proctocolectomy and ileal pouch-anal anastomosis	Pouch twisting leading to ischemia or obstruction, obstruction at site of defunctioning loop ileostomy, pelvic collection
Bariatric	Gastric band	Migration, erosion
	Duodenal switch	Anastomotic leak, bowel obstruction, pancreatitis
Gynecology	Radical hysterectomy (Wertheim)	Ureteric injury, bleeding from bladder or pelvic side wall

1.6.6 Surgical Material Left in Error

Robust operating theater procedures incorporating repeated swab, sharps, and instrument counts should prevent this complication, but the radiologist must consider the possibility of retained surgical material when abnormalities that do not immediately configure to expected intra-abdominal anatomy or postoperative complications are encountered. Almost by definition, this is not an expected diagnosis for the referring clinician, and it is often very helpful to show them the "stigmata" to remove any doubts they may have that the diagnosis is correct.

1.6.7 Retained Foreign Material

A retained surgical swab or sponge may lead to either aseptic or septic complications if not recognized. Sometimes referred to as a gossypiboma, this term is coined from an unlikely combination of Latin – gossypium (cotton) and Swahili – boma – (place of concealment). An alternative term occasionally used is a textiloma.

Where retained material remains sterile, there may be a prolonged time interval between surgery and any subsequent swab-related complication when an indolent foreign body response may lead to fibrosis, adhesions, and occasionally internal fistula formation. On CT, a soft tissue mass with internal gas bubbles (retained between the cotton fibers) and an enhancing rim is the typical finding (Manzella et al. 2009). Gas trapped between the threads of a surgical swab can last for weeks or months and can mimic the appearance of retained Surgicel. Identifying the wavy internal high-density radiopaque marker will help differentiate, as these should be incorporated in all surgical swabs to assist identification (Fig. 1.29). Examination for signs of fistula formation between the mass and the adjacent GI tract is important. Where infection develops, a more exudative response occurs with abscess formation (Fig. 1.30). As gas foci and an enhancing margin are found in sterile and infected gossypibomas, it can be difficult to confirm or

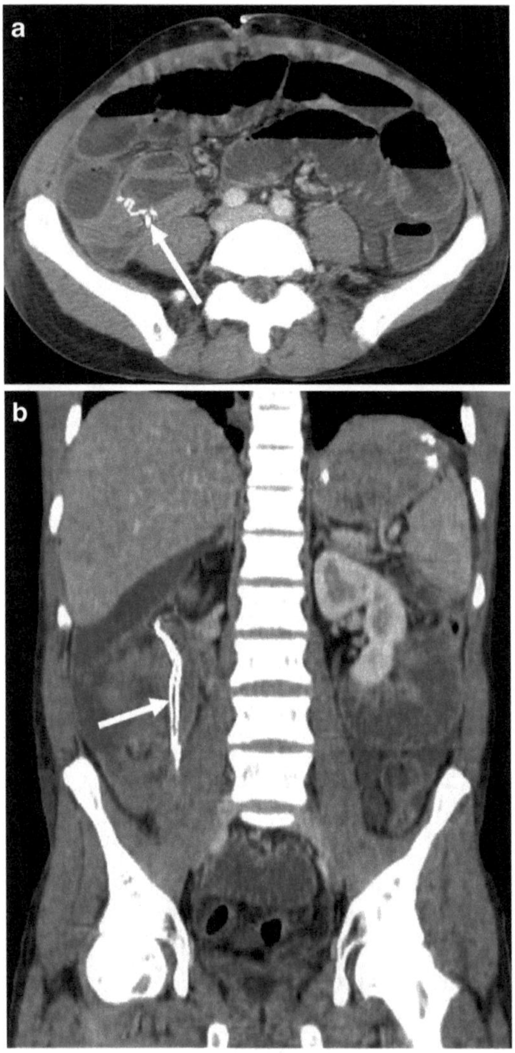

Fig. 1.29 Retained surgical swab. Patient presented with small bowel obstruction following surgery for Crohn disease. (**a**) Axial CT section showing a high-density serpiginous structure in the right iliac fossa (*arrow*). (**b**) Coronal image (*arrow*) increases confidence that this is not a normal staple line, leading to a diagnosis of a retained surgical swab

exclude infection on imaging grounds alone. In any case, the swab should be removed, assuming it is clinically appropriate, to prevent further complications.

Retained surgical instruments rarely lead to any difficulty with diagnosis and are usually made of metal. Plastic instruments are much more difficult to demonstrate and may be of soft tissue or fat density.

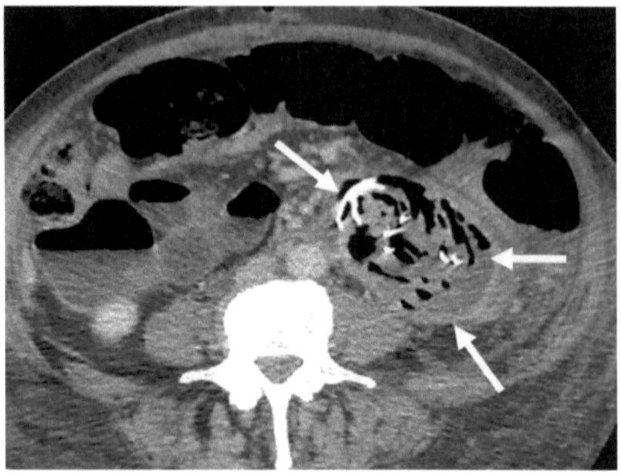

Fig. 1.30 Retained surgical swab. Ten days post-Hartmann procedure, hysterectomy, and unilateral oophorectomy for advanced rectal carcinoma with signs of sepsis. CT demonstrates a well-demarcated, left-sided abdominal mass with an enhancing margin, internal gas densities, and serpiginous high-density ribbon, consistent with a retained surgical swab (*arrows*). The volume and distribution of gas suggests infection, but as internal gas is common with retained cotton based material, differentiating infected from noninfected swabs can be difficult

1.7 Complications Related to Laparoscopic Surgery

1.7.1 General Surgical Principles of Laparoscopic Surgery

Laparoscopic gastrointestinal surgery has rapidly progressed over the last two decades. It is ideally suited for the morbidly obese in bariatric surgery and is associated with reduced pain, shorter hospital stays, and reduced incisional hernia rates in all branches of GI surgery. Now that a laparoscopic approach has been proven to be feasible and safe, there is an exciting trend toward fewer laparoscopic ports and even better cosmesis. It is worth remembering, however, that laparoscopic surgery in certain groups remains just as challenging as for open surgery (Del Rio et al. 2010). Recurrent surgery (e.g., recurrent inflammatory bowel disease or adhesional obstruction), malignancy, emergency surgery, trauma, and active inflammation will almost always make the surgery more challenging and increase the risk of complications and hence the likely need for radiological input.

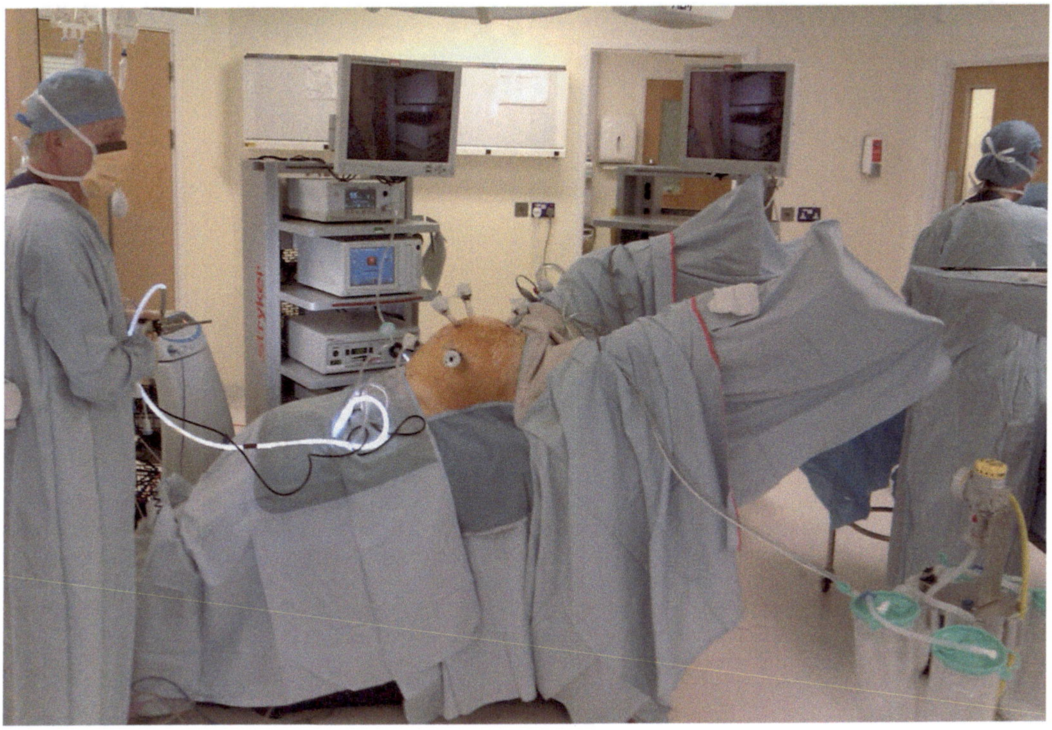

Fig. 1.31 Modified Lloyd-Davis position. Note the position of the 5 laparoscopic port sites in the abdomen

Robotic surgery has gained acceptance worldwide with a new study of rectal surgery being commenced (ROLAAR). Its cost remains the major barrier to widespread use; its "stable platform" in terms of the optical image ("steadier than the assistant"), and the 7 degrees of freedom (four robotic arms each with 90 degrees of articulation) makes suturing much easier in confined spaces. The same laparoscopic ports are still required for surgery in the abdomen, however.

The use of single-port surgery (SILS) allows the optical port and other working ports to be delivered via a single 2 cm (often transumbilical) incision. Natural orifice surgery (NOTES) uses endoscopic technology with entry into the abdominal cavity via the stomach, vagina, and, now, the colon. Specimen retraction is achieved through these same orifices (stomach, vagina, and colon), leaving no scars on the abdomen, but these orifices now need to be considered when reviewing postoperative imaging in such cases. Future technology may see miniature robots inserted via the natural orifice routes, while magnets are already employed to aid retraction. Nanotechnology will aid the reduction in the size of the operating instruments; the size of the tumor specimen being resected will likely remain the main barrier to truly scarless surgery. For example, the spleen can be broken up intracorporeally preextraction, but a donor nephrectomy or a malignant colonic resection specimen needs to be removed intact.

Laparoscopic abdominal surgery almost always requires general anesthesia, and patients are usually assessed preoperatively to assess their fitness for surgery. During surgery, the patient is carefully positioned to enable a steep table position to aid retraction. Laparoscopic anterior resection, for example, requires the patient to be placed in the modified Lloyd-Davis position, very steeply head down with maximal right side down tilt (Fig. 1.31). This position moves the small bowel superiorly and to the right, providing clear identification of the inferior mesenteric pedicle and minimizing injury to small bowel loops. Poor positioning and long operating times can lead to

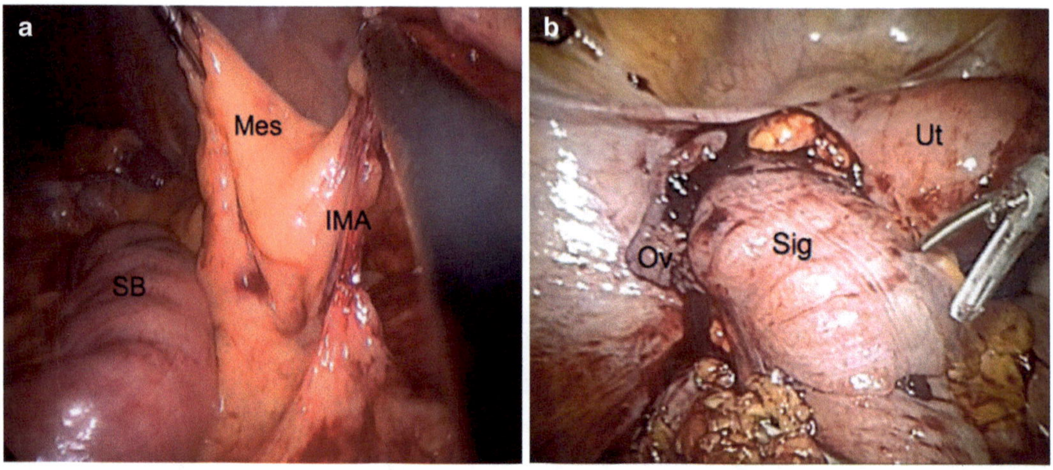

Fig. 1.32 Potential for laparoscopic iatrogenic injury during surgery for diverticular disease. (**a**) The small bowel (*SB*) naturally lies on *top* of the *left* colonic mesentery. Retraction of the SB medially and the colonic mesentery (*Mes*) anterolaterally and tilting of the patient are required to minimize the risk of iatrogenic injury during ultrasonic dissection of the inferior mesenteric artery pedicle (*IMA*). (**b**) Sigmoid colon (*Sig*) is densely adherent to the left pelvic side wall, left ovary (*Ov*), and uterus (*Ut*). Left ureter (*not shown*) has already been delineated at the pelvic brim before further dissection off the side wall is attempted; the iliac vessels are also at risk with such distorted anatomy

cerebral edema due to cerebral venous stasis, skin pressure problems at contact points on the right side of the patient or compartment syndrome in the calves. Reducing the laparoscopic pressure from 15 mmHg to 12 mmHg can reduce some of the pressure-related problems (e.g., diaphragmatic splinting and poor venous return) that can give anesthetic instability during surgery. Despite changing the patient's positioning, occasionally, the anatomy will be unfavorable. Figure 1.32 demonstrates small bowel loops impinging on the inferior mesenteric pedicle which are at risk from thermal injury from the ultrasonic scalpel.

Surgical success is dependent on "good optics" and effective pneumoperitoneum to delineate the tissue planes and anatomy. Pneumoperitoneum remains an essential aspect of laparoscopic surgery, and without it surgery cannot be undertaken. A Veress needle is inserted into the left upper quadrant provided there is no clinical evidence of splenomegaly. The Veress needle can also be placed "blind" at the umbilicus aiming down into the pelvis to avoid aortic puncture. The disadvantage with puncturing blind is that rarely a small bowel loop may be adherent to the umbilicus, resulting in an inadvertent enterotomy and possible postoperative peritonitis. Therefore, the surgeon usually will view the umbilical needle puncture from one of the other laparoscopic ports.

For many surgeons, the Hassan technique remains the safest way to enter the abdomen. The abdomen is entered under direct vision often paraumbilically and then pneumoperitoneum established. A middle ground is the use of optical ports; the camera being inserted inside the port and the abdomen entered under vision. Once again, the left upper quadrant is employed most commonly for this, but adhesions or omental bleeding can impair the surgeon's view. Injuries to structures such as the small bowel are still possible using this technique. The number of additional ports depends on the operation undertaken and the operator's preferences. The use of 5-mm ports technically reduces the risk of port site complications and improves cosmesis, but certain instruments (e.g., laparoscopic staplers used for bowel anastomoses or vessel ligation) will not fit down them so a balance must be struck. Depending on the surgeon, all or none of the 10-mm port sites will be formally closed at the end of a procedure; 5-mm ports do not require closure. The "bladeless trocar" technology now available does appear to reduce the size of the defects and the trauma caused to subcutaneous tissues.

1.7.2 Patterns of Complications

Despite all the proven benefits of laparoscopic surgery, complications still occur. Bleeding can occur from any port site either at the time of trocar insertion or withdrawal. Most will settle either spontaneously or with suture control. Injury to the inferior epigastric vessels must be controlled properly as this can be life threatening. Omental bleeding can be brisk and if it occurs at the start of the procedure can hamper views of tissue planes and anatomy.

Veress needles have been associated with injuries to intraperitoneal and retroperitoneal structures. While optical ports and the Hassan technique have reduced these risks overall, Veress needles remain safe in experienced hands, but it remains possible with any technique to inadvertently damage a small bowel loop adherent to the anterior abdominal wall or damage a major vessel (e.g., aorta or IVC) during port insertion. A through-and-through injury to the small bowel with the port traversing both walls can be very challenging to spot laparoscopically. The defect is usually only apparent via other ports prior to port removal or in the postoperative period if peritonitis ensues. Aggressive grasping or tearing of the small bowel can cause inadvertent injuries, while late thermal injuries related to energy sources (diathermy, ultrasonic dissections) are well recognized.

When reporting preoperative CT examinations, the radiologist should highlight any vascular tree abnormality, for example, abdominal aortic aneurysm (AAA). This is because of the recognized increased risk of aortic aneurysm rupture during abdominal surgery and to prevent a trocar injury to the aorta.

Bladder perforation can also occur during insertion of the suprapubic port in cases during laparoscopic appendicectomy and transperitoneal inguinal hernia repairs (TEPP). Asking patients to void prior to theater or placement of indwelling urethral catheters reduces these risks. Solid organ injury is unusual but reported. The liver parenchyma can be injured during laparoscopic cholecystectomy if the gallbladder lies partially or completely embedded in the liver, for example, intrahepatic gallbladder. The spleen can be damaged during port site insertion in the left upper quadrant or during mobilization of the splenic flexure during left-sided colonic resections during laparoscopic adrenalectomy. The kidney can be mobilized and damaged during right or left colonic mobilization if the wrong surgical plane is inadvertently dissected.

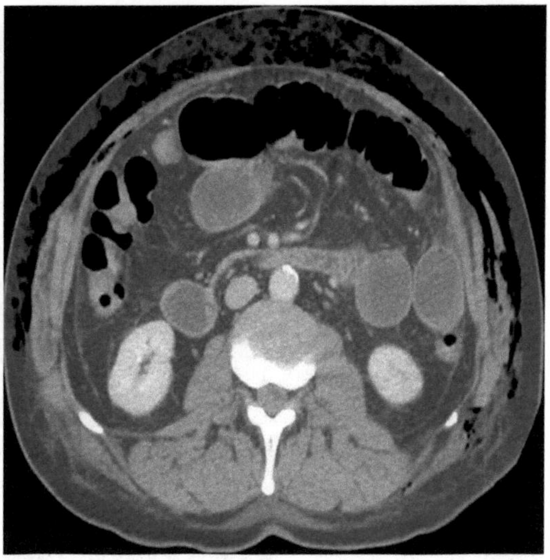

Fig. 1.33 Excessive gas deposition in the subcutaneous tissues of the anterior abdominal wall due to preperitoneal insufflation during laparoscopy (rather than necrotizing fasciitis)

Other aspects of laparoscopic surgery can make postoperative radiological interpretation more difficult. Preperitoneal insufflation may be a particular problem with obese patients where gaining access to the peritoneal cavity can be difficult for the surgeon but rarely leads to any problem for the patient. On CT, linear and punctate gas foci may be seen tracking to a variable extent within the subcutaneous fat and extraperitoneal tissue planes (i.e., surgical emphysema) (Fig. 1.33). This needs to be distinguished from gas foci seen in necrotizing fasciitis, although the clinical findings (necrotic patch of skin) and the patient's systemic condition will differentiate.

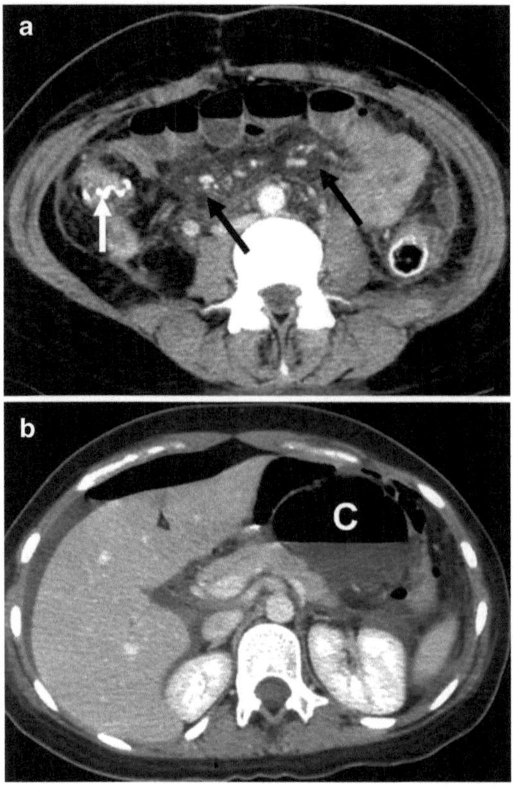

Fig. 1.34 Small bowel injury post–laparoscopic right hemicolectomy. (**a**) Normal CT appearances of the anastomosis (*white arrow*) but with increased density of the fat within the central small bowel mesentery (*black arrows*). (**b**) A more cephalad image shows pneumoperitoneum and a large collection (*C*) within the lesser sac. At subsequent laparotomy, a perforated jejunal loop was identified some distance from the anastomosis and considered secondary to laparoscopic bowel injury

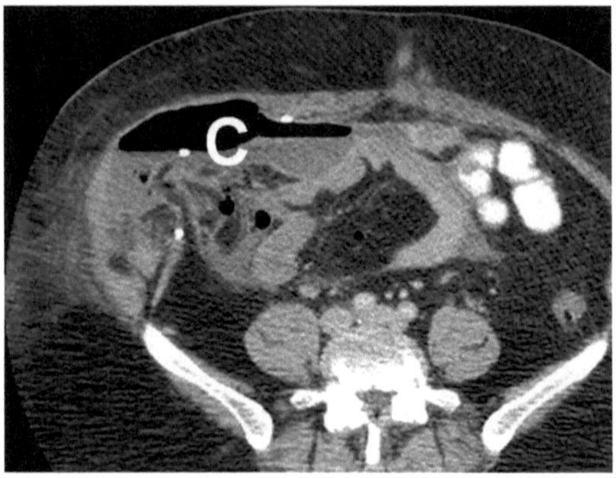

Fig. 1.35 Four days post–laparoscopic incisional hernia repair. Axial CT shows a large collection (*C*) containing gas and fluid crossing the permeable mesh (indicated by high density rivets). At subsequent laparotomy, a hole in the adjacent colon was identified

As already mentioned, vascular injury is a feared complication although, if controlled at the time, it does not always necessitate immediate conversion to open laparotomy. Major injuries to the aorta, IVC, and iliac vessels still account for a significant percentage of laparoscopic surgical deaths and might be masked at the time by tamponade from its retroperitoneal location, raised intra-abdominal pressure from pneumoperitoneum, and inaccessibility to the laparoscope. Injuries to other vessels are classified as minor (a classification of the vessel size rather than indicating the severity of risk) with the inferior epigastric vessels being the most commonly injured, although the volume of blood loss can still be life threatening if not detected early. Direct cannulation of a major vessel followed by CO_2 insufflation can lead to serious consequences including death if not immediately appreciated. Bowel trauma may present late with signs of sepsis or peritonism and well-established contamination (Figs. 1.34 and 1.35). When colonic injury is suspected, water-soluble contrast enema or CT may help confirm or exclude a leak.

Diathermy has revolutionized surgery and minimized blood loss, but in generating the energy and heat to coagulate tissues, it does risk surrounding structures if they come into contact with the working tip or blade. Monopolar currents are most likely to cause damage, although the bipolar tips are also very hot, and the new ultrasonic dissectors also reach extremely high temperatures. The small bowel, for example, is at high risk of damage if not adequately retracted away from the surgical field during colonic resection (Fig. 1.34). Bladder injury can result from access-related events or diathermy (Fig. 1.36), whereas pancreatic injury (Fig. 1.37) typically occurs during colonic or upper GI tract mobilization. Late common bile duct injury can occur if excessive energy is transferred via the cystic duct as it is dissected. Care must also be taken to place the earthing pad away from sites of metalwork, such as joint prostheses, and on a surface area wide enough to safely carry the energy away from the patient.

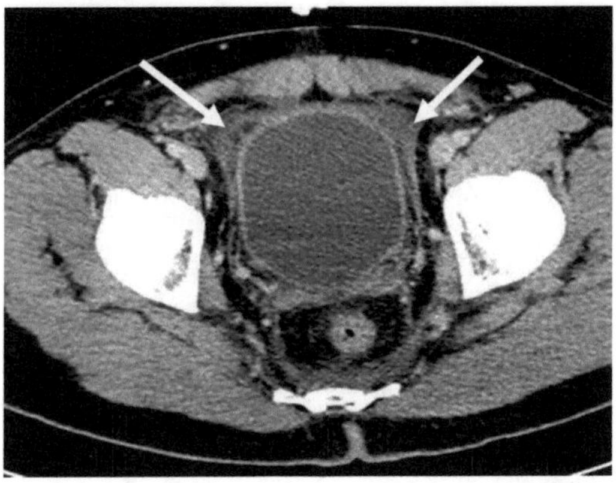

Fig. 1.36 Bladder injury post–laparoscopic appendicectomy. Note fluid (urine) in the anterior perivesicular space (*arrows*)

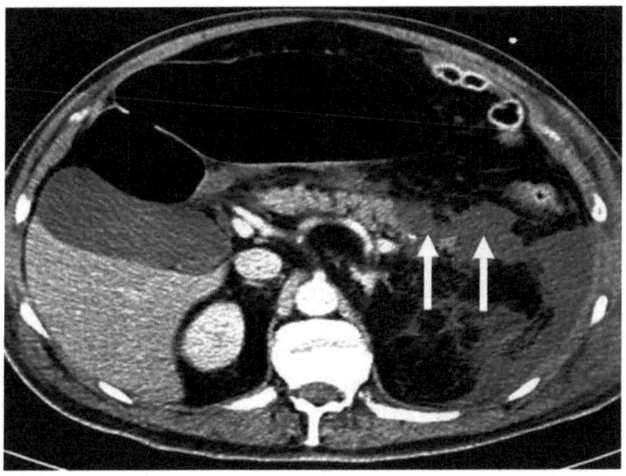

Fig. 1.37 Pancreatic injury post–laparoscopic subtotal colectomy. There is pancreatic fluid tracking from the pancreatic tail (*arrows*) to the left paracolic gutter

1.7.3 Specific Complications

1.7.3.1 Port Site Hernia

Where port site incisions of 7 mm or greater are made, there is a recognized risk of omentum or small bowel herniating through the defect if port site closure is suboptimal (Fig. 1.38). 5-mm incisions are rarely associated with port site problems (Bevan et al. 2010). As new bladeless trocars cause less damage to the fascial layers, some surgeons do not routinely close 10-mm laparoscopic ports. Other surgeons are selective (closing the umbilical port which is a common site of herniation), while others are scrupulous in closing all ports greater than 5 mm. Single-port surgery has the additional benefit of only having one port to close. It is possible to undertake a subtotal colectomy and end ileostomy via a single port in the right iliac fossa, which eventually becomes the stoma site.

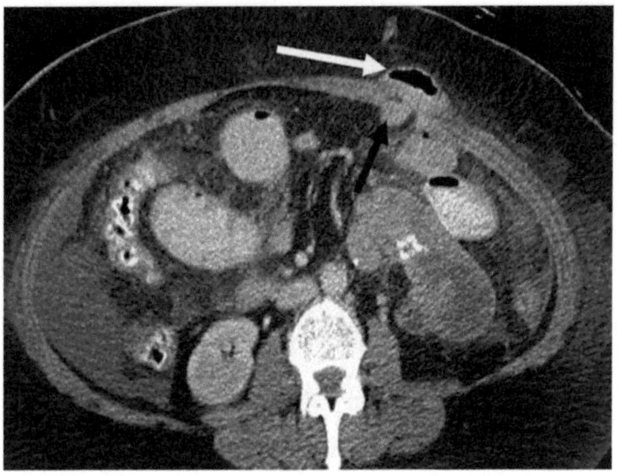

Fig. 1.38 Small bowel obstruction secondary to a port site hernia post–gastric bypass surgery. Axial CT demonstrates dilated loops of small bowel and ascites with a point of transition at the anterior abdominal wall due to prolapse of bowel through a port site defect (*white arrow*). Collapsed efferent loop (*black arrow*). Ischemic small bowel was present at surgery

Herniation of small bowel into a port site may cause bowel obstruction and even ischemia due to impairment of its blood supply. A Richter hernia can also occur in which the antimesenteric wall of the small bowel loop herniates through the defect. Although this does not cause bowel obstruction, it can lead to ischemia and strangulation. The patient can simply appear nonspecifically unwell or just "slow to improve." Occasionally, drains are inserted down port sites, and if a 10-mm port site has been used, there is an increased risk of herniation through that drain site (Fig. 1.39).

1.7.3.2 Retained Tissues or Objects

The most common retained objects are surgical clips, which generally lead to no adverse consequences for the patient. We have seen one case where a dropped clip acted as a focus for small bowel obstruction. Retained or dropped stones postcholecystectomy are known to become a nidus for infection, and so every attempt is made to remove the gallbladder intact usually within a

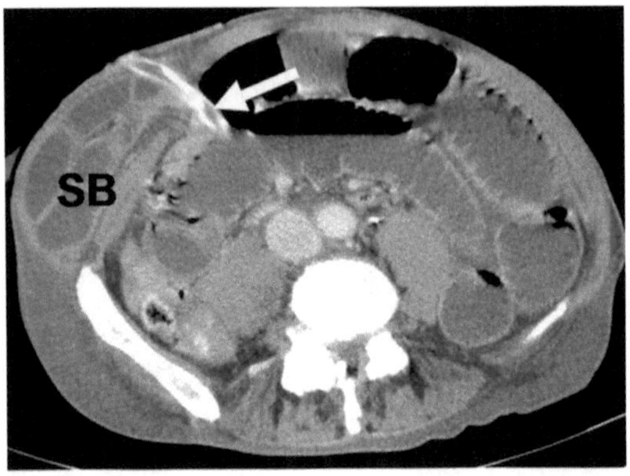

Fig. 1.39 Port site hernia. Use of a laparoscopic port site for surgical drain placement (*arrow*) complicated by herniation of small bowel (*SB*) and subsequent obstruction

specimen retraction bag to minimize risk of spillage (Sect. 5.4.7). A retained appendicolith in cases of perforated appendicitis is well known as a cause of subsequent postoperative collections, typically in the pelvis or right iliac fossa.

1.8 Wound Complications

Wound sepsis in isolation is not a common indication for CT in the postoperative patient. Edema in the abdominal wall, hematoma, seroma, and cellulitis are frequently encountered in the immediate postoperative period. Infected wounds are generally managed without any need for imaging, but superficial discrete collections are readily assessed by ultrasound.

Necrotizing fasciitis is a life-threatening condition, which requires immediate and aggressive surgical intervention. If untreated, the condition is associated with mortality rates of up to 75%. Necrotizing fasciitis involves the skin, subcutaneous tissues, and fascia and occurs either spontaneously or following surgery. The precipitating injury can be trivial or even unrecognized. Differentiating early necrotizing fasciitis from normal postoperative changes can be difficult particularly where there has been preperitoneal insufflation with surgical emphysema (Fig. 1.33): close clinicoradiological correlation is required in this setting (Figs. 1.40 and 1.41). Unfortunately, the early CT signs can be

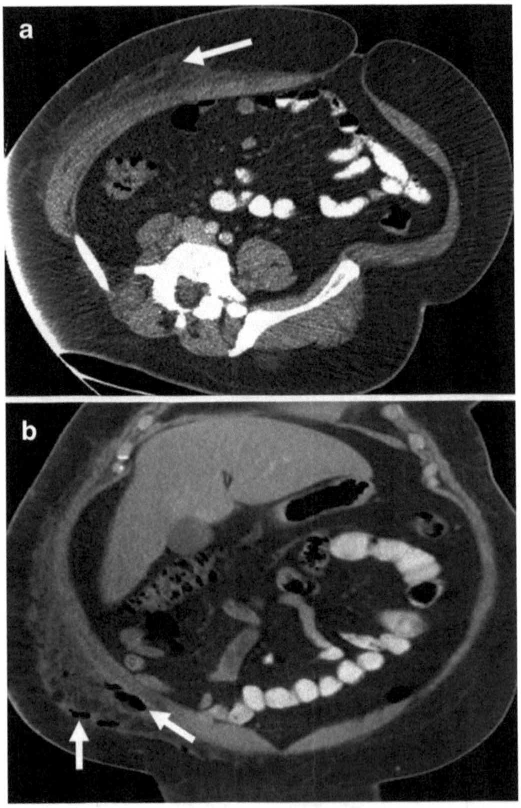

Fig. 1.40 (**a**, **b**) Necrotizing fasciitis. Early changes. Initial CT from a patient presenting with a groin infection. Note edematous changes in the subcutaneous fat of the right flank (*arrow*). (**b**) Follow-up coronal CT 3 days later showing interval development of gas (*arrows*) within the subcutaneous fat. Patient underwent extensive debridement

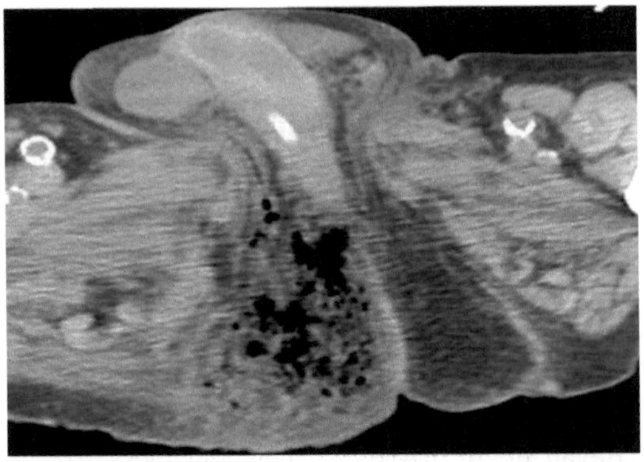

Fig. 1.41 Unenhanced axial CT from a patient presenting with sepsis and an ischiorectal fossa abscess 2 months following what was thought an uncomplicated low anterior resection. There is extensive necrosis raising concerns for necrotizing fasciitis. However, at surgery, there was a small anastomotic disruption (*not shown*), leak, and sepsis with no evidence of necrotizing fasciitis

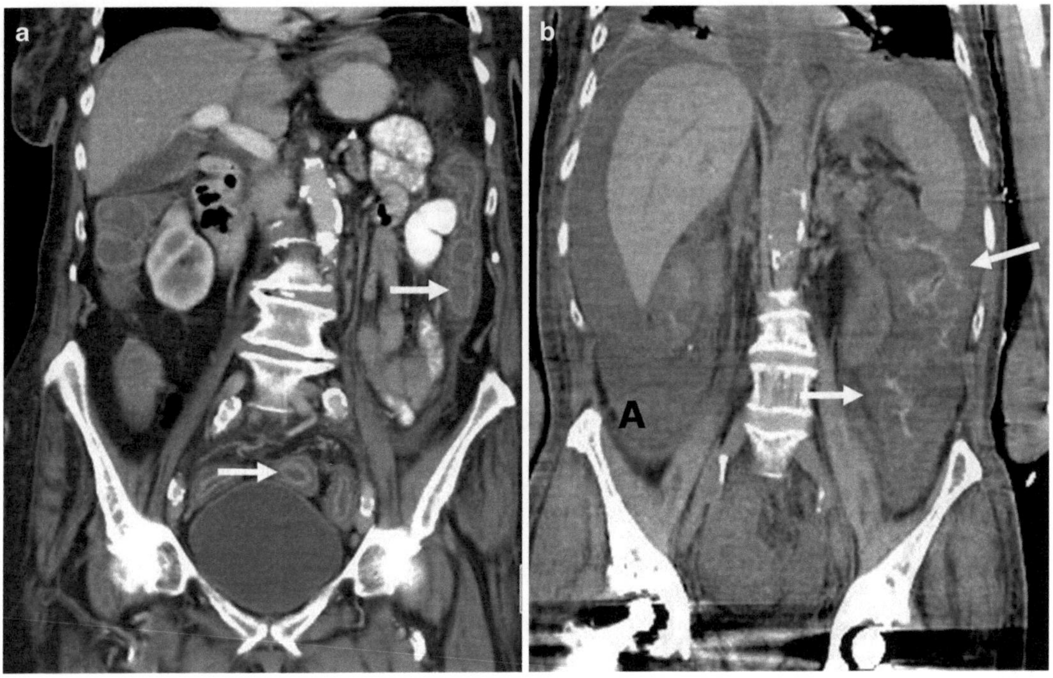

Fig. 1.42 Pseudomembranous colitis in two different patients. (**a**) Coronal CTs show a pancolitis with intense mucosal enhancement (*arrows*) and only traces of ascites. (**b**) Extreme low-density mural thickening (*arrows*) and large-volume ascites (*A*)

minimal, but unexpected foci of gas in the soft tissues should be sought. Gadolinium-enhanced T1W MR sequences have been recommended as a reliable means of identifying those patients with enough tissue necrosis to warrant immediate aggressive surgical debridement.

1.9 Assorted Problems in the Postoperative Abdomen

1.9.1 Acute Colitis

In a postoperative patient with no previous history of inflammatory bowel disease, colitis may be due to infection or ischemia.

1.9.1.1 Infective (Pseudomembranous) Colitis

This is responsible for an increasing morbidity and mortality in postoperative patients as well as the general hospital population. It is most commonly but not exclusively due to infection with *Clostridium difficile* and is almost always related to prior antibiotic history. Colitis can develop after or during a conventional course of antibiotics but is a recognized complication after a single dose and can manifest after a significant delay.

CT findings include:

- Segmental or pan colitis (Fig. 1.42).
- Mural thickening that is characteristically greater than for other causes of colitis (10 mm or more). Mucosal hyperenhancement.
- Mural thickening is typically low attenuation, but a range of densities can be encountered.
- Low-volume ascites is a frequent finding.
- Rarely, the inflammatory process extends into the distal ileum, resulting in pseudomembranous enteritis.
- Toxic megacolon can develop if not promptly treated.

Whenever CT reveals colitis, it is important to recommend evaluation for diarrheal and antibiotic history as well as recommending *C. difficile* toxin assessment.

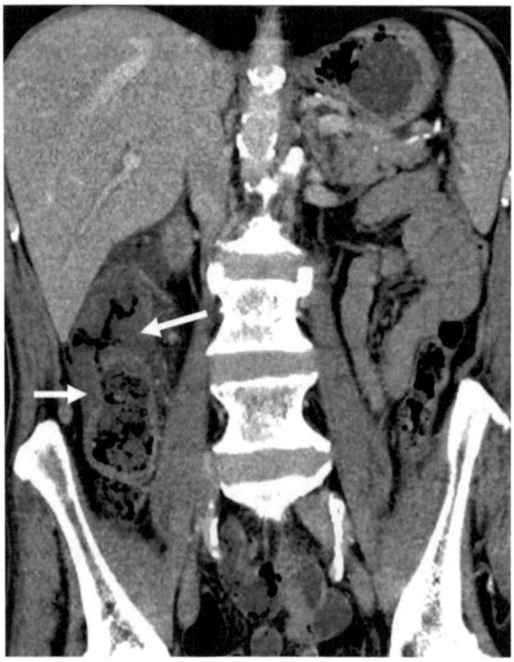

Fig. 1.43 Coronal CT image showing an ischemic segment affecting the proximal ascending colon (*arrows*) secondary to hypoperfusion. Compare poor enhancement with other sections of the colon that show normal wall appearances

1.9.1.2 Acute Ischemic Colitis

This can be secondary to arterial or venous compromise and may arise in the following instances:

- A complication in a patient with established arteriopathy
- Resulting from low flow status (hypotension/hypoperfusion often compounded by high-dose inotropes causing mesenteric vasospasm) (Fig. 1.43)
- As an embolic complication secondary to a cardiac dysrhythmia (e.g., atrial fibrillation).
- Occurs rarely in patients with vasculitis

CT signs to look for include (Taourel et al. 2008):

- Mural thickening – varying degrees can be found due to wall edema but characteristically less than that found with pseudomembranous colitis (Fig. 1.44). This may result in thickening of the haustral folds producing thumb printing.
- Mural density – can be reduced or increased (due to capillary leakage of blood or contrast).
- Ascites – often associated but may be minimal or absent in some cases.
- Occlusion of mesenteric arteries or veins.
- Pneumatosis coli.
- Portal venous gas – look for gas in branches of mesenteric veins, splenic vein, and portal vein. Intrahepatic gas will typically be located at the periphery of liver and will often give the characteristic "bird claw" branching appearance. Biliary tree gas by comparison rarely reaches the periphery and is usually found in the more central biliary ducts.

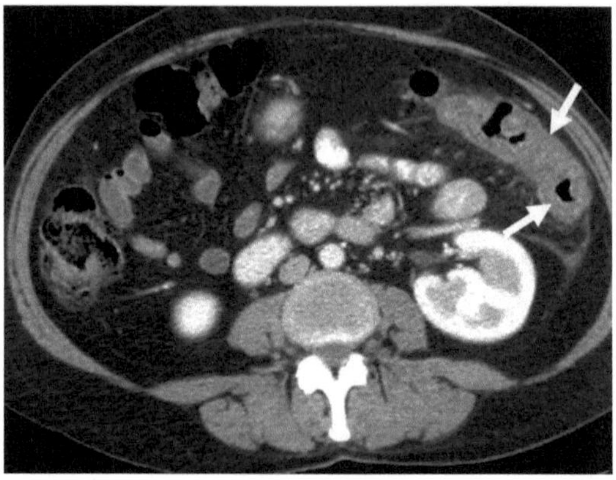

Fig. 1.44 Left colon mural thickening with poor enhancement confirmed as ischemic colitis involving the splenic flexure and proximal descending colon (*arrows*)

1.9.2 Small Bowel Ischemia

In the postoperative patient, the most common etiology is strangulated small bowel obstruction secondary to adhesions/hernia. Low cardiac output and post surgical hypercoagulable states are additional risk factors. Look for mural thickening, changes in mural enhancement (Fig. 1.45), pneumatosis (Fig. 1.46), and portal venous gas as well as ensuring assessment of both mesenteric arteries and veins (Fig. 1.47).

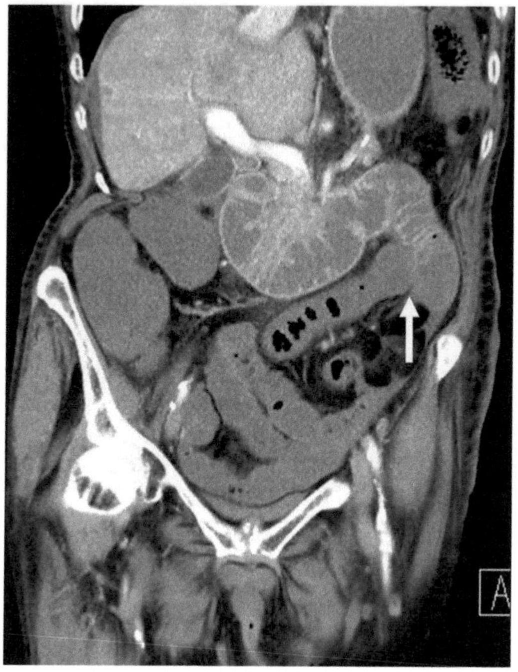

Fig. 1.45 Ischemic small bowel. Coronal projection clearly shows the cutoff (*arrow*) between viable and severely ischemic small bowel

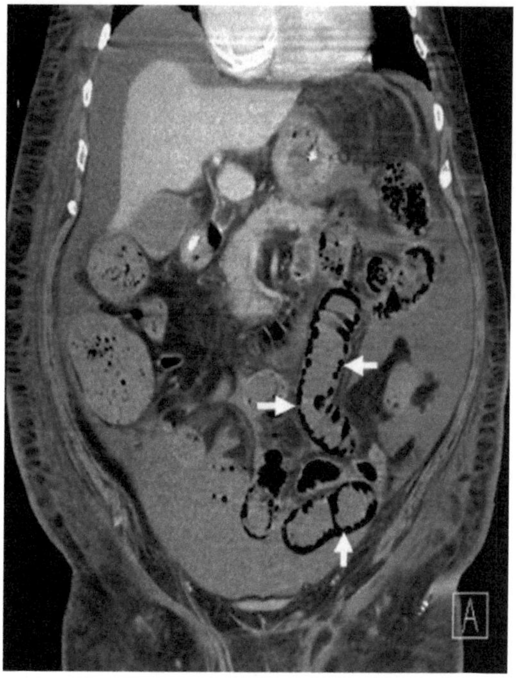

Fig. 1.46 Ischemic small bowel. Example showing extreme small bowel pneumatosis (*small arrows*) in a patient with unexplained sepsis following coronary artery bypass surgery

1.9.2.1 Caveats When Diagnosing Small or Large Bowel Ischemia

- When considering a diagnosis of large or small bowel ischemia, guard against overcalling both mural thickening and mural hyperenhancement when the small or large bowel loops under review are collapsed. Try to identify an adjacent segment of colon or small bowel with better gaseous distension. If the wall of that distended segment is thickened, it is more likely to reflect significant pathology.
- Both colonic and small bowel loops immediately adjacent to a focal inflammatory process (e.g., an acutely inflamed gall bladder) may exhibit secondary mural thickening or hyperenhancement due to spreading inflammation that should not be misinterpreted as representing primary bowel pathology.
- The cecum is the most readily distensible segment of colon and as such can become markedly distended when colonic obstruction is established, and the ileocecal valve is competent, preventing small bowel reflux of gas. Changes that suggest mural necrosis and impeding perforation may be imminent include mural irregularity and pericecal edema. As discussed

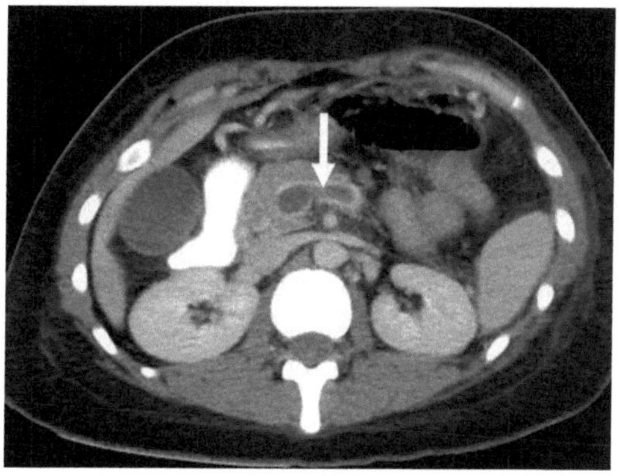

Fig. 1.47 Postoperative spontaneous venous thrombosis involving the portal venous confluence (*arrow*)

previously regarding large bowel obstruction, air trapping behind viscous colonic contents can closely mimic gas in the colon wall. To reiterate, always check the interface between aerated and fluid-filled lumen. If the apparent "mural" gas stops at the air fluid interface, air trapping by bowel content is more likely (Fig. 1.22). Where curvilinear gas densities extend beyond this interface, true mural gas is present, and ischemia must be considered.

1.9.3 Portal Vein Thrombosis (PVT)

Thrombosis of the portal venous system has a plethora of etiologies including cirrhosis, hypercoagulable states, intra-abdominal malignancy, and abdominal inflammatory conditions such as appendicitis, pancreatitis, and diverticulitis. PVT can therefore be found incidentally when scanning the postoperative abdomen for another reason. Spontaneous portal vein thrombosis is a recognized, albeit uncommon, complication of abdominal surgery. This may result in one of the following complications:

- Portal hypertension (and cavernous transformation of the portal vein)
- Mesenteric ischemia/infarction
- Hepatic infarction

The management of PVT is difficult and guided by the patient's comorbidity and postoperative recovery. Some clinicians may consider anticoagulation or even intravascular thrombolysis; particularly in the setting of ischemia related to acute thrombosis, and in this setting, a vascular radiology opinion is essential. However, where cavernous transformation of the portal vein is recognized, this implies portal vein occlusion occurred weeks or months previously (i.e., it is not a current acute event). This observation may be very important to guide clinicians in their choice of patient management, particularly since anticoagulation may carry significant risks in patients soon after surgery.

1.9.4 Neutropenic Enterocolitis

This diagnosis should always be considered in immunocompromised postoperative patients or those undergoing chemotherapy (Fig. 1.48). Neutropenic enterocolitis, sometimes referred to as typhlitis, is a common cause of an acute abdomen in this patient group and most often produces right colonic mural thickening, pericolonic stranding, ascites, cecal pneumatosis, and associated small bowel thickening (the presence of the latter two signs is used in differentiating from pseudomembranous colitis) (Vogel et al. 2010).

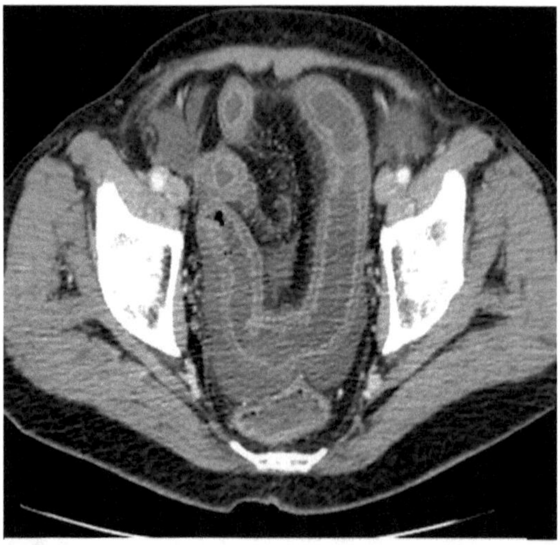

Fig. 1.48 Neutropenic enteritis. Patient with gastric carcinoma who developed an acute neutropenic enteritis after a single cycle of chemotherapy

1.9.5 The Other Postoperative "-itis's"

A detailed review of these topics is outside the brief of this chapter, and the reader is referred to appropriate general radiology textbooks and review articles. Acute appendicitis and acute diverticulitis are common causes of an acute abdomen and are as likely to develop in the postoperative abdomen as in the general population. Acute pancreatitis may follow a direct intraoperative injury to the pancreas or occur in a patient with established biliary tract disease (e.g., following laparoscopic cholecystectomy for cholelithiasis). Gallbladder disease however is worthy of particular evaluation.

1.9.5.1 Acute Cholecystitis

Variants include:

- Acute calculus cholecystitis
- Acute acalculous cholecystitis

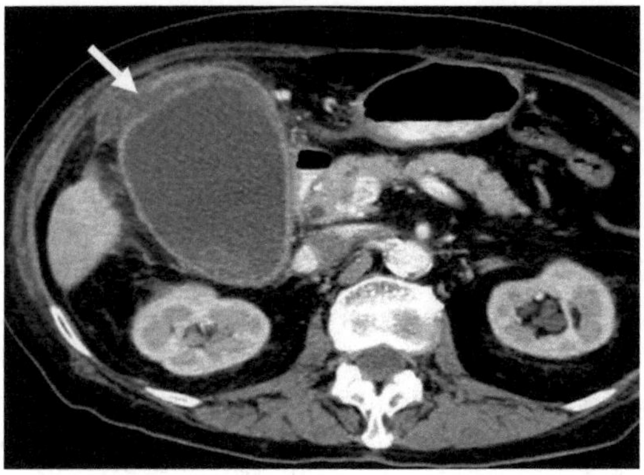

Fig. 1.49 Perforated gallbladder and biliary peritonitis. CT shows a small fundal perforation (*arrow*). Early percutaneous cholecystostomy can prevent this complication

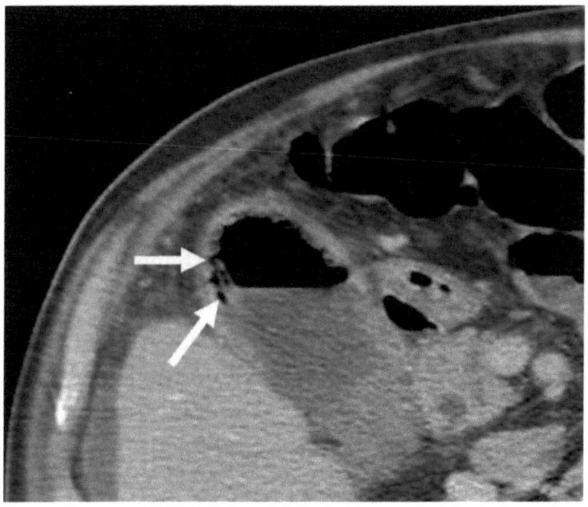

Fig. 1.50 Emphysematous cholecystitis. Coned CT view of the gallbladder showing an air/fluid level and mural gas (*arrows*)

- Gangrenous cholecystitis
- Emphysematous cholecystitis

Gallstones can occlude the cystic duct in any patient in the postoperative period, leading to acute cholecystitis. When the postoperative clinical picture is confusing and cholecystitis has not have been considered by referring clinicians, CT requested for an alternative suspected diagnosis may reveal the typical features of acute gallbladder inflammation. These include:

- A distended thick-walled gallbladder
- Hyperdense gall stones – however, ultrasound is more sensitive
- Pericholecystic inflammatory changes
- Complications including gallbladder perforation (Fig. 1.49), pericholecystic abscess and emphysematous cholecystitis (Fig. 1.50) (which is usually associated with diabetes), and gangrene (Fig. 1.51)

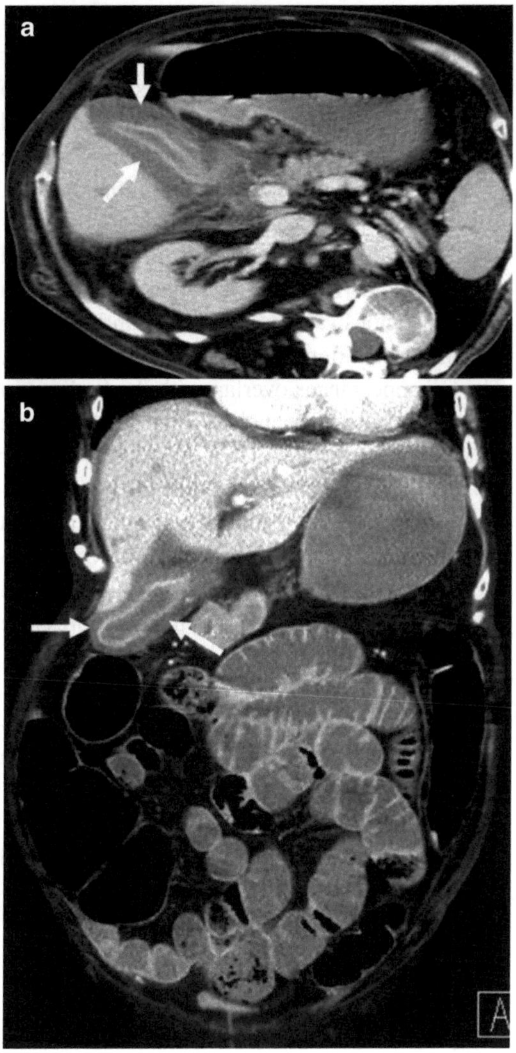

Fig. 1.51 Gangrenous cholecystitis. (**a**) Axial and (**b**) coronal CT images of patient with a surgically proven gangrenous cholecystitis. Note marked gallbladder wall thickening (*arrows*), associated ileus and spinal deformity

Where cholecystitis is the favored primary clinical diagnosis, abdominal ultrasound should be the initial imaging choice rather than CT. If jaundice develops and ultrasound cannot confirm or exclude common duct calculi or biliary dilatation, magnetic resonance cholangiopancreatography (MRCP) should be considered assuming the patient does not have a contraindication to MRI.

Acalculous cholecystitis is encountered in postoperative patients with severe burns or major trauma. It is estimated to be responsible for up to 90% of all postoperative acute cholecystitis and is thought to be due to a combination of the presence of systemic mediators of inflammation, biliary stasis and ischemia. The risk of complications, including gallbladder wall necrosis and subsequent perforation, is greater than with calculus cholecystitis. A significantly higher mortality rate often reflects a delayed diagnosis. The CT appearances overlap with the findings in conventional calculus cholecystitis, but the degree of gallbladder wall distension is often greater with the acalculous variant. When necrosis develops, mural irregularity, hypoenhancement, and intramural gas may be found. Progression to mural necrosis can be averted by image-guided percutaneous cholecystostomy to decompress the gallbladder.

Gangrenous cholecystitis usually develops as a complication of untreated cholecystitis and typically results from gallbladder wall ischemia developing secondary to excessive gallbladder distension. CT signs to look for include:

- Absent, discontinuous, or irregular mural enhancement
- Intraluminal membranes that appear as linear densities within the gallbladder lumen
- Gas within the gallbladder wall or lumen

1.10 Image-Guided Drainage

There are several causes of sepsis in the postoperative period:

- Anastomotic failure and leak
- Infected abdominal or pelvic fluid collections
- Peritonitis
- Infected ascites
- Obstructed kidney
- Gallbladder empyema
- Pneumonia
- Lung empyema

CT is often requested in patients who develop pyrexia, who have raised inflammatory markers, or who are slow to recover in the postoperative period. When a fluid collection is identified on imaging, it is important to liaise with the surgeon to correlate this with the clinical status of the patient and the likelihood that this may be infected.

Image-guided drainage of intra-abdominal collections or sources of sepsis is extremely important. Reoperating on a sick patient in order to drain a septic focus is associated with significant morbidity due to the risks of anesthesia and impaired postoperative bowel function. Wherever possible, the reporting radiologist should offer to drain a postoperative collection or, if they feel unable, to obtain an opinion from an interventional radiology colleague who can.

1.10.1 Route of Access

There are multiple anatomical routes for drainage:

- Pelvic collections – transrectal, transvaginal, or transgluteal
- Gallbladder empyema – transhepatic or direct puncture
- Lesser sac collections – transgastric via endoscopic ultrasound (EUS) or transabdominal route
- Lung empyema – pleural drainage

1.10.2 Choice of Modality

Ultrasound and CT can be used to guide percutaneous drainage. The choice depends on local practice and departmental design (e.g., a dedicated interventional ultrasound room can remove pressure from overburdened CT departments).

Advantages of ultrasound include:

- Its ability to characterize the content of fluid collections and to determine the presence of septations.
- Real-time ability to guide needle placement.
- Portability which is invaluable in draining collections in patients on intensive care/high dependency wards who are too unwell to travel to the radiology department.
- Access to particular cavities (e.g., transrectal, transvaginal, or EUS transgastric).

- Less dependence on the axial plane (cf. CT guided).
- Transducer pressure may displace overlying bowel loops.
- No radiation exposure.

Disadvantages of ultrasound include:

- Difficulties in draining deeper abdominopelvic and retroperitoneal collections
- Problems distinguishing gas/fluid-filled collections from atonic bowel
- Limited views in patients with dressings, surgical drains, and a "gassy" abdomen

Advantages of CT include:

- Accurate needle placement with visualization of adjacent and deeper structures, thus avoiding injury to bowel and organs.
- Facilitates drainage of deep abdominal, pelvic, and retroperitoneal collections.
- Oral contrast can be given to distinguish bowel from a collection.

Disadvantages include:

- Radiation exposure.
- Time-consuming, particularly if needle positioning is difficult due to the location of critical strictures in relation to the collection. This can be limited by access to CT fluoroscopy but will inevitably delay under pressure CT lists.
- Not portable.

1.10.3 Consent

Best practice dictates that the person performing the intervention should counsel the patient regarding the risks and benefits of any intervention. This assumes that the patient is competent to give their consent and understand the advantages and risks of the procedure. This presents difficulties in a number of scenarios including patients with preexisting cognitive impairment, patients with acute confusion related to systemic sepsis, and patient on intensive care with altered conscious levels. In these situations, it is important that any discussion is led by the clinical team since they will be best able to judge a patients competence to give informed consent or failing that to enable the patient's next of kin to be involved in any decision making.

When providing consent for any procedure, potential complications should be discussed. These should be events that are either common or severe/life threatening. There is very little consensus about what precisely should be included in consent for any particular procedure, but it should be remembered that inadequate consent is a common source of litigation, and that time spent in discussion and written recording of the consent process will limit the chances that legal action will be either necessary or succeed.

It is helpful during consent to explain the procedure in a step by step fashion so that the patient understands what to expect at each stage of the process, particularly as most image-guided intervention is performed without sedation. The patient should be told what to expect at the end of the procedure, and it is relevant to tell them whether they should expect postprocedure discomfort (e.g., following transgluteal drainage or where a drain lies against the diaphragm). When covering the risks of the procedure, the following main areas should be covered: bleeding, perforation (hollow viscus puncture or pneumothorax), and infection as well as the risks of not performing the procedure at all. This discussion should ideally take place in advance of the procedure in a quiet private environment to allow confidential discussion and an opportunity to ask questions.

1.10.4 Assessment of Coagulation Status

Routine measurement of clotting times and platelet levels is advised prior to drainage of fluid collections since these can be deranged if the patient is septic or has a relevant comorbidity, for example, where liver synthetic function is abnormal. There is no consensus on upper limits of clotting values above which drainage should not occur, and this will depend on personal practice and the method of drainage (e.g., transhepatic cholecystostomy or percutaneous transhepatic biliary drainage versus a superficial abdominal collection).

It is also important to consider the patients other medications, which may have important interactions with coagulation. These include the use of warfarin and heparin. Warfarin should be stopped prior to any procedure and converted to short-acting heparin that can be stopped just prior to the procedure (since it has a short half-life). Prophylactic low-molecular-weight heparin (dose 5,000 i.u) is not a contraindication to intervention, but therapeutic doses (e.g., >10,000 i.u) should be stopped 24 h prior. Cardiology patients are often on a combination of aspirin and clopidogrel, which are both antiplatelet agents. While many interventional radiologists are happy to continue aspirin, clopidogrel is usually stopped 7–10 days before any planned procedure. However, this may not be possible if the patient has recently undergone coronary artery stenting, for example, due to risk of stent occlusion. These decisions should be resolved on a case-by-case basis.

Personal practice varies, but the authors practice is to attempt drainage of easily accessible abdominal collections if the INR is less than 2 when the platelet count is normal (although many radiologists would only accept a lower INR threshold of 1.5 or less). Above this level, intravenous vitamin K can be administered, but this takes several hours to take effect and relies on good liver synthetic function; where this fails, fresh frozen plasma may be required. In clinical situations where immediate intervention is required in a patient with markedly deranged clotting, prothrombin agents such as Beriplex (CSL Behring, UK) can be used. In all such cases, discussion with a hematologist is advised.

1.10.5 Drainage Technique

1.10.5.1 Cleaning Solution

The skin at the site of intended needle puncture is initially cleaned with agents such as alcohol, chlorhexidine, or iodine. Chlorhexidine is associated with less allergic reactions than iodine-based solutions. The site of needle entry should be cleansed in a slightly abrasive manner (to ensure adequate sterilization), starting centrally and working systematically outward in a circular fashion (in order not to contaminate a clean area with skin commensal organisms).

1.10.5.2 Local Anesthetic

Lidocaine is the most commonly used agent. Its duration of action is approximately 1 h. Lidocaine is available in 1% or 2% concentration and has a maximum dose of 20 or 10 ml, respectively (for a 70-kg patient = 3 mg/kg), since doses above this carry a risk of cardiotoxicity. Mixing adrenaline with lidocaine can double its duration of action by inducing local vessel vasoconstriction and reduced systemic absorption. This also allows a greater dose to be used (7 mg/kg). Bupivacaine has a longer duration of action (approximately 12 h) and can be used in procedures where prolonged anesthesia may be required, for example, following transgluteal drainage.

Skin anesthesia is usually achieved with a 21 G or 23 G needle forming a large superficial "bleb." Deeper anesthesia is obtained with a larger diameter needle (19 G), aspirating prior to injecting and to ensure that injection into a vessel does not occur. It is important to inform the patient that they will experience a second "sting" when the needle comes into contact with the peritoneum. At this point, administration of a generous quantity of local anesthetic is advised as passage of dilators and drains through the peritoneal lining can be painful.

1.10.5.3 Technique

Collections can be drained by either a "single-stab" or Seldinger technique. The "single-stab" method can be employed when the collection is large, superficial, or if it is being drained under ultrasound guidance. The editors favor the Seldinger technique as this provides more secure access and is performed over a guidewire (usually a J-wire). CT or ultrasound images of the wire within the collection are reassuring but not always required as long as the initial cannula needle puncture position is confirmed in the center of the collection and fluid is easily aspirated. It is important to remember that it may not be possible to aspirate very viscous fluid despite a well-sited cannula, and proceeding to drain placement will usually yield fluid.

When advancing dilators over the wire to allow subsequent drain placement, it is important to advance the dilator in the direction of the initial puncture to avoid an acute kink forming in the wire. This also occurs if the wire is coiled within the collection or a loop forms in the soft tissues between the skin and target cavity, and the same point on the wire is repeatedly stretched on a bend. When this occurs, salvage of the procedure requires careful thought. In most cases, if the kink is within the collection, a large dilator may be left in the collection (e.g., 8–10 Fr) and the wire pulled back firmly and then exchanged for a new one. If the kink is within the soft tissues, this is more problematic. If lots of wire is looped within the collection, then it may be possible to withdraw the wire so that this kink lies "outside" the patient. It may then be possible to advance a thinner more flexible dilator or the plastic sheath of the puncture needle across the kink into the collection, without displacing the wire, to allow safe exchange for a new wire. Where this maneuver fails, a new puncture of the collection will be required.

The drainage catheter contains an internal stiffener cannula of either plastic or metal, and both are advanced through the skin and subcutaneous tissues and just into the collection. The cannula is then unlocked from the drain and the drain advanced into the collection over the wire. If both the stiffener and the catheter are advanced as a single unit into the collection, there is a chance that the catheter can pass through the posterior part of the collection. The editors favor use of larger diameter drains (10–12-Fr pigtail catheters) if the fluid is turbid with 8-Fr drains reserved for more serous fluid collections. This can usually be judged by the fluid content aspirated at the initial puncture. Occasionally, multiple drains are required if there is more than one fluid collection or if the collection is septated or loculated. If the collection is surrounded by bowel, turning the patient into an oblique or lateral position can move bowel away from the line of access. Traversing small bowel is not an absolute contraindication to percutaneous drainage particularly if the patient is too unwell for surgical intervention.

When the drain is sited, the collection should be aspirated to dryness using a three-way tap into the drainage bag and then left on free drainage. Generous dressings are also applied to prevent drains dislodging on the ward. Depending on the location of the drain, the underlying cause for the collection forming and difficulty of the procedure, it may be appropriate to perform imaging prior to drain removal. In some cases where no further fluid is draining (e.g., in the pelvis), retraction of the drain into a more superficial locule will be successful and prevent the patient undergoing a second potentially unnecessary procedure. It is therefore important to indicate this clearly in the patient record to prevent inappropriate drain removal on the ward.

1.11 Principles of Fluoroscopy and Ultrasound in the Postoperative Patient

1.11.1 Fluoroscopy: General Considerations

Fluoroscopic examinations provide real-time functional assessment and familiar images for surgical colleagues to interpret compared with other modalities. However, they rely on a patient being able to cooperate with the procedure and in particular to move while on a fluoroscopy machine (e.g., into a decubitus position for rectal catheter placement) or to drink liquid for upper GI contrast studies. The radiologist who performs these studies often best appreciates these human factors (i.e., to know what is and is not possible for a particular patient). A patient's mobility, presence of obesity, requirement for respiratory support, number and position of drains, catheters, intravenous infusion lines, and whether they have access to analgesia influence this. Fluoroscopy is therefore usually reserved for patients that are not critically ill (where CT provides a more rapid global assessment).

1.11.1.1 Contrast Selection

When selecting a contrast agent, it is important to remember that barium has a very limited role. Water-soluble iodinated contrast agents are typically chosen because of the risk of barium peritonitis from a barium leak. Barium is not easily reabsorbed when a leak occurs into the thorax or mediastinum, and there will be artifact if CT scans are required. In addition, administering barium to a patient with bowel obstruction or ileus may result in barolith formation and make a bad problem worse. A double-contrast study is not required in the postoperative assessment, and the mucosal coating that barium provides is generally not needed.

When selecting an iodinated contrast agent, the choice is of either a nonionic or an ionic agent. If there is any possibility of aspiration of contrast (i.e., for upper GI contrast studies), then nonionic contrast is required since aspiration of ionic contrast can result in severe pneumonitis. The authors have now moved to using only nonionic contrast for these examinations. A high iodine concentration is usually required (300 mg/ml) for upper GI contrast studies or where small volumes on contrast are being used to allow adequate visualization (e.g., cutaneous fistula assessment). Lower iodine concentration (150 mg/ml) may be used where larger volumes on contrast are needed such as for postoperative examinations of the lower GI or urinary tract. Ionic contrast may be used in these cases without the concerns regarding risk of aspiration, and it may be cheaper to use in the volumes that are needed for these studies. The miscellaneous "problem-solving" examinations often asked of fluoroscopy, such as evaluation of abdominal fistulas and confirming position of drains, may be performed with either ionic or nonionic contrast.

There are two areas where barium may still have a role. The first is in assessment of patients after esophagectomy. A minority of departments choose to follow an initial normal assessment of the anastomosis with iodinated contrast with a final check with barium since its superior mucosal coating can detect very subtle anastomotic defects. Second is in the assessment of a patient with a "battlefield abdomen" from previous surgeries with multiple abdominal wall fistulas. In this setting, a combination of fistulography may be coupled with a barium small bowel meal-type examination. Often, water-soluble contrast agents become too dilute to give accurate anatomic detail of the small bowel, and in these long-term hospital inpatients that have had surgery many months earlier, there is no longer concern for peritoneal leak since the small bowel loops are cocooned in adhesions.

1.11.1.2 Therapeutic Effects

Water-soluble fluoroscopic examinations can have a dual role. As well as excluding pathology, they can also have an important therapeutic effect on the intestine. Postoperative small bowel contrast studies after administration of 50–150 ml iodinated contrast, in the presence of ileus or obstruction of the small bowel seen on CT, have been shown to reduce the need for surgery and predict success of conservative management (Catena et al. 2011). Similarly, large bowel ileus often responds well to a water-soluble enema, which may be performed to exclude an obstructing lesion in a collapsed segment of distal colon demonstrated at CT.

1.11.1.3 Integration with CT

A final consideration is that fluoroscopic evaluation can be coupled with subsequent CT scanning. This is particularly important where the postoperative anatomy is distorted, and there is doubt at the end of the examination whether a leak is present or not. An immediate unenhanced CT can quickly resolve any doubt. The presence of high-strength oral contrast does not prevent accurate detection of leaks as the area of concern can be viewed with a widened CT window. In certain cases, the editors use fluoroscopy less frequently and perform CT with higher-strength contrast to detect postoperative leaks, for example, 8% Omnipaque 300 mg/ml (20 ml mixed with 250 ml of water).

1.11.2 Ultrasound: General Considerations

The outstanding attributes of ultrasound are its portability and real-time evaluation (Sect. 1.10.2). In the assessment of a postoperative patient, there are clear roles where ultrasound is an appropriate first diagnostic tool. These include the evaluation of the renal tract for obstruction, assessment of vessel patency in the liver transplantation, exclusion of deep vein thrombosis, as well as for directing image-guided intervention. However, there may be a role of ultrasound in other situations where CT is deemed inappropriate, for example, where a patient is deemed too unstable for transfer outside a critical care ward so that although the exclusion value may be more limited, it can still direct patient care.

Where ultrasound assessment is determined to be the most appropriate examination, the patient must be appropriately prepared. This should involve removal of as many dressings as possible to allow access to the abdomen or site of interest, and liaison with ward nursing staff is very important in this regard. However, some dressings cannot be removed so easily and so must be worked around (e.g., those related to vacuum packing devices). Similarly, an open abdominal wound or presence of stoma bags will further exacerbate problems with access.

Ultrasound probes should have a disposable probe cover placed on it as part of a good hospital infection control strategy as well as thorough cleaning of the probe at the end of the procedure with antiseptic wipes to reduce risk of spread of infection.

A gas-filled abdomen can make assessment very difficult. However, a rigorous assessment for ultrasound "windows" can achieve the diagnosis. In this setting, it is important that any urinary catheters are clamped so that the full bladder can be used to assess the pelvis. It is also important that additional support staff are available to help turn and support the patient to allow assessment of the retroperitoneum and pleural spaces. In patients with peritonism or severe abdominal pain, probe pressure may make the examination intolerable. Planning prior analgesia administration can assist and reduce delays for it taking effect.

Where there is a high index of suspicion that a collection is present, it is often better to anticipate this by planning intervention at the same visit and bringing all relevant equipment where a portable examination is being performed. This minimizes delay and is a most time effective. To enable this, remember to ensure that coagulation has been assessed (and is normal) and that the supervising clinician is happy for you to proceed before leaving the department.

References

Bader FG, Schröder M, Kujath P, Muhl E, Bruch HP, Eckmann C. Diffuse postoperative peritonitis – value of diagnostic parameters and impact of early indication for relaparotomy. Eur J Med Res. 2009;14: 491–6.

Bevan KE, Venkatasubramaniam A, Mohamed F, Moran BJ, Cecil TD. Respect for the laparoscopic port site: lessons in diagnosis, management, and prevention of port-site hernias following laparoscopic colorectal surgery. J Laparoendosc Adv Surg Tech A. 2010;20: 451–4.

Catena F, Di Saverio S, Kelly MD, Biffl WL, Ansaloni L, Mandala V, Velmahos GC, Sartelli M, Tugnoli G, Lupo M, Mandala S, Pinna AD, Sugarbaker PH, Van Goor H, Moore EE, Jeekel J. Bologna guidelines for diagnosis and Management of Adhesive Small Bowel Obstruction (ASBO): 2010 Evidence-Based Guidelines of the World Society of Emergency Surgery. World J Emerg Surg. 2011;6:5.

Del Rio P, Dell'Abate P, Gomes B, Fumagalli M, Papadia C, Coruzzi A, Leonardi F, Pucci F, Sianesi M. Analysis of risk factors for complications in 262 cases of laparoscopic colectomy. Ann Ital Chir. 2010;81:21–30.

Earls JP, Dachman AH, Colon E, Garrett MG, Molloy M. Prevalence and duration of postoperative pneumoperitoneum: sensitivity of CT vs left lateral decubitus radiography. AJR Am J Roentgenol. 1993;161:781–5.

Elsayes KM, Menias CO, Smullen TL, Platt JF. Closed-loop small-bowel obstruction: diagnostic patterns by multidetector computed tomography. J Comput Assist Tomogr. 2007;31:697–701.

Ergün T, Lakadamyal H. The CT frequencies of various non-traumatic acute abdominal emergencies in hemodialysis, peritoneal dialysis patients and the general population. Eur J Radiol. 2012;81:13–20.

Frager DH, Baer JW, Rothpearl A, Bossart PA. Distinction between postoperative ileus and mechanical small-bowel obstruction: value of CT compared with clinical and other radiographic findings. AJR Am J Roentgenol. 1995;164:891–4.

Gayer G, Jonas T, Apter S, Amitai M, Shabtai M, Hertz M. Postoperative pneumoperitoneum as detected by CT: prevalence, duration, and relevant factors affecting its possible significance. Abdom Imaging. 2000; 25:301–5.

Kerr SF, Hyland R, Rowbotham E, Chalmers AG. Postoperative omental infarction following colonic resection. Clin Radiol. 2012;67:134–9.

Manzella A, Filho PB, Albuquerque E, Farias F, Kaercher J. Imaging of gossypibomas: pictorial review. AJR Am J Roentgenol. 2009;193:S94–101.

Ott V, Groebli Y, Schneider R. Late intestinal fistula formation after incisional hernia using intraperitoneal mesh. Hernia. 2005;9:103–4.

Singh AK, Gervais DA, Lee P, Westra S, Hahn PF, Novelline RA, Mueller PR. Omental infarct: CT imaging features. Abdom Imaging. 2006;31:549–54.

Taourel P, Aufort S, Merigeaud S, Doyon FC, Hoquet MD, Delabrousse E. Imaging of ischemic colitis. Radiol Clin North Am. 2008;46:909–24.

Vogel MN, Goeppert B, Maksimovic O, Brodoefel H, Faul C, Claussen CD, Horger M. CT features of neutropenic enterocolitis in adult patients with hematological diseases undergoing chemotherapy. Rofo. 2010;182(1):76–81.

Young ST, Paulson EK, McCann RL, Baker ME. Appearance of oxidized cellulose (Surgicel) on postoperative CT scans: similarity to postoperative abscess. AJR Am J Roentgenol. 1993;160:275–7.

Zielinski MD, Eiken PW, Bannon MP, Heller SF, Lohse CM, Huebner M, Sarr MG. Small bowel obstruction-who needs an operation? A multivariate prediction model. World J Surg. 2010;34:910–9.

The Esophagus

2

Damian J.M. Tolan, Keith M. Harris, Deepak Prasad, and Samir P. Mehta

Contents

2.1	**Introduction**	41
2.1.1	General Considerations	41
2.2	**Esophageal Resection**	42
2.2.1	Clinical Indications	42
2.2.2	Surgical Techniques and Postoperative Anatomy	42
2.2.3	Normal Postoperative Imaging	44
2.2.4	Postoperative Complications	46
2.2.5	Role of Image-Guided Intervention	57
2.3	**Esophageal Bypass and Substitution**	58
2.3.1	Clinical Indications	58
2.3.2	Choice of Conduit/Substitute and Position	58
2.3.3	Normal Postoperative Imaging	59
2.3.4	Postoperative Complications	61
2.4	**Heller Myotomy**	65
2.4.1	Clinical Indication and Surgical Technique	65
2.4.2	Postoperative Imaging	66
2.4.3	Postoperative Complications	66
2.5	**Teaching Points**	68
References		69

D.J.M. Tolan, MBChB, MRCP, FRCR (✉)
Department of Clinical Radiology, Leeds Teaching Hospitals NHS Trust, Lincoln Wing, St James's University Hospital, LS9 7JT, Leeds, UK
e-mail: damian.tolan@leedsth.nhs.uk

K.M. Harris, FRCSEd, FRCR
Department of Clinical Radiology, Leeds Teaching Hospitals NHS Trust, Bexley Wing, St James's University Hospital, LS9 7JT, Leeds, UK

D. Prasad, MBBS, MRCP, FRCR
Department of Radiology, Bradford Teaching Hospitals NHS Trust, Bradford Royal Infirmary, Duckworth Lane, Bradford, BD9 6RJ, UK

S.P. Mehta, MA, DM (Oxon), FRCS
Department of Upper Gastrointestinal Surgery, Leeds Teaching Hospitals NHS Trust, Bexley Wing, St James's University Hospital, LS9 7JT, Leeds, UK

2.1 Introduction

Esophageal surgery is performed for both benign and malignant diseases and ranges in complexity depending on the degree of access required to the thorax and mediastinum and whether anastomoses are formed. Radical esophageal resection carries a significant mortality and morbidity. Radiology has an important role in both patient selection for surgery and the assessment and treatment of postoperative complications. A thorough understanding of operative procedures and normal postoperative anatomy is key to ensure that imaging techniques are optimized to detect these complications and guide management.

2.1.1 General Considerations

Patient care within the radiology department is of primary importance. Depending on the operation, patients may have chest drains, abdominal drains, urinary catheters, central venous access

J. Brittenden, D.J.M. Tolan (eds.), *Radiology of the Post Surgical Abdomen*,
DOI 10.1007/978-1-4471-2775-8_2, © Springer-Verlag London 2012

catheters, nasogastric tubes, and sometimes feeding jejunostomies. They may also require ventilatory support. This combination adds greatly to the complexity of patient preparation and transfer to and from the radiology department. It is therefore essential that adequate staffing is available to assist in transfers and proper care is taken to ensure that catheters and drains are not displaced.

2.2 Esophageal Resection

2.2.1 Clinical Indications

Esophageal resection is typically reserved for malignancy and less commonly required for non-malignant diseases, where it is usually reserved for treatment of intractable benign strictures unresponsive to balloon dilatation or stenting. Recognized indications for esophageal resection include:

- Esophageal malignancy
- High-grade dysplasia in Barrett's esophagus
- Strictures due to reflux, radiation, or caustic ingestion
- Neuromotor dysfunction from end-stage achalasia or scleroderma
- Iatrogenic perforation
- Spontaneous perforation (Boerhaave's syndrome)

2.2.2 Surgical Techniques and Postoperative Anatomy

Part or all of these operations may be performed laparoscopically depending on local expertise. Minimally invasive surgery has the benefit of improved short-term outcomes following resection, including reduced hospital stay, lower postoperative blood loss, and fewer overall complications (Verhage et al. 2009).

2.2.2.1 Ivor Lewis (Lewis-Tanner) Esophagectomy

This is a two-stage procedure commonly performed for mid-esophageal malignancy and benign disease affecting the mid- to distal esophagus.

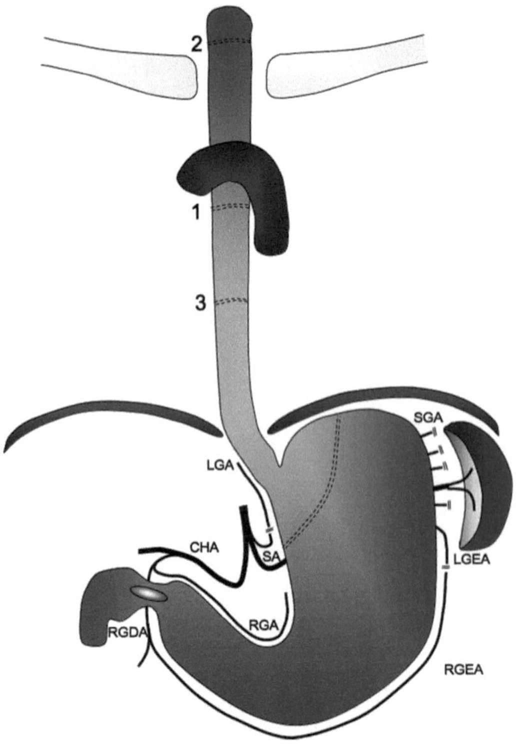

Fig. 2.1 Overview of resections. Resection of the esophagus involves dissection within the abdomen and thorax with potential to extend into the neck. The abdominal stage of esophagectomy procedures involves midline incision and division of the short gastric (*SGA*), left gastroepiploic (*LGEA*), and left gastric (*LGA*) arteries, leaving the right-sided vessels (right gastric (*RGA*) and right gastroepiploic (*RGEA*) from the right gastroduodenal artery (*RGDA*) as the dominant arterial supply to the stomach tube and the spleen and splenic artery (*SA*) and common hepatic artery to liver (CHA) intact. The tube is fashioned by stapling from the lesser curve toward the fundus. A pyloroplasty is performed to facilitate gastric emptying as the vagus nerve fibers to the pylorus are sacrificed. Depending on the extent of resection required, the anastomosis is then made to mid-esophagus (*1* Ivor Lewis esophagectomy), cervical esophagus (*2* either Lewis-McKeown or transhiatal esophagectomy), or more distal esophagus (*3* thoracoabdominal esophagectomy)

First, the accessible parts of the lower esophagus, stomach, and duodenum are fully mobilized via an abdominal approach (Fig. 2.1) accompanied with lymphadenectomy focusing upon the coeliac axis and its branches. Depending on local practice, a pyloroplasty is performed at this time to facilitate gastric emptying (as the vagus nerves that relax the pylorus are

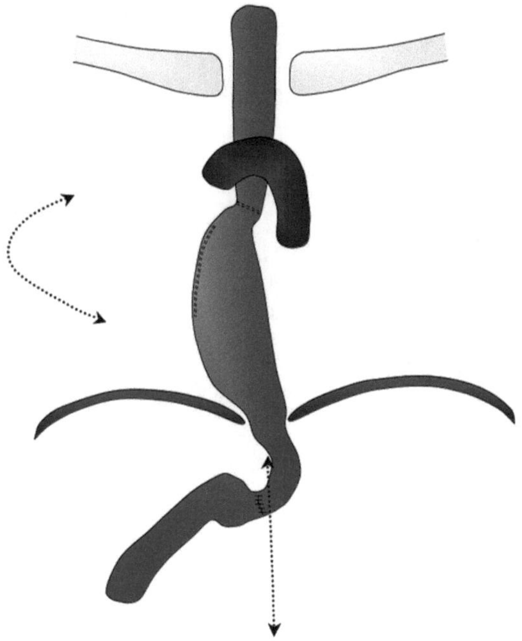

Fig. 2.2 Ivor Lewis procedure. After abdominal dissection, the thorax is opened via the 4th or 5th intercostal space (*arrows*) following collapse of the right lung. The esophagus is dissected to the level of the aortic arch, and the diseased esophagus and cardia are removed. The gastric tube is delivered into the thorax, and the fundus is anastomosed to the remnant esophagus below the aortic arch

sacrificed when the lesser curve and fundus are transected with esophagus). The abdomen is then closed.

The second stage enters the right chest via the fourth or fifth rib interspace. The esophagus is mobilized with an extensive lymphadenectomy, and the tumor is resected with a wide tumor-free margin. A gastric tube is created out of the mobilized stomach by resection of the greater curve (usually with a linear stapler) and a stapled end-to-end or end-to-side anastomosis made from the gastric conduit to the remaining esophagus at the approximate level of the aortic arch (Figs. 2.2 and 2.3a–c).

2.2.2.2 Three-Stage (Lewis-McKeown) Esophagectomy

In addition to the Ivor Lewis procedure, this technique employs a neck dissection as a third stage (Fig. 2.1). This allows an esophagogastric anastomosis to be fashioned in the neck (Fig. 2.4) to allow resection of the esophageal segment from the thoracic inlet to the aortic arch and results in a more extensive esophageal resection and lymphadenectomy.

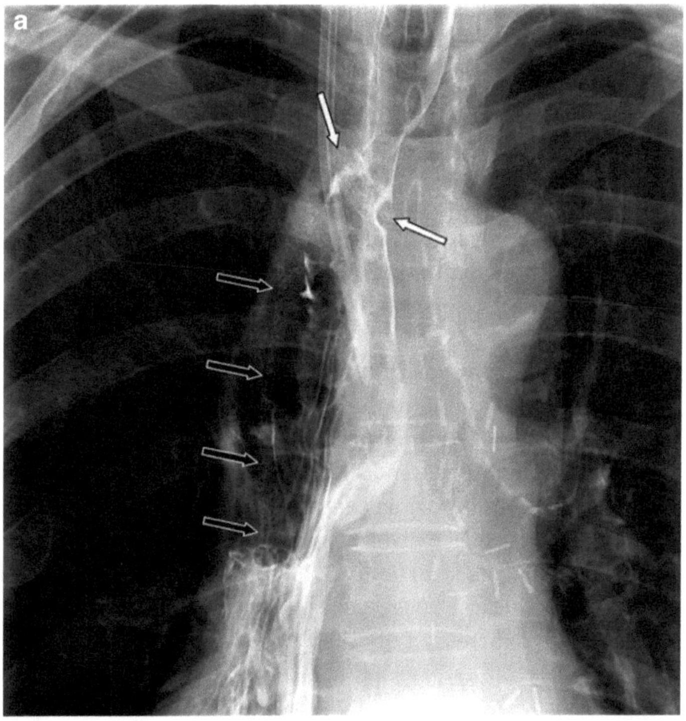

Fig. 2.3 Normal postoperative evaluation following Ivor Lewis esophagectomy. (**a**) Proximal esophagogastric anastomosis indicated by oblique staple line (*white arrows*) and gastric tube stapled anastomosis (*black arrows*). (**b**) The gastric tube is clearly defined and intact (*black arrows*). The right chest drain (*C*) and right internal jugular line are normally placed postoperatively. (**c**) Prompt emptying of the antrum (*A*) into the duodenum (*D2*) with no sign of pyloroplasty leak (*arrow head*)

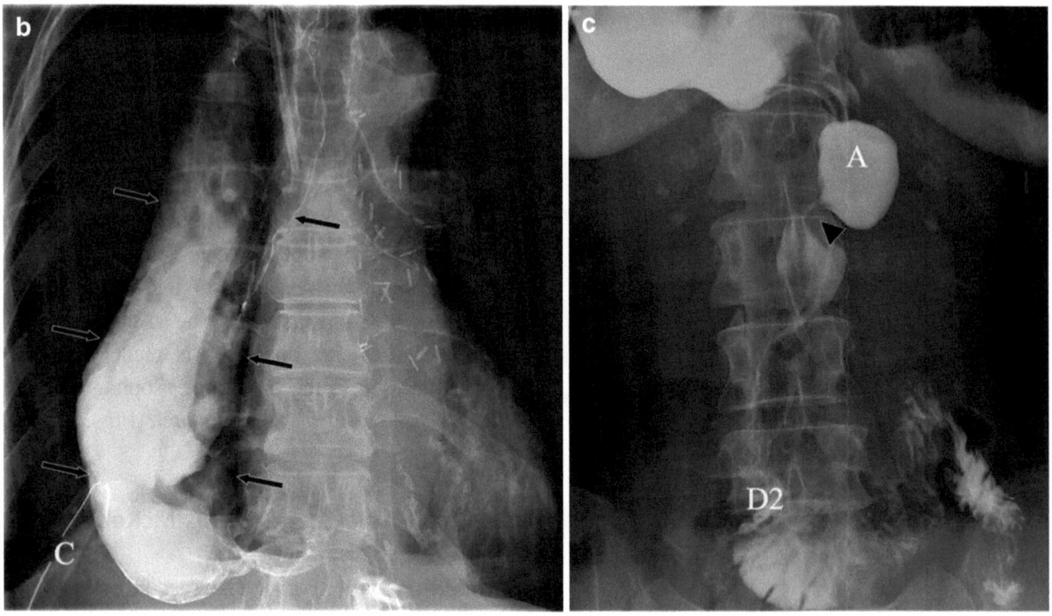

Fig. 2.3 (continued)

2.2.2.3 Transhiatal Esophagectomy Without Thoracotomy

The stomach and esophagus are first mobilized from below by dissection through the esophageal hiatus and then from above through the neck (Fig. 2.1). The esophageal anastomosis to the gastric tube is made in the neck after delivering the tube through the posterior mediastinum (Figs. 2.5 and 2.6). By avoiding a thoracotomy, this procedure is usually reserved for patients with poor respiratory function and/or patients with very early stage malignancy, as an extensive lymphadenectomy is not feasible. It has also been used for curative and palliative resections of thoracic and cervicothoracic esophageal malignancy.

2.2.2.4 Left Thoracoabdominal Approach

The abdominal and posterior mediastinal dissections can be undertaken through a single incision along the left sixth or seventh intercostal space. A gastric tube is fashioned and anastomosed in a similar manner to the Ivor Lewis resection (Fig. 2.7). Although less favored than the Ivor Lewis and transhiatal esophagectomy, it continues to be used in the treatment of esophageal or gastric tumors near the gastroesophageal junction.

2.2.3 Normal Postoperative Imaging

2.2.3.1 Upper GI Contrast Studies

Water-soluble contrast studies are performed 5–10 days postoperatively, depending on local preference. While they are a standard part of postoperative care in the majority of surgical units, they are not performed routinely in all in which case they are reserved for patients in whom there is clinical concern for leak (Hogan et al. 2008). Their role is to assess for anastomotic integrity and to look for the presence of leaks before removal of chest drains and nasogastric tubes and before commencing oral intake. Ionic or nonionic iodinated contrast may be used. An advantage of nonionic contrast is that where aspiration occurs, there is no risk of chemical pneumonitis that may occur with ionic agents. Dilute barium contrast has been recommended for use after an initial negative water-soluble evaluation to detect subtle anastomotic leaks and increase sensitivity (Swanson et al. 2003; Tanomkiat and Galassi 2000). This is not our routine practice.

It is important to obtain control radiographs at the level of the anastomosis to identify the

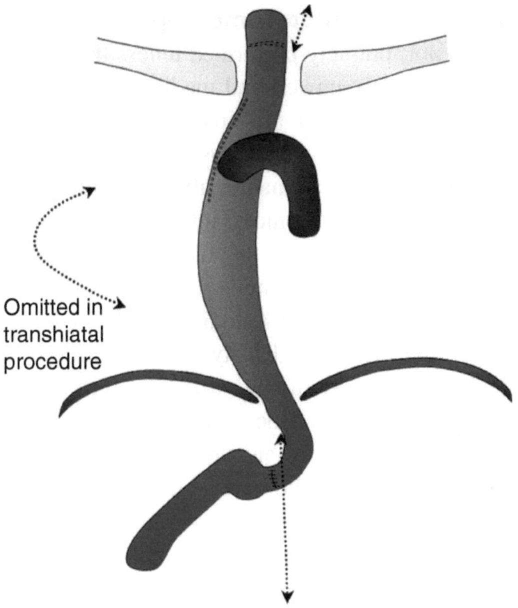

Fig. 2.4 Lewis-McKeown procedure. The thorax is usually entered first (*arrows*), followed by the abdomen with dissection of the neck at the end of the procedure via a left cervical incision (*arrows*) where the gastroesophageal anastomosis is formed. This allows resection of more proximal tumors and more extensive lymphadenectomy. Transhiatal procedure. Thoracic incision is avoided. Gastric dissection is continued into the posterior mediastinum to the level of the carina after the hiatus is widened. The left side of the neck is then opened (*arrows*), and the more proximal esophagus ics dissected down to the carina from above. The cervical esophagus is divided and the esophagus removed. The gastric tube is finally maneuvered through the posterior mediastinum for anastomosis to the cervical esophagus (see Fig. 2.6)

rows of surgical sutures and the volume of effusions present. This also aids subsequent interpretation to allow differentiation of surgical clips from small leaks and detect increased density of pleural effusions or along drains when an occult leak is present. Normally there is free flow of contrast across the esophagogastric anastomosis with no holdup. It is also essential that the patient takes an adequate amount of contrast with each swallow as small leaks may be missed if sufficient distension is not achieved with contrast. It is important to ensure that all potential sites of leak are examined in turn during the examination (Sect. 2.2.4.2).

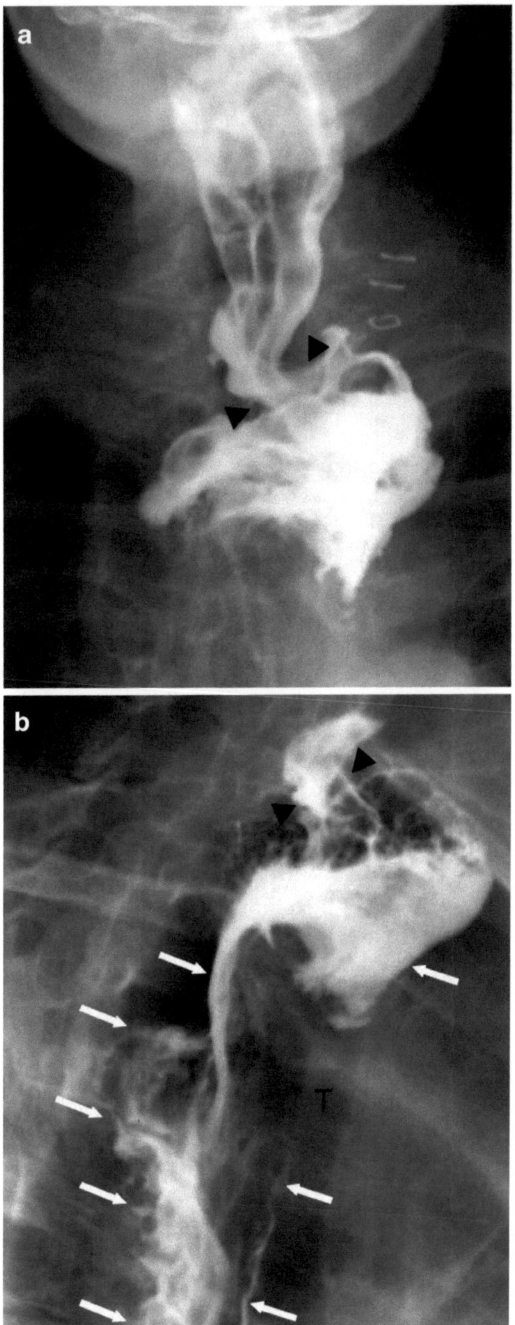

Fig. 2.5 (**a**, **b**) Normal esophagogastric anastomosis in the neck just above the thoracic inlet (*arrowheads*) following three-stage esophagectomy. Staples are related to closure of the cervical dissection. The gastric tube (*arrows*) abuts the trachea (*T*)

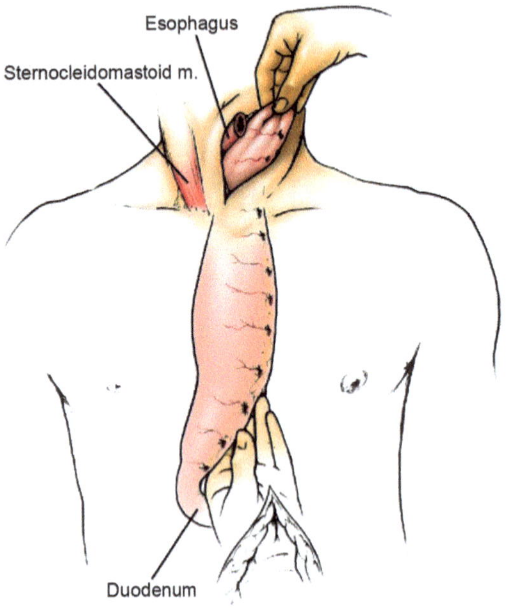

Fig. 2.6 Transhiatal esophagectomy. The esophagus is delivered into the neck from the abdomen without thoracotomy

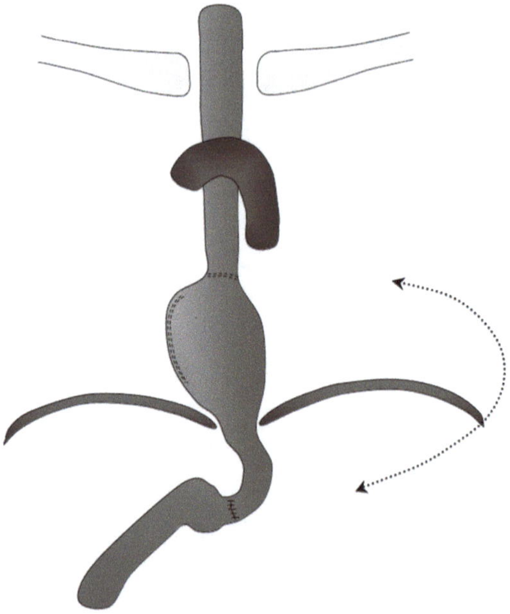

Fig. 2.7 Thoracoabdominal procedure. The thorax and abdomen are both opened through a single extended intercostal incision to include the left diaphragm (*arrows*). Since the descending aorta limits access to the esophagus, dissection is more limited and the anastomosis is more caudal

2.2.3.2 Computed Tomography (CT)

CT is not routinely performed unless the patient is systemically unwell and mediastinal and thoracic complications are suspected. When performed, water-soluble contrast media given orally just before the examination allows simultaneous assessment of anastomotic integrity. Many radiologists advocate use of higher-concentration oral contrast for these studies, which is our practice (e.g., 500 ml of 8% nonionic iodinated contrast); the increased density aids detection of a leak without producing artifacts. Intravenous contrast should also be administered to clarify mediastinal anatomy and to allow detection of other important pathologies such as pulmonary embolism. The anastomosis should be in continuity with absence of extraluminal gas or fluid collections, and an intact staple line should be present. Stranding in the fat around the anastomosis is normal in the early postoperative period, and pulmonary atelectasis is frequently present.

2.2.4 Postoperative Complications

The frequency of postoperative complications is high in this group of patients, ranging from 40% to 60%, and influenced by choice of technique and patient factors (e.g., minimal vs. open, smoker vs. nonsmoker) (Griffin et al. 2002; Veeramootoo et al. 2009; Verhage et al. 2009). Although there are variations in the surgical technique for esophagectomy, the main categories of complications are similar. Certain complications occur either during or very soon after surgery and are detected and treated by experienced clinical teams without recourse to complex radiological investigation. These include:

- Tracheal injury (1%) (Gupta et al. 2009)
- Mediastinal vascular injury (3%)
- Gastric tube necrosis (1–2%) (Sect. 2.2.4.3)

They are usually recognized at the time of surgery or in the early postoperative period (1–2 days), precipitating an immediate return to theater (Sarela et al. 2008; Griffin et al. 2002).

Recurrent laryngeal nerve palsy is uncommon (<3%), arising as a result of retraction of tissues

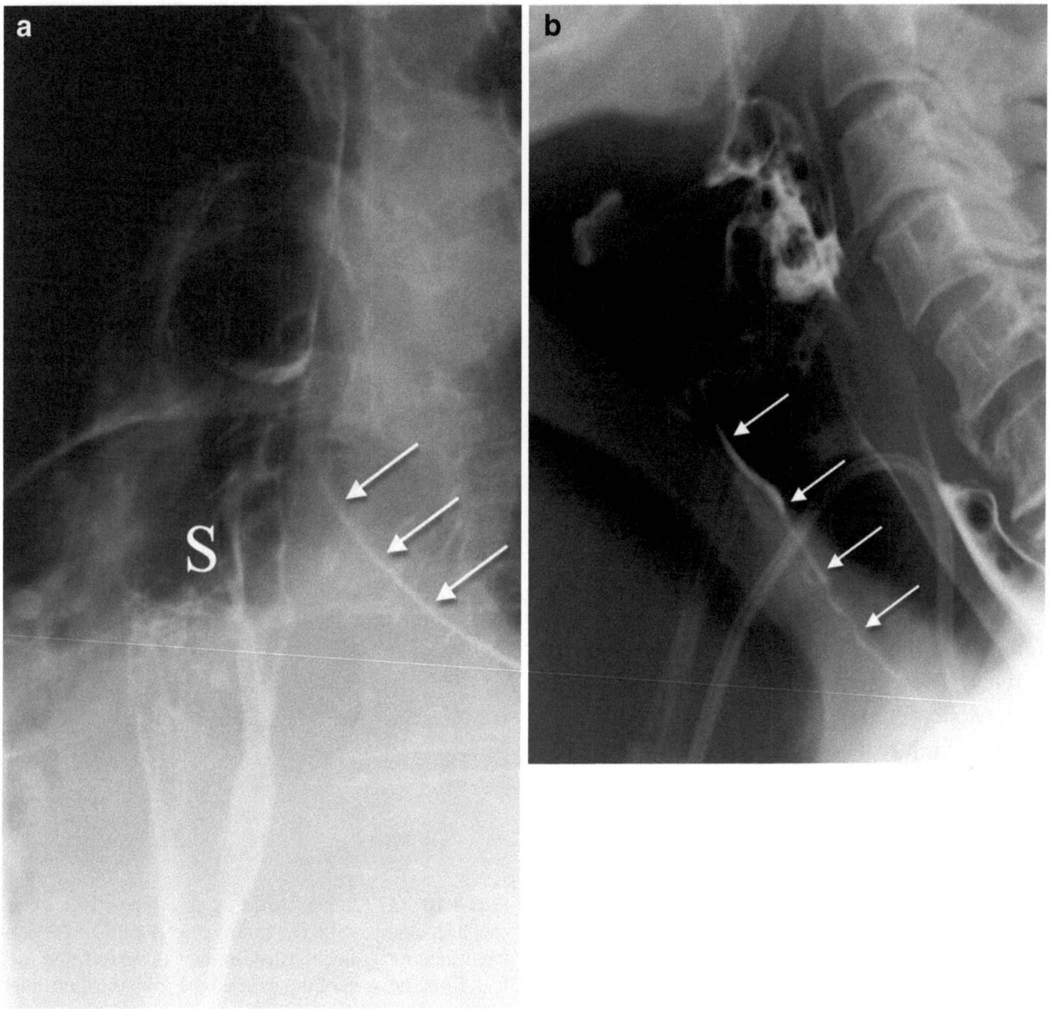

Fig. 2.8 Aspiration: a potential pitfall. (**a**) Transhiatal esophagectomy with contrast within the left lower lobe bronchus (*arrows*) raises possibility of esophagotracheal fistula despite normal assessment of anastomosis and gastric tube (*S*). (**b**) However, assessment of the pharynx reveals gross aspiration of contrast (*arrows*), subsequently determined as due to recurrent laryngeal nerve palsy

during dissection for cervical anastomosis, particularly in transhiatal surgery, with little role for radiology in the diagnosis or management. This is usually transient, but in a minority, it may persist. The main clinical relevance is the loss of airway protection and increased risk of aspiration (Fig. 2.8).

We will now deal with those more common complications or those where radiology has input in diagnosis and management.

2.2.4.1 Pulmonary and Pleural Complications

These are the most common complications of esophagectomy, and major complications occur in up to 20% of patients (Verhage et al. 2009; Griffin et al. 2002) with risk increased in smokers and those undergoing thoracotomy. They fall into two groups: general complications of thoracic surgery such as atelectasis, pneumonia, aspiration, pulmonary embolism, and respiratory

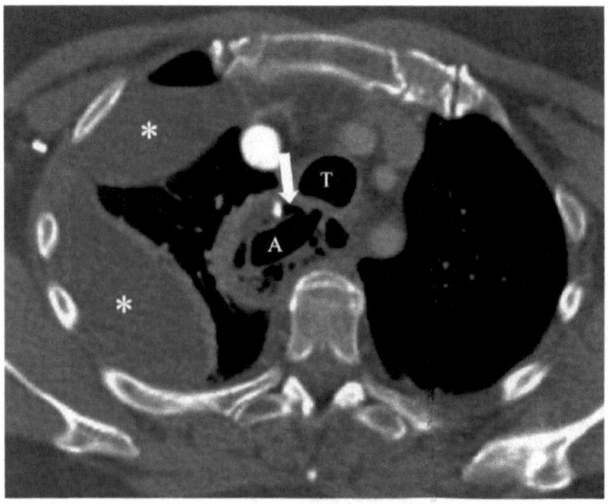

Fig. 2.9 Breathless and poor progress with a large right effusion on radiograph 2 weeks post-Ivor Lewis esophagectomy. Small defect in the anastomosis (*A*) medial to the staple line filled with gas (*arrow*), producing a large loculated right hydropneumothorax (*asterisks*)

failure and those that are specific to esophageal surgery. These specific complications also fall into two categories: those arising as a consequence of injury to a structure, such as to the thoracic duct (producing a chyle leak and chylothorax in1% of cases) or blood vessels (hemothorax), or those resulting from loss of integrity of the gastric tube or anastomoses (empyema, pneumothorax, fistula etc.).

Plain film radiography has an important role in the rapid initial evaluation of these complications, in conjunction with monitoring of type and volume of output from chest drains (e.g., enteric vs. chylous vs. blood) and the patient's clinical status. Ultrasound or CT may be employed to assess for loculation of effusions, but CT is also able to assess for pulmonary embolism that may complicate the postoperative patient and explain sudden respiratory compromise while also allowing a more global assessment including the mediastinum and anastomoses and should be considered the main diagnostic tool (Fig. 2.9). It can also plan intervention, such as to target loculated pleural collections distant to surgical postoperative drains for image-guided drainage, which may be carried out with either CT or ultrasound.

Fistulas are an additional complication and may extend from the gastric tube to bronchus (less commonly trachea) or the pleural space.

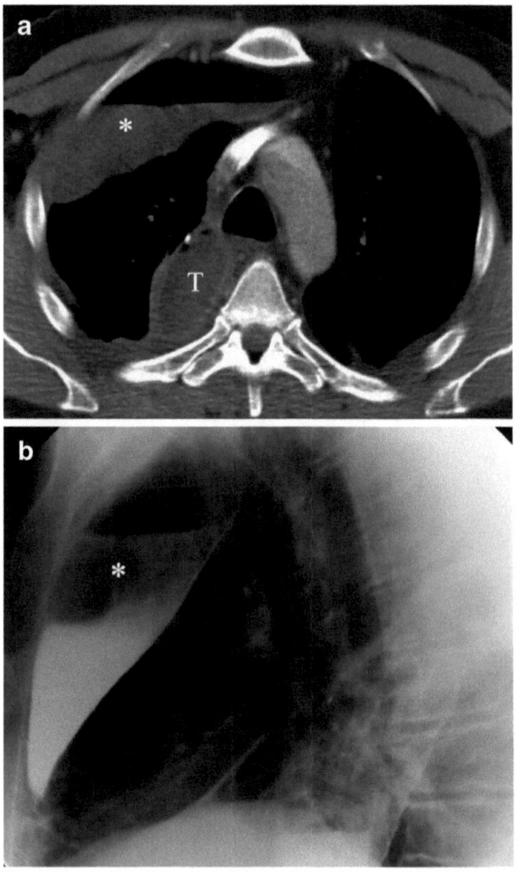

Fig. 2.10 (**a**) CT performed on day 4 post-Ivor Lewis esophagectomy with respiratory deterioration. A loculated anterior collection has formed (*asterisk*) due to a leak from the apex of the gastric tube from the fluid-filled gastric tube (*T*). (**b**) Confirmed on contrast swallow

Oral contrast can confirm that a fistula is present by filling a collection or, to define the course of fistula and site of fistulation, by filling the tract. For this purpose, both real-time fluoroscopy and CT are complementary modalities. Patients with a normal or difficult-to-interpret fluoroscopic examination can have the diagnosis clarified with immediate CT and vice versa (Fig. 2.10). In some cases, fistulas may develop many months after initial surgery due to pathology affecting the tube, such as deep ulceration (Nakagawa et al. 2005) (Fig. 2.11).

2.2.4.2 Anastomotic Leak

Anastomotic leak is one of the major postoperative complications following esophagectomy,

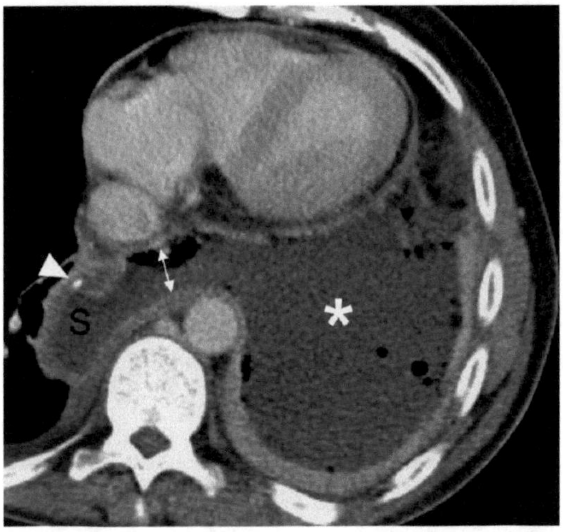

Fig. 2.11 One year following Ivor Lewis esophagectomy with sepsis and respiratory symptoms. The gastric tube (*S*) (staple line – *arrowhead*) has ulcerated on the medial wall (*arrow*), producing a wide defect resulting in an empyema in the left pleural space (*asterisk*)

carrying significant morbidity. With modern surgical management of intrathoracic leaks, the mortality can be as low as 3.3%, in some series having no impact on long-term survival (Sarela et al. 2008), while other series report higher mortality (Griffin et al. 2001). The site of anastomosis also influences the leak rate (cervical 15.5% vs. thoracic 4.2%) (Turkyilmaz et al. 2009). Predictors of poor outcome after leak include advancing age, cervical rather than thoracic anastomosis, presence of necrosis, and presentation of leak (clinical worse than radiological) (Alanezi and Urschel 2004; Turkyilmaz et al. 2009).

Clinical features range from signs of sepsis to increased chest drain output, to respiratory compromise, to surgical emphysema, while other patients have few or no clinical signs.

It may occur in the early postoperative period (2–3 days) due to technical failure or later (3–7 days) commonly due to ischemia. About half of intrathoracic leaks are subclinical, and most subclinical leaks heal without any treatment. Upper GI contrast study may demonstrate a minor leak with contrast collecting around the anastomotic site (Figs. 2.12 and 2.13) or uncontained leak with contrast material flowing freely

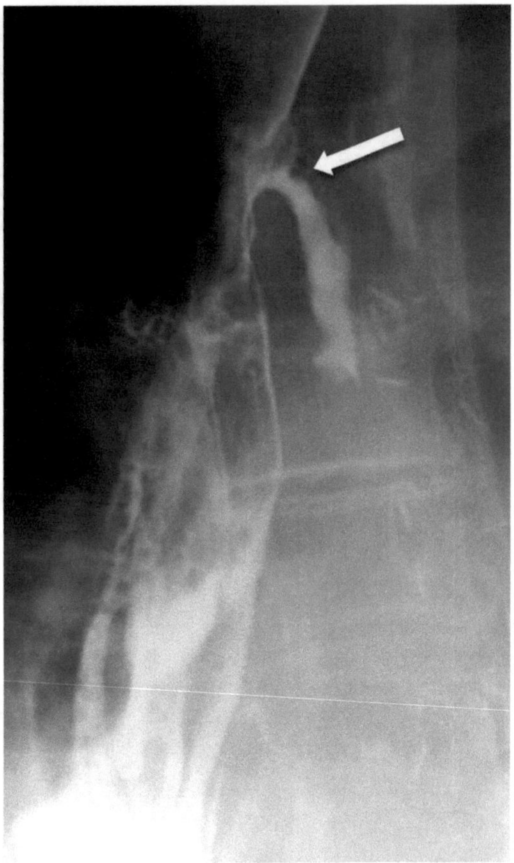

Fig. 2.12 Small contained anastomotic leak (*arrow*) from the esophagogastric anastomosis following Ivor Lewis esophagectomy

into the pleural cavity (Fig. 2.14). It is important that the "apex" of the gastric tube has been fully filled with contrast or a leak at this location will be overlooked. The apex of the tube usually lies more cranial than the anastomosis and lying the patient flat and even prone may be required to achieve complete filling of this recess (Fig. 2.15). It is true to say that fluoroscopic examinations do not have 100% sensitivity or specificity. Indeed, some authors propose that it is not a useful routine procedure and that clinical assessment is more valuable, particularly with cervical anastomoses (Boone et al. 2008).

On CT, gas and fluid collections around the anastomotic site are usually seen when a leak is present, but these findings are not specific (Upponi et al. 2008). Extraluminal contrast

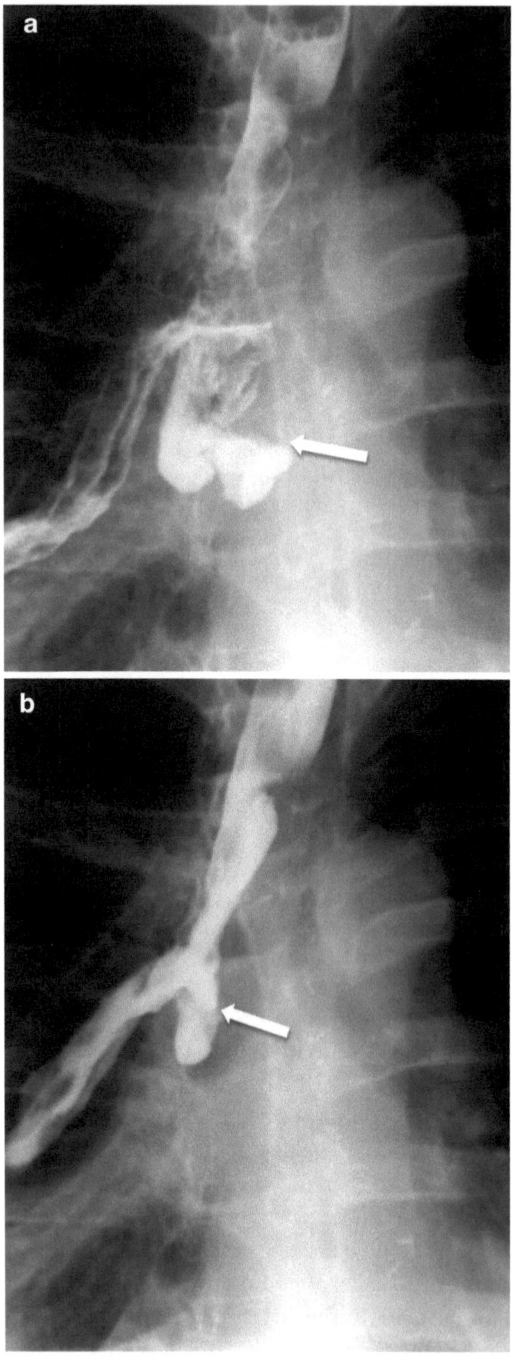

Fig. 2.13 (**a**) Contained 3-cm mediastinal leak (*arrow*) from the esophagogastric anastomosis following Ivor Lewis esophagectomy. (**b**) Reduction in size on subsequent examination 2 weeks later

confirms the presence of leak, and oral contrast should be administered where possible, which increases the sensitivity of the examination

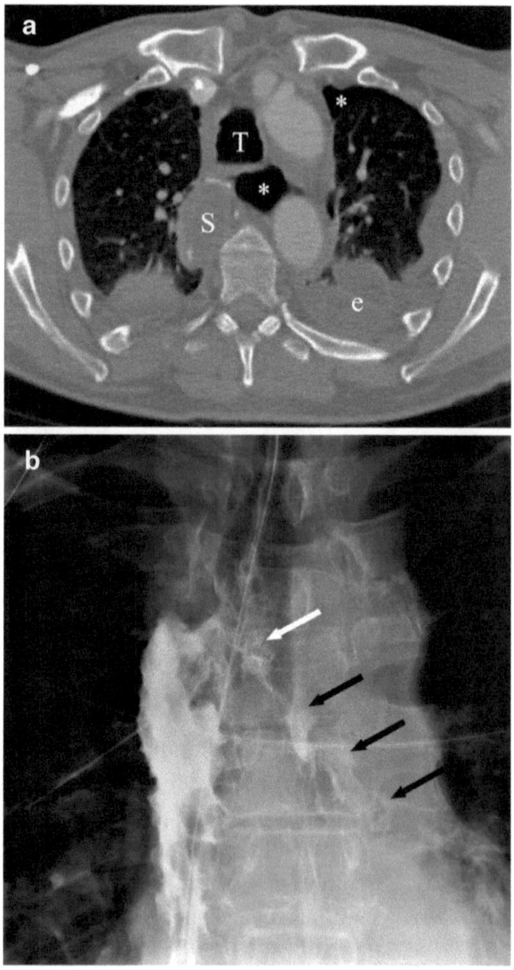

Fig. 2.14 (**a**) CT for postoperative sepsis and bilateral pleural effusions after esophagectomy. CT shows mediastinal gas and left pneumothorax (*asterisk*) and moderate left effusion (*e*). Gastric tube (*S*), trachea (*T*). (**b**) Water-soluble swallow identifies an uncontained anastomotic leak (*white arrow*) tracking into the left pleural cavity (*black arrows*)

beyond fluoroscopy (100% vs. 67%) and patients find CT a more tolerable examination (Upponi et al. 2008) (see Sect. 2.2.3.2). Discontinuity of the anastomosis may be seen if there has been complete disruption.

Anastomotic leak can occur at any of the various sites depending on the type of the operation the patient has undergone. These, in order of frequency, are:

- Esophagogastric anastomosis (Figs. 2.16 and 2.17)
- Gastric tube leak

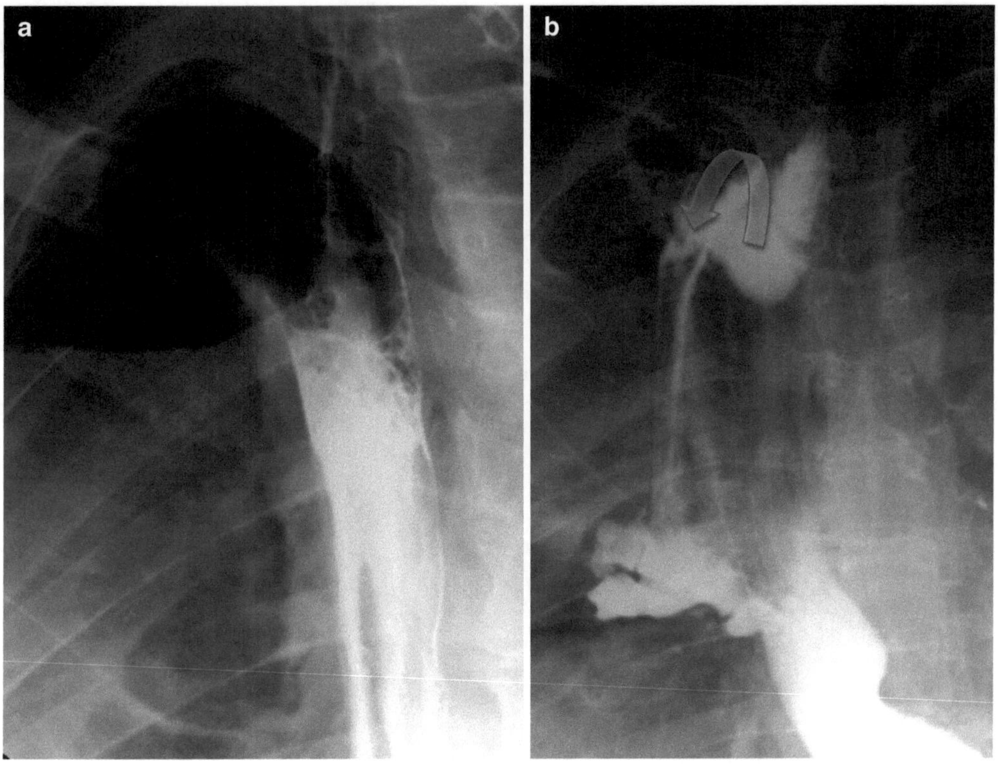

Fig. 2.15 Post Ivor Lewis esophagectomy day 7 routine swallow. (**a**) Erect swallow is normal. (**b**) Patient lying supine, leading to overflow of contrast via leak at apex of gastric tube into the pleural cavity (*curved arrow*)

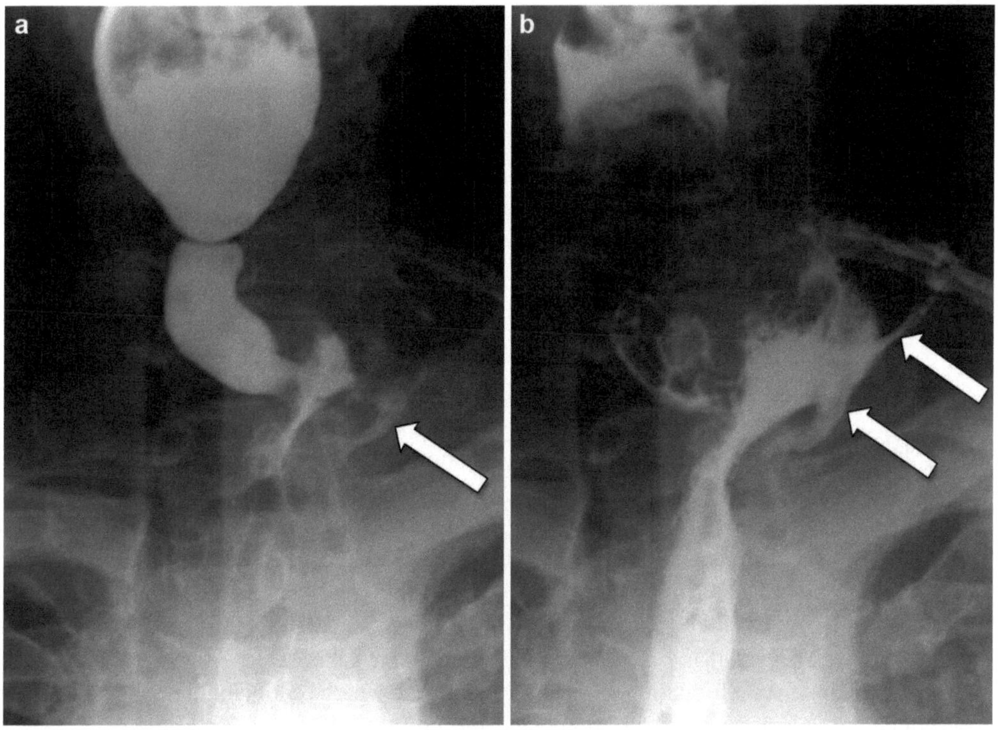

Fig. 2.16 (**a**, **b**) Leak at cervical anastomosis after transhiatal esophagectomy into a contained cavity at the apex of the left lung (*arrows*)

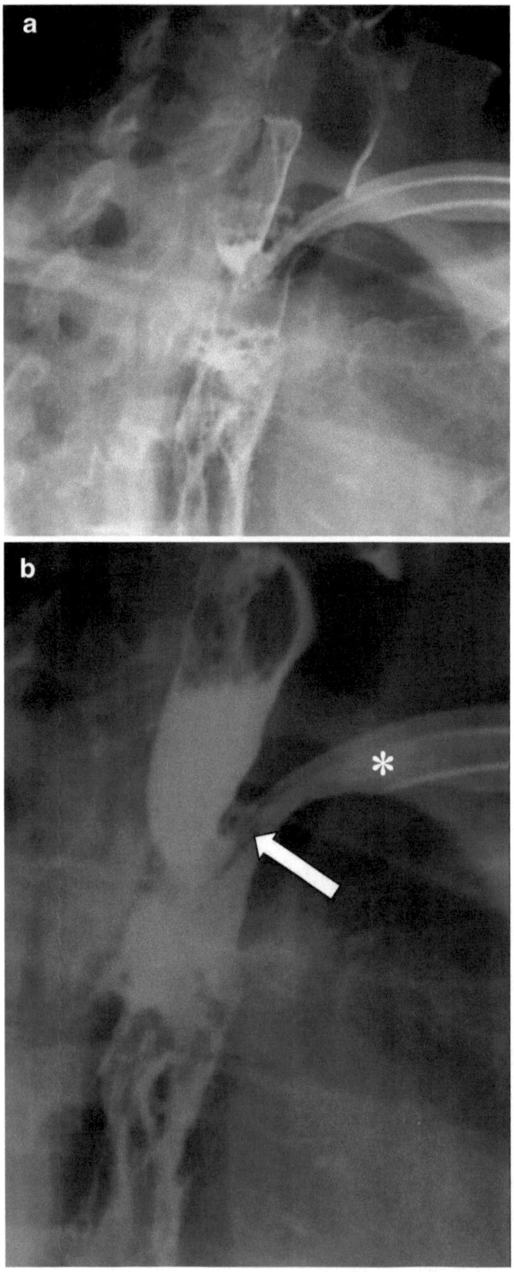

Fig. 2.17 (**a**, **b**) Transhiatal esophagectomy with corrugated drain at cervical anastomosis (*arrow*). Careful inspection on the delayed images shows increased density from contrast within the drain due to a small anastomotic leak (*asterisk*)

- Gastric tube apex leak (Fig. 2.15)
- Pyloroplasty leak (Fig. 2.18)

A leak can lead to fistula formation with adjacent anatomic structures, such as the bronchial

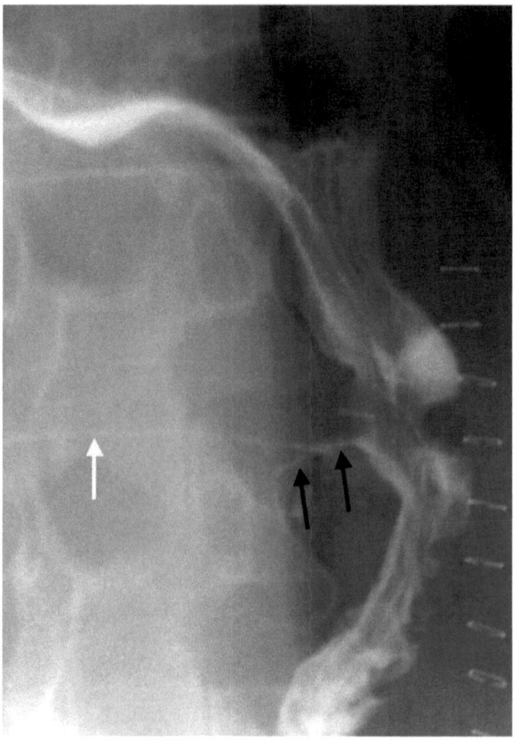

Fig. 2.18 Asymptomatic small pyloroplasty leak (*black arrows*) on routine postoperative assessment – healed with conservative management (surgical drain (*white arrow*))

tree, pleura, or skin. Patients who develop leaks are also at increased risk of eventual fibrotic stricture formation (see Sect. 2.2.4.5).

Mediastinitis and sepsis secondary to anastomotic leaks are the most severe complications and result in serious postoperative morbidity and mortality. These require drainage by either image-guided or surgical approaches, depending on the location and accessibility.

In some instances, leaks may be managed with self-expandable metallic stents, with some series demonstrating success rates of up to 92% (Leers et al. 2009), although our own experience has not always been so positive (Fig. 2.19). Others have used endoscopically placed fibrin glue (Nakagawa et al. 2005) or other novel devices to seal fistulas (Green et al. 2010). However, where there are more extensive leaks, revisional surgery is required, which is not without risk and additional mortality (Griffin et al. 2001).

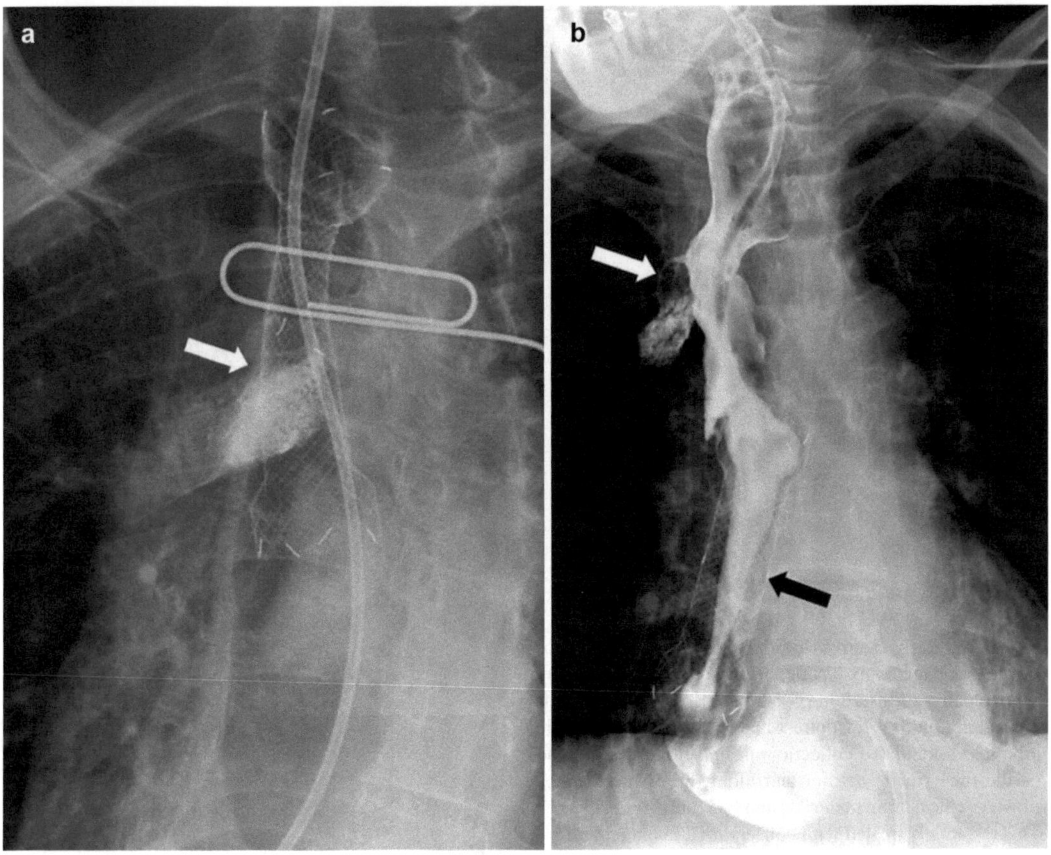

Fig. 2.19 Decision for conservative treatment of anastomotic leak post-Ivor Lewis. (**a**) A covered esophageal stent was placed across the leak (*arrow*) under fluoroscopic guidance. (**b**) Planned follow-up swallow shows persistent large defect (*white arrow*) with distal migration of stent into gastric tube (*black arrow*)

2.2.4.3 Tube Necrosis/Ischemia

The vascular supply to the stomach is reduced when mobilized from its abdominal position. The short gastric, left gastric, and left gastroepiploic arteries are sacrificed, leaving the right gastric and right gastroepiploic arteries providing arterial inflow to the gastric tube (Fig. 2.1). The gastric fundus and cardia staple line (anastomotic site and resection margin, respectively) are most distant from the inflow. When a cervical anastomosis is formed, where the gastric tube is stretched further toward the thoracic inlet, the tension on the arterial supply is greater.

Graft ischemia fortunately occurs only in a minority of cases (1–2%) but carries a significant morbidity and mortality (Griffin et al. 2002; Alanezi and Urschel 2004).

Clinically, patients present with signs of sepsis accompanied by metabolic acidosis and persistently elevated inflammatory markers within the first week following surgery. Unfortunately, imaging is suboptimal in the diagnosis of ischemia, with a disappointingly low sensitivity (33%) when compared with endoscopic evaluation (Veeramootoo et al. 2009). Where clinical features are equivocal, then endoscopy has an important role with very high accuracy in the diagnosis or exclusion of acute tube necrosis and ischemia (Maish et al. 2005; Veeramootoo et al. 2009). However, where clinical suspicion is high, many surgeons will take the patient to theater for exploration of the tube rather than delay for additional investigation.

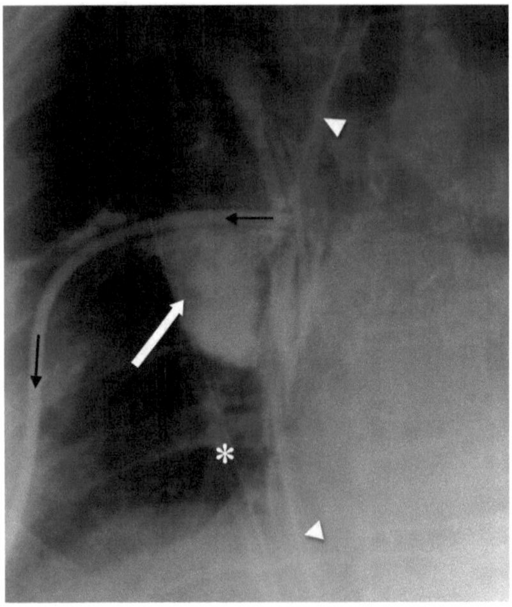

Fig. 2.20 Early necrosis of the gastric tube post Ivor Lewis esophagectomy – patient returned to theater on day 2 for repair and insertion of T-tube. High output via left chest drain on day 7. Contrast is leaking from the gastric tube into a loculated collection around the proximal end of the tube (*white arrow*) and along the T-tube (*black arrows*). Chest drain (*asterisk*) and NG tube (*arrowheads*). This eventually healed with conservative management

When tube necrosis is demonstrated on imaging, a leak is usually present either at the anastomosis or the tube staple line due to breakdown of the gastric wall (Fig. 2.20). The main role of imaging is in follow-up assessment for complications.

2.2.4.4 Torsion of Tube

During creation of the anastomosis, care is taken to ensure that the gastric tube is not twisted before being anastomosed. It is a particular risk of transhiatal surgery where the tube is negotiated to the thoracic inlet blind (Fig. 2.21). As well as the mechanical effects of torsion causing gastric obstruction, it places strain on the vascular supply and may precipitate ischemia and necrosis.

2.2.4.5 Anastomotic Stricture

Stricturing in the early days of the postoperative period is due to impaired wound healing, and the

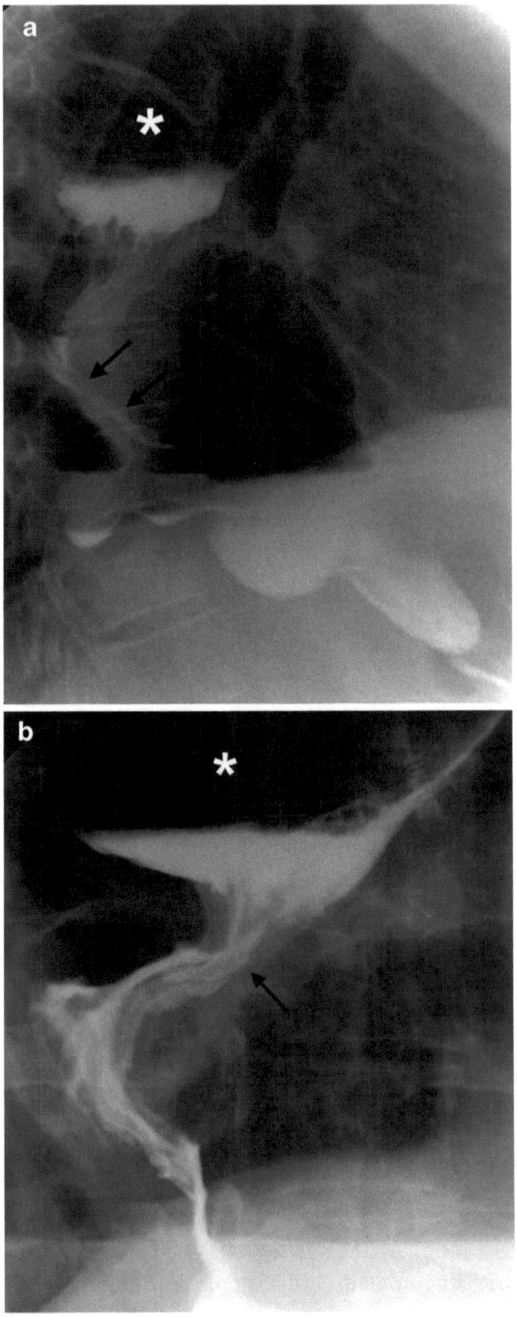

Fig. 2.21 (**a**, **b**) Tube twist in transhiatal esophagectomy. Routine day 7 postoperative swallow. There is a narrowing at the midpoint of the gastric tube (*arrow*), indicating a twist in the tube – the partial twist did not cause long-term functional problems despite some proximal dilatation (*asterisk*). A complete twist is a major complication that frequently causes obstruction, ischemia, and necrosis

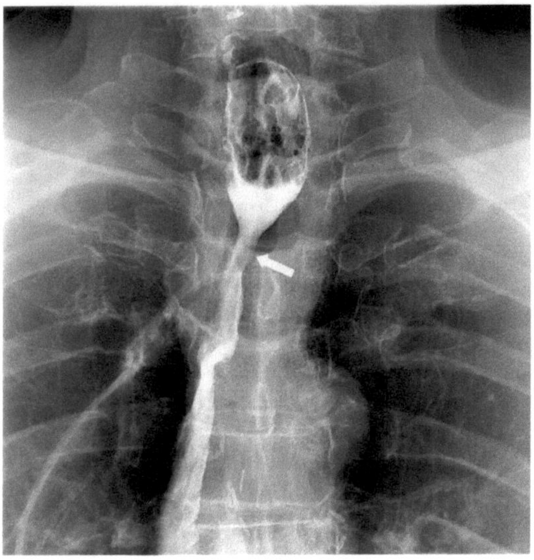

Fig. 2.22 Tight cervical esophageal benign anastomotic stricture (*arrow*) following three-stage esophagectomy for cancer complicated by leak (*not shown*). Serial balloon dilatations required for relief of symptoms

risk increases if there has been an anastomotic leak (Fig. 2.22). These can be treated effectively with balloon dilatation, particularly if they are short (Figs. 2.23 and 2.24). Strictures resistant to balloon dilatation may require placement of retrievable endoluminal stents or even surgery in a small minority of cases, which is more likely where ischemia results in a long stricture and may require creation of an esophageal bypass or substitution (see Sect. 2.3.1).

2.2.4.6 Chylothorax

Chyle leak and thoracic duct injury is a potential complication of all types of esophagectomy due to the proximity of the duct to the esophagus, with a higher prevalence in transthoracic than in transhiatal surgery. Chest tube drainage greater than 200–400 ml every 12 h for a period greater than 48 h indicates thoracic duct injury. The role of radiology is generally to exclude other complications such as anastomotic leak. Management options range from conservative treatment (drainage of effusion, parenteral nutrition) to open or minimally invasive thoracic surgery with clipping, suturing, or fibrin glue injection of the thoracic duct injury (Hayden et al. 2007).

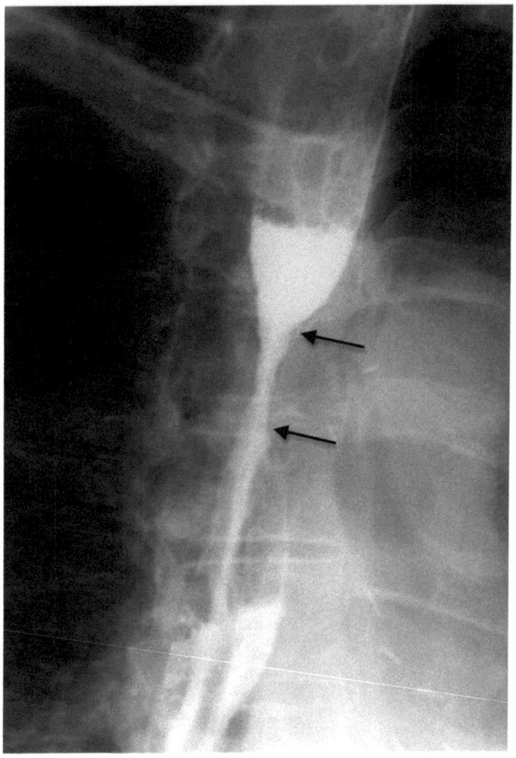

Fig. 2.23 Delayed anastomotic stricture (*black arrows*) requiring balloon dilatation 8 months post-Ivor Lewis esophagectomy

2.2.4.7 Delayed Emptying

This can occur due to lack of a pyloric drainage procedure, wall edema following pyloroplasty (probably the most common cause (Fig. 2.25)), obstruction at the level of hiatus, or a redundant intrathoracic stomach with consequent twisting or kinking (see Sect. 2.2.4.4). A large air-fluid level in the gastric tube is an indicator of delayed emptying. This is often subclinical, as not all patients vomit, and the volume of residual gastric content can make assessment of gastric emptying and anastomoses difficult as a result of dilution. In such cases, clinical correlation is required, and where necessary, endoscopic evaluation or further water-soluble swallow may be appropriate to reassess before normal diet is resumed (Fig. 2.26).

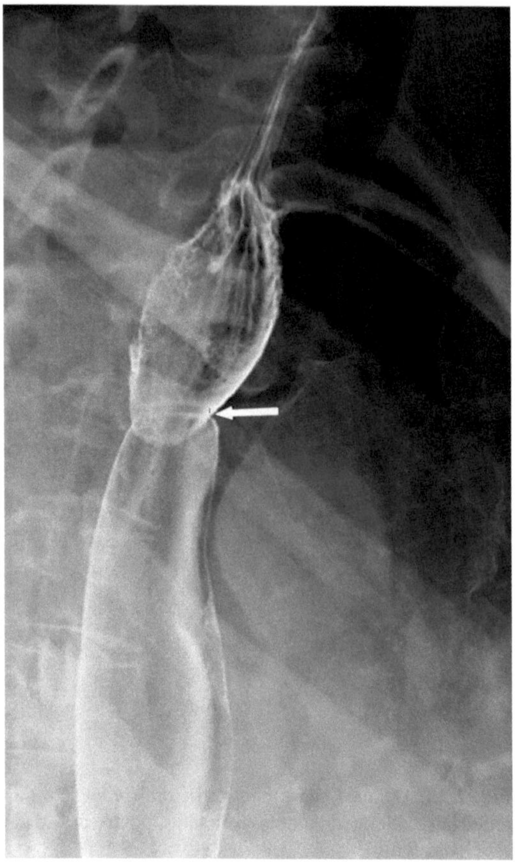

Fig. 2.24 Limited esophageal resection for repair of H-type tracheoesophageal fistula in infancy. Repeated episodes of food bolus obstruction due to short anastomotic stricture (*arrow*) presenting 30 years after initial surgery

2.2.4.8 Hiatus and Diaphragmatic Hernias

Gastric mobilization and widening of the hiatus increase the risk of diaphragmatic hernia which may occur in 2–3% of cases, with most cases developing within 1 year of surgery, although some occur much later despite closure of the defect (Vallböhmer et al. 2007; Vyas et al. 2009). Depending on the volume of abdominal content herniating, the width of the diaphragmatic defect, and associated respiratory or intestinal symptoms (such as obstruction), surgical repair is usually attempted to close the defect, which may involve synthetic mesh (Vyas et al. 2009) (Fig. 2.27). Occasionally, herniation or failure of mesh repair may be precipitated by vomiting or coughing (Fig. 2.28).

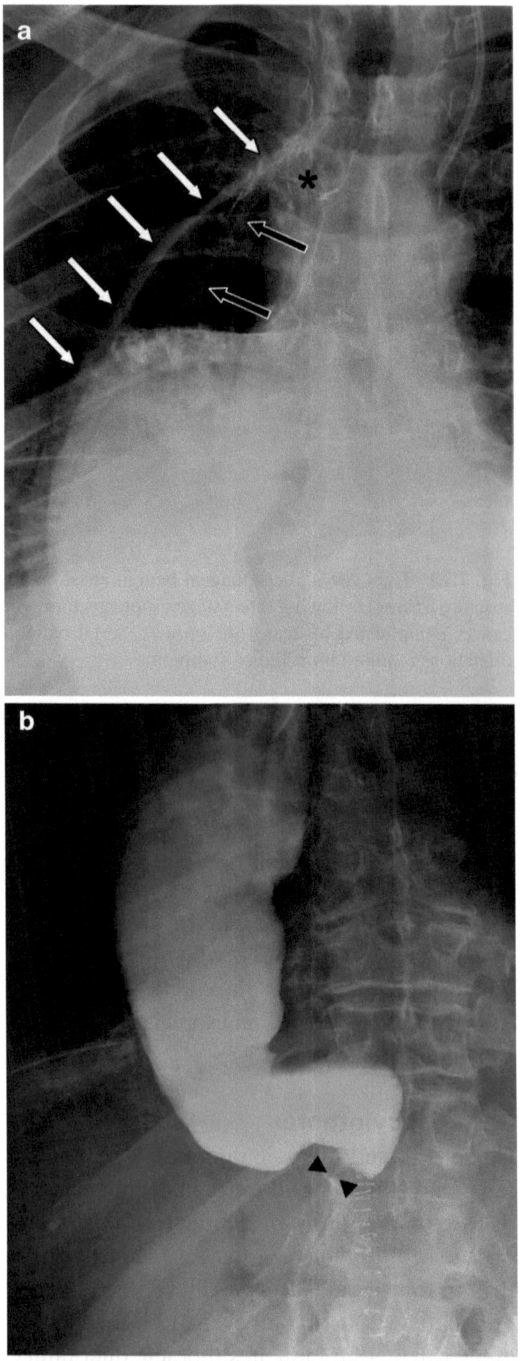

Fig. 2.25 Vomiting day 6 post Ivor Lewis esophagectomy. (**a**) The wall of the dilated tube is clearly demonstrated against the surrounding lung (*white arrows*) with no proximal anastomotic leak (*asterisk*) and intact tube staple line (*black arrows*). (**b**) Tight stenosis at the pylorus (*arrowheads*) despite pyloroplasty – often due to postoperative edema. This resolved without intervention

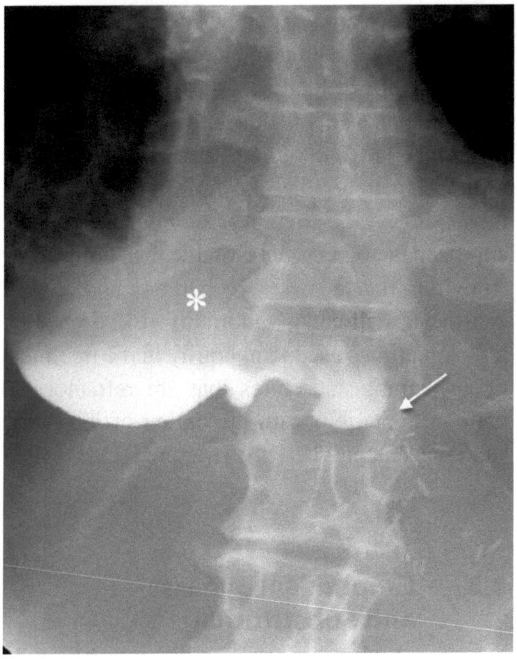

Fig. 2.26 Delayed emptying of the tube (*asterisk*) due to stenosis at the pylorus (*white arrow*) 21 days after Ivor Lewis esophagectomy. This is most often from edema but occasionally requires endoscopic dilatation as in this case

2.2.4.9 Cardiovascular Complications

Most cardiovascular complications are related to peri- and postoperative hemorrhage. Meticulous surgical technique now frequently results in less than 500 ml of blood loss from surgery (Griffin et al. 2002). Delayed bleeding usually requires reoperation rather than interventional radiology for bleeding control and manifests with hypotension and tachycardia, sometimes accompanied by hemothorax and blood in chest drains. Imaging rarely has a role. Rare complications result from delayed ulceration from the tube into the mediastinal structures and fistulation to pericardium (Kato et al. 2010) and right ventricle (Rana et al. 2010) with fatal consequences.

2.2.5 Role of Image-Guided Intervention

2.2.5.1 Drain Insertion

Surgically placed drains in the right thorax in the postoperative period generally deal with collections that develop as a consequence of leak. Occasionally, more loculated collections in the right thorax or those that track into the left thorax (Fig. 2.14) will require image-guided drain insertion, or when the thoracotomy has not been performed (e.g., transhiatal approach). While ultrasound can deal with predominantly fluid collections, more loculated, gas-containing, or difficult-to-access collections may require CT-guided drainage (Fig. 2.10). Minimally invasive tech-

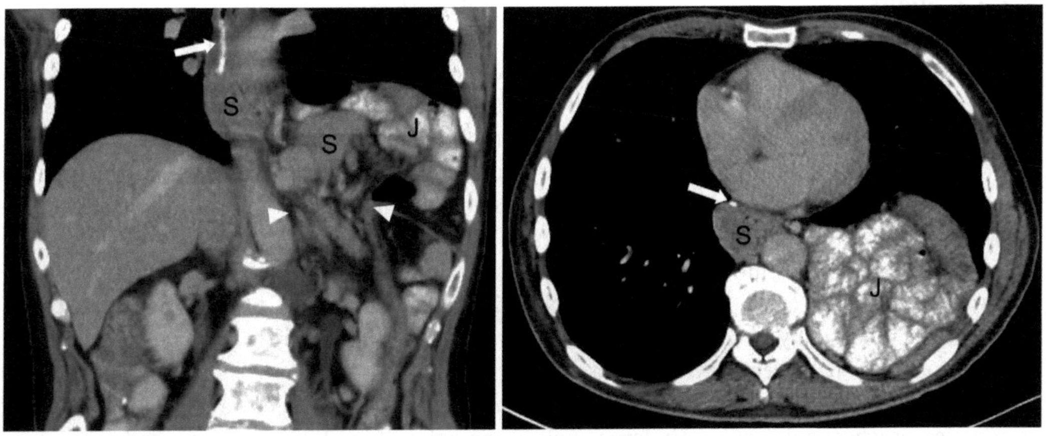

Fig. 2.27 Three weeks post transhiatal distal esophagectomy for Barrett's esophagus with severe dysplasia presenting with vomiting and weight loss (*arrow* – staple line). The stomach (*S*) and proximal jejunum (*J*) have herniated across a wide diaphragmatic defect (*arrowheads*) requiring surgical mesh repair

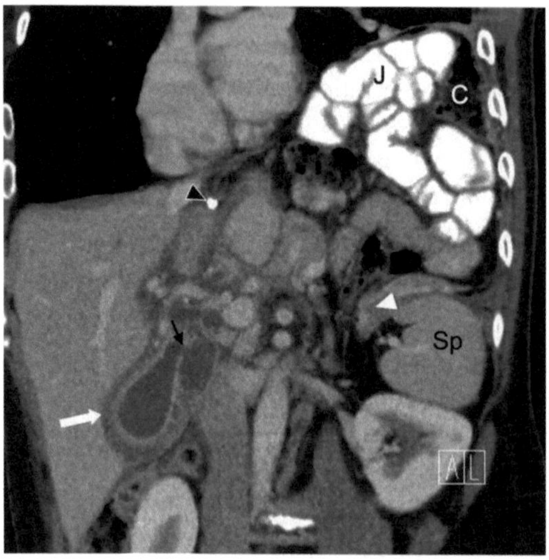

Fig. 2.28 Previous mesh repair of diaphragmatic hernia following transhiatal esophagectomy. Two days of right-sided abdominal pain with perforation (*black arrow*) of inflamed gallbladder (*white arrow*) followed by vomiting and breathlessness. The hernia repair has failed with a wide defect at the hiatus (*arrowheads* – (*black*) rivet on right crus and (*white*) on left diaphragm). Jejunum and colon have herniated into right chest. Spleen remains in the abdomen (*Sp*)

niques have an important role to play to minimize morbidity resulting from leaks (Sarela et al. 2008). Usually, small-caliber drains (8Fr–12Fr) are sufficient to manage most collections, with the authors favoring a Seldinger technique.

2.2.5.2 Stents

Stents are also an adjunct to dealing with anastomotic leaks. Generally, covered stents are deployed with a wide enough diameter to grip the wall and prevent migration (up to 3 cm diameter – wider than those typically used for management of malignancy). The success rate varies between series but is not 100%, a recent series with 59% success rate mirroring the author's experience (D'Cunha et al. 2011). Endoscopic assistance is not usually necessary, particularly when a road map has been provided by a prior contrast study, but can be helpful where anatomy is complex or where a defect is very large, making wire manipulation past the leak difficult. Migration does occur in a significant proportion of cases, requiring further stent placement.

It is important to acknowledge that stents are also associated with a small but significant number of serious or fatal complications that include aortic fistula, stent erosion, and even enlargement of a leak (D'Cunha et al. 2011). However, in a group of patients that are frail, having endured major surgery, an attempt at a minimally invasive approach is often more favorable than proceeding straight to theater where reoperation and general anesthesia will carry a mortality risk. Stents are also sometimes used temporarily in the treatment of anastomotic strictures that are refractory to balloon dilatation, with the option of long-term stent placement where the stricture recurs.

2.3 Esophageal Bypass and Substitution

Esophageal bypass surgery may be performed with or without esophageal resection and provides an alternative pathway for passage of food.

2.3.1 Clinical Indications

- Gastric conduit failure post-esophagectomy
- Carcinoma of the esophagus
- Severe stricture, e.g., corrosive ingestion
- Neuromuscular disorders
- Tracheoesophageal fistula

While the most common indication is failure of gastric conduit (Dowson et al. 2007), in some situations, the stomach may not be suitable to form a conduit for esophagectomy, for example, after previous gastric surgery, in which case a substitute may be chosen.

2.3.2 Choice of Conduit/Substitute and Position

A variety of substitutes have been used, including colon (Fig. 2.29), jejunum, and myocutaneous or fasciocutaneous flaps to construct a neo-esophagus in the context of cervical esophageal resection for tumors of or those invading

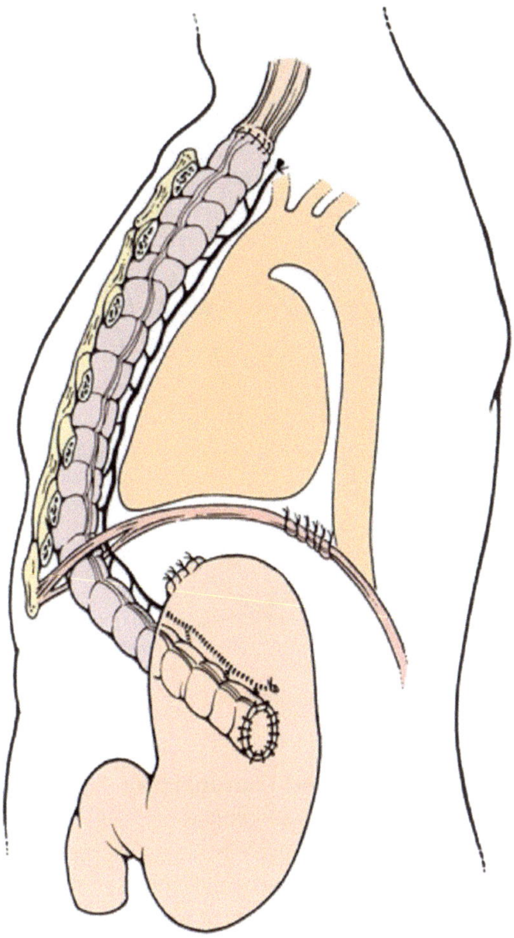

Fig. 2.29 Position of a substernal colon bypass. The right colon or transverse colon may be used. Emptying is accomplished predominantly by gravity. Colon bypasses are durable procedures that are associated with low anastomotic stricture rates and surprisingly few symptoms. They may also be positioned in subcutaneous or retrocardiac positions

the cervical esophagus (e.g., laryngeal carcinoma) (Disa and Cordeiro 2001). The conduit may be placed in a cervical, intrathoracic/retrocardiac, substernal, or rarely presternal/subcutaneous position. The substernal route is most commonly employed where the thoracic esophagus is being replaced.

The length of reconstruction governs the choice of conduit as well as whether a free (usually jejunum – Fig. 2.30) (Ascioti et al. 2005) or pedicled conduit (colon or jejunum – Fig. 2.31) is required. While the jejunum retains its peristaltic action, the colon generally relies on gravity for passage of luminal contents. This type of surgery is technically challenging, particularly where microvascular anastomoses are formed for free flaps, which are usually formed to internal mammary or cervical arteries and veins. Timing is also a consideration as in some patients, a delay is required when the surgery is for conduit failure after esophagectomy. This delay allows treatment of sepsis or optimization of nutrition to maximize the chances of graft function. In experienced hands, technical success rates are high (>90%) with acceptably low complication rates (Ascioti et al. 2005; Poh et al. 2011).

Myocutaneous (e.g., pectoralis major) or fasciocutaneous flaps can also be created from graft sites in the arm (e.g., radial forearm) or leg (e.g., anterolateral thigh). These are harvested to produce a flap of skin along with supplying nerves, arteries and veins, and deeper tissue depending on the type of flap (muscle or fascia) and either harvested and grafted onto neck vessels (fasciocutaneous) or rotated into its new position (pectoralis major flap). Muscle tends to be used where a large defect needs to be filled with tissue. These form a functionally flexible graft that can be fashioned into either a U shape or a tube to recreate the pharynx or cervical esophagus with an epithelialized lining and excellent functional outcomes (Murray et al. 2008). A further advantage is that the abdomen is not opened.

2.3.3 Normal Postoperative Imaging

2.3.3.1 Upper GI Contrast Studies

Contrast studies elegantly demonstrate the postoperative anatomy and the esophageal substitute. Normal anatomy of the conduit will vary, with haustrations in the colon (Fig. 2.32), valvulae conniventes in jejunum (Fig. 2.33), and relatively smooth featureless mucosal in myocutaneous flaps (Fig. 2.34). The colon may temporarily "jejunalize" in the first months after surgery (Agha and Orringer 1984), and spasm may also be evident in this period, which is usually temporary and does not necessarily imply pathology.

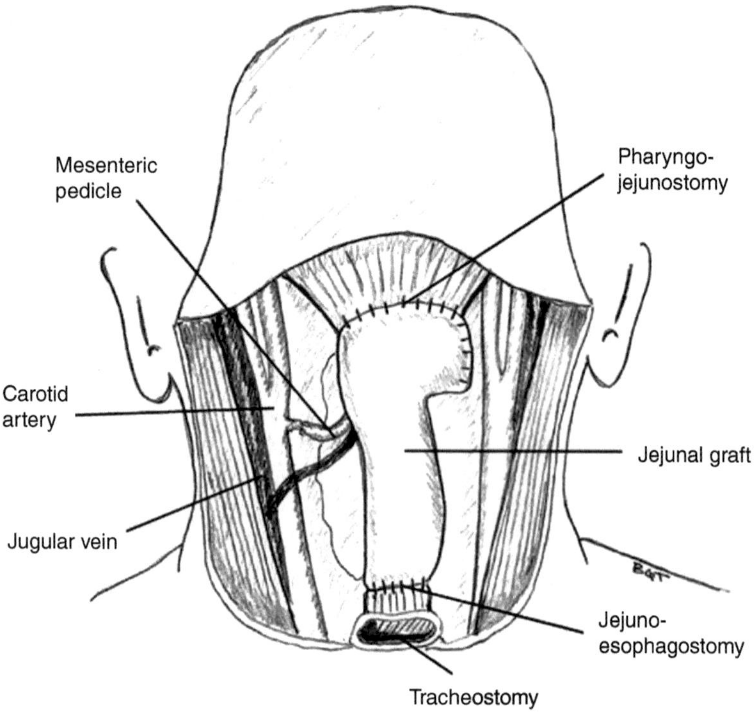

Fig. 2.30 Free jejunal graft used as an interposition after pharyngolaryngoesophagectomy with microvascular anastomoses to recipient vessels. A jejunal segment, 15–20 cm long with a suitably long mesenteric pedicle, is harvested via a midline abdominal incision and subsequently used as an interposition

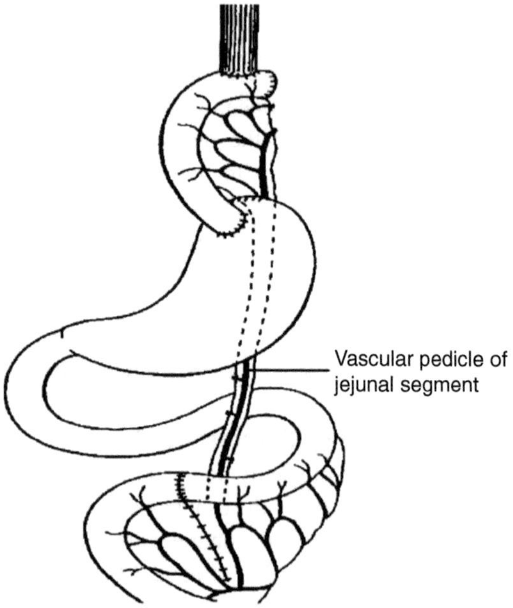

Fig. 2.31 Jejunal interposition: the Merendino procedure. Both anastomoses are performed in an end-to-side fashion using circular staplers; the jejunogastrostomy is placed to the posterior wall of the stomach. A longer jejunal segment may be used to replace the whole esophagus either on a mobilized pedicle or as a supercharged free flap

2.3.3.2 Computed Tomography

CT shows the neo-esophagus as well as any extraluminal pathology. When a substernal route has been employed, particular attention must be paid as the vascular pedicle of the neo-esophagus is at risk of compromise due to venous compression, particularly at the level of xiphoid process and narrow thoracic inlet. Indeed, in some cases, the manubrium is excised to increase the space for the graft and mitigate against this potential complication.

It is important to consider the abdominal component of the operation when the clinical concern is a search for occult sepsis since enteroenteric and coloenteric anastomoses may have been formed during harvesting of the conduit, which are also at risk of leak as well as the anastomoses in the thorax.

Myocutaneous and fasciocutaneous flaps obviously recreate normal anatomy to a degree. However, particularly with reference to fasciocutaneous flaps, there is fat surrounding the cutaneous tube, which has a distinctive appearance. Since there is normally relatively little fat adjacent to the central structures of the neck, this may be disconcerting when first

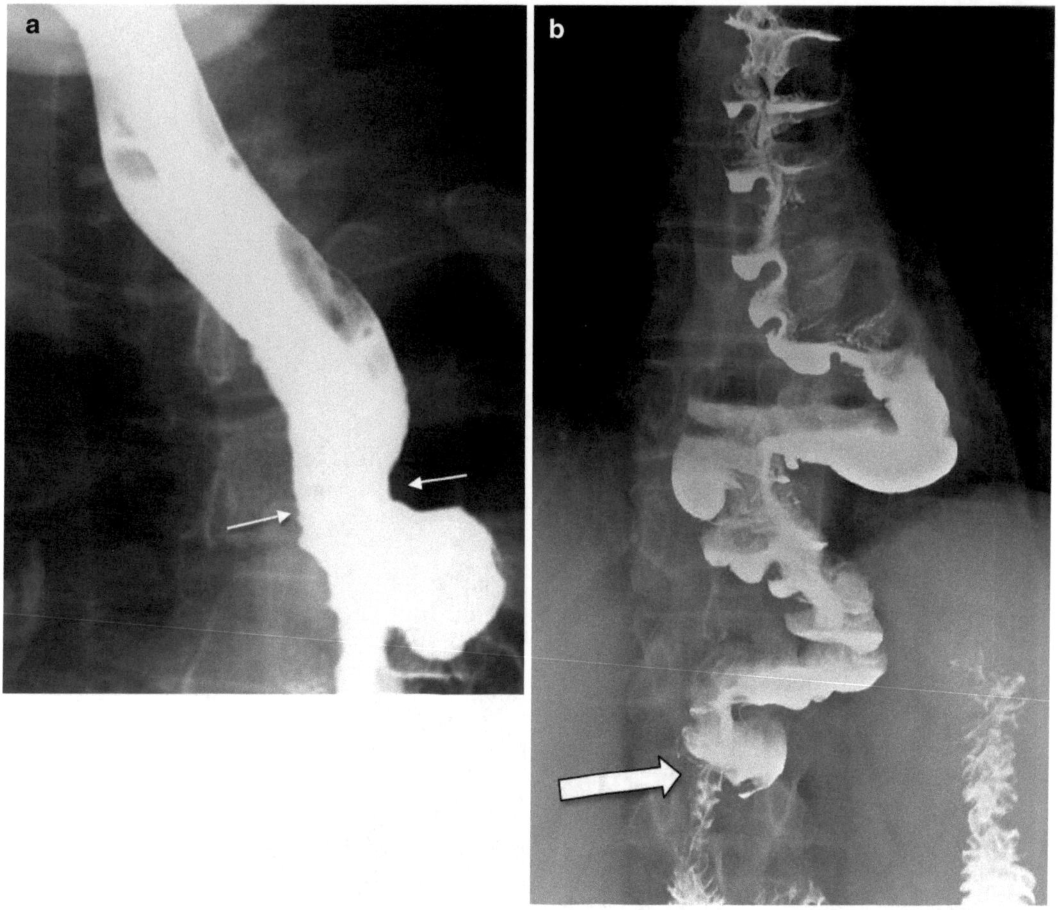

Fig. 2.32 (**a**, **b**) Colonic interposition after gastric tube necrosis following Ivor Lewis esophagectomy. Normal appearances of proximal (*thin arrows*) and distal ends (*thick arrow*) of the transverse colon graft from proximal esophagus to small bowel

encountered. Where there is inadequate clinical information or radiological experience of assessing these grafts, the authors suggest that the referring clinician reviews the scan with the radiologist to explain the composition of the graft, particularly where this is being developed as a new technique.

2.3.4 Postoperative Complications

2.3.4.1 Conduit Necrosis/Ischemia and Anastomotic Leak

While gastric tube ischemic complications are infrequent (1%), there is a higher rate for jejunum (11.3%) and colon (13.3%) (Moorehead and Wong 1990). Risk factors include longer length of conduit, route of passage, and neck anastomosis compared with thoracic anastomosis. This complication carries a significant mortality and is usually heralded by signs of sepsis, elevated inflammatory markers, and acidosis and sometimes associated with anastomotic or graft leak. As with gastric tube necrosis, a high index of suspicion is essential with the diagnosis made by a combination of endoscopy and contrast swallow (Wormuth and Heitmiller 2006). To reduce the risk of necrosis to jejunal grafts, microvascular anastomoses are created (e.g., to internal mammary vessels) to augment the inflow from the mobilized jejunal branch supply of the superior mesenteric artery, so-called supercharging.

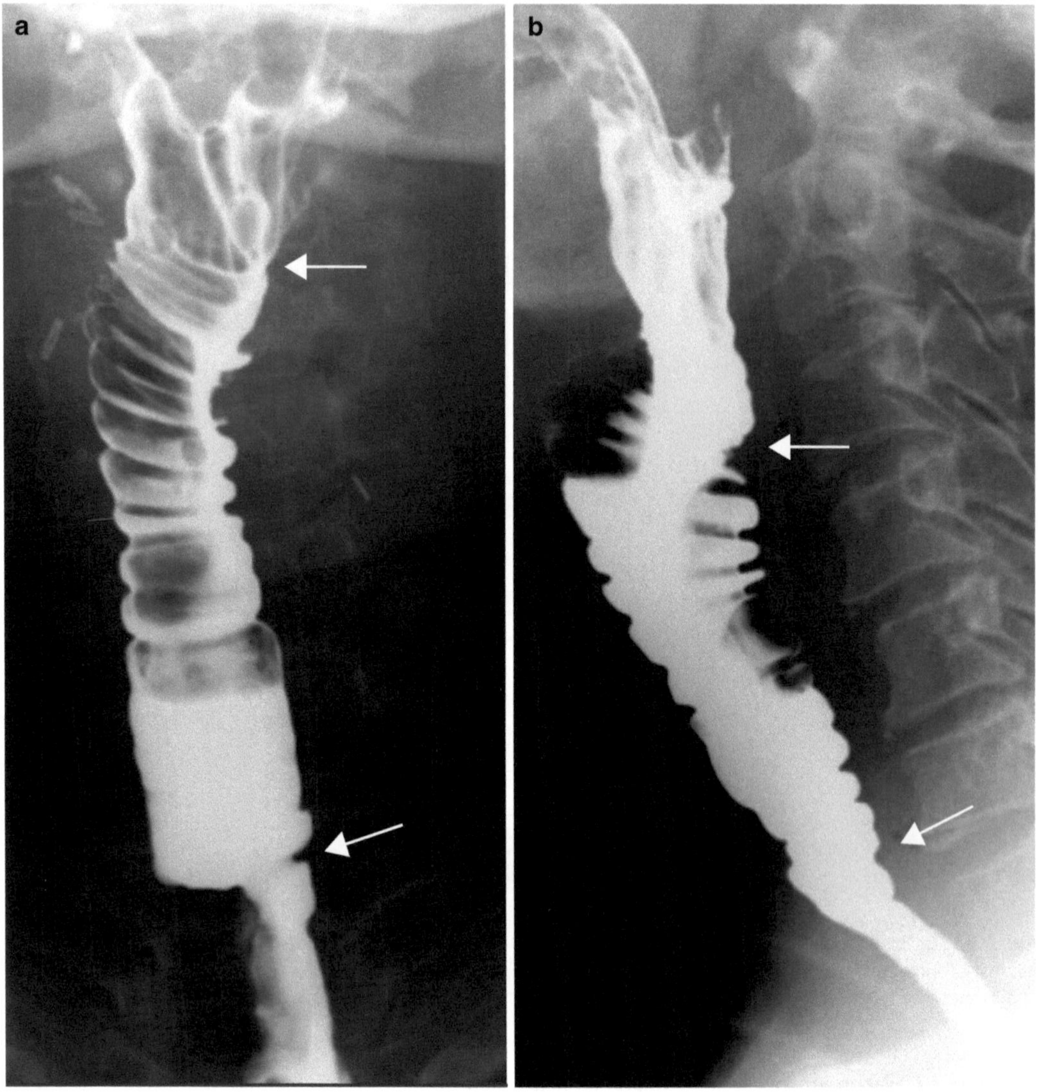

Fig. 2.33 (**a**, **b**) Normal free jejunal interposition flap following resection of cervical esophagus. Note normal pattern of valvulae conniventes and the anastomosis to hypopharynx and thoracic esophagus (*arrows*). (**c**) (overleaf) It is important not to misdiagnose concertinaed folds as a leak (*arrow*)

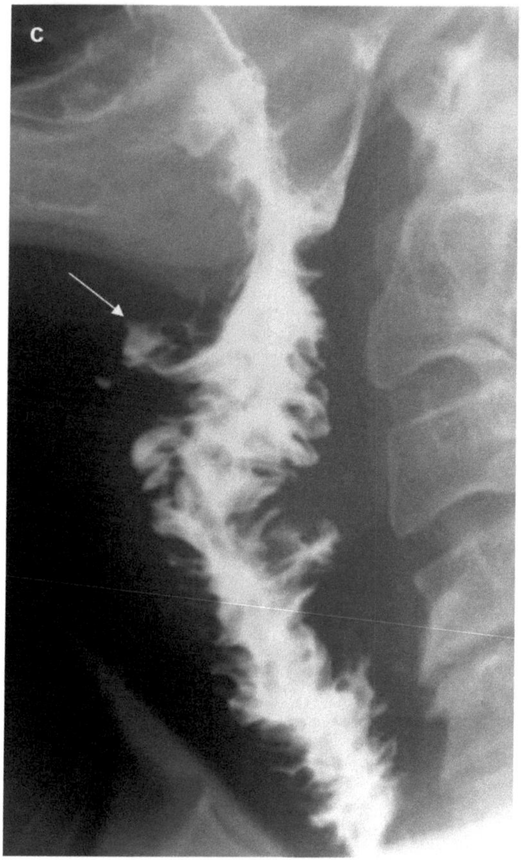

Fig. 2.33 (continued)

Specific imaging features depend on the type of esophageal reconstruction. Radiology is not generally used to diagnose necrosis but rather than to search for an explanation for clinical deterioration, such as anastomotic leak. With bowel segments, there is a loss of the normal fold pattern with thickening, distortion, and ulceration, and this may be accompanied by anastomotic breakdown or perforation of the conduit itself (Fig. 2.35).

Myocutaneous and fasciocutaneous flap necrosis may also be accompanied by anastomotic leak on contrast studies, while CT may show surgical emphysema and either increased or decreased enhancement of the flap with excessive fat stranding and swelling of soft tissues (Figs. 2.36 and 2.37).

When either necrosis or ischemia is diagnosed, the management varies according to severity. In mild cases, management may involve supportive care, while more severe ischemia and necrosis may require resection of part or all of the tube, or replacement with a new conduit with or without creation of a defunctioning proximal cervical stoma.

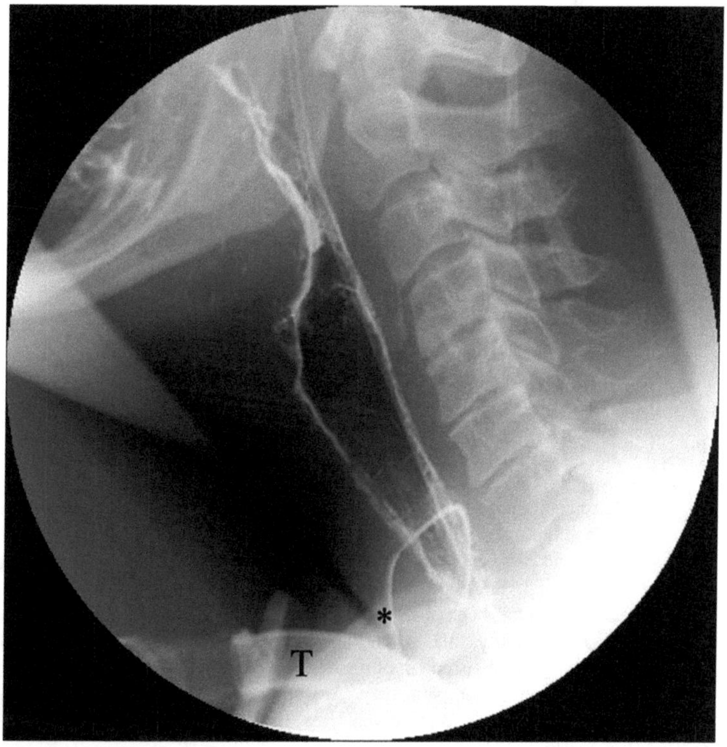

Fig. 2.34 Normal evaluation after fasciocutaneous flap following laryngopharyngoesophagectomy for cancer. Smooth mucosa (skin from graft) and multiple small high-density clips from tissue dissection (tracheostomy (*T*), surgical drain (*asterisk*))

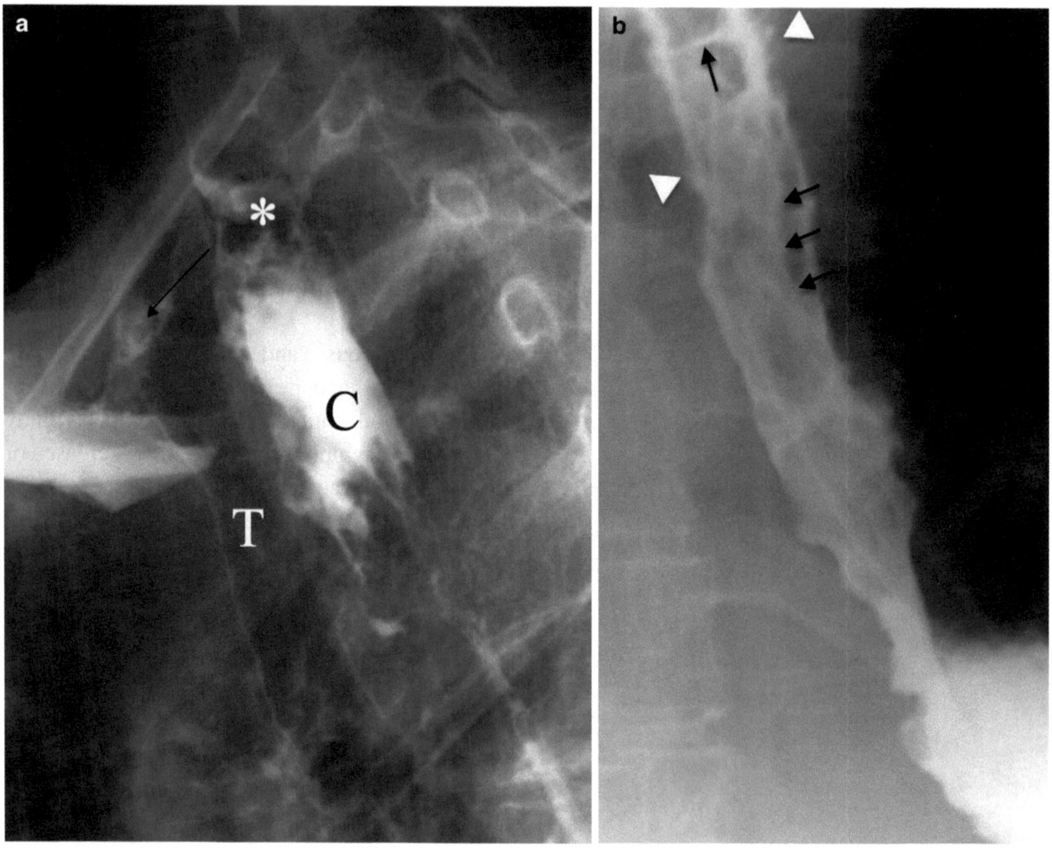

Fig. 2.35 Anastomotic leak from colonic tube ischemia. (**a**) Defect at the anastomosis (*asterisk*) of the colonic tube (*C*) with contrast tracking into cavity (*arrow*) anterolateral to trachea (*T*). (**b**) Note that the tube has lost the normal haustral pattern and developed an irregular outline (*arrowheads*). Linear mucosal pattern from ischemic ulceration (*arrows*)

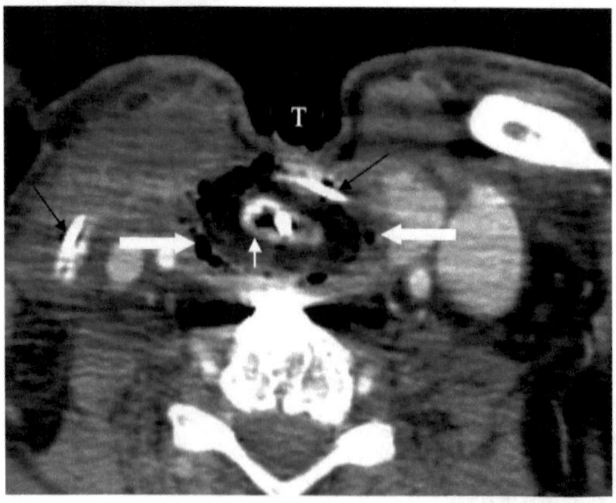

Fig. 2.36 Fasciocutaneous flap necrosis. Failure to progress with rising inflammatory markers day 5 post–cervical esophagectomy and laryngectomy for esophageal carcinoma with lateral thigh flap reconstruction and NG tube in lumen. Surgical drain has been placed (*thin black arrow*). Localized surgical emphysema around the flap (*thick white arrow*) and hyperenhancement of the mucosa (*small white arrow*) indicate major pathology. At surgery, an ischemic flap was resected, and jejunal free flap was inserted (tracheostomy (*T*))

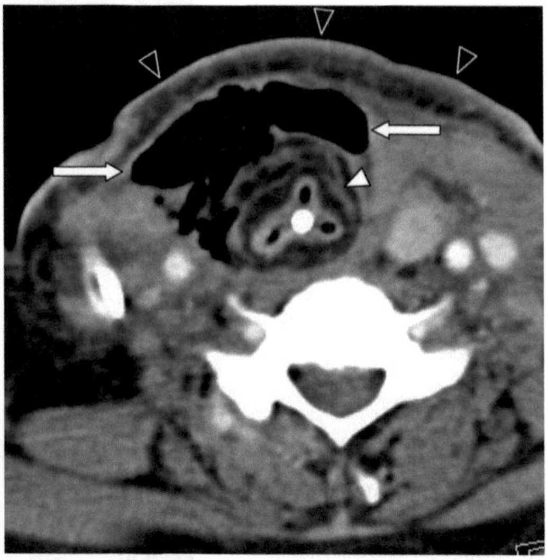

Fig. 2.37 Fasciocutaneous radial forearm flap reconstruction of cervical esophagus with skin erythema and concern for abscess. Marked surgical emphysema (*arrows*) with stranding and induration of the fat related to the flap (*white arrowhead*) and skin (*black arrowheads*) due to ischemia requiring flap excision

2.3.4.2 Conduit Leak

Leaks may occur at either end of the anastomosis but most often at the cervical anastomosis (Ascioti et al. 2005). Although leaks are associated with necrosis, this is not always the case (Figs. 2.35a, b and 2.38). It is important not to confuse bunching of jejunal mucosa with a leak, which can be difficult where a free graft is used for cervical esophageal reconstruction (Fig. 2.33c). Fasciocutaneous flaps have leak or fistula rates of 13% (Murray et al. 2008).

2.3.4.3 Other Conduit Complications

There are three main additional complications that may be encountered. These are stricture, reflux, and graft redundancy.

Anastomotic strictures may form with any conduit affecting enteric or fasciocutaneous interpositions, particularly at sites of previous leak or as a consequence of graft ischemia (Fig. 2.39) (Murray et al. 2008). As with esophagogastric strictures, these frequently require balloon dilatation (Renzulli et al. 2004) or even stent placement as nonoperative techniques.

Strictures may also develop in one or more points along the graft away from the anastomosis, most likely as a result of ischemia (Li et al 2007; Agha and Orringer 1984). It is also important to remember that a harvested bowel segment may develop complications related to underlying disease, with diverticulitis recognized in colonic segments (Cheng et al. 2006).

Reflux is a potential problem with any long esophageal replacement conduit but particularly nonperistaltic colonic grafts. This is exacerbated by graft redundancy where the conduit elongates and dilates over time after placement, resulting in kinking and retention of food within the graft. This may affect both colonic and jejunal grafts (Ascioti et al. 2005; Strauss et al. 2008). This gives rise to symptoms due to mass effect on adjacent organs in the thorax, which can be very unpleasant. This usually requires surgical revision to refashion the conduit to the correct length.

2.3.4.4 Donor Site Complications

Where jejunum or colon has been mobilized, there is clearly a risk of complication related to the anastomosis performed to restore intestinal continuity. Perforation and anastomotic leak are usually heralded by development of abdominal symptoms. Anastomotic leaks are fortunately rare. Morbidity from cutaneous graft sites is also low.

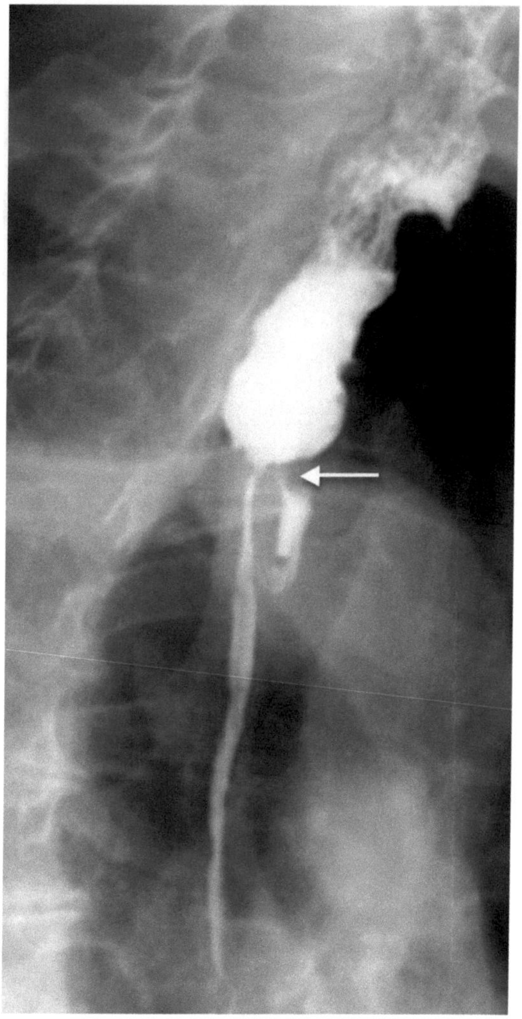

Fig. 2.38 Small contained distal jejunoesophageal anastomotic leak (*arrow*). Healed without intervention

2.4 Heller Myotomy

2.4.1 Clinical Indication and Surgical Technique

Achalasia is an idiopathic condition producing inadequate relaxation of the lower esophageal sphincter. This causes delayed esophageal transit, reflux, chest discomfort, and respiratory complications from aspiration. While there was a vogue

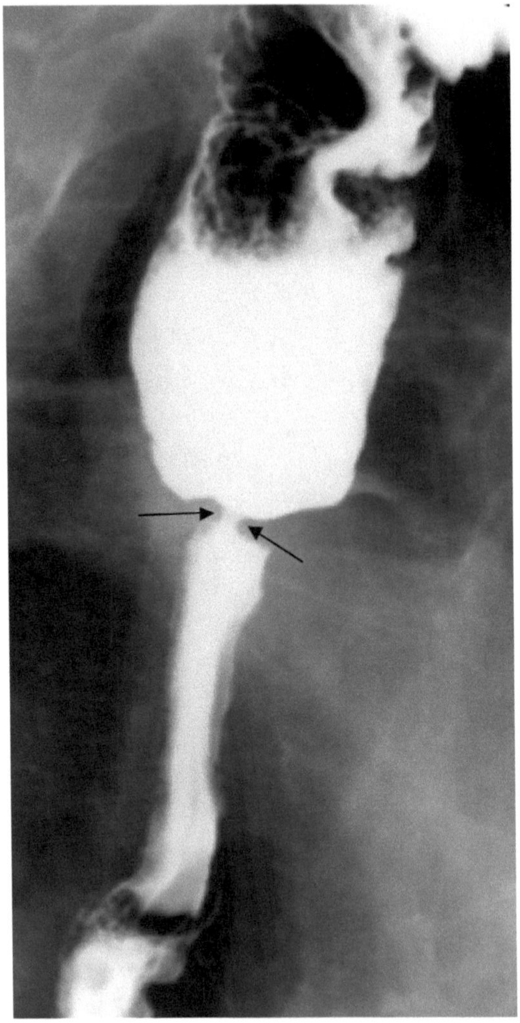

Fig. 2.39 Jejunal interposition with tight distal anastomotic stricture (*black arrows*) 2 months after surgery requiring course of endoscopic balloon dilatation

for nonsurgical techniques such as balloon dilatation and botulinum toxin injection, the technical success rates are considered inferior to surgery, particularly in young men. In addition, where surgery takes place after these interventions, some series have noted a higher complication rate (Smith et al. 2006). Now, laparoscopic Heller myotomy is the primary treatment for patients presenting with achalasia that are fit for surgery in many centers, reserving nonsurgical management only for more frail individuals, although the optimal treatment remains a controversial topic (Richter and Boeckxstaens 2011).

Heller myotomy involves division of the lower esophageal sphincter along its full length, extending to the cardia where the circular muscle terminates. This is a full-thickness division of the muscle down to the submucosal layer and performed laparoscopically (Fig. 2.40a). Defunctioning of the circular muscle predisposes to reflux (in 20–30% of cases), and so the operation is now usually accompanied by fundoplication. Any of the different forms of fundoplication may be performed depending on local preference, but the Dor procedure has been shown to produce the most satisfactory combination of reflux protection and lower incidence of dysphagia (Fig. 2.40b) (Rebecchi et al. 2008). The operation is often performed as a day case procedure and has a low complication rate, particularly in the immediate postoperative period. However, achalasia symptoms may recur, usually within 12 months, requiring additional intervention either with redo surgery or dilatation (Zaninotto et al. 2008).

2.4.2 Postoperative Imaging

Imaging has a limited role in the postoperative evaluation of these cases as the complication rate is so low. Where there is clinical concern for perforation, then water-soluble swallow is indicated, but most complications are delayed, presenting weeks and months after surgery, and require functional assessment of the esophagus. In this situation, barium may be used safely.

In a normal evaluation, there should be no holdup of contrast at the gastroesophageal junction, a normal diameter esophageal lumen (i.e., no dilatation), and no evidence of esophageal dysmotility. There will also usually be signs of distortion of the fundus resulting from fundoplication. Cross-sectional imaging is seldom required.

2.4.3 Postoperative Complications

2.4.3.1 Esophagotomy and Leak

The esophageal mucosa may be inadvertently damaged during the myotomy. This is usually

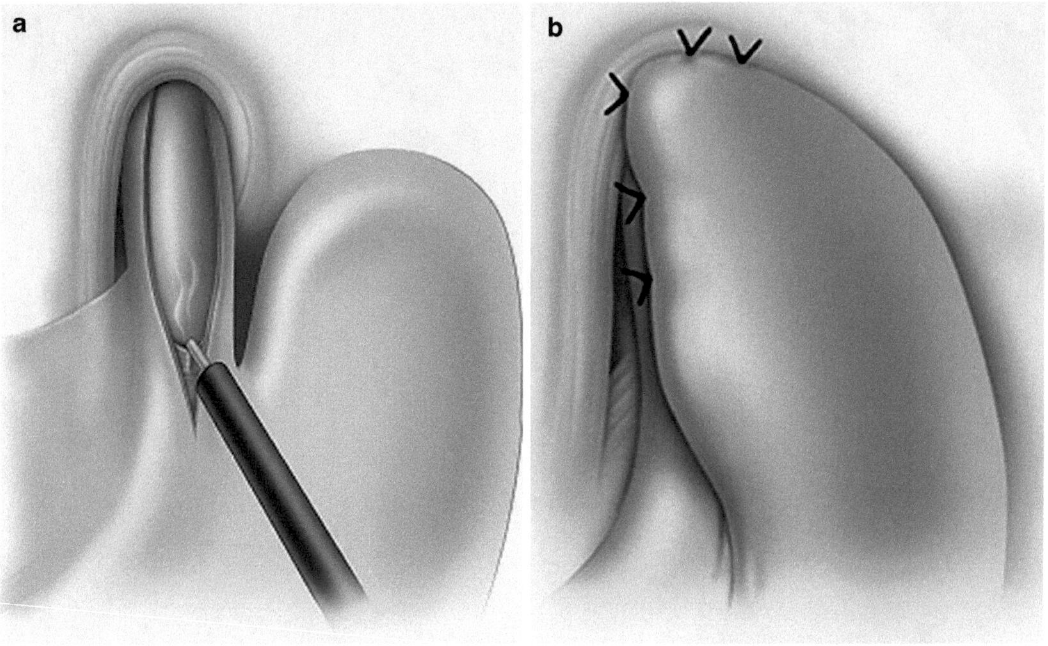

Fig. 2.40 (**a**) Completed myotomy. After reaching the submucosal plane, the myotomy is then extended for about 6 cm upward and onto the gastric wall. (**b**) Completed Dor fundoplication. Sutures are placed between the gastric fundus and the rim of the esophageal hiatus

identified and repaired at the time of surgery and is more likely where previous intervention has taken place, with an incidence varying from 5% to 25% depending on the series (Rosemurgy et al. 2005; Finan et al. 2009). Leak, however, is a very uncommon complication, occurring in less than 1% of cases. Leak will occur at the gastroesophageal junction. Management will depend on the size of leak and whether associated collections are present.

2.4.3.2 Postoperative Dysphagia – Recurrent Achalasia, Stricture, or Fundoplication Complication?

While a majority of patients have good sustained symptomatic relief following surgery, 10% will develop postoperative dysphagia (Zaninotto et al. 2008). The three main etiologies for this are related to inadequate division of the lower esophageal sphincter (recurrent achalasia), postoperative fibrosis producing a stricture, and the fundoplication wrap causing extrinsic compression on the lower esophagus (Iqbal et al. 2006). An inadequate division of the sphincter may be indicated by a short mucosal bulge (rather than a longer bulge which is expected postoperatively) (Fig. 2.41a, b), although this is not reliably demonstrated when a fundoplication has also been performed.

The main role of imaging with contrast swallow is to confirm that there is functional obstruction at the gastroesophageal junction and to reassess esophageal motility. Poor contractility of the esophagus with dilatation may be the cause of dysphagia but is not always due to failed surgery and functional obstruction (from the causes listed above) since sometimes the surgery may have been performed for end-stage achalasia, with the dilatation merely indicating a failure of recovery of normal esophageal contractility (Fig. 2.42). On the other hand, tertiary contractions and spasm are typically associated with functional obstruction. In either situation, endoscopy is normally performed to evaluate the degree of stenosis, if present, with the option of performing balloon dilatation to either loosen the wrap, treat a fibrotic stricture, or augment the myotomy when due to incomplete muscle division, with balloon dilatation being effective in 75% of cases (Zaninotto et al. 2008).

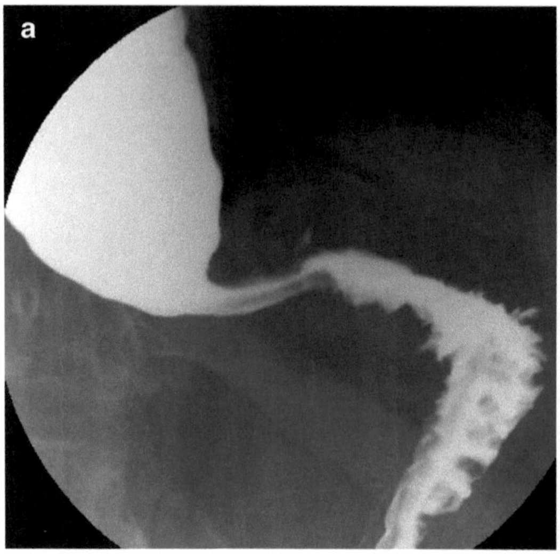

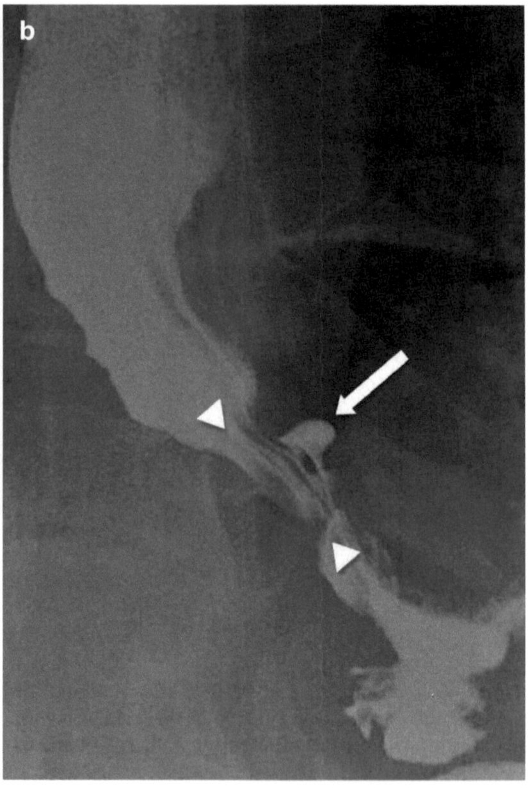

Fig. 2.41 (**a**) Achalasia in 26-year-old male with typical rat tail tapering of distal esophagus on initial barium study. (**b**) Continued dysphagia following Heller myotomy. Repeat swallow shows delayed esophageal emptying and mucosal bulge (*arrow*) not extending along the length of the GOJ (*between arrowheads*), indicating incomplete division of the lower esophageal sphincter

Dysphagia may also develop as a consequence of hiatus hernia, particularly where the fundoplication migrates into the thorax. Diagnosing wrap migration on a contrast study is important since this will not respond to dilatation and may require surgical repair. In this situation, the addition of effervescent granules may provide the requisite gastric distension to demonstrate the hernia.

Where endoscopic techniques fail, further surgical revision may be necessary either to complete the myotomy, revise the fundoplication or event, or resect the esophagus (Iqbal et al. 2006).

2.4.3.3 Reflux

Reflux is a major complication of Heller myotomy when performed alone (20–30%) but also complicates a smaller number of cases where fundoplication has been performed (5%). Contrast swallow will confirm the presence of reflux and assess the adequacy of esophageal motility and the anatomy of the wrap (whether complete or not and the presence of hiatus hernia), which aids surgical planning for patients in whom acid suppression fails to control symptoms.

2.5 Teaching Points

- Successful outcomes from esophageal surgery require significant support from radiologists who must have a thorough understanding of the range of operations being performed.
- Contrast swallow and CT are both first-line investigations depending on clinical indication – usually swallow for leak or stricture and CT for sepsis. Both may be required in more complex cases.

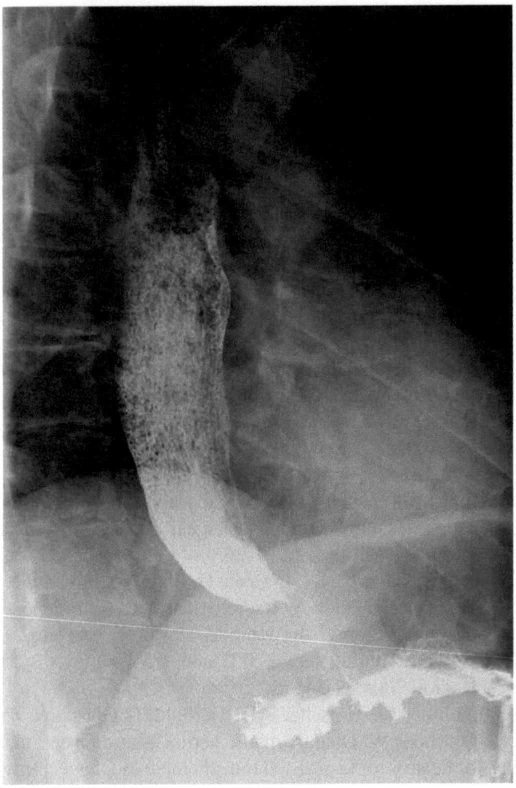

Fig. 2.42 Failed Heller myotomy. Persistent esophageal dilatation with mottled food debris in esophagus despite laparoscopic Heller myotomy for achalasia 4 months earlier

- Conduit anatomy may be very complex, requiring assistance from the surgeon or clinical records to determine the form of reconstruction.
- Many of the most life-threatening complications are diagnosed and managed surgically without need for radiological evaluation (tube necrosis, chyle leak, postoperative hemorrhage).
- Despite cross-sectional imaging advances, fluoroscopic contrast studies will continue to play a major role in the evaluation of early and late complications of esophageal surgery.

References

Agha FP, Orringer MB. Colonic interposition: radiographic evaluation. AJR Am J Roentgenol. 1984;142: 703–8.

Alanezi K, Urschel JD. Mortality secondary to esophageal anastomotic leak. Ann Thorac Cardiovasc Surg. 2004; 10:71–5.

Ascioti AJ, Hofstetter WL, Miller MJ, Rice DC, Swisher SG, Vaporciyan AA, Roth JA, Putnam JB, Smythe WR, Feig BW, Mansfield PF, Pisters PW, Torres MT, Walsh GL. Long-segment, supercharged, pedicled jejunal flap for total esophageal reconstruction. J Thorac Cardiovasc Surg. 2005;130:1391–8.

Boone J, Rinkes IB, van Leeuwen M, van Hillegersberg R. Diagnostic value of routine aqueous contrast swallow examination after oesophagectomy for detecting leakage of the cervical oesophagogastric anastomosis. ANZ J Surg. 2008;78:784–90.

Cheng YJ, Li HP, Kao EL. Perforated diverticulum: rare complication of interposed substernal colon. Ann Thorac Surg. 2006;82:717–9.

D'Cunha J, Rueth NM, Groth SS, Maddaus MA, Andrade RS. Esophageal stents for anastomotic leaks and perforations. J Thorac Cardiovasc Surg. 2011;142:39–46.

Disa JJ, Cordeiro PG. Reconstruction of the hypopharynx and cervical esophagus. Clin Plast Surg. 2001;28:349–60.

Dowson HM, Strauss D, Ng R, Mason R. The acute management and surgical reconstruction following failed esophagectomy in malignant disease of the esophagus. Dis Esophagus. 2007;20:135–40.

Finan KR, Renton D, Vick CC, Hawn MT. Prevention of post operative leak following laparoscopic Heller myotomy. J Gastrointest Surg. 2009;13:200–5.

Green DA, Moskowitz WB, Shepherd RW. Closure of a broncho-to-neoesophageal fistula using an Amplatzer Septal Occluder device. Ann Thorac Surg. 2010;89: 2010–2.

Griffin SM, Lamb PJ, Dresner SM, Richardson DL, Hayes N. Diagnosis and management of a mediastinal leak following radical oesophagectomy. Br J Surg. 2001;88:1346–51.

Griffin SM, Shaw IH, Dresner SM. Early complications after Ivor Lewis subtotal esophagectomy with two-field lymphadenectomy: risk factors and management. J Am Coll Surg. 2002;194:285–97.

Gupta V, Gupta R, Thingnam SK, Singh RS, Gupta AK, Kuthe S, Gupta NM. Major airway injury during esophagectomy: experience at a tertiary care center. J Gastrointest Surg. 2009;13:438–41.

Hayden JD, Sue-Ling HM, Sarela AI, Dexter SP. Minimally invasive management of chylous fistula after esophagectomy. Dis Esophagus. 2007;20:251–5.

Hogan BA, Winter DC, Broe D, Broe P, Lee MJ. Prospective trial comparing contrast swallow, computed tomography and endoscopy to identify anastomotic leak following oesophagogastric surgery. Surg Endosc. 2008;22:767–71.

Iqbal A, Tierney B, Haider M, Salinas VK, Karu A, Turaga KK, Mittal SK, Filipi CJ. Laparoscopic re-operation for failed Heller myotomy. Dis Esophagus. 2006;19:193–9.

Kato T, Mori T, Niibori K. A case of gastropericardial fistula of a gastric tube after esophagectomy: a case report and review. World J Emerg Surg. 2010;5:20.

Leers JM, Vivaldi C, Schäfer H, Bludau M, Brabender J, Lurje G, Herbold T, Hölscher AH, Metzger R. Endoscopic therapy for esophageal perforation or anastomotic leak with a self-expandable metallic stent. Surg Endosc. 2009;23:2258–62.

Li DX, Levine MS, Rubesin SE, Laufer I. Nonanastomotic Strictures After Colonic Interposition. AJR Am J Roentgenol. 2007;189:30–4.

Maish MS, DeMeester SR, Choustoulakis E, Briel JW, Hagen JA, Peters JH, Lipham JC, Bremner CG, DeMeester TR. The safety and usefulness of endoscopy for evaluation of the graft and anastomosis early after esophagectomy and reconstruction. Surg Endosc. 2005;19:1093–102.

Moorehead RJ, Wong J. Gangrene in esophageal substitutes after resection and bypass procedures for carcinoma of the esophagus. Hepatogastroenterology. 1990;37:364–7.

Murray DJ, Novak CB, Neligan PC. Fasciocutaneous free flaps in pharyngolaryngo-oesophageal reconstruction: a critical review of the literature. J Plast Reconstr Aesthet Surg. 2008;61:1148–56.

Nakagawa M, Seki M, Koike J, Kanai T. Gastric tube-to-pleural fistula seventeen months after esophagectomy: successful endoscopic treatment of an unusual complication. Jpn J Thorac Cardiovasc Surg. 2005;53: 569–72.

Poh M, Selber JC, Skoracki R, Walsh GL, Yu P. Technical challenges of total esophageal reconstruction using a supercharged jejunal flap. Ann Surg. 2011;253: 1122–9.

Rana ZA, Hosmane VR, Rana NR, Emery DL, Goldenberg EM, Gardner TJ. Gastro-right ventricular fistula: a deadly complication of a gastric pull-through. Ann Thorac Surg. 2010;90:297–9.

Rebecchi F, Giaccone C, Farinella E, Campaci R, Morino M. Randomized controlled trial of laparoscopic Heller myotomy plus Dor fundoplication versus Nissen fundoplication for achalasia: long-term results. Ann Surg. 2008;248:1023–30.

Renzulli P, Joeris A, Strobel O, Hilt A, Maurer CA, Uhl W, Büchler MW. Colon interposition for esophageal replacement: a single-center experience. Langenbecks Arch Surg. 2004;389:128–33.

Richter JE, Boeckxstaens GE. Management of achalasia: surgery or pneumatic dilation. Gut. 2011;60:869–76.

Rosemurgy A, Villadolid D, Thometz D, Kalipersad C, Rakita S, Albrink M, Johnson M, Boyce W. Laparoscopic Heller myotomy provides durable relief from achalasia and salvages failures after botox or dilation. Ann Surg. 2005;241:725–33.

Sarela AI, Tolan DJ, Harris K, Dexter SP, Sue-Ling HM. Anastomotic leakage after esophagectomy for cancer: a mortality-free experience. J Am Coll Surg. 2008;206:516–23.

Smith CD, Stival A, Howell DL, Swafford V. Endoscopic therapy for achalasia before Heller myotomy results in worse outcomes than Heller myotomy alone. Ann Surg. 2006;243:579–84.

Strauss DC, Forshaw MJ, Tandon RC, Mason RC. Surgical management of colonic redundancy following esophageal replacement. Dis Esophagus. 2008;21: E1–5.

Swanson JO, Levine MS, Redfern RO, Rubesin SE. Usefulness of high-density barium for detection of leaks after esophagogastrectomy, total gastrectomy, and total laryngectomy. AJR Am J Roentgenol. 2003; 181:415–20.

Tanomkiat W, Galassi W. Barium sulfate as contrast medium for evaluation of postoperative anastomotic leaks. Acta Radiol. 2000;41:482–5.

Turkyilmaz A, Eroglu A, Aydin Y, Tekinbas C, MuharremErol M, Karaoglanoglu N. The management of esophagogastric anastomotic leak after esophagectomy for esophageal carcinoma. Dis Esophagus. 2009;22:119–26.

Upponi S, Ganeshan A, D'Costa H, Betts M, Maynard N, Bungay H, Slater A. Radiological detection of post-oesophagectomy anastomotic leak - a comparison between multidetector CT and fluoroscopy. Br J Radiol. 2008;81:545–8.

Vallböhmer D, Hölscher AH, Herbold T, Gutschow C, Schröder W. Diaphragmatic hernia after conventional or laparoscopic-assisted transthoracic esophagectomy. Ann Thorac Surg. 2007;84:1847–52.

Veeramootoo D, Parameswaran R, Krishnadas R, Froeschle P, Cooper M, Berrisford RG, Wajed SA. Classification and early recognition of gastric conduit failure after minimally invasive esophagectomy. Surg Endosc. 2009;23:2110–6.

Verhage RJ, Hazebroek EJ, Boone J, Van Hillegersberg R. Minimally invasive surgery compared to open procedures in esophagectomy for cancer: a systematic review of the literature. Minerva Chir. 2009;64: 135–46.

Vyas S, Sarkar S, Mitchell I, Stoker D. Delayed transhiatal herniation of the small bowel after Ivor Lewis esophagectomy. Minerva Chir. 2009;64:427–9.

Wormuth JK, Heitmiller RF. Esophageal conduit necrosis. Thorac Surg Clin. 2006;16:11–22.

Zaninotto G, Costantini M, Rizzetto C, Zanatta L, Guirroli E, Portale G, Nicoletti L, Cavallin F, Battaglia G, Ruol A, Ancona E. Four hundred laparoscopic myotomies for esophageal achalasia: a single centre experience. Ann Surg. 2008;248:986–93.

The Stomach and Duodenum

3

Damian J.M. Tolan, Keith M. Harris, Deepak Prasad, and Samir P. Mehta

Contents

3.1 **Introduction** 72

3.2 **Gastroesophageal Reflux Surgery** 72
3.2.1 Clinical Indications 72
3.2.2 Fundoplication: Principles and Types 72
3.2.3 Normal Postoperative Imaging 72
3.2.4 Postoperative Complications 73
3.2.5 Relevant Historic Antireflux Procedures 76

3.3 **Hiatus Hernia Repair** 77
3.3.1 Clinical Indication 77
3.3.2 Surgical Technique 77
3.3.3 Postoperative Complications and Imaging 78

3.4 **Gastric Resections and Surgery for Peptic Ulcer Disease** 78
3.4.1 Clinical Indications 78
3.4.2 Surgical Techniques 78
3.4.3 Normal Postoperative Imaging 82
3.4.4 Postoperative Complications 82
3.4.5 Tumor Recurrence 91
3.4.6 Additional Operations for Peptic Ulcer Disease 91

3.5 **Bariatric Surgery** 92
3.5.1 Introduction 92
3.5.2 Restrictive Surgery 93
3.5.3 Combined Restrictive and Malabsorptive 95
3.5.4 Normal Postoperative Imaging 97
3.5.5 Postoperative Complications 100

3.6 **Radiological Insertion of Gastrostomy (RIG)** 115
3.6.1 Indications 115
3.6.2 Nonradiological Techniques for Gastrostomy 115
3.6.3 Technique for RIG 115
3.6.4 Complications of RIG 117

3.7 **Duodenal Resection and Surgery for Peptic Ulcer Disease** 117
3.7.1 Pancreas Preserving Total Duodenectomy (PPTD) and Segmental Duodenectomy (SD) 117
3.7.2 Duodenal Ulcer Surgery 118
3.7.3 Duodenal Obstruction and Palliation 122

3.8 **Teaching Points** 123

References 124

D.J.M. Tolan, MBChB, MRCP, FRCR (✉)
Department of Clinical Radiology,
Leeds Teaching Hospitals NHS Trust,
Lincoln Wing, St James's University Hospital,
LS9 7JT Leeds, UK
e-mail: damian.tolan@leedsth.nhs.uk

K.M. Harris, FRCSEd, FRCR
Department of Clinical Radiology,
Leeds Teaching Hospitals NHS Trust,
Bexley Wing, St James's University Hospital,
LS9 7JT, Leeds, UK

D. Prasad, MBBS, MRCP, FRCR
Department of Radiology, Bradford Teaching Hospitals
NHS Trust, Bradford Royal Infirmary,
Duckworth Lane, Bradford, BD9 6RJ, UK

S.P. Mehta, MA, DM (Oxon), FRCS
Department of Upper Gastrointestinal Surgery,
Leeds Teaching Hospitals NHS Trust,
Bexley Wing, St James's University Hospital,
LS9 7JT, Leeds, UK

J. Brittenden, D.J.M. Tolan (eds.), *Radiology of the Post Surgical Abdomen*,
DOI 10.1007/978-1-4471-2775-8_3, © Springer-Verlag London 2012

3.1 Introduction

Over the last 15 years, there has been a dramatic increase in the number and range of indications for gastric surgery as a consequence of the introduction of laparoscopic techniques, changes in the incidence and location of gastric cancer, and the burgeoning demand for bariatric surgery. As these techniques have developed, some older surgical procedures have now been superseded or abandoned altogether. However, radiologists need to be aware of the whole gamut of surgical procedures on the stomach, including those that are no longer performed, in order to identify normal postoperative anatomy and also any complications from historical procedures, particularly when medical records may no longer be available. We will address this chapter by indication for surgery: gastroesophageal reflux and hiatus hernia, gastric resection, other gastric surgery for peptic ulcer disease, bariatric surgery, duodenal resections, and surgery for peptic ulcer disease.

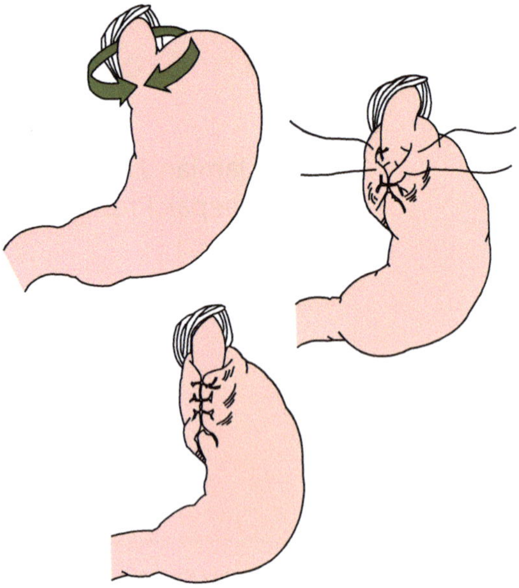

Fig. 3.1 Nissen fundoplication. The wrap is created around gastroesophageal junction using the fundus, which is passed posteriorly

3.2 Gastroesophageal Reflux Surgery

3.2.1 Clinical Indications

- Gastroesophageal reflux disease refractory to medical therapy
- Reflux symptoms with or without the presence of a hiatus hernia
- Other symptoms of reflux, including cough and asthma
- Adjunct to Heller myotomy (see Sect. 2.4)

3.2.2 Fundoplication: Principles and Types

In this procedure, the fundus of the stomach is wrapped posteriorly (or less commonly anteriorly) around the distal esophagus and lower esophageal sphincter. This is to augment the lower esophageal sphincter, providing compression in order to minimize reflux. The fundus is often sutured anteriorly, making a complete 360° wrap. The wrap extends for 2–3 cm, encircling the lower esophageal sphincter, and lies below the level of the diaphragm. At least one of the sutures usually involves the esophageal wall to prevent slippage into the thorax. This procedure is known as a Nissen fundoplication. Occasionally, the surgeon may decide to perform a partial posterior wrap known as a Toupet fundoplication. During antireflux surgery, the crura are always approximated to further prevent reflux symptoms (Canon et al. 2005).

Depending on the extent of wrap, different types of fundoplication are described:

- Nissen – 360° posterior wrap (Fig. 3.1)
- Toupet – 270° posterior wrap
- Dor (less commonly performed) – 180° anterior wrap (Fig. 2.40b)

3.2.3 Normal Postoperative Imaging

As complications are uncommon and seldom occur in the immediate postoperative period, routine imaging is not indicated unless there is clinical concern for a complication (such as vomiting or complete dysphagia).

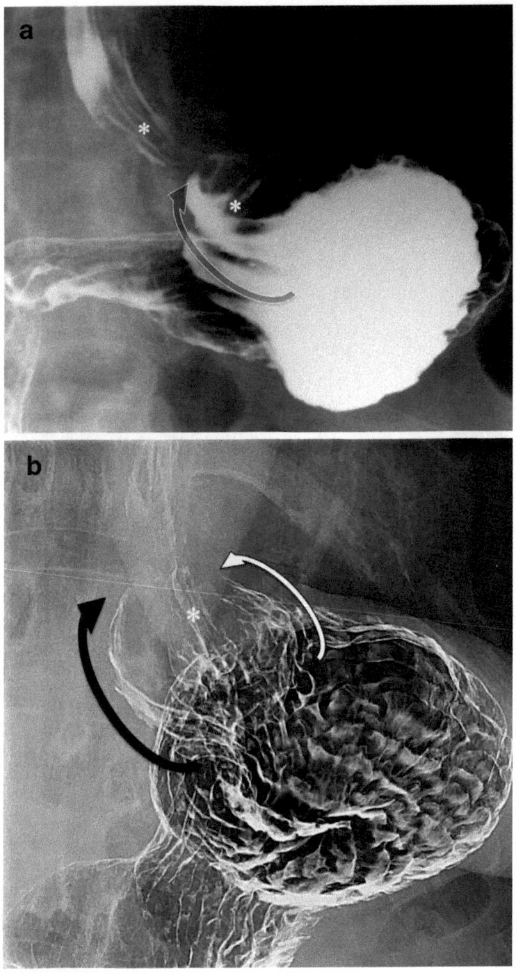

Fig. 3.2 Normal Nissen fundoplication. (**a**) Single contrast and (**b**) double-contrast examinations. Part of the posterior fundus is pulled posteriorly to the left (*black arrow*), while the anterior fundus is wrapped anteriorly (*white arrow*) to completely encircle the lower esophagus (*asterisk*)

3.2.3.1 Contrast Swallow

In the immediate postoperative period, water-soluble contrast is used to exclude a leak; subsequently, barium is used. Normally, the tapered narrowing of the distal esophagus and gastroesophageal junction extends over 2–3 cm. The wrapped segment should be below the diaphragmatic hiatus (Canon et al. 2005) (Fig. 3.2a, b).

3.2.3.2 CT

The wrap should be positioned below the diaphragmatic hiatus. "Thickening" at the gastroesophageal junction from fundoplication is not always evident.

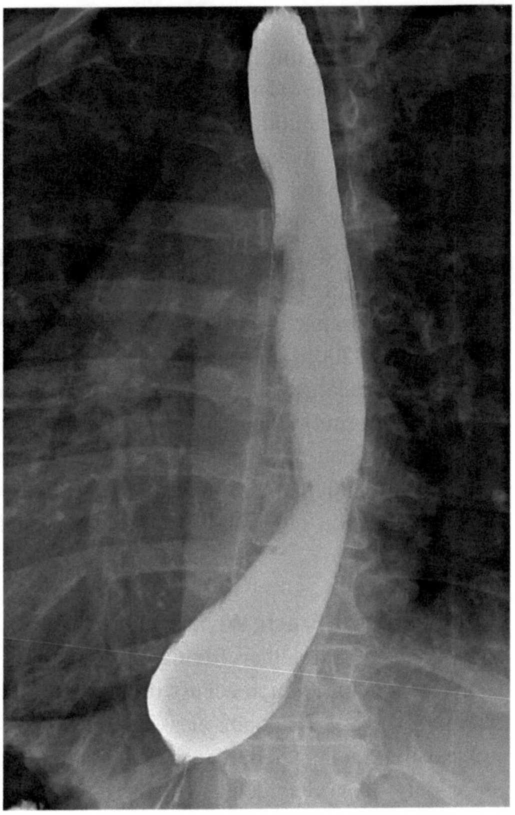

Fig. 3.3 Nissen wrap over restriction. Aperistaltic esophagus on prone swallow, due to over restriction following redo fundoplication

3.2.4 Postoperative Complications

3.2.4.1 Tight Wrap: Dysphagia and Dysmotility

High-grade holdup can occur as the esophagus passes through the wrap (Canon et al. 2005). While mild transient holdup, due to postoperative edema, may settle spontaneously in the immediate postoperative period, more significant persistent holdup may require endoscopic balloon dilatation or even revision. This may be associated with esophageal dysmotility ranging from a weak or inadequate primary stripping wave to overcome the stenosis to tertiary contractions or even a dilated atonic esophagus, termed secondary achalasia (Wehrli et al. 2007). The latter may occur in more chronic cases. Major postoperative dysmotility is fortunately an uncommon complication (Fig. 3.3).

3.2.4.2 Wrap Migration/Slipped Wrap

This occurs when the fundoplication slips distally to encircle the stomach rather than the gastroesophageal junction, due to failure of the sutures holding the wrap to the esophagus (Hatfield and Shapir 1985). Sudden postoperative deterioration may occur and may be indicated on plain film radiography with a dilated gastric bubble (Fig. 3.4a). Contrast swallow confirms dilated stomach folds superior to the wrap (Canon et al. 2005) and sometimes, where the slip is bigger, a larger dilated gastric tube with an hourglass deformity (the transition point may not be demonstrated due to gastric contents) (Fig. 3.4b) (Hatfield and Shapir 1985). This is a rare complication but usually requires surgical correction.

3.2.4.3 Intrathoracic Wrap Herniation

The stomach can either herniate through the esophageal hiatus, which occurs in up to 30% of patients at 1 year (Hainaux et al. 2002). This is not usually accompanied by recurrent symptoms, since only 36% of patients with herniation are symptomatic (Hainaux et al. 2002). When herniation does occur, the wrap may pass alongside the lower esophagus with the GOJ remaining in a normal position (paraesophageal-type hernia – 70% of hernias) (Fig. 3.5) or in a "sliding" configuration with proximal migration of the GOJ (30% of hernias) due to the wrap being too loose or if the hiatus is wide open (Figs. 3.6 and 3.7) (Hainaux et al. 2002; Canon et al. 2005). While CT does not provide functional information, the abnormal position of the wrap can often be demonstrated and should be assessed in any postoperative patient. Such patients can present with chest pain, mimicking cardiorespiratory disor-

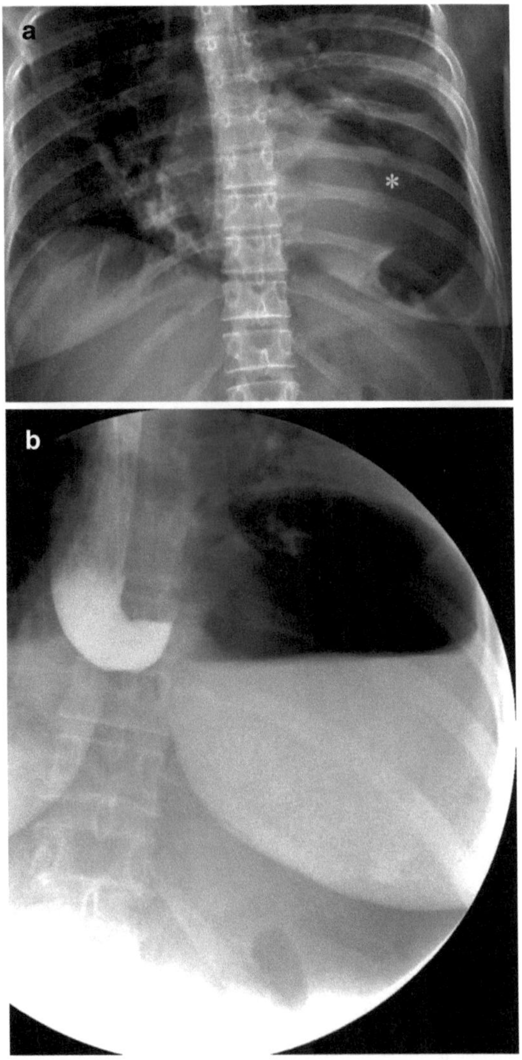

Fig. 3.4 Acute respiratory deterioration with vomiting, day 2 post Nissen fundoplication. (**a**) Dilated gastric bubble (*asterisk*) on the chest radiograph indicates significant abnormality. (**b**) Contrast swallow indicates obstruction below the expected position of the wrap, in the region of the mid gastric body. Patient returned to theater for immediate revision of the fundoplication

Fig. 3.6 (**a**) Nissen wrap migration. Dysphagia 8 months post fundoplication. Barium meal shows the fundal wrap (*curved arrow*) around the cardia (*straight arrows*) now lies above the diaphragmatic hiatus, which required surgical revision. (**b**) Toupet fundoplication (*curved arrows*) with migration above the hiatus (*black arrow*) on double-contrast examination

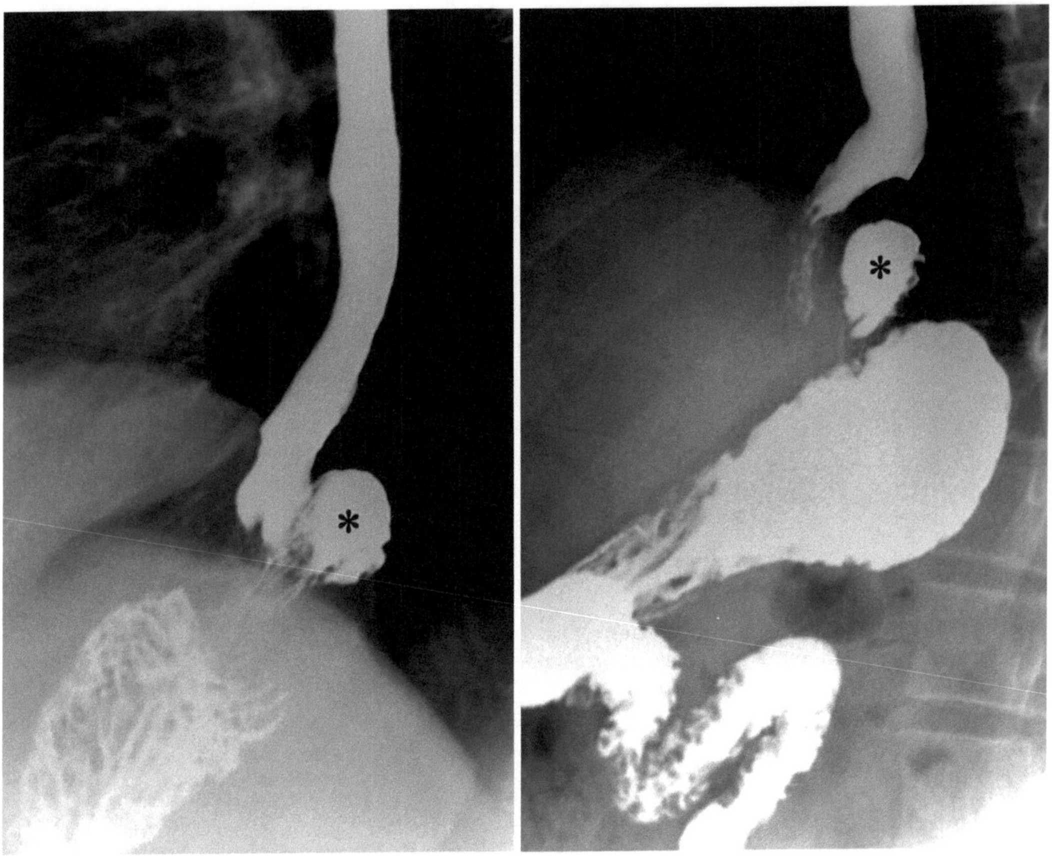

Fig. 3.5 Paraesophageal hernia post fundoplication with a segment of fundus (*asterisk*) alongside the distal esophagus and normally positioned GOJ

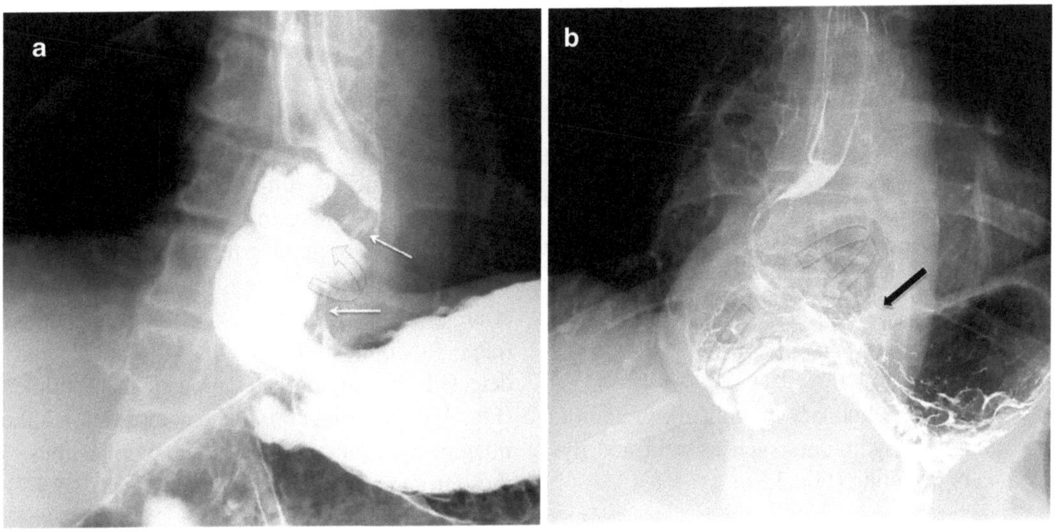

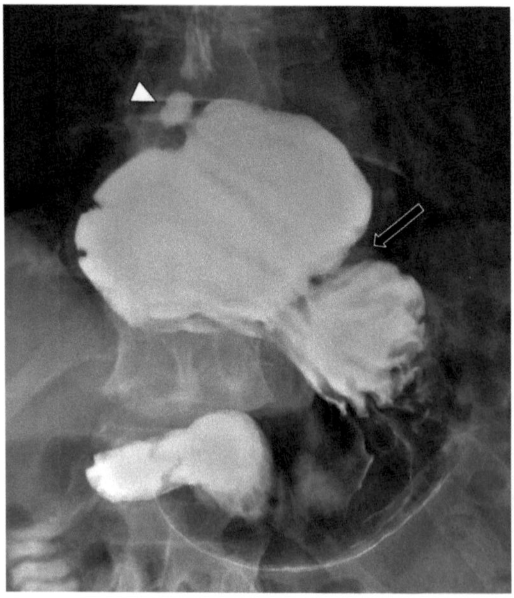

Fig. 3.7 Nissen fundoplication recurrent hiatus hernia. Upper stomach has passed through hiatus (*arrow*). Plication of fundus is incomplete (*arrowhead*)

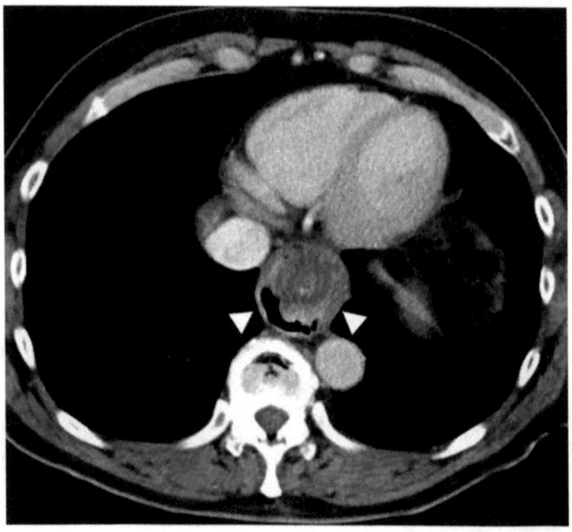

Fig. 3.8 Nissen wrap migration CT Patient 2 weeks post fundoplication with severe epigastric pain and vomiting. CT shows a "doughnut" of soft tissue around the lower esophagus (*arrowheads*) from migration of the wrap due to incomplete closure of the hiatal defect

ders (such as pulmonary embolism), in addition to abdominal symptoms such as pain and dysphagia or vomiting (Fig. 3.8).

3.2.4.4 Fundoplication Dehiscence

On barium swallow, there is no typical tapering of the gastroesophageal junction or filling defect in the fundus to suggest fundoplication. A completely dehisced fundoplication often mimics normal findings in a healthy patient who has not undergone any operation, and typically, there is associated gastroesophageal reflux (Thoeni and Moss 1979; Canon et al. 2005).

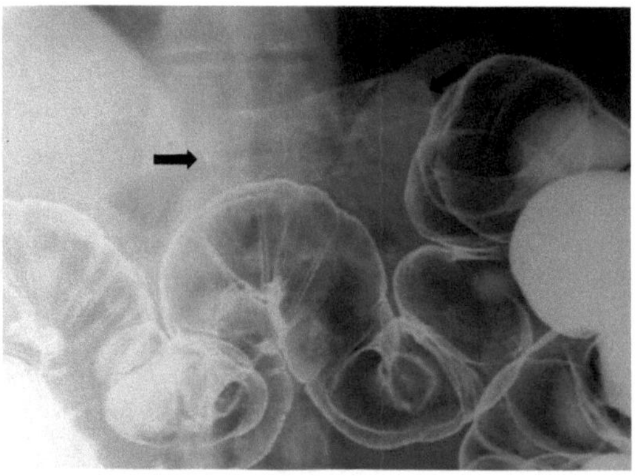

Fig. 3.9 Angelchik antireflux device. Incidental finding on barium enema examination (*arrows*). Note similar appearance to laparoscopic gastric balloon for obesity but without tube or reservoir

3.2.5 Relevant Historic Antireflux Procedures

3.2.5.1 Angelchik Antireflux Prosthesis

In the 1970s and 1980s, this device was placed for treatment of reflux. Functioning in a similar mechanism to a laparoscopic gastric band for obesity, it consisted a silicone-filled C-shaped balloon tied around the gastroesophageal junction (but without any reservoir for adjustment – an important clue to differentiate from a gastric band). It is no longer in widespread use, despite being effective in treating reflux, due to problems with erosion, fracture, gas bloating (Burhenne et al. 1984), and the success of other techniques (e.g., fundoplication). It may be incidentally detected on imaging evaluation of the abdomen (Fig. 3.9) or to diagnose a late complication – the imaging appearances mimicking complications of those from gastric band placement (Sect. 3.5.5.7).

3.2.5.2 Belsey Mark IV Repair

This is another procedure that has been superseded by newer techniques. The lower 4 cm of

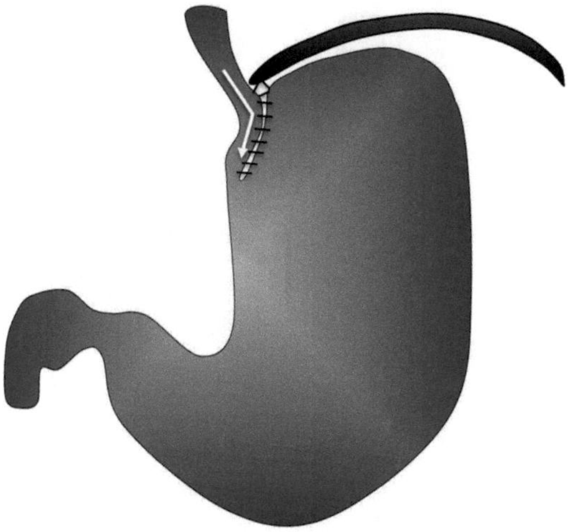

Fig. 3.10 Belsey Mark IV repair. By suturing the fundus to the abdominal esophagus, an angle is created (*arrow*) to prevent reflux. This is then fixed with a suture to the diaphragm

esophagus were sutured to the adjacent gastric fundus, altering the angulation of the abdominal portion of the distal esophagus by making the lowest portion deviate medially to create a "valve" to prevent reflux. This was then fixed to the adjacent diaphragm to prevent proximal migration (Fig. 3.10) (Hatfield and Shapir 1985). Radiographic features of surgical failure were associated with transhiatal migration or loss of the angulation between the thoracic and intra-abdominal portions of the distal esophagus (Orringer et al. 1972). The Hill repair followed similar principles but with posterior diaphragmatic defect repair which is indistinguishable from the Belsey repair on imaging. These procedures are now only encountered in evaluation of patients with new symptoms and a history of surgery performed decades previously.

3.3 Hiatus Hernia Repair

3.3.1 Clinical Indication

- Paraesophageal hernia (symptomatic or nonsymptomatic)
- Addition to fundoplication
- Repair of defects from surgery of the esophagus where the hiatus is widened (e.g., transhiatal esophagectomy)

Intrathoracic stomach is often discovered in elderly patients (e.g., on CT scans), and many individuals are asymptomatic. Chronic symptoms may include reflux-type symptoms such as heartburn, regurgitation, and dysphagia but also obstructive symptoms such as chest pain and vomiting. These latter symptoms may often fail to respond to medical therapy or conservative measures. Consequently, elective repair may be undertaken with symptom relief in 80–90% of patients with low operative mortality and morbidity (Dallemagne et al. 2011; Louie et al. 2011; Furnée et al. 2011). Acute repair is warranted in patients who present with an acute gastric volvulus (mesenteroaxial volvulus carrying the highest risk) often with a higher risk of morbidity and mortality (Louie et al. 2011).

3.3.2 Surgical Technique

Where hiatus hernia repair is performed for intrathoracic stomach (usually defined as >30% of the stomach within the thorax), the hernia sac is resected, and the stomach is reduced into the abdomen. This may be performed laparoscopically. In the preoperative workup, the presence or absence of esophageal shortening is assessed either by barium swallow or by endoscopy, as this has implications on the surgical technique. Where shortening is demonstrated, a *gastroplasty* may be performed to "lengthen" the esophagus by creating additional length from the gastric cardia (e.g., *Collis gastroplasty* – Fig. 3.11) (Canon et al. 2005).

The stomach is reduced into the abdomen and any volvulus corrected. The hernia sac is then resected and the hiatal defect closed. This may be performed with nonabsorbable sutures or mesh (Mitiek and Andrade 2010). The best method or hernia repair remains controversial. There is some evidence to suggest that mesh might reduce radiological recurrence, but it is associated with other complications such as higher dysphagia rates (Watson 2011) and in addition the risk of mesh erosion into the esophagus. Addition of fundoplication to the procedure often reduces symptomatic postoperative reflux (Furnée et al. 2011; Mitiek and Andrade 2010).

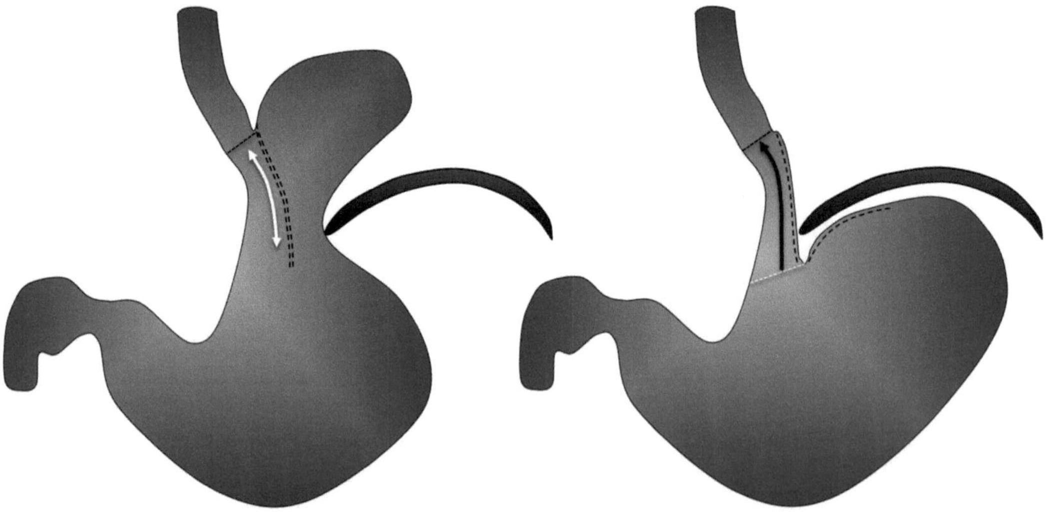

Fig. 3.11 Collis gastroplasty. Where the esophagus is shortened and the GOJ is pulled proximally, the esophagus may be lengthened by stapling to divide the fundus from the cardia to produce a short gastric tube. The new GOJ now extends below the hiatus (*broken white line*). This procedure may be augmented by fundoplication

3.3.3 Postoperative Complications and Imaging

Complications are usually related to failure of hiatus hernia repair. While the radiological recurrence rate can be as high as 66%, most patients with a degree of recurrence have an improved quality of life and less reflux (Dallemagne et al. 2011) and 81% of patients are symptom free (Louie et al. 2011). Clinically significant hernias occur in 5% of cases (Watson 2011) and very few patients require repeat surgical repair (Dallemagne et al. 2011).

Routine postoperative imaging is not usually required unless there is a suspicion of a leak or if the patient is symptomatic. Symptoms of immediate hiatal hernia recurrence may include heartburn, regurgitation, dysphagia, or vomiting. A functional assessment with contrast swallow is usually the most appropriate first evaluation, reserving water-soluble contrast for exclusion of leak or where high-grade obstruction is suspected. Metallic rivets might indicate a mesh repair (Fig. 3.12a). An advantage of cross-sectional imaging is to define the size of the defect and presence or absence of other viscera within the hernia. Both contrast swallow and CT can provide useful information when complex hernias are present (Figs. 2.27, 2.28, and 3.12b).

3.4 Gastric Resections and Surgery for Peptic Ulcer Disease

3.4.1 Clinical Indications

- Carcinoma
- Gastrointestinal stromal tumor
- Complicated peptic ulcer disease
- Prophylactic for hereditary diffuse gastric cancer

3.4.2 Surgical Techniques

3.4.2.1 Billroth I Partial Gastrectomy

Now seldom performed, the distal stomach is resected and the proximal stomach anastomosed directly to the first part of the duodenum (Fig. 3.13a). With a small resection, the stomach can look remarkably normal on contrast studies but is reduced in size and without a clearly defined pylorus.

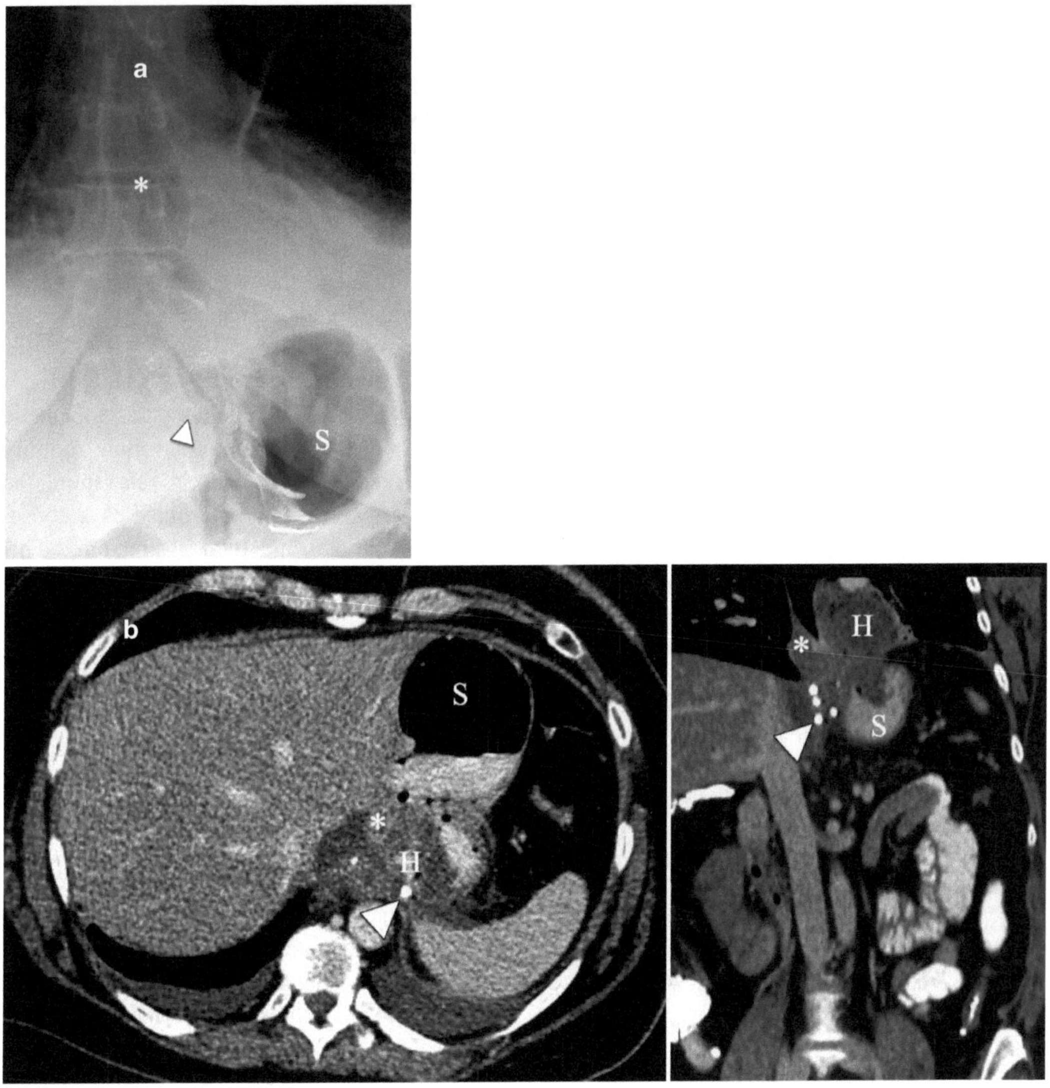

Fig. 3.12 (**a**) Repair of massive hiatus hernia (intrathoracic stomach) with rivets from mesh to repair the hiatal defect (*arrowhead*). (**b**). Patient returned with severe epigastric pain and vomiting. CT with positive oral contrast in the stomach (*S*) and normal position of the esophagus (*asterisk*) shows a rolling paraesophageal hernia (*H*) has formed despite rivets anchoring mesh (*arrowhead*) requiring further surgery

3.4.2.2 Billroth II/Polya Partial Gastrectomy

Here the distal stomach is resected with closure of the duodenal stump. A gastroenterostomy is then created to the remaining proximal stomach, which restores continuity. The loop of jejunum is placed in either a retrocolic or an antecolic position and can be anastomosed in either an iso- (Fig. 3.13b) or antiperistaltic direction. This procedure is again becoming historical as many surgeons now favor the subtotal gastrectomy with Roux loop reconstruction (Fig. 3.14).

3.4.2.3 Subtotal Gastrectomy with Roux Loop Reconstruction

The distal stomach is resected and the duodenal stump closed, as with a Polya partial gastrectomy, but continuity is restored with a Roux loop reconstruction.

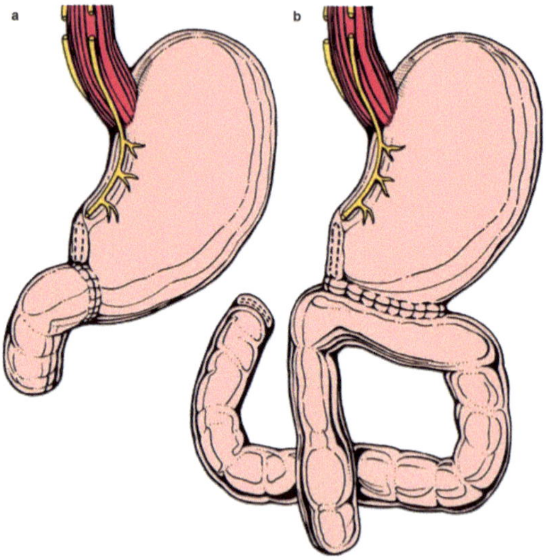

Fig. 3.13 Distal gastrectomy (and truncal vagotomy) with either (**a**) gastroduodenostomy – Billroth I or (**b**) gastrojejunostomy – Billroth II (also known as Polya)

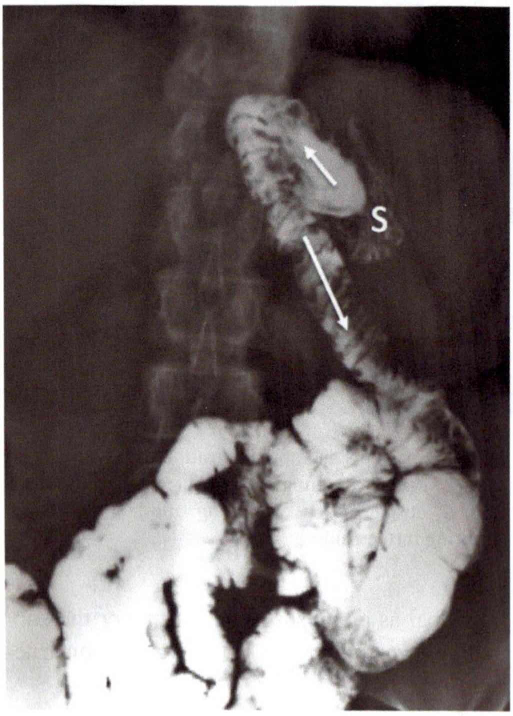

Fig. 3.14 Small bowel meal showing normal postoperative appearance following partial gastrectomy with Roux loop reconstruction. Contrast exits via the efferent jejunal limb (*arrows*) from the proximal stomach (*S*)

3.4.2.4 Total Gastrectomy

Usually performed for gastric malignancy. The whole stomach is resected with lymphadenectomy. The duodenal stump is stapled closed and/or over sewn. A Roux loop is brought up and anastomosed (usually end to side) to the distal esophagus, with a blind limb of varying length. There is a further jejunojejunal anastomosis 50–60 cm distal to the esophagojejunal anastomosis (Figs. 3.15 and 3.16a, b).

3.4.2.5 Truncal Vagotomy

Since the vagus nerve supplies parasympathetic innervation to the stomach, controlling motility and acid secretion and pyloric relaxation, the vagus nerves are usually sacrificed as a consequence of subtotal and total gastrectomy. This procedure is also performed as part of the management of duodenal ulceration and accompanied by pyloroplasty (Sect. 3.4.6.2).

3.4.2.6 Wedge Resection

In some instances, wedge resection may be appropriate, for example, for resection of a small gastrointestinal tumor that is ulcerated and causing anemia, where lymphadenectomy is not required for oncologic clearance. This may be performed laparoscopically or as an open procedure (Lee et al. 2011). The operation carries far less morbidity than either partial gastrectomy or total gastrectomy, and no anastomoses are formed which also reduces the risk of complication (Goh et al. 2010).

3.4.2.7 Gastroenterostomy

This is performed to overcome gastric outlet obstruction. Historically, this was as an alternative to pyloroplasty in order to improve drainage of the stomach following truncal vagotomy. The first accessible jejunal loop is anastomosed side to side to the stomach. This loop can be brought onto the stomach in front of the transverse colon (antecolic) or through the transverse mesocolon onto the posterior wall of the stomach (retrocolic). The development of bile gastritis and an increased risk of gastric cancer are long-term potential complications. Most surgeons now favor Roux loop

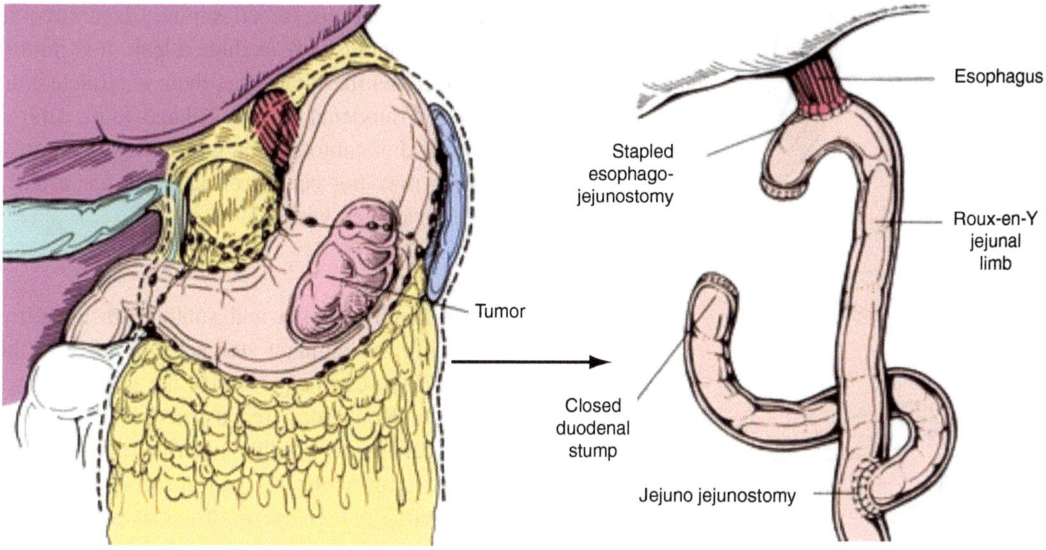

Fig. 3.15 Total gastrectomy. The stomach is resected with the greater omentum along with lymph node dissection along the celiac axis and gastrohepatic ligament. The stomach is then anastomosed to a jejunal Roux loop

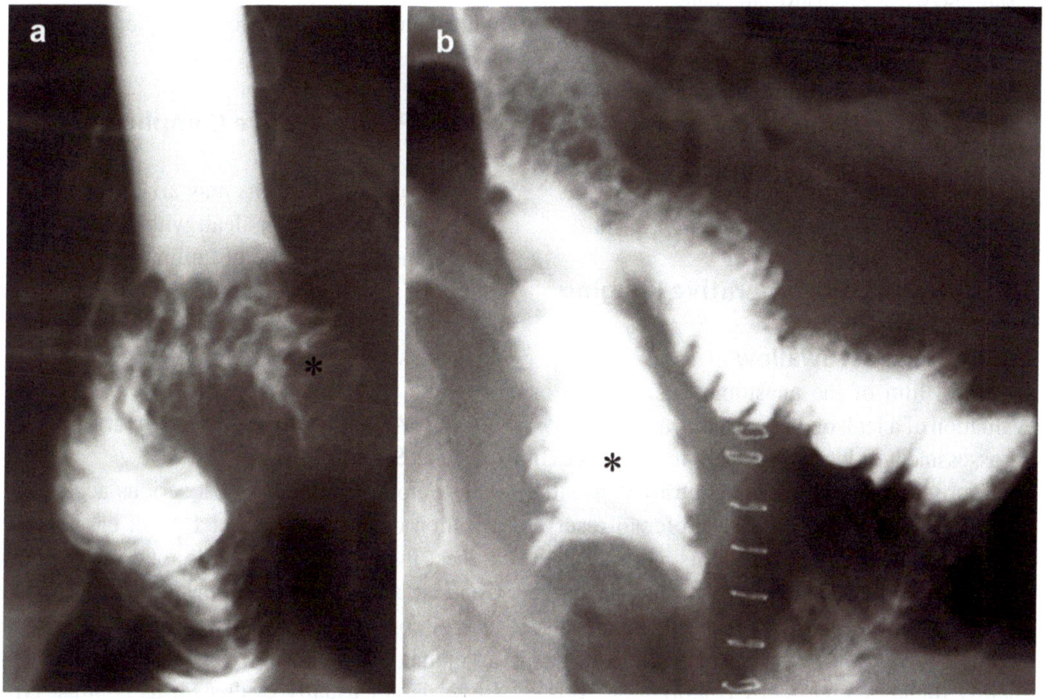

Fig. 3.16 Total gastrectomy normal OJ anastomosis. The blind limb of the esophagojejunal anastomosis (*asterisk*) can lie either (**a**) right or (**b**) left and can vary in length. Excessively long limbs may result in an afferent limb syndrome

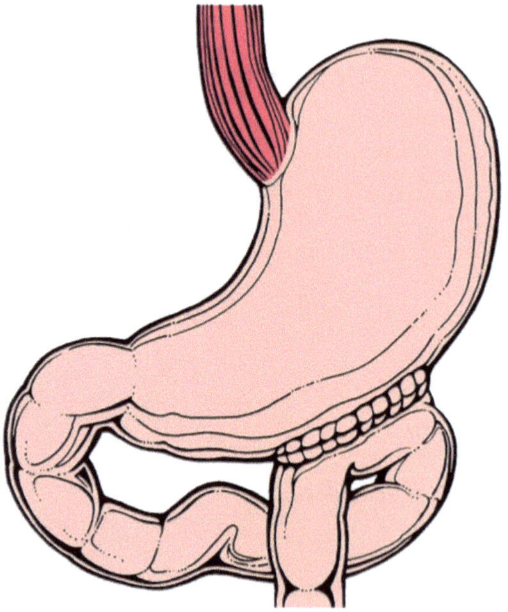

Fig. 3.17 Gastroenterostomy. The jejunum is anastomosed in either a retrocolic or antecolic position to the greater curve to allow drainage of gastric content. This is now usually reserved as a palliative procedure

reconstruction for anything other than short-term palliation (e.g., for malignant gastric outflow obstruction), since a Roux loop of adequate length prevents bile entering the stomach (Fig. 3.17).

3.4.3 Normal Postoperative Imaging

3.4.3.1 Contrast Swallow

A control film of the anastomotic site helps in evaluation of a leak on the postcontrast image. As for assessment of leaks elsewhere in the upper GI tract, an initial water-soluble contrast is usually performed, but some surgeons prefer to reserve contrast studies only for patients with clinical suspicion of leak, since contrast studies detect small subclinical leaks in 7% while being false negative in some cases where leaks are subsequently found on endoscopy (Lamb et al. 2004). Where no leak is identified, barium may be used, depending on local preference, but this is not the author's practice due to problems with related artifacts with CT or angiography in these patients as well as the small risk of barium peritonitis. The examination is performed with the patient in multiple positions (erect, supine, decubitus) in order to conclusively exclude a leak. It is important to remember that when there is clinical concern for duodenal stump leakage (e.g., after a Billroth II or subtotal/total gastrectomy), contrast studies may not be appropriate and are usually better evaluated with CT.

3.4.3.2 CT

For Billroth II/Polya and subtotal gastrectomy, following the remnant stomach inferiorly to the jejunal loop can help identify the gastrojejunostomy. In Roux loop reconstruction, the jejunal limbs can be seen either anterior (antecolic) or posterior (retrocolic) to the transverse colon with the distal jejunojejunal anastomosis usually indicated by a staple line. The duodenum serves as a landmark to locate the proximal end of the biliary limb and is also indicated by a staple line; this limb lies posterior to the superior mesenteric vessels. The duodenum should be specifically evaluated for abnormal fluid or gas collections that may indicate duodenal stump leak (see Sect. 3.4.4.1).

3.4.4 Postoperative Complications

A range of complications may arise from gastric resection. These will be dealt with in turn. Some are common to any type of luminal surgery, such as leak or stricture, while others are more specific to gastric surgery. Partial gastrectomy complications are summarized in Fig. 3.18.

3.4.4.1 Anastomotic and Duodenal Stump Leak

Anastomotic leak is the most serious acute complication occurring in about 10% of cases and is highest in patients undergoing total gastrectomy. Contrast studies will demonstrate extraluminal leak of contrast from the esophagojejunal or gastrojejunal anastomoses. However, the duodenal stump is not usually evaluated, as contrast typically fails to enter the biliary limb after a Roux-en-Y reconstruction or the afferent jejunal limb following a Billroth II (Fig. 3.19). It is important to assess position of drains – rarely drains migrate into the lumen which can lead to diagnostic pitfalls (Fig. 3.20).

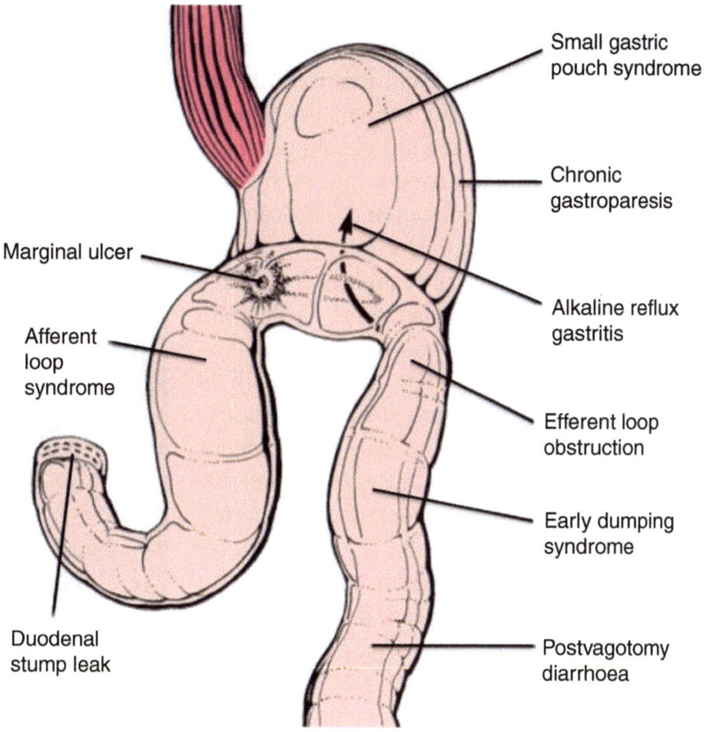

Fig. 3.18 Post partial gastrectomy complications. Billroth II- and Roux-en-Y-related complications include duodenal stump leak and afferent loop syndrome (less common in Roux loop reconstruction). Other symptoms related to the residual stomach and efferent loop are also shared

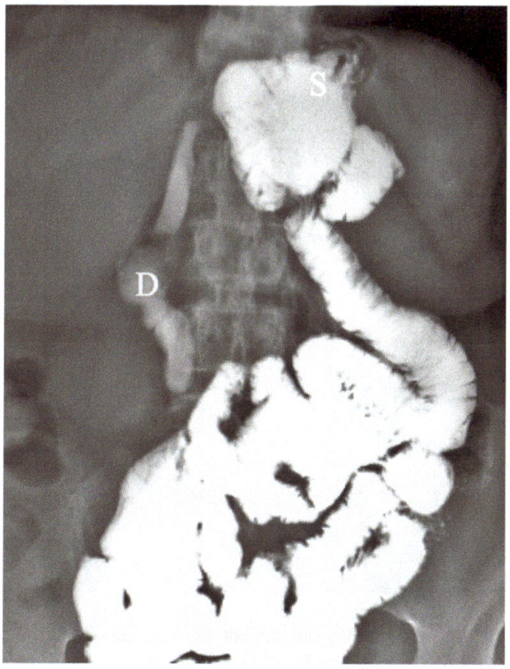

Fig. 3.19 Incidental reflux to the afferent loop following Billroth II reconstruction. A small volume of contrast has passed into the duodenum (*D*) from the stomach (*S*)

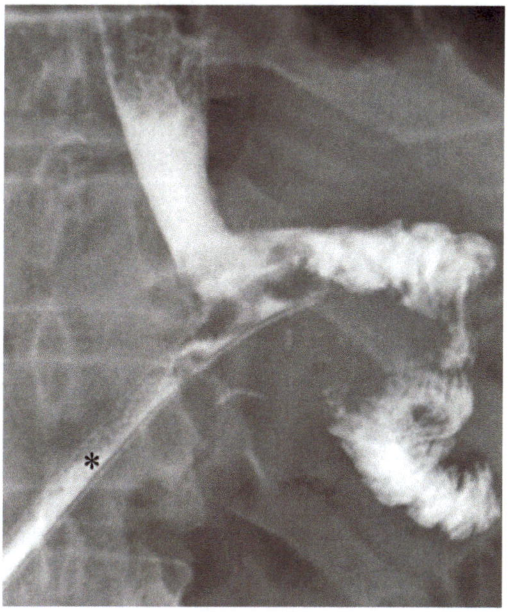

Fig. 3.20 Interpretation pitfall. Day 7 post total gastrectomy contrast study first reported as showing no leak. Note contrast in surgical drain (*asterisk*) indicating that a leak is in fact present due to drain migration into the lumen

With gross anastomotic dehiscence CT demonstrates pneumoperitoneum, extraluminal accumulation of contrast and free fluid. It can be difficult to detect more subtle leaks without positive oral contrast, and this should generally be administered unless there is a contraindication. It is extremely important to evaluate for collections and where present to indicate whether and how they can be drained with image guidance. The normal anatomical barriers are disrupted due to transection of peritoneal ligaments and mesenteries from gastric mobilization at surgery and, consequently, collections can develop at unusual or unexpected locations. After total gastrectomy and when the collection is small, it will usually accumulate in the left subphrenic space (Fig. 3.21). Conservative management of leaks and abscesses with gut rest and drainage of collections is the usual approach and successful in a majority of cases, even when leaks are large (Fig. 3.22). Superficial collections can be imaged with ultrasound, particularly where they relate to port sites (if the surgery has been performed laparoscopically). It is important to differentiate a port site hernia from a collection or hematoma (Fig. 3.23). However, CT is also a useful modality in this setting, and probably more able to provide a

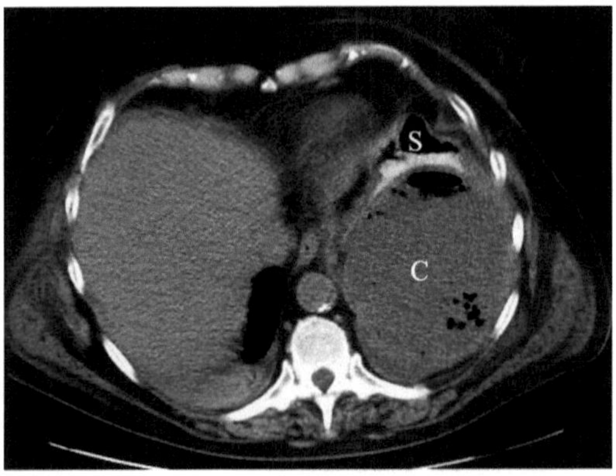

Fig. 3.21 Failure to progress with sepsis and nausea. Day 10 post partial gastrectomy and splenectomy for malignant GIST. A large infected splenic bed collection (*C*) is demonstrated compressing the proximal stomach (*S*) that resolved after ultrasound-guided drain insertion

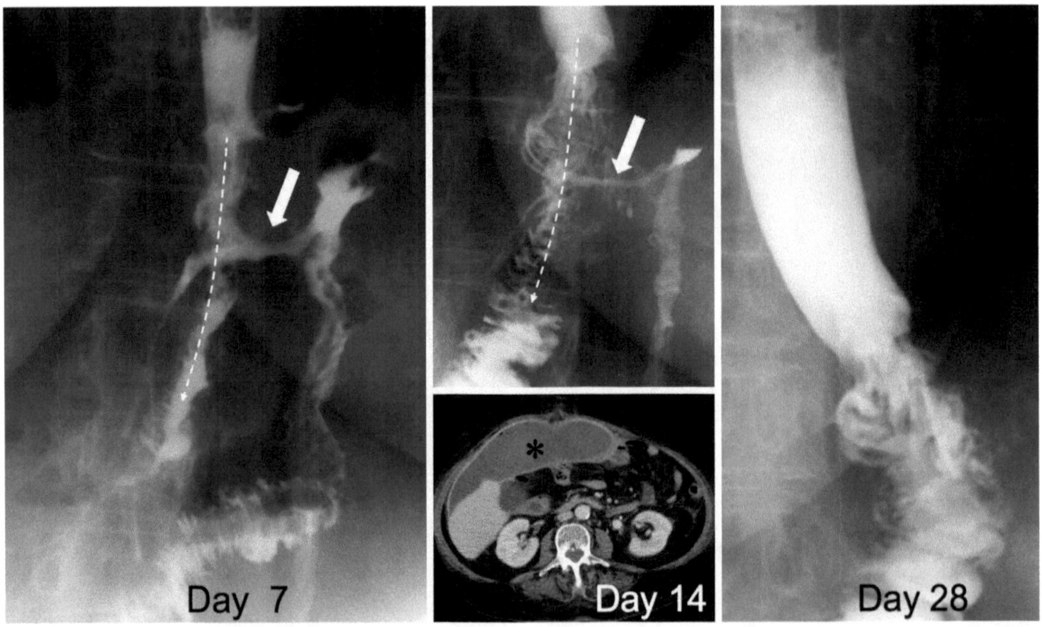

Fig. 3.22 Successful outcome after large leak following total gastrectomy. Large defect identified at routine postoperative swallow on day 7 (*white arrow*) with contrast lying outside the jejunal loop (*broken arrow*). Follow-up on day 14 showed ongoing leak with a smaller defect (*white arrow*), but the patient became septic and CT showed a large right subhepatic abscess (*asterisk*), drained using ultrasound guidance. By day 28, the predischarge contrast swallow shows the leak has sealed

Radiology of the Post Surgical Abdomen

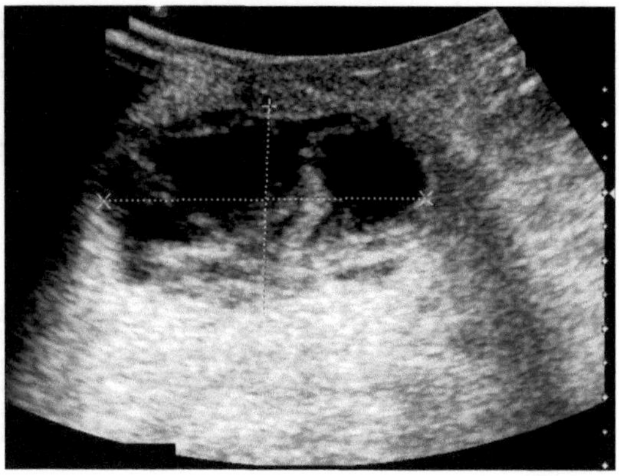

Fig. 3.23 Day 6 post laparoscopic gastrectomy. Localized pain and erythema over a left-sided abdominal port site raising concern for post site bowel hernia. Ultrasound shows a 4 cm × 3 cm septated subcutaneous collection related to infected hematoma treated with incision and drainage

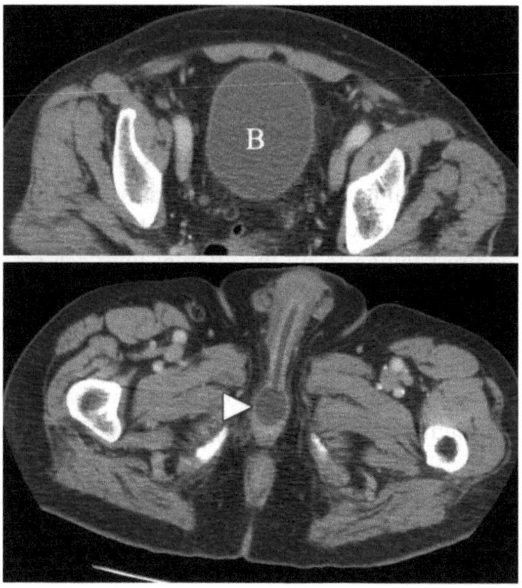

Fig. 3.24 Importance of comprehensive review. CT for sepsis and reduced urine output day 2 post total gastrectomy. On the most distal CT slice, the Foley catheter balloon is malpositioned in the membranous urethra (*arrowhead*) explaining poor urine output with distended bladder (*B*)

global assessment in the postoperative period (e.g., in a search for sites of sepsis – Fig. 3.24) or to problem solve where the ultrasound findings are equivocal (Fig. 3.25).

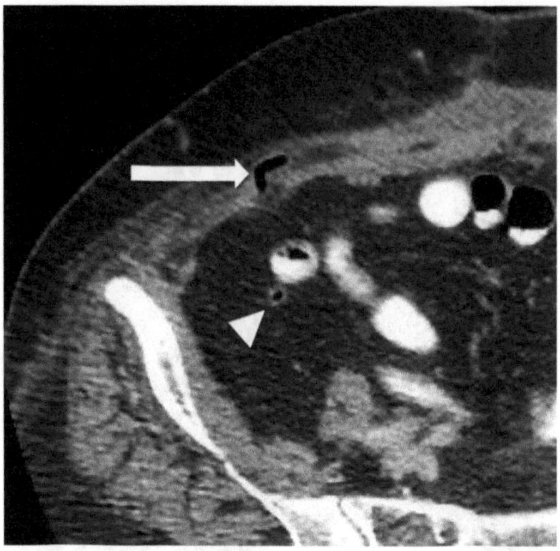

Fig. 3.25 Readmission with right iliac fossa pain CT scan 3 weeks post laparoscopic gastrectomy. The appendix (*arrowhead*) has herniated through the port site defect (*arrow*)

Duodenal stump leak on CT usually localizes into the right subhepatic space as a fluid collection with varying quantities of gas (Fig. 3.26). Although it can occur without a precipitant, it is often predisposed by afferent loop obstruction (see Sect. 3.4.4.2) or biliopancreatic limb proximal to the jejunojejunal anastomosis of a Roux loop (0.2% cases) due to anastomotic stricture or internal hernia (Aoki et al. 2010). This should not be mistaken for resolving postoperative fluid or hematoma, and the radiologist should have a high index of suspicion for this complication, as it is difficult to diagnose clinically (unless the surgical drain adjacent to the oversewn duodenal stump produces a high output of effluent). A further indication is disruption of the duodenal stump metal staple line (Fig. 3.27). Where there is doubt, image-guided aspiration and repeat CT after a short delay are both relevant options depending on the clinical status of the patient – a duodenal stump leak will generally increase without intervention. Image-guided drainage, where possible, prevents unnecessary surgical intervention (Fig. 3.28).

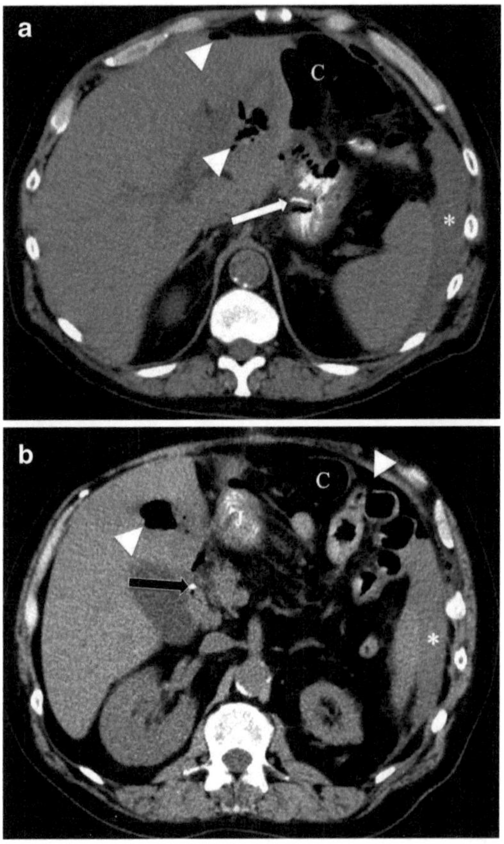

Fig. 3.26 (**a**, **b**) Total gastrectomy duodenal stump leak. Sepsis day 10 post total gastrectomy for cancer. Left perisplenic collection (*asterisk*) and excessive pneumoperitoneum (*arrowheads*) particularly in the periportral space. The gastrojejunal anastomosis is intact (*white arrow*) with no leak of positive oral contrast. Subsequent CT-guided aspiration of the collection aspirated bile, confirming suspicion of duodenal stump leak (*black arrow*). Patient returned to theater for washout and placement of a surgical drain at top of duodenal stump (*C* colon, *J* Roux loop)

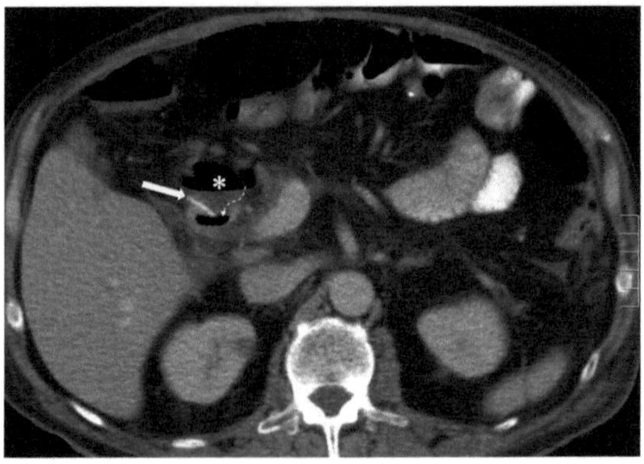

Fig. 3.27 Small duodenal stump leak following partial gastrectomy. The duodenal staple line (*arrow*) is "open" at the medial end (*curved arrow*) allowing pancreatic and biliary secretions to leak and form the collection anterior to D2 (*asterisk*)

3.4.4.2 Afferent Loop Obstruction/Syndrome

Afferent loop obstruction causing afferent loop syndrome is an uncommon complication associated with Billroth II gastrectomy and gastrojejunostomy and affects 1% of patients. It occurs due to complete or partial obstruction of the afferent limb at the gastroenterostomy site, which may result from adhesions, or twisting of the bowel proximal to the gastric anastomosis. Acute obstruction is a surgical emergency as this may lead to duodenal stump blow out, whereas chronic partial obstruction still requires intervention but without the same urgency. An afferent limb longer than 30–40 cm and antecolic gastrojejunostomy increase the risk of this complication. Patients can present with nonspecific symptoms such as nausea and bloating, epigastric pain, vomiting (when the obstruction is relieved), or signs of malnutrition due to bacterial overgrowth. Contrast studies are of limited benefit, since contrast failing to fill the afferent limb can be a normal finding. However, CT demonstrates a fluid-filled dilated afferent limb, including the duodenum, and is usually associated with biliary dilatation, due to obstruction to outflow by raised intraluminal pressure (Gayer et al. 2002; Smith et al. 1994).

Treatment usually involves either surgical revision (from Billroth II to Roux-en-Y anastomosis) or treatment of the underlying cause (e.g., reduction of internal hernia, adhesiolysis, etc.).

3.4.4.3 Other Anastomotic Complications

Stricture formation may affect the anastomosis for any of the surgical procedures, affecting the esophagojejunal anastomosis in 4–6% (Fig. 3.29a) (Fukagawa et al. 2010; Kim et al. 2009), up to 20% of Billroth I (Fig. 3.30), and 6% Billroth II/Roux-en-Y procedures (Fig. 3.31) (Takahashi et al. 1992). Anastomotic strictures may be managed successfully with balloon dilatation, but this does carry a small risk of perforation and resteno-

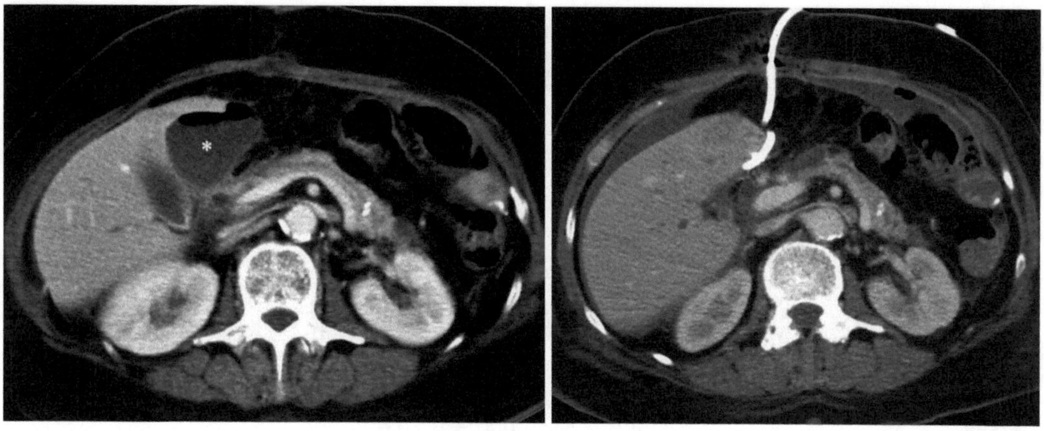

Fig. 3.28 Duodenal stump leak after Billroth II gastrectomy with right subhepatic collection (*asterisk*). A 10Fr catheter was placed with CT guidance, and the collection was aspirated to dryness

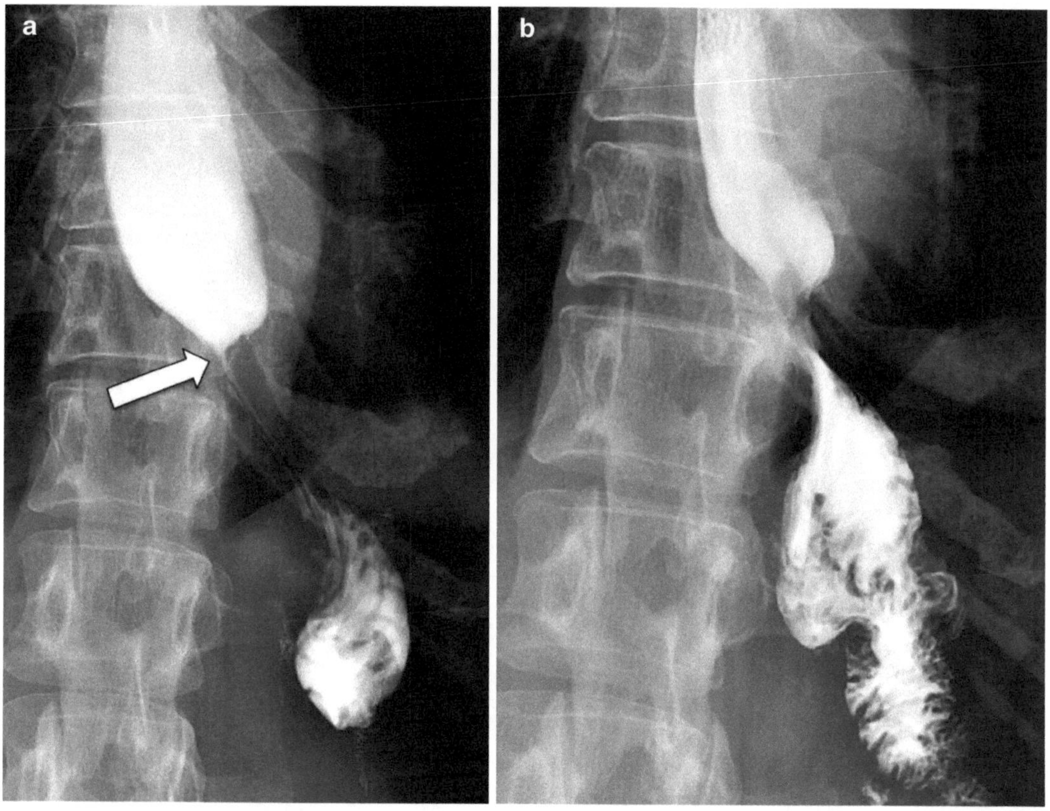

Fig. 3.29 Total gastrectomy anastomotic stricture with complication of balloon dilatation. (**a**) Postoperative vomiting related to tight anastomotic stricture (*arrow*). (**b**) Initially treated successfully with balloon dilatation to allow passage of contrast into the jejunal Roux loop. (**c**) The esophagojejunal stricture has been ruptured following repeated dilatation for recurrent anastomotic stricture with contrast extravasating (*arrowhead*) from the normal lumen (*black arrow*). (**d**) Contrast injected via a catheter (*arrow*) following placement of a covered stent shows the successfully occluded

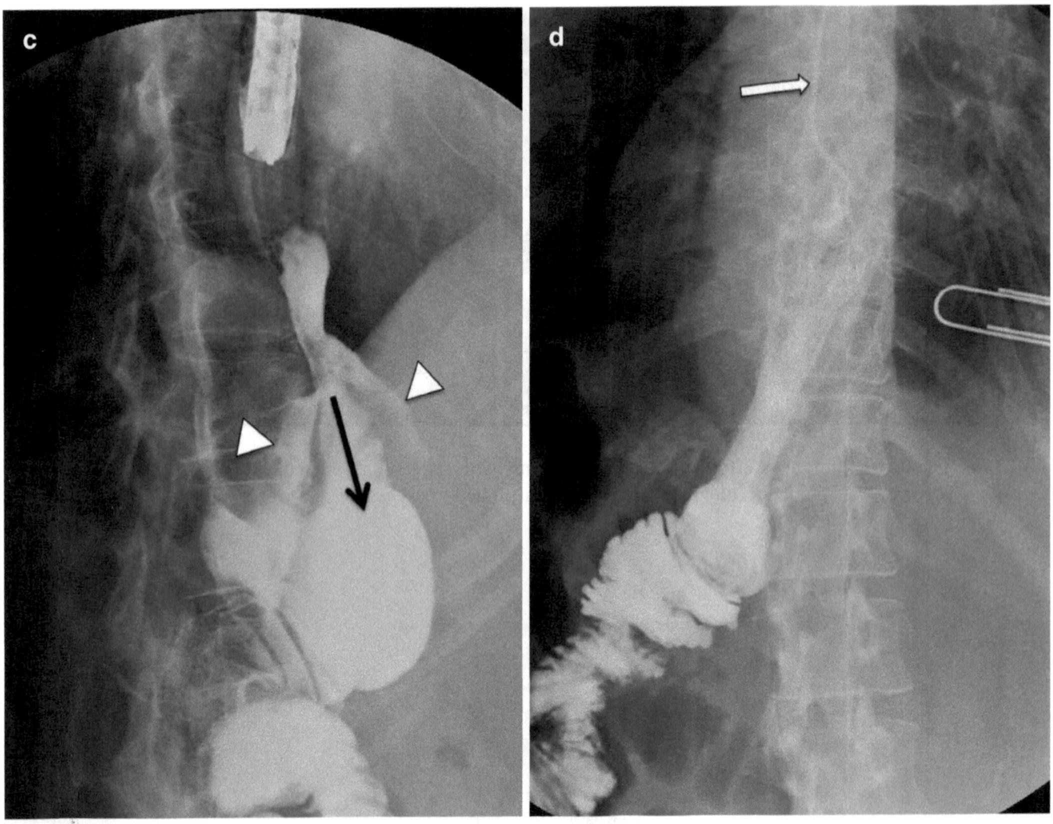

Fig. 3.29 (continued)

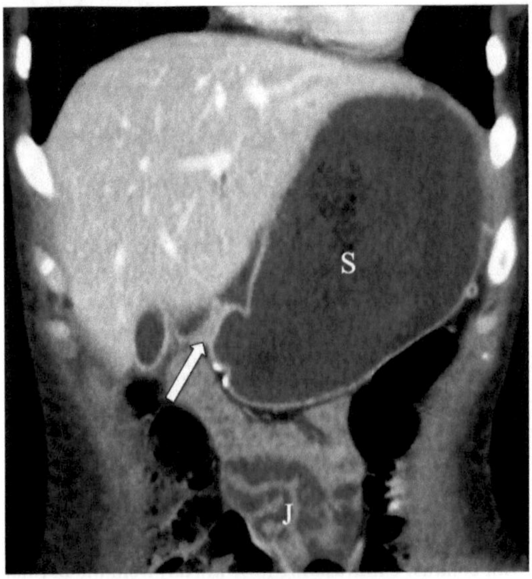

Fig. 3.30 Billroth I anastomotic stricture reconstruction after antrectomy for bleeding GIST with early satiety. Anastomotic stricture (*arrow*) at gastrojejunal anastomosis producing gastric outflow obstruction (*S* stomach, *J* jejunum)

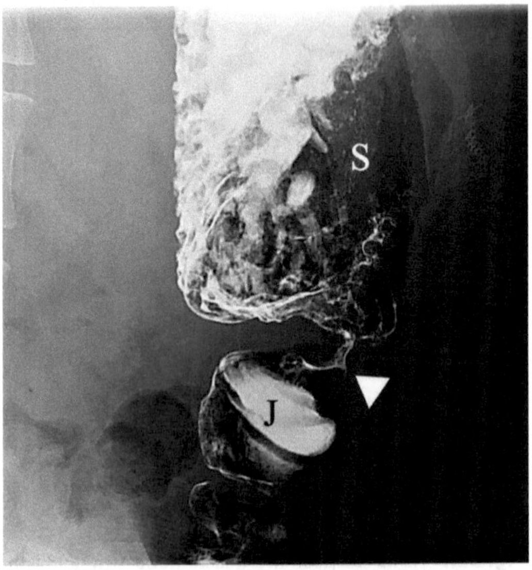

Fig. 3.31 Distal gastrectomy with Roux loop reconstruction with vomiting 6 weeks postoperative. Tight gastrojejunal anastomotic stricture (*arrowhead*) on barium swallow: resolved following endoscopic balloon dilatation (*S* stomach, *J* jejunum)

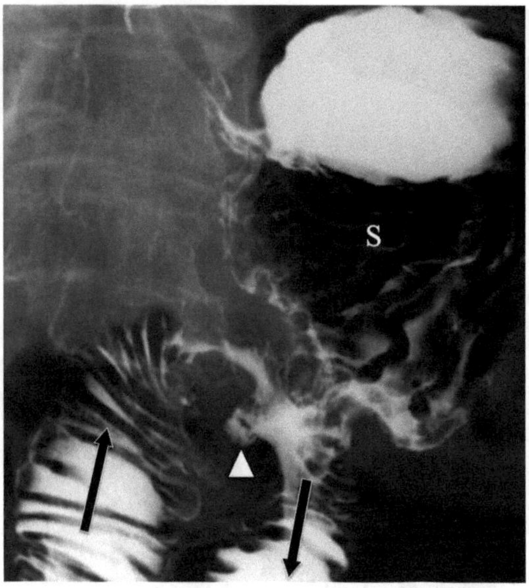

Fig. 3.32 Deep parastomal jejunal ulcer (*arrowhead*) several years after Polya gastrectomy. Note the gastric remnant (*S*) and direction of flow of bowel content along jejunal loop (*arrow*)

sis (Fig. 3.29b, c) (Kim et al. 2009). Perforation may be treated with placement of a covered metallic stent (Ustündag et al. 2001) (Fig. 3.29d).

Parastomal ulceration is a consequence of acid secretion on the jejunal anastomosis. It was previously a very prevalent complication most commonly affecting the gastroenterostomy or the efferent limb producing clinical symptoms of dyspepsia, nausea, postprandial pain, or GI bleeding (Cleator et al. 1974). In the majority of cases, these patients are diagnosed at endoscopy and there is no requirement for radiology. However, it is important to be aware of this complication. Superior mucosal definition is provided by barium rather than water-soluble contrast, and a double-contrast technique will provide the best opportunity to make the diagnosis (Fig. 3.32) (Smith et al. 1994). Very rarely gastrojejunal ulceration can progress to gastrojejunocolic fistula (Cleator et al. 1974). Management requires control of hemostasis for bleeding and treatment of the ulcer with medical therapy, reserving surgery for mechanical complications such as secondary stricture or fistula formation.

3.4.4.4 Gastric Remnant Complications

Bile reflux gastritis is a complication of the Billroth I and II reconstructions, due to free reflux of duodenal contents in type I anastomoses, or mixing of duodenal contents with stomach juice at the jejunostomy in type II. Gastric remnant inflammation is exacerbated by helicobacter pylori infection (Li et al. 2008). A long Roux loop is protective against bile reflux, which is a reason why this form of reconstruction is now routinely performed.

Gastroparesis is a common postoperative complication. Generally, this resolves in the early postoperative period but may persist in patients with gastric atony preoperatively (from chronic dilatation) where there may be a role for radionuclide emptying studies to confirm delayed emptying.

Since the resection removes part of the stomach, a small gastric pouch is an expected outcome. Limiting gastric capacity produces early satiety, seen in 43% at 3 months and 16% at 5 years (Pedrazzani et al. 2007) (an effect harnessed therapeutically for bariatric surgery).

By removing the body of the stomach, where intrinsic factor is produced by parietal cells, patients may develop vitamin B12 deficiency and are usually treated prophylactically with replacement therapy.

Gastric remnant malignancy is commonest at the anastomosis (69%) and usually occurs many years after the initial surgery (mean 32 years) (Mezhir et al. 2011). Risk is increased irrespective of whether the initial surgery was for benign or malignant disease (Ahn et al. 2008). Radiologists evaluating patients with such a history must be highly vigilant; malignancy can be very difficult to diagnose on cross-sectional imaging or where there is suboptimal distension or coating of the remnant on barium meal examinations (Fig. 3.33).

3.4.4.5 Efferent Complications

Efferent loop obstruction causing abdominal pain, nausea, and vomiting may be caused by adhesions (Fig. 3.34), local recurrence of malignancy (Kim et al. 2002), intussusception (jejunogastric or jejunojejunal) (Reyelt and Anderson

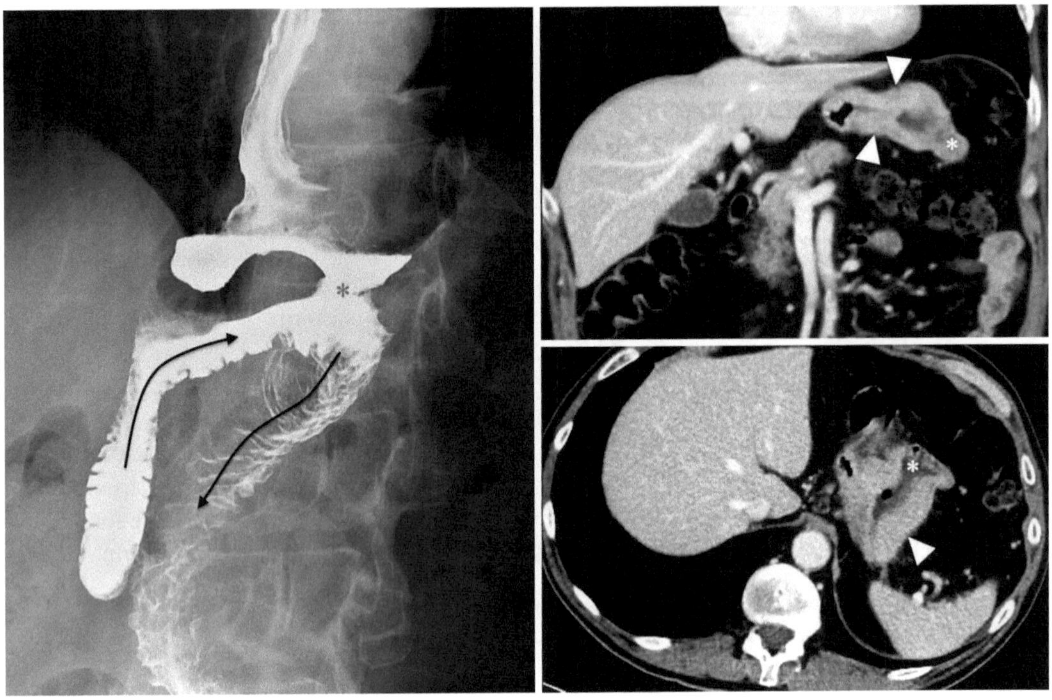

Fig. 3.33 Tumor in gastric remnant. Barium and CT examinations in a patient with vomiting, 40 years post Billroth II for duodenal ulcer. The anastomosis remains patient (*asterisk*), but there is diffuse thickening of the gastric remnant (*arrowheads*) from linitis plastica. Note the distortion and poor pouch volume on barium examination as the only clue to abnormality. *Arrow* denotes the flow of contrast in afferent and efferent limbs

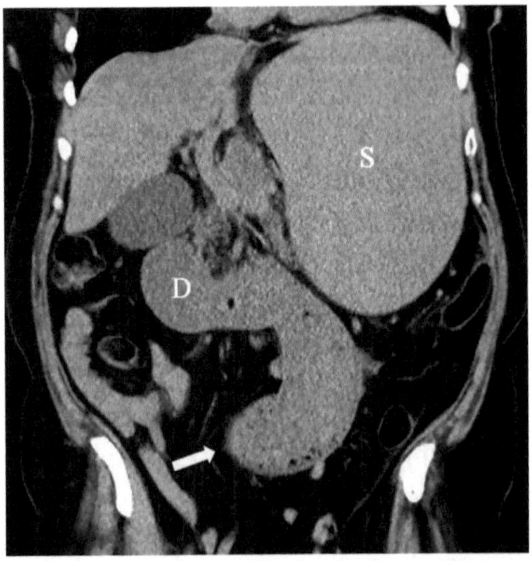

Fig. 3.34 Billroth 1 adhesive SBO. Gastric outflow obstruction 23 years post Billroth I gastrectomy for antral ulcer. CT demonstrates dilated stomach (*S*) and duodenum (*D*). Jejunal adhesions divided at the transition (*arrow*) at later laparotomy

1964; Kwak et al. 2010), or internal hernia (see Sect. 3.5.5.4). Hiatus hernia may also occur, promoting reflux and dysfunction of the gastric remnant or esophagojejunal anastomosis (Fig. 3.35). Early Dumping results from rapid transit of undigested food into the jejunum causing fluid shift into the lumen due to the hyperosmolarity of the gastric contents and affects up to two thirds of patients (Mine et al. 2010) with symptoms settling with time in the majority (Pedrazzani et al. 2007). The risk is lower in older patients as well as patients undergoing partial or subtotal gastrectomy (Mine et al. 2010). Clinical symptoms develop soon after eating and include nausea, bloating, vomiting, and diarrhea with treatment centered on dietary modification with small frequent meals.

Late dumping usually occurs within 3 h of a meal and is related to relative hypoglycemia from oversecretion of insulin in response to rapid carbohydrate loading of the small intestine. Dietary modification to limit carbohydrate intake is an important

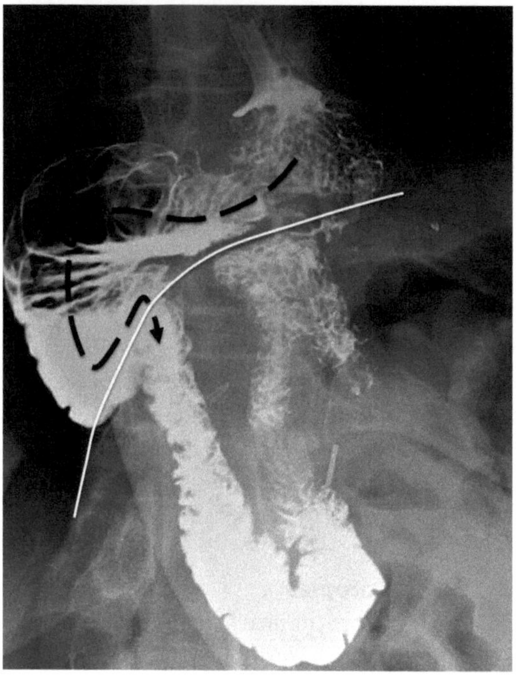

Fig. 3.35 Total gastrectomy with transhiatal dissection for gastric cancer with new obstructive symptoms. Acute angulation of the jejunal loop as it enters the abdomen (*arrow*) due to combination of adhesion and herniation above the diaphragm (*white line*)

aspect of treatment. Rapid gastric emptying in patients with a remnant stomach may be indicated by barium contrast examinations or radionuclide gastric emptying studies (Hejazi et al. 2010). In both cases, revision surgery is reserved for patients with intractable symptoms, where Roux loop reconstruction may be offered, for example, to patients after unsuccessful Billroth II surgery.

Postvagotomy diarrhea is uncommon and often related to the dumping syndrome. Division of the vagus nerve increases gut peristalsis, which is why highly selective vagotomy is preferred to truncal vagotomy where possible, thus maintaining innervation to the duodenum. Management is usually supportive (Cuschieri 1990).

3.4.5 Tumor Recurrence

The pattern of recurrent adenocarcinoma and distortion of postoperative anatomy can make the diagnosis of tumor recurrence challenging. CT is the primary modality for follow-up of cases for this indication. It is particularly important to diagnose recurrent or metastatic disease in symptomatic patients, in order to plan treatment through either surgery (e.g., completion gastrectomy) or palliative chemotherapy where appropriate or indeed to plan other interventions such as endoluminal stenting. Vigilance should be particularly heightened in cases with adverse features at resection (positive nodal status, locally advanced tumor >T2, poor cell differentiation, positive resection margin). In the early postoperative period, recurrence is unlikely, but as time progresses, malignancy becomes a more likely cause for pathologies such as small bowel obstruction. In particular, cases should be carefully evaluated for nodal, peritoneal, or serosal deposits, but also local recurrence in the surgical bed or anastomosis as well as distant spread to liver, lungs, and other organs (Kim et al. 2002).

Gastrointestinal stromal tumors rarely metastasize to lymph nodes but may spread via peritoneum and to the liver. Since these are typically hypervascular tumors, arterial phase CT imaging is a useful adjunct to the portal venous phase. PET-CT is also sensitive in the detection of recurrence. It is important to remember that imatinib therapy can produce dramatic changes to the character of residual malignant disease (with a cystic homogeneous hypoattenuating appearance on contrast-enhanced CT or lack of FDG uptake on PET-CT) while the size of a lesion itself remains static (Hong et al. 2006). These require careful evaluation in the follow-up period to assess for change in character that may indicate disease progression without alteration in the size of the lesion.

3.4.6 Additional Operations for Peptic Ulcer Disease

3.4.6.1 Highly Selective Vagotomy

This operation was developed in the era prior to effective medical treatment for duodenal ulceration and helicobacter pylori eradication. The procedure

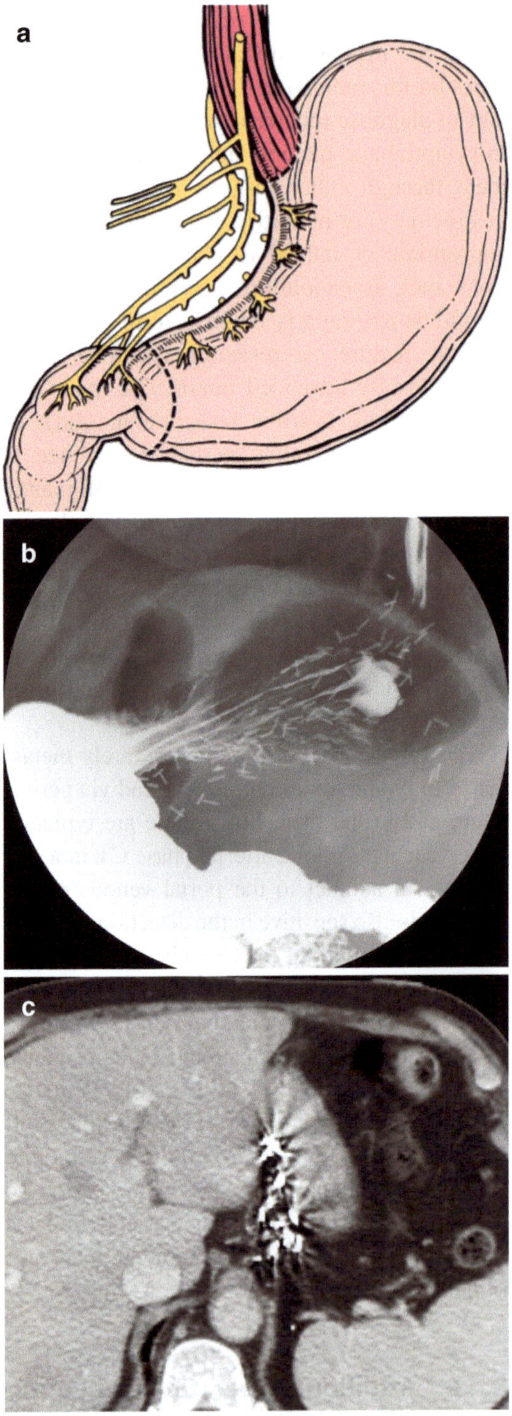

Fig. 3.36 (**a**) Highly selective vagotomy: the acid secreting parietal cells are denervated by division of the vagus nerve along the lesser curve, while maintaining normal function of the pylorus to limit side effects. (**b**) Barium swallow and (**c**) CT demonstrate multiple clips along the lesser curve of the stomach. None of the stomach has been resected. The multiplicity and density of clips is in this position is characteristic of a highly selective vagotomy

denervates the gastric parietal cells while maintaining normal vagal innervation and contractility to the pylorus, thereby reducing the potential for postvagotomy dumping syndrome, which was a common problem following truncal vagotomy. The procedure involved intricate dissection of the lesser omentum from the lesser curvature of the stomach in order to protect the main anterior and posterior branches of the vagus nerve, leaving innumerable metal clips as the telltale sign of this surgery but without any gastric resection (Fig. 3.36a, b, c). Although it provided symptomatic relief in 85% of cases, the overall recurrence rate of 15% and in addition the development of postvagotomy symptoms meant that it passed out of favor, and is now seldom performed (Macintyre et al. 1990).

3.4.6.2 Pyloroplasty

Pyloroplasty is performed to assist gastric emptying and is usually performed in the setting of esophagectomy with gastric pull up (e.g., Ivor Lewis or Lewis-McKeown procedures), for gastroparesis or accompanying truncal vagotomy for complicated peptic ulcer disease (e.g., duodenal ulceration). The procedure may also be performed following emergency surgery for a bleeding peptic ulcer. The pyloroplasty is made longitudinally through the muscle and then sewn closed in a perpendicular direction. This is known as the Heineke-Mikulicz technique and is limited to the pylorus (Fig. 3.37). Rarely, a more extensive Finney pyloroplasty may be performed, when the duodenum is scarred, to create a wider side-to-side gastroduodenal anastomosis. Complications requiring imaging are uncommon and centered on leaks from the pyloroplasty site (Fig. 2.18) or obstruction from edema (Fig. 2.26).

3.5 Bariatric Surgery

3.5.1 Introduction

Morbid obesity is an epidemic in Western society. As the number of morbidly obese patients increases (BMI greater than 40), the demand for bariatric surgery is increasing. In some surgical departments, the demand for weight loss operations outstrips demand for other more traditional workload

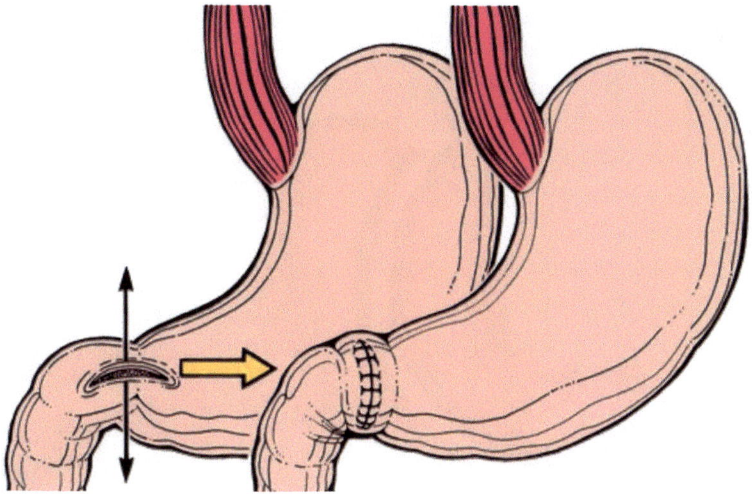

Fig. 3.37 Heineke-Mikulicz pyloroplasty. The pyloric sphincter is cut longitudinally and the defect closed in a perpendicular orientation to open the pylorus for drainage

for upper GI surgeons. Weight loss from surgery reduces long-term morbidity relating to morbid obesity, including cardiovascular disease, diabetes, sleep apnea, and asthma despite the increased mortality risk associated with surgery in such a high-risk group (Sjöström et al. 2007). It also provides definitive sustained weight reduction compared with dietary management.

The types of surgery available may be categorized as either restrictive, wherein the capacity of the stomach is reduced which, in turn, provides early satiety, or a combination of restrictive and malabsorptive effects. Procedures with both malabsorptive and restrictive components tend to provide greater weight loss than restrictive procedures alone (Sjöström et al. 2007).

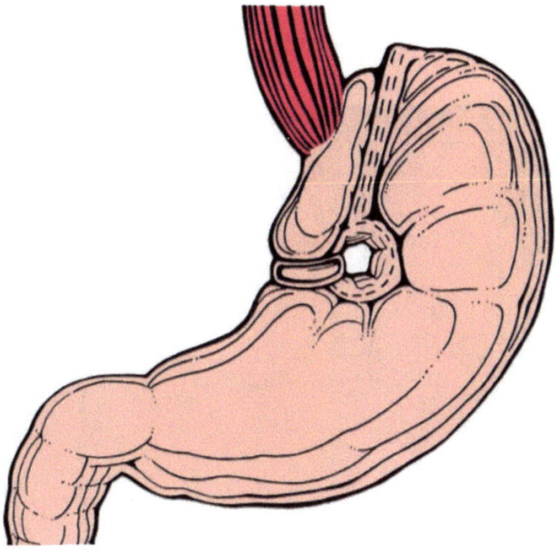

Fig. 3.38 Vertical banding gastrostomy. A vertical staple line runs inferiorly parallel to the lesser curve creating a pouch with a silicone band at its inferior end to create restriction of the outlet

3.5.2 Restrictive Surgery

3.5.2.1 Vertical Banded Gastroplasty

Similar to the Magenstrasse and Mill procedure (see Sect. 3.5.2.4) but in addition a synthetic band is placed around the gastric tube to augment restriction (Fig. 3.38) (Trenkner 2009; Smith et al. 1984). This has also been superseded by other techniques.

3.5.2.2 Sleeve Gastrectomy

A narrow gastric tube of reduced capacity is created along the lesser curve by stapling along the length of the stomach (Fig. 3.39a, b). The excluded stomach segment including the greater curve is removed (Trenkner 2009; Quigley et al. 2011).

3.5.2.3 Laparoscopic Adjustable Gastric Band (LAGB)

An inflatable synthetic band is placed laparoscopically just below the gastroesophageal junction, thereby creating a small gastric pouch above (Fig. 3.40). The band is connected by tubing to a subcutaneous port on the anterior abdominal wall enabling, under aseptic conditions, easy adjustment of the volume within the band and thereby the degree of restriction. Care must be taken to use dedicated atraumatic needles for band adjust-

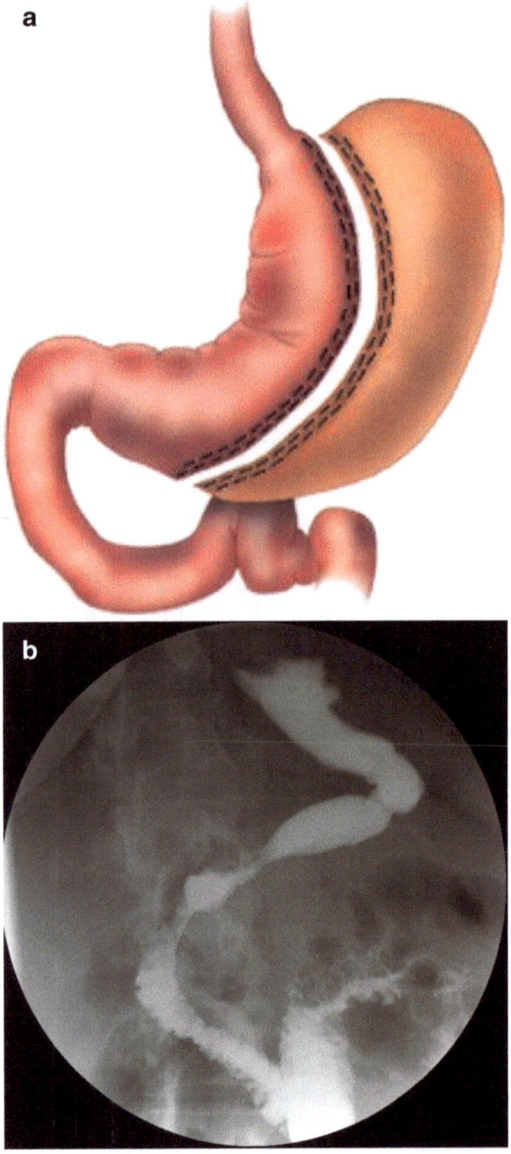

Fig. 3.39 Sleeve gastrectomy. (**a**) A vertical staple line resects the fundus and greater curve of the stomach creating a narrow proximal aperture at the gastroesophageal junction for restriction, along with a reduction of gastric volume. (**b**) Normal appearance on contrast examination demonstrating the slender gastric tube

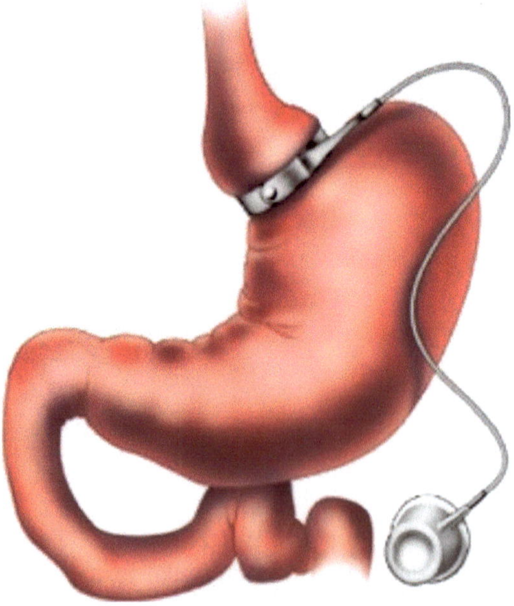

Fig. 3.40 Gastric band. The band is placed at the gastroesophageal junction to produce adjustable restriction

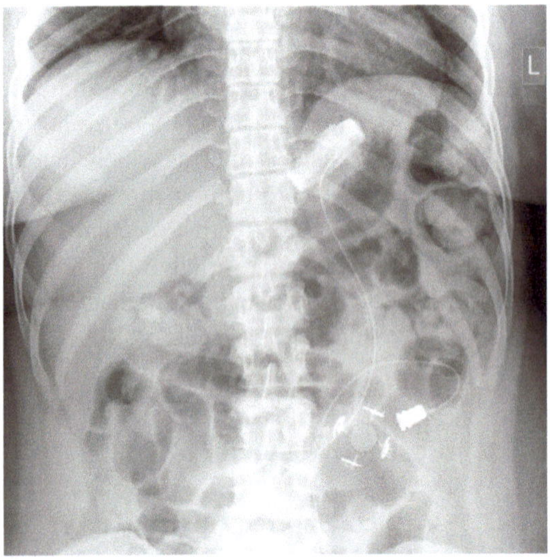

Fig. 3.41 Gastric band normal AXR. Note that the band is normally oriented at approximately 45° with an unbroken line connecting to the reservoir in the mid abdomen

ment to prevent damage to the membrane of the port. There are several different manufacturers of bands with a variation in the appearances of the band, the reservoir, and the band volume (Wiesner et al. 2000; Mehanna et al. 2006; Quigley et al. 2011; Mortelé et al. 2001). The band should normally be positioned below the hiatus, orientated at an angle, approximately 45° to horizontal (to indicate a satisfactory position at the GOJ) with all components of the band properly connected (Fig. 3.41).

3.5.2.4 Magenstrasse and Mill Procedure (M&M)

A narrow gastric tube is created by stapling from the antrum up to the fundus, thereby functionally excluding the majority of the stomach. The Magenstrasse (or street of the stomach) is the long narrow tube fashioned from the lesser curvature, which conveys food from the esophagus to the antral "Mill" (Figs. 3.42 and 3.43) (Johnston et al. 2003). Gastric juices can exit the excluded stomach into the small common distal antrum. Normal antral grinding of solid food and antro-pyloro-duodenal regulation of gastric emptying and secretion are preserved.

A drawback of this technique is that over time the Magenstrasse can dilate, thereby removing the restriction and precipitating weight gain (Fig. 3.44). This procedure is no longer frequently performed since the development of other techniques

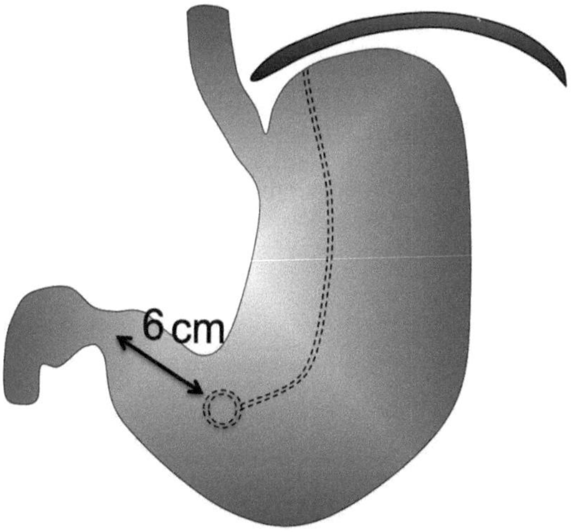

Fig. 3.42 Magenstrasse and Mill. A linear staple line extends toward the antrum from the cardia and is completed by a circular staple line, dividing the stomach into two compartments

3.5.3 Combined Restrictive and Malabsorptive

3.5.3.1 Roux-en-Y Gastric Bypass (RYGB)

A small volume gastric pouch is fashioned from the proximal stomach just below the gastroesophageal junction. The majority of stomach is thereby excluded from food. A Roux loop is brought up and anastomosed, either end-to-side or side-to-side, onto this small gastric pouch (Figs. 3.45 and 3.46) and may be placed in an antecolic or retrocolic position (through the transverse mesocolon) (Fig. 3.47). The comparative lengths of the components of the Roux loop reconstruction dictate how much of a malabsorptive effect the procedure will produce in addition to the restrictive effects of the small gastric pouch. The more distal the enteroenteric anastomosis, the less area for mixing food from the gastric limb with digestive enzymes from the pancreaticobiliary limb to allow absorption and the greater the malabsorptive effect (Scheirey et al. 2006; Quigley et al. 2011).

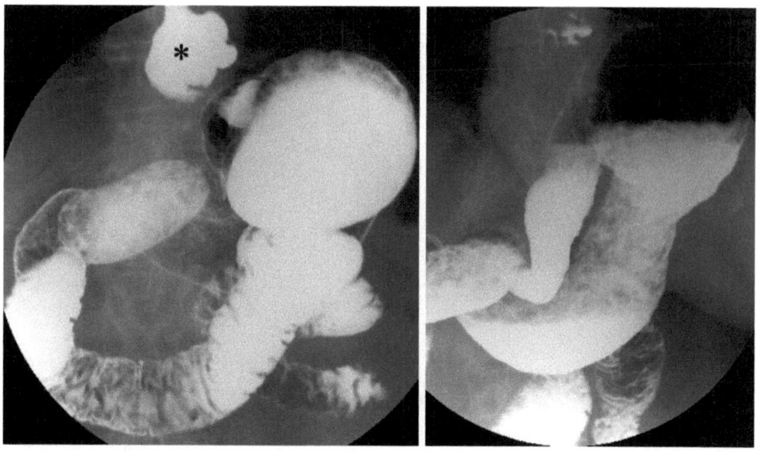

Fig. 3.43 History of previous gastric surgery many years earlier for obesity but unknown type – persistent reflux. The anatomy only becomes clear with change in position from supine to erect indicating M&M and hiatus hernia (*asterisk*)

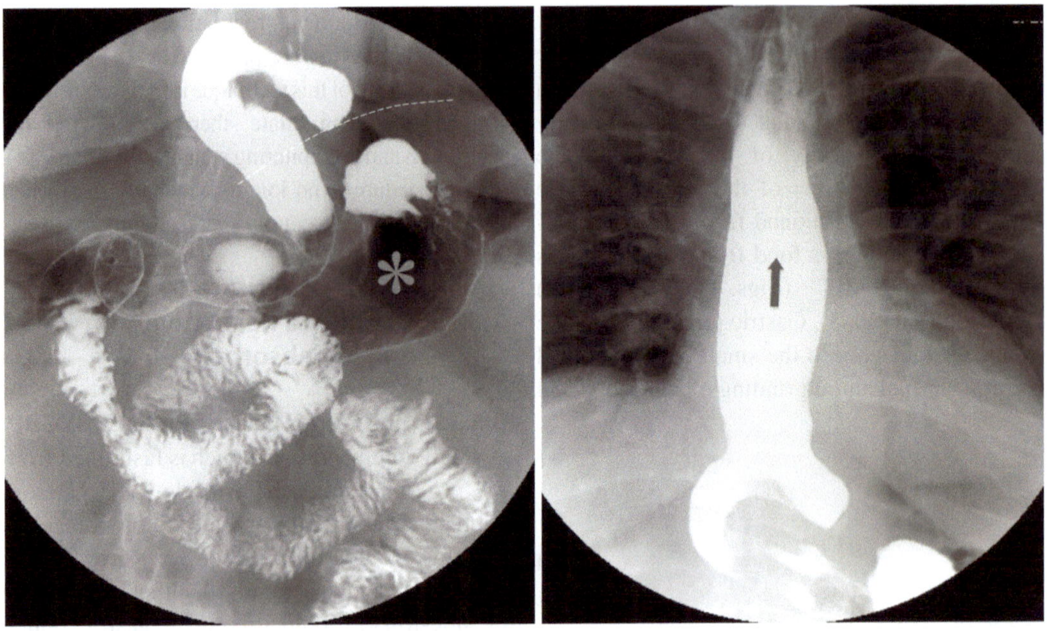

Fig. 3.44 M&M hiatus hernia 5 years post M&M for obesity. Now intractable reflux symptoms and weight gain. The gastric remnant remains in a normal position (*asterisk*). The gastric tube intermittently herniates across the diaphragm (*broken white line*) producing severe reflux (*arrow*)

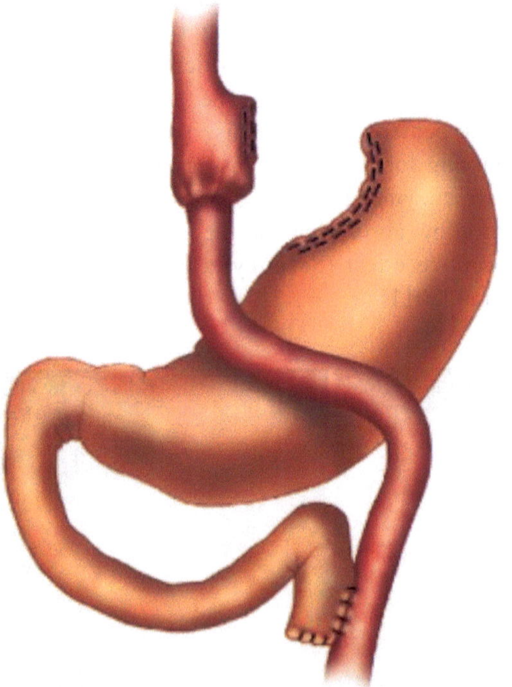

Fig. 3.45 RYGB. The stomach is transected to produce a small pouch of cardia separate from the rest of the stomach. This is then anastomosed to a jejunal Roux loop. The distance from the jejunojejunal anastomosis to the terminal ileum is adjusted to influence the degree of malabsorption

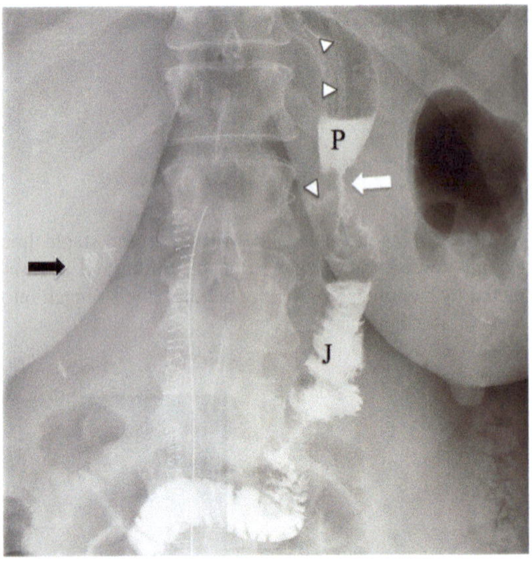

Fig. 3.46 Normal post RYGB with pouch (*P*) anastomotic restriction (*white arrow*) and unobstructed jejunal loop (*J*). Note clips from prior cholecystectomy (*black arrow*) and staple line (*arrowheads*) to form excluded stomach

3.5.3.2 Duodenal Switch with Biliopancreatic Diversion

This is a complex procedure, where the distal small bowel is directly anastomosed onto the

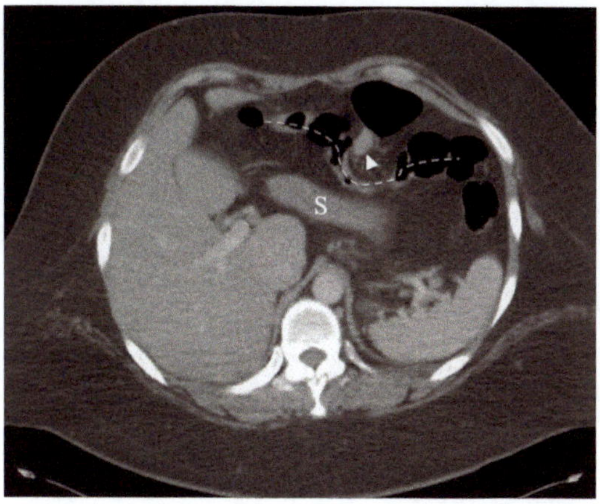

Fig. 3.47 RYGB normal CT. The Roux loop (*arrowhead*) lies in front of the transverse colon (*dotted line*) and excluded stomach (*S*)

disconnected duodenum. The remainder of the small bowel is reanastomosed distally, producing a largely malabsorptive procedure. This is frequently combined with a sleeve gastrectomy as an additional restrictive component, which may be performed as an initial primary procedure before a second operation for the switch (Fig. 3.48) (Trenkner 2009; Quigley et al. 2011).

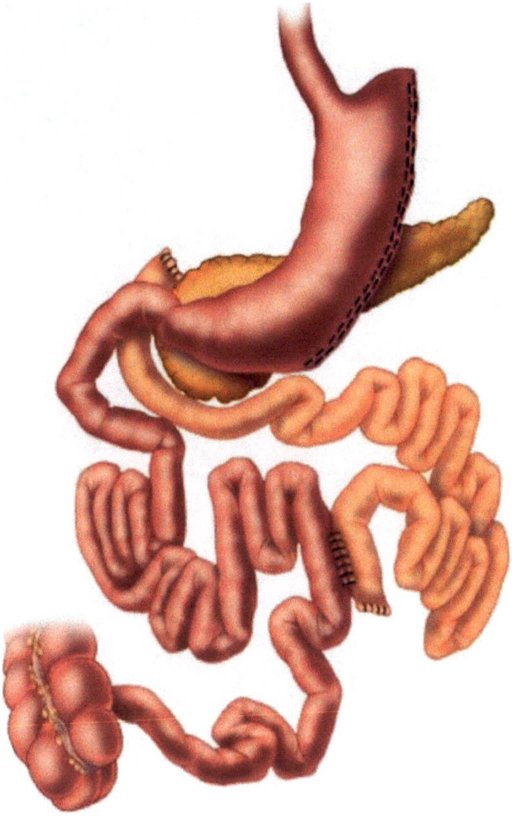

Fig. 3.48 Duodenal switch with biliopancreatic diversion. Sleeve gastrectomy for restriction is coupled with division of the first part of the duodenum. This is then anastomosed to a long Roux loop, which joins the biliary pancreatic limb distally to induce malabsorption

3.5.4 Normal Postoperative Imaging

3.5.4.1 General Considerations for Obese Patients

The weight limit and aperture of fluoroscopy and CT equipment are important considerations prior to undertaking imaging for patients with morbid obesity. While some patients may not exceed the weight limit of equipment (often up to 200 kg), their wide girth may preclude access to the CT gantry, for example. Equipment manufacturers are providing scanners with wider bore (for CT and MRI) and higher tube current loading (for CT) to allow for this and maintain image quality. It is likely that departments performing high volumes of these procedures will need to invest in equipment that will tolerate this caseload.

Where the weight limit of fluoroscopy equipment is exceeded, it is possible to perform examinations with the footrest of the table removed and the patient standing on the floor. Obviously, this limits the assessment (since supine evaluation is not possible), but diagnostic studies may be performed with this modification. The tube limit should also be considered when performing examinations as beam attenuation can cause tube overloading, particularly where a “run” of exposures is being performed (e.g., 2 frames per s). Using a larger field of view and single exposures will avoid this complication, which is a particular problem with older equipment.

3.5.4.2 Fluoroscopy

Unless in the immediate postoperative period, an upper GI contrast examination can be performed with barium.

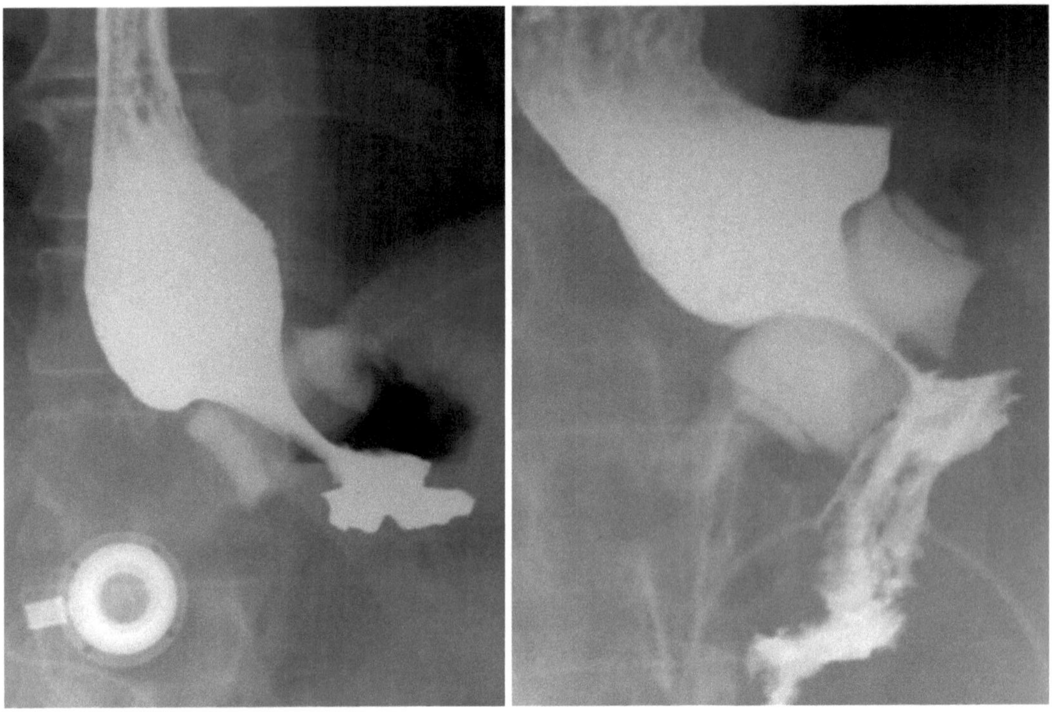

Fig. 3.49 Normal appearance after LAGB in two patients. A small focal proximal pouch should form from dilatation of the GOJ due to restriction

LAGB

A control radiograph should always be performed on which the band should be orientated perpendicular to the gastroesophageal junction (Fig. 3.41). The tubing should be assessed for any discontinuity and the port for rotation or inversion – the port should normally appear as a circular structure (Figs. 3.41 and 3.49). An oval shape indicates abnormal orientation. On ingestion of contrast, the band position is assessed in anteroposterior or right posterior oblique position because if the patient is turned to the left, contrast in the fundus can obscure it. Adequate restriction is indicated by formation of a small pouch proximal to the balloon (Fig. 3.49), and no signs of dysmotility. Free passage of contrast without dilatation suggests under restriction.

LAGB Adjustment Technique for Radiologists

Most gastric band adjustments can be performed in the surgical clinic without the aid of imaging, using water to test the functional result. However, patients with unexplained symptoms (e.g., lack of restriction despite apparently adequate filling, or nausea/other obstructive symptoms despite minimal restriction) or difficulty in accessing the port (e.g., deep port due to obesity or possible rotation) require image-guided adjustment.

The initial assessment requires an erect contrast swallow to evaluate the degree of restriction at baseline (too much or too little) and to ensure that the band is in a normal position. The patient is then laid supine, and the skin over the port site prepared using aseptic technique with cleaning solution (e.g., chlorhexidine) and an adhesive sterile drape to maintain an aseptic field (that will be maintained with change in position). Local anesthetic is not normally required. The port site position can be confirmed by palpation or using imaging guidance to confirm the position with a metal object on the skin (e.g., towel clip). The port is then fixed between thumb and index finger with the left hand to prevent movement and displace soft tissue while an atraumatic needle (e.g., Huber needle) is inserted into the reservoir through the membrane. *A normal beveled needle should not ever be used as this damages the membrane and promotes leakage.* Successful needle puncture feels similar to a lumbar puncture procedure, with gripping of the advancing needle followed by a gentle "give" when the needle is within the port reservoir. If the needle hits and slides off a hard surface, it has probably glanced off the port casing – the needle should be withdrawn into the subcutaneous fat (without pulling out of the skin and causing a second skin puncture), the angle slightly adjusted and a further pass attempted. If necessary, needle position relative to the port can be rechecked with fluoroscopy.

When within the port, the needle is then connected to an empty syringe. The volume of aspirate is carefully noted to calculate the degree of adjustment required. Adjustments in 0.5–1 ml increments from the baseline volume (up or down depending on whether more or less restriction is needed) are usually appropriate but will vary depending on the type of band and balloon volume. We inject contrast (200 mg/ml iodine) into the reservoir, which allows us to confirm balloon filling, and to exclude tube leaks. With each adjustment, the needle is quickly removed, and the patient is then tilted erect and a barium swallow performed to assess the constriction of the GOJ (hence need for adherent drapes). If further adjustment is required, the patient is placed supine again, needle reinserted in the reservoir, and more contrast injected or withdrawn until a satisfactory result achieved with one or more check swallows.

Difficult port access – the technique described above may be adjusted when port access is difficult. Once the port is punctured, the Huber needle is attached to a connecting tube and aspirated and adjusted as described above before the connecting tube is clamped/occluded to prevent the port emptying into the syringe (which can then be disconnected). The needle may then be left in the port and the patient tilted semierect (e.g., 45–60°) and the check swallow performed in this position. As a note of caution in obese patients, the weight of fat may displace the needle by this change in position, particularly when it has been placed in a deep subcutaneous pocket. This should be carefully monitored during the change to semierect position and the needle position confirmed and position rechecked (and repositioned if necessary) before further volume adjustment in the supine position.

Other Bariatric Operations

A frontal control radiograph should be performed to demonstrate the position of a band or the staple lines depending on the procedure (Trenkner 2009). It is important to evaluate the surgical site properly because a break in the staple line may be difficult to see once barium has filled the pouch and the remainder of the stomach. Radiologists should always be vigilant of focal dilatation of small bowel loops or an excluded stomach that may herald obstruction.

Good technique with correct orientation is essential (Jha et al. 2006). Examinations are usually performed semi-upright or erect, in a right posterior oblique (RPO) position, since overlapping of bowel can make assessment of leaks and strictures difficult with a straight anterior projection. This is good for evaluating both the integrity of the staple line and the diameter of the stoma. Additional left posterior oblique or even lateral projections may be performed to clarify anatomy. Sometimes the addition of supine positioning can assist in the demonstration of normal postoperative anatomy to either fill with contrast or to unravel the overlap of structures with the weight of barium (such as following VBG or M&M operations) – this is particularly useful in a patient being worked up for revision surgery where the question is "what operation was performed in the past?" (Fig. 3.43). A change of position may also unmask complications not demonstrated on erect imaging alone (Fig. 3.50).

In the postoperative period, water-soluble contrast studies may struggle to diagnose a leak from the distal jejunojejunal anastomosis in RYGB due to dilution of contrast; where there is doubt, CT can provide additional confirmation.

3.5.4.3 CT

CT is usually reserved for assessment of the point and cause of efferent loop obstruction, to assess for a source of sepsis, and for general problem solving in patients failing to progress adequately after surgery (Yu et al. 2004; Blachar et al. 2002). Intravenous and positive oral contrast are important to delineate normal anatomy. Such complications usually arise from resectional restrictive surgery or combined operations rather than LAGB placement, but it may be valuable in selected patients with severe or unexplained symptoms after LAGB (Blachar et al. 2007). As with assessment of the duodenal stump, CT is superior in the evaluation of the biliopancreatic limb, since contrast studies will seldom reflux contrast proximally to allow a diagnosis to be made.

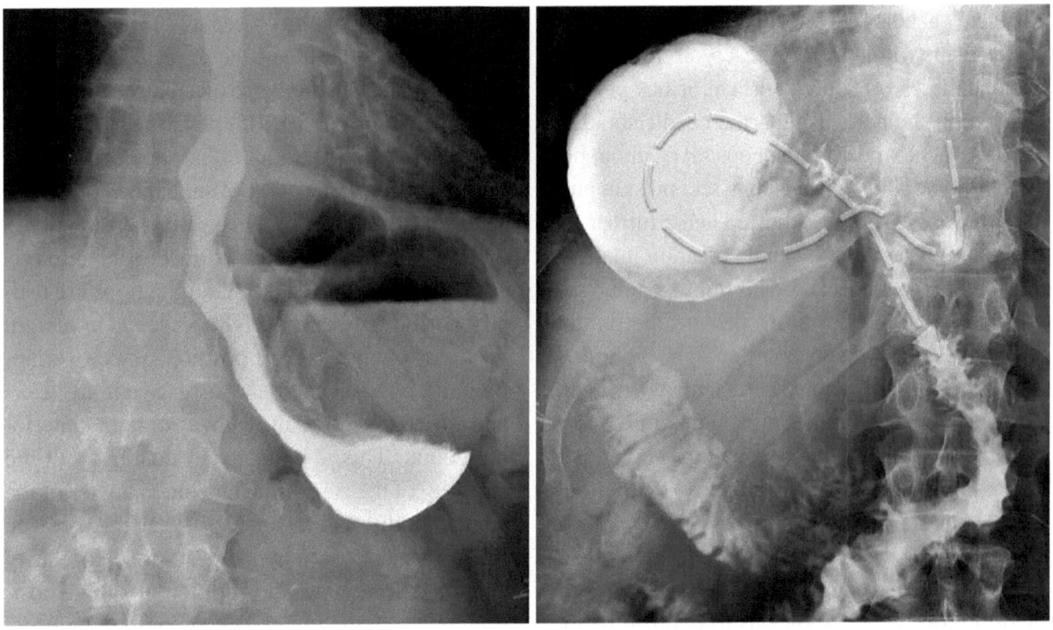

Fig. 3.50 Intermittent vomiting after RYGB. The residual gastric pouch herniates up and right and twists through the hiatus (*dashed arrow*) with change in position from erect (*left*) to supine (*right*)

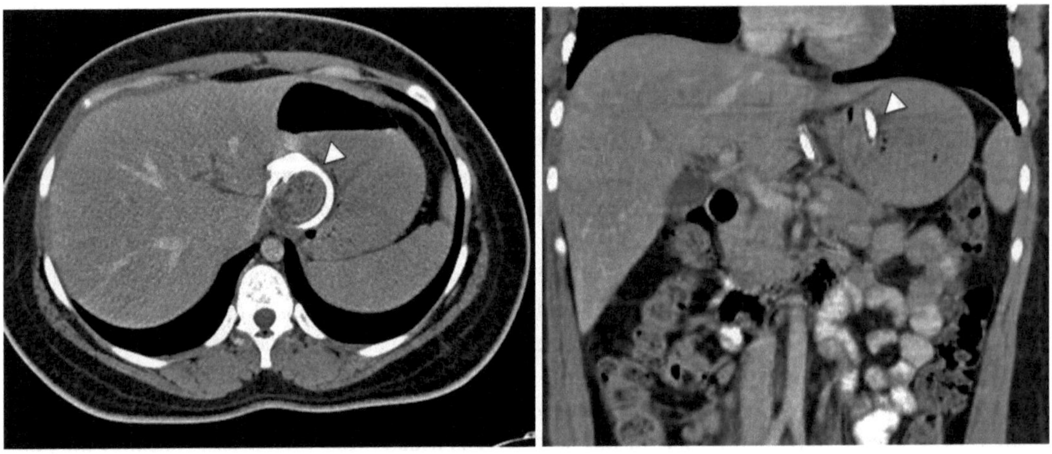

Fig. 3.51 Vomiting following LAGB. Pitfall: positive oral contrast has become dilute within the stomach and isodense to the wall (compared to denser contrast in the jejunum). The scan was reported to demonstrate band erosion into the lumen of the stomach, although with hindsight the wall is just visible lateral to it (*arrowhead*) and confirmed on contrast swallow (*not shown*)

It is important to be aware of a diagnostic pitfall arising from oral contrast producing an isodensity to soft tissue, which may lead to incorrect interpretation (Fig. 3.51). This is a benefit of utilizing denser positive contrast (e.g., 8%). The excluded stomach after RYGB may also be misinterpreted as a postoperative collection in the setting of sepsis – it will continue to contain some fluid from gastric secretions (Fig. 3.52).

3.5.5 Postoperative Complications

3.5.5.1 Anastomotic Leaks (Roux-en-Y Gastric Bypass and Sleeve Gastrectomy)

Proximal

Early postoperative leaks occur in less than 5% of patients, with the majority related to the gastrojejunostomy in RYGB (Blachar et al.

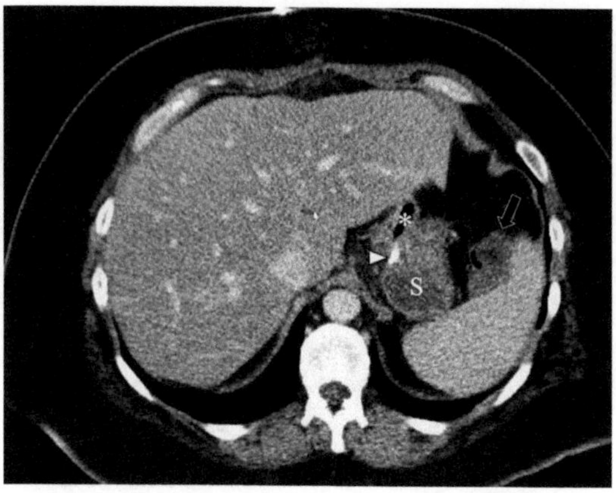

Fig. 3.52 Pitfall: post Roux-en-Y gastric bypass with postoperative pyrexia. The excluded stomach (*S*) containing fluid should not be mistaken for collection (*arrow*), since it abuts the staple line (*arrowhead*) which excludes the gastric pouch (*asterisk*). This resolved with antibiotics alone

2002). It is important to differentiate a leak from a plication defect (Trenkner 2009). Plication defects occur in predictable locations and tend to fill and empty under fluoroscopic observation. Leaks persist and get more obvious with time due to increasing amounts of leaked contrast. Occasionally, the gastric remnant will leak due to disruption of the staple line – CT is required to detect this complication since it will not be filled with oral contrast (Blachar et al. 2002).

In the authors' experience, sleeve gastrectomy leaks tend to occur from the proximal end of the staple line, close to the gastroesophageal junction (Fig. 3.53). These may be managed with covered stent placement, but our personal experience of this method is disappointing (Fig. 3.54).

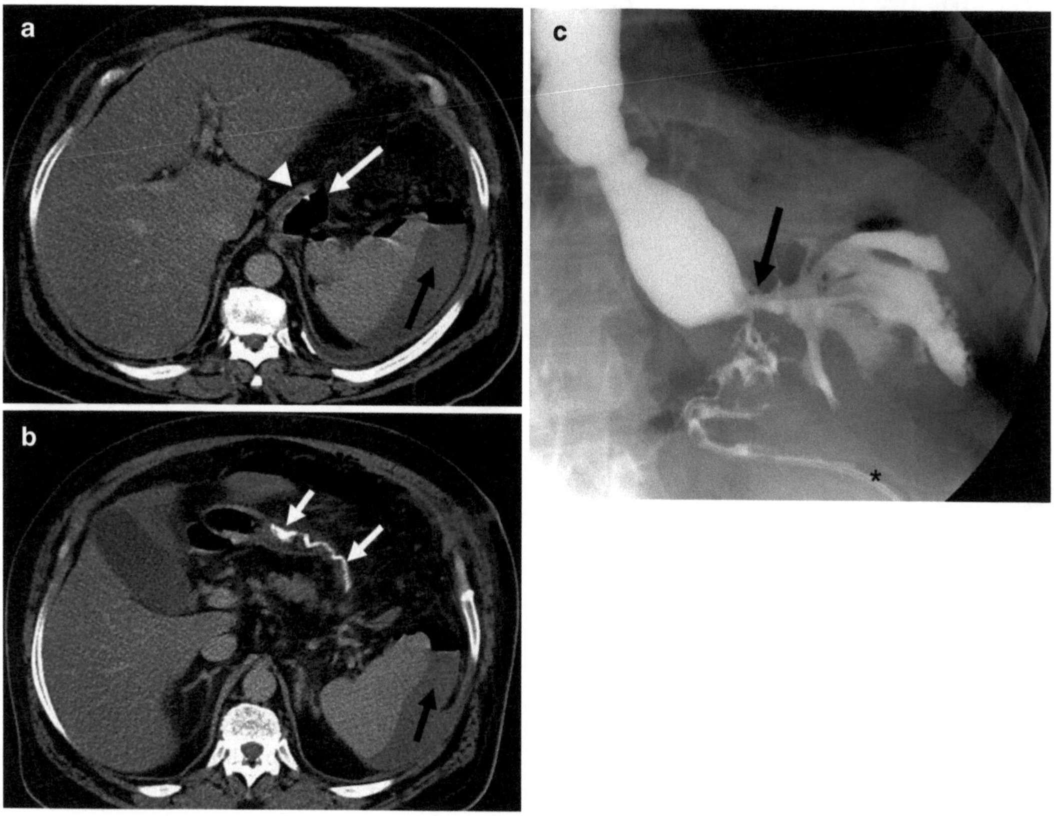

Fig. 3.53 Sleeve gastrectomy leak. (**a**) CT for pyrexia 1 week post sleeve gastrectomy with gas collection (*white arrow*) just posterior to gastric tube (*arrowhead*) and large left subdiaphragmatic collection (*black arrow*). (**b**) The dense staple line (*white arrows*) running along the body of the gastric remnant is intact. (**c**) Subsequent swallow shows contrast leak (*arrow*) from the fundal end of the staple line toward the surgical drain (*asterisk*) – the typical location for leaks

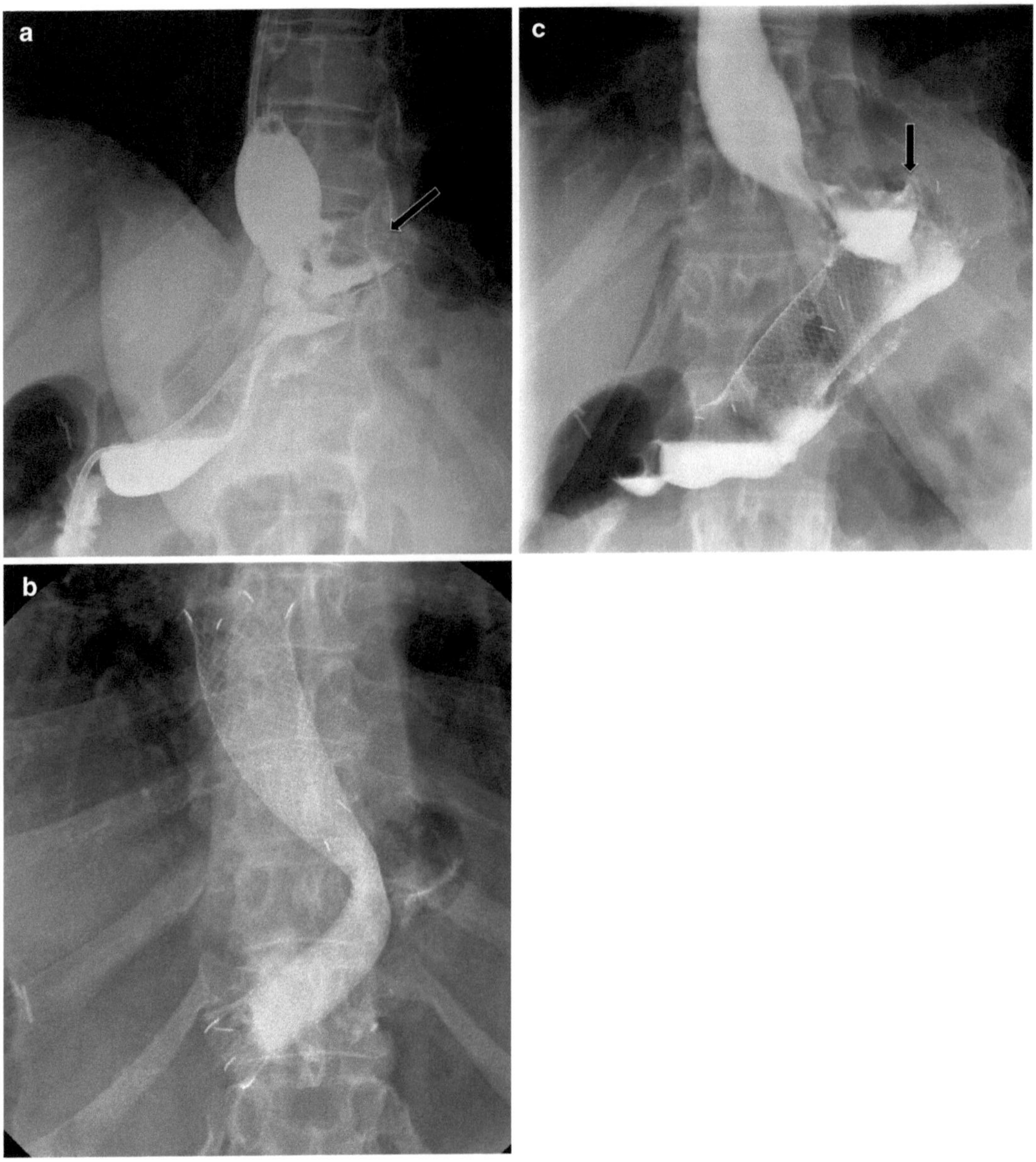

Fig. 3.54 Sleeve gastrectomy stent migration. (**a**). Leak at the proximal end of the gastric tube (*arrow*) after sleeve gastrectomy (NJ tube in situ). (**b**) Stent successfully placed. (**c**) The stent migrated with the proximal end holding open the disrupted staple line (*arrow*) and could not be retrieved

Distal

The jejunal anastomosis is an uncommon site for leak. In general, water-soluble postoperative studies only examine the proximal anastomosis. Where there is a high index of suspicion, delayed imaging is required to ensure that the whole of the jejunal Roux loop is opacified (Fig. 3.55). CT with positive oral contrast (or following the initial proximal assessment with fluoroscopy) can be helpful.

3.5.5.2 Fistula to Excluded Stomach (RYGB, VBG, M&M)

This occurs due to staple line dehiscence, which may occur in the early postoperative period due to mechanical failure of staples (Fig. 3.56) or late when patients usually present with either weight gain (Fig. 3.57) or with other symptoms such as pain (Fig. 3.58). On barium swallow, the contrast follows an unusual course or forms a second

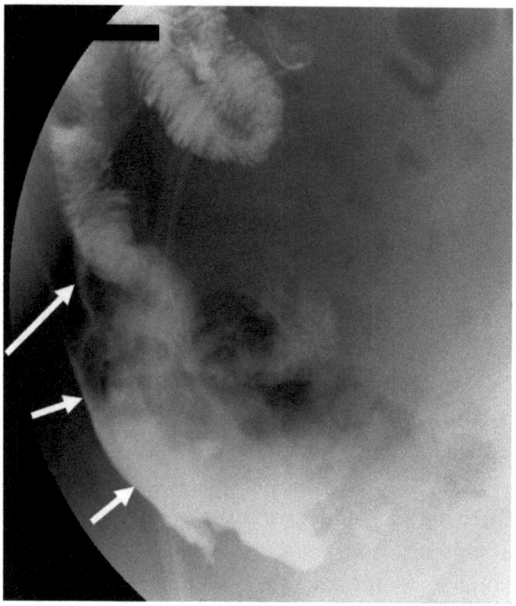

Fig. 3.55 RYGB distal anastomotic leak. Gross leak of contrast adjacent to jejunojejunal anastomosis after Roux-en-Y gastric bypass with free spill on contrast into peritoneum (*arrows*)

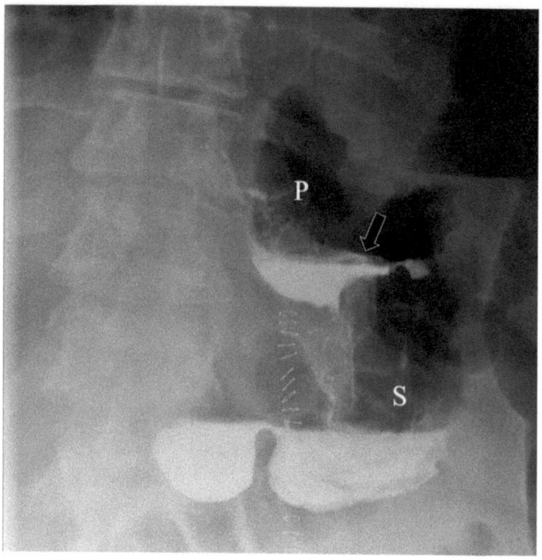

Fig. 3.56 RYGB pouch disruption. Day 2 postoperative. The staple line dividing pouch (*P*) from excluded stomach (*S*) is disrupted (*arrow*) with all contrast entering stomach and no Roux loop filling

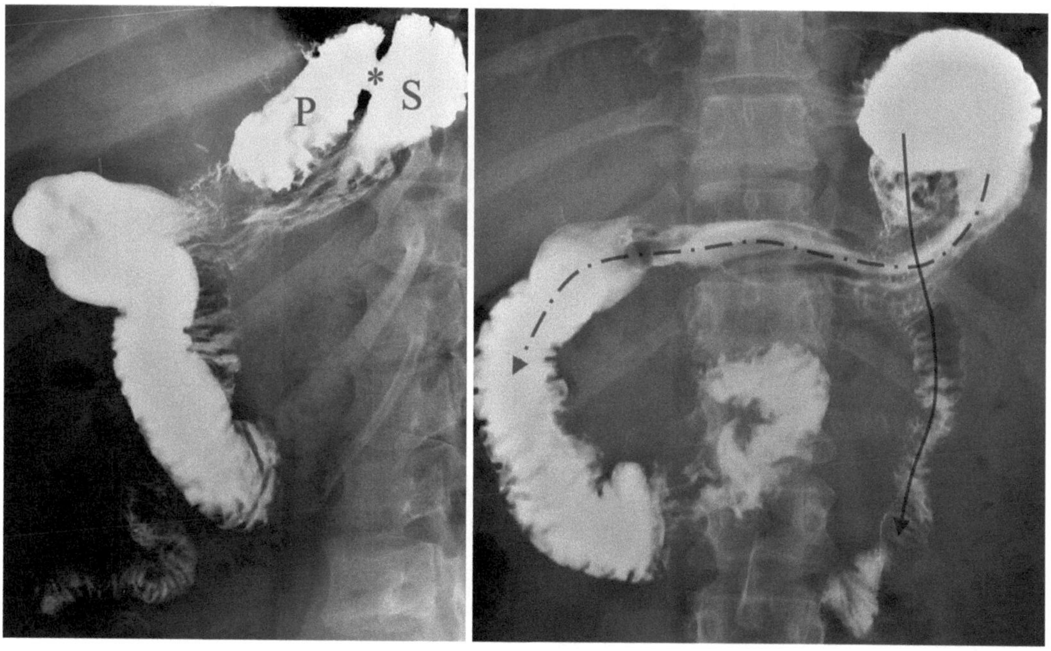

Fig. 3.57 RYGB fistula. There is communication between the gastric pouch (*P*) and stomach (*S*) via a fistula (*asterisk*). Consequently, contrast preferentially exits via the stomach (*broken arrow*) since there is restriction at the gastrojejunal anastomosis entering the Roux loop (*continuous arrow*)

channel leading from the proximal pouch. The dehiscence can be narrow, or there may be complete disruption of staple lines. It is important to review the pattern of oral contrast on CT – no contrast should normally reside within the remnant stomach, unless there has been reflux up the

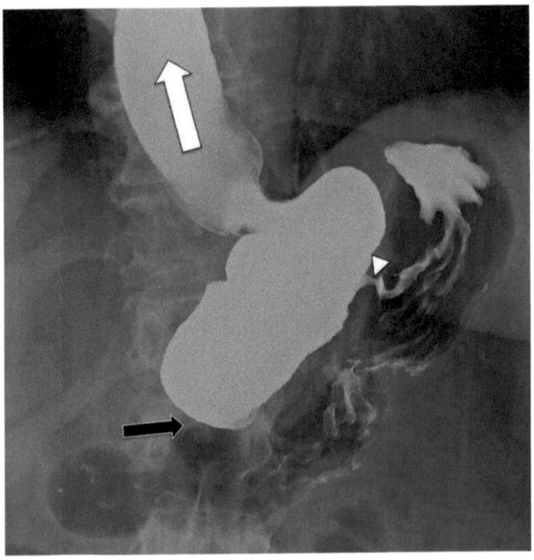

Fig. 3.58 VBG obstruction and fistula: previous VBG with reflux symptoms. Reflux confirmed (*white arrow*) due to tight restriction by band (*black arrow*). The staple line to the excluded stomach is disrupted (*arrowhead*) with filling of the fundus

biliopancreatic limb. Where contrast is present (with none in the duodenum), a gastrogastric fistula should be suspected (Trenkner 2009).

3.5.5.3 Gastric Channel and Gastric Outlet Obstruction (VBG, Sleeve Gastrectomy, M&M, RYGB)

An appropriate gastric channel size to balance adequate food intake and controlled weight loss is in the range of 10–12 mm, although some patients might tolerate smaller sized channels. When strictured, the obstruction may produce vomiting in the acute stage, which may cause either immediate or delayed staple-line rupture (Fig. 3.58). Other strictures develop months after surgery and give rise to bloating, reflux symptoms, and nausea (Fig. 3.59a, b). Water-soluble contrast agents should be aspirated if possible (with an NG tube) after the examination in order to prevent pulmonary aspiration

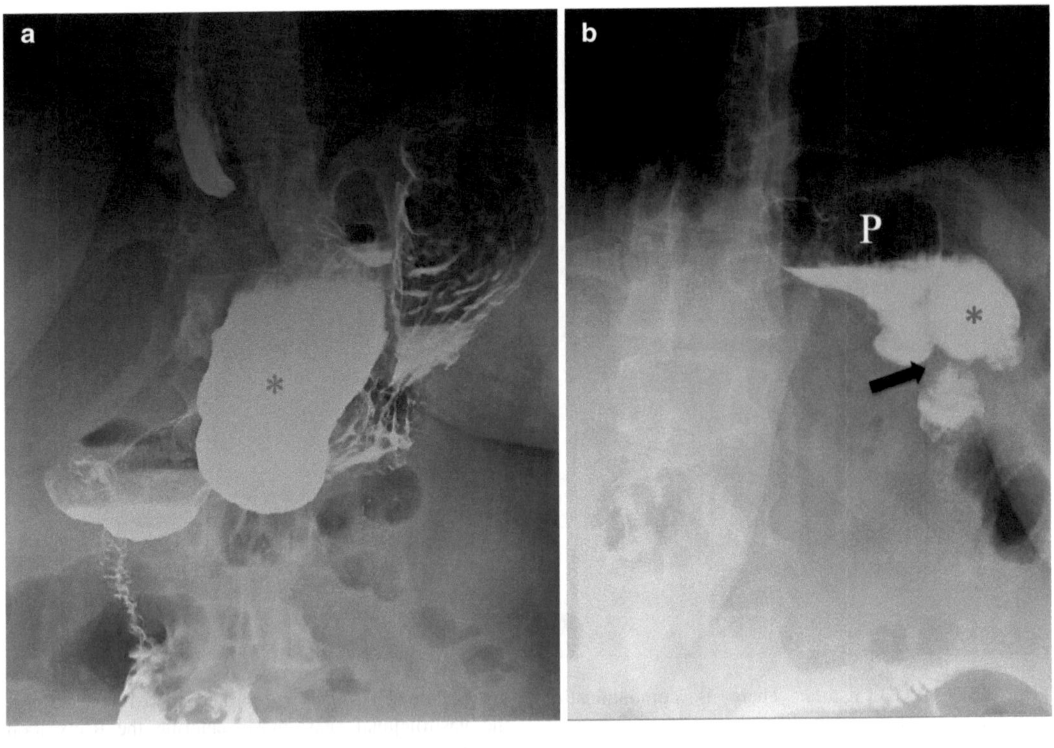

Fig. 3.59 Gastric obstruction. (**a**) Recurrent vomiting 10 years after VBG. The band is causing over restriction and gross dilatation of the pouch (*asterisk*). The band had eroded into gastric wall requiring partial gastrectomy and RYGB reconstruction. (**b**) Excessive weight loss post RYGB. The pouch (*P*) and blind end of Roux loop (*asterisk*) are dilated due to stricture (*arrow*) requiring resection and revision of the anastomosis

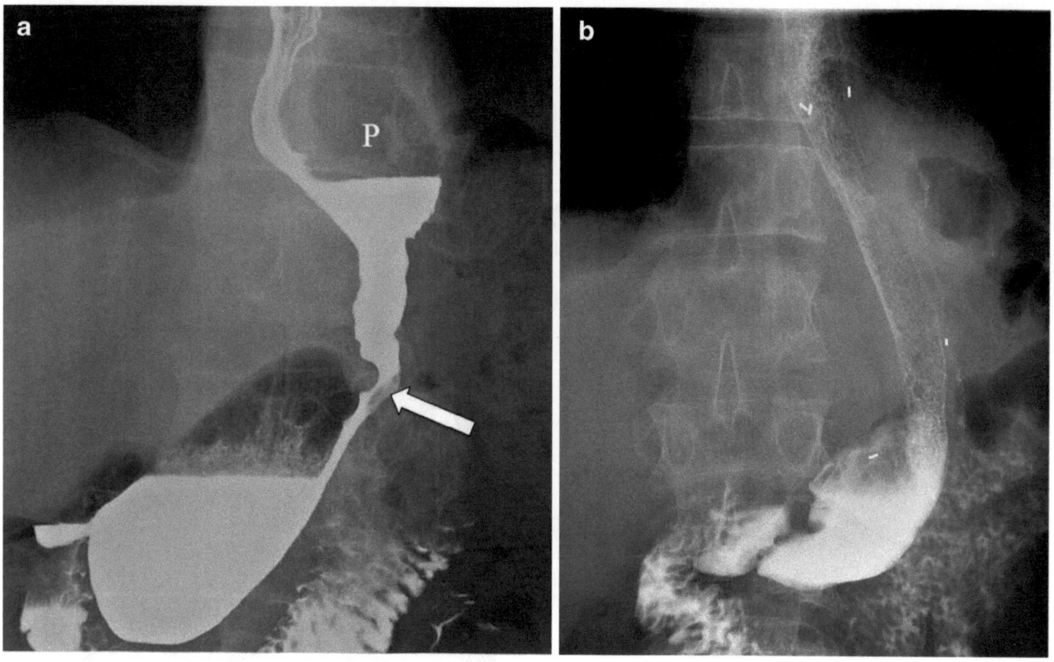

Fig. 3.60 Sleeve gastrectomy stricture. (**a**) Vomiting 4 years post sleeve gastrectomy. Mid gastric stricture (*arrow*) after sleeve gastrectomy, unresponsive to repeat endoscopic dilatation with a proximal pouch forming (*P*). (**b**) Temporary placement of retrievable stent resulted in sustained dilatation of the stricture and resolution of symptoms

particularly when high-grade obstruction is demonstrated.

Usually, obstruction requires revisional surgery (normally conversion to RYGB or revision of RYGB), but balloon dilatation and stent placement are sometimes successful less invasive alternatives (Fig. 3.60) (unless VBG has been performed, as the band restriction will not resolve with these interventions).

3.5.5.4 Efferent Loop Obstruction (RYGB)

CT is the best modality for indicating the cause and site for obstruction. Where possible, conservative management is chosen (e.g., for adhesive obstruction), but early surgical intervention is required for more serious forms of obstruction (internal hernia, incisional hernia).

Internal Hernia

Internal hernia can either be an early or late complication and should be considered in a patient with Roux-en-Y bypass who presents with abdominal pain or obstructive symptoms. Three types of hernias (small bowel herniation) are described (Fig. 3.61a):

- Through the transverse mesocolon (Fig. 3.61b)
- Through the defect in small bowel mesentery at the jejunojejunostomy
- Petersen hernia (herniation behind Roux loop, Fig. 3.61c)

A cluster of small bowel loops on the left side of abdomen demonstrated on CT or small bowel follow-through suggests internal herniation (Fig. 3.61c) (Blachar et al. 2002). In mesocolic herniation, multiple small bowel loops are present cephalad to the transverse mesocolon, rather than just the single Roux loop. Other signs described are mesenteric swirl sign (swirl of engorged mesenteric vessels, Fig. 3.61b) (Trenkner 2009) and pinch sign (where the Roux limb is "pinched" as it passes through the defect in transverse mesocolon and allows accurate

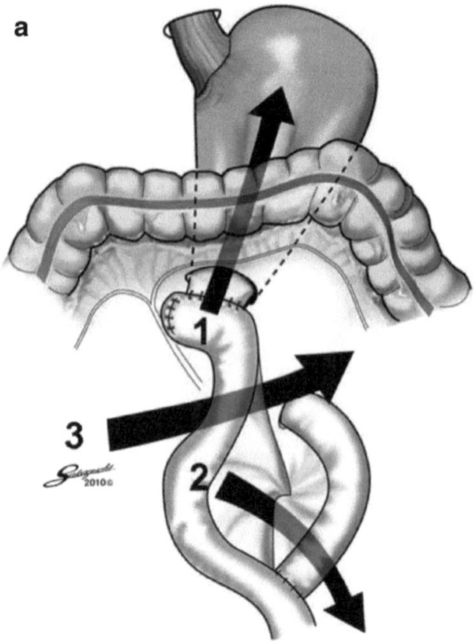
a
1
2
3
2010©

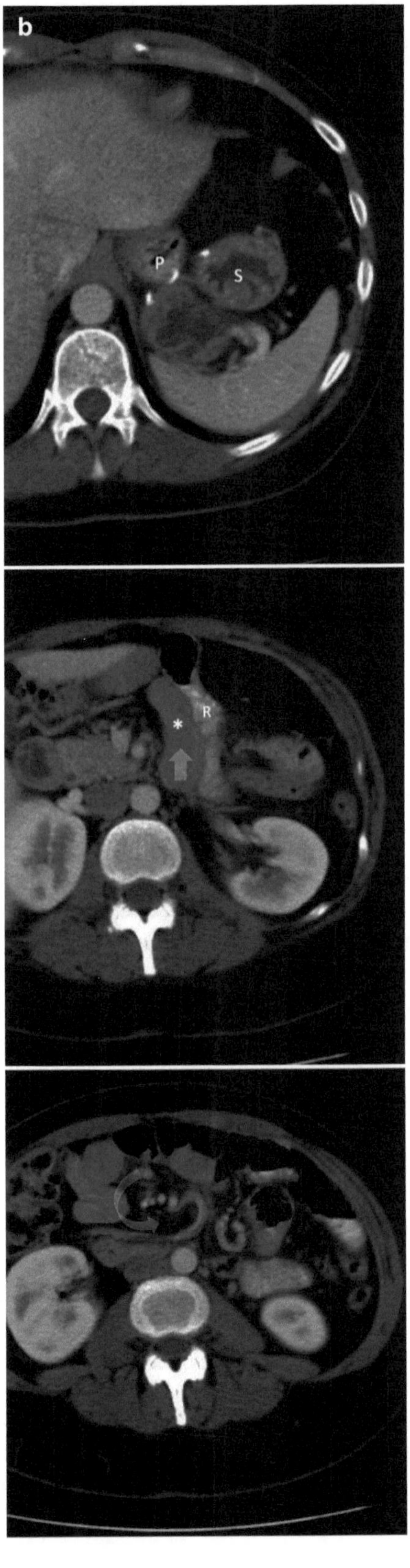
b
P
S
R
*

Fig. 3.61 (continued)

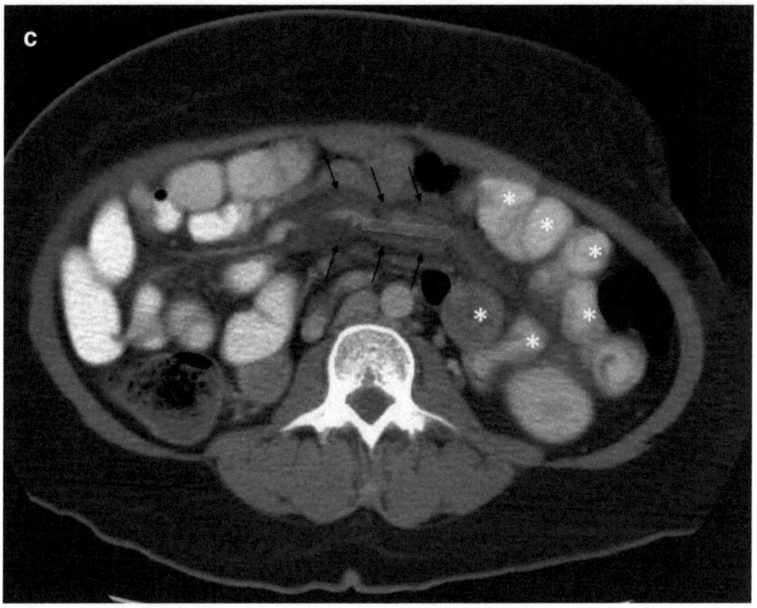

definition of the amount of small bowel cephalad to the defect) (Yu et al. 2004). To reduce the likelihood of internal herniation, defects are usually closed at the time of surgery, and the retrocolic Roux loop is less favored due to the higher rate of internal hernia.

Port Site/Incisional Hernia

Hernias are not always clinically palpable because of abdominal fat, and clinical symptoms may be vague since the efferent limb will produce relatively little secretion from such a small pouch and may not present with proximal small bowel obstruction if the patient is nil by mouth. Contrast studies may indicate obstruction, but retained fluid in the loop may not demonstrate the point or cause of obstruction. In this regard, CT is clearly superior (Fig. 3.62).

Adhesive Obstruction and Distal Anastomotic Stricture

It is again important to be vigilant for dilated gas-filled bowel loops when performing routine postoperative contrast studies of the proximal anastomosis that may give a clue to subclinical/asymptomatic efferent loop obstruction. An abrupt transition at the jejunojejunal staple line indicates anastomotic stricture either from adhesion (Fig. 3.63) or from stricture formation (Fig. 3.64). Again, CT is probably better than fluoroscopy at discriminating the cause of obstruction.

Fig. 3.61 (**a**) Post RYGB internal herniation occurs in one of three places after retrocolic reconstruction: *1* mesenteric defect of the transverse mesocolon, *2* jejunal mesenteric space at the jejunojejunostomy, *3* Petersen's space, between the mesentery of the alimentary limb and transverse mesocolon. (**b**) 1 year post RYGB with vague symptoms. Pouch (*P*) and stomach (*S*) are normal. However, a jejunal loop (*asterisk*) has herniated alongside the retrocolic Roux loop (*R*) through the transverse mesocolon (*arrow*). Note accompanying twist in the mesenteric vessels (*curved arrow*). (**c**) Petersen's hernia with edematous mesentery (*black arrows*) from herniation of jejunal loops (*asterisks*) to the left of midline through the mesenteric defect (*large arrow*)

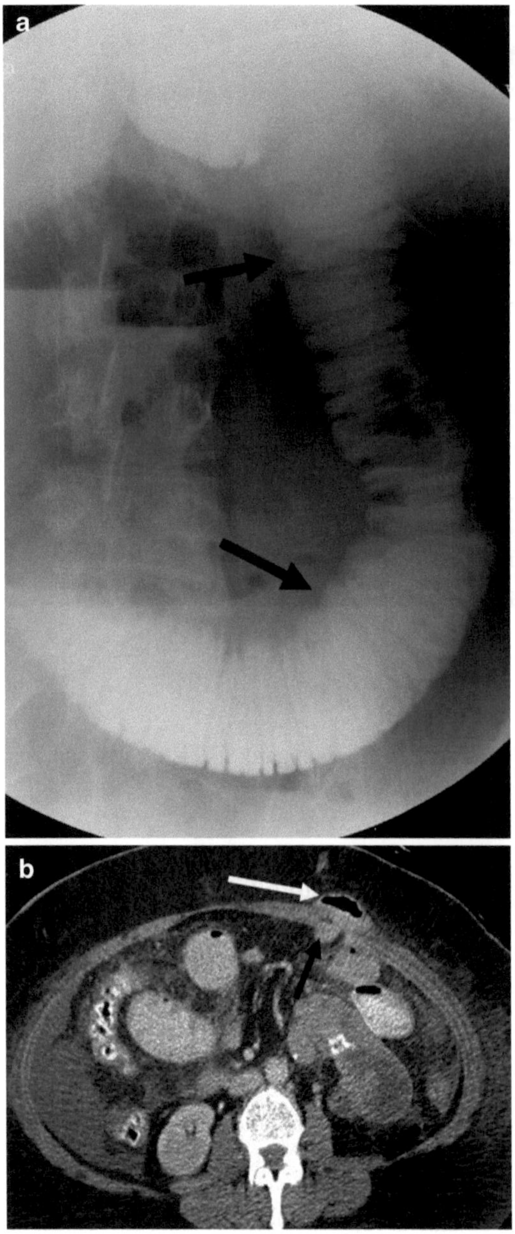

Fig. 3.62 (**a**) Recurrent vomiting following laparoscopic RYGB. (**a**) The roux loop is dilated (*arrows*), but the transition point is not identified. (**b**) CT shows an abrupt transition point from port site hernia in the left abdominal wall (*white arrow*) with a collapsed distal loop (*black arrow*)

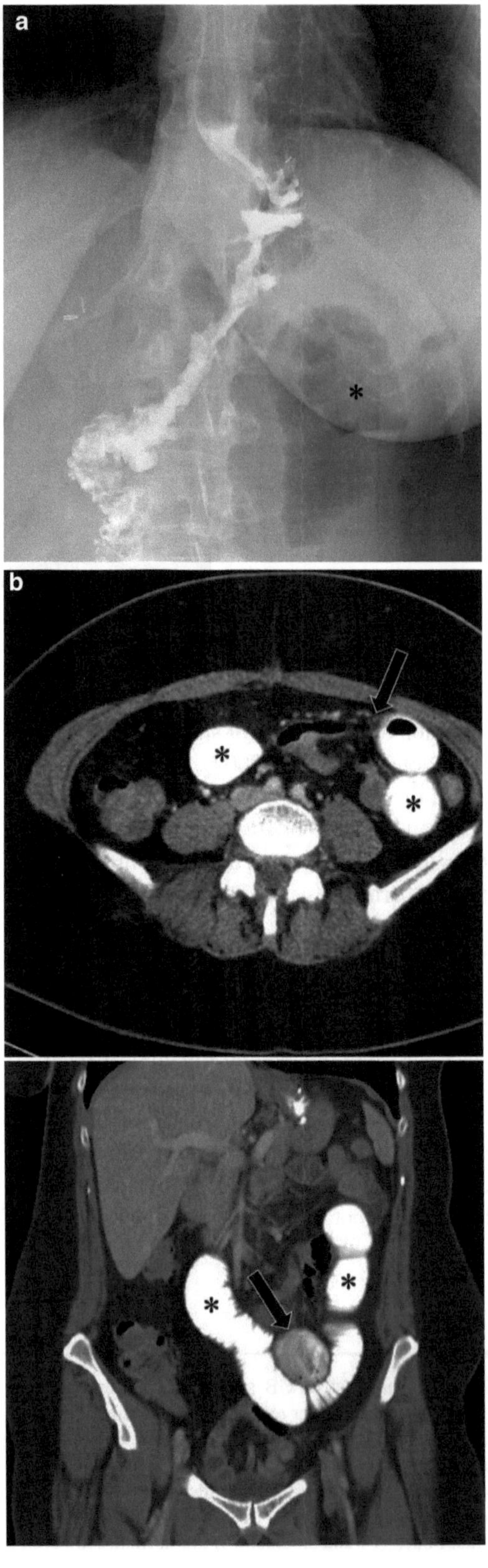

Fig. 3.63 RYGB adhesive obstruction – persistent nausea 1 week after RYGB. CT and fluoroscopy are complementary. (**a**) Water-soluble swallow: the pouch and Roux loop look normal with no obstruction. However, a dilated small bowel loop is present (*asterisk*). (**b**) CT 1 h later shows a dilated contrast-filled jejunal tube (*asterisk*) due to adhesive obstruction proximal to the jejunojejunal anastomosis (*arrow*)

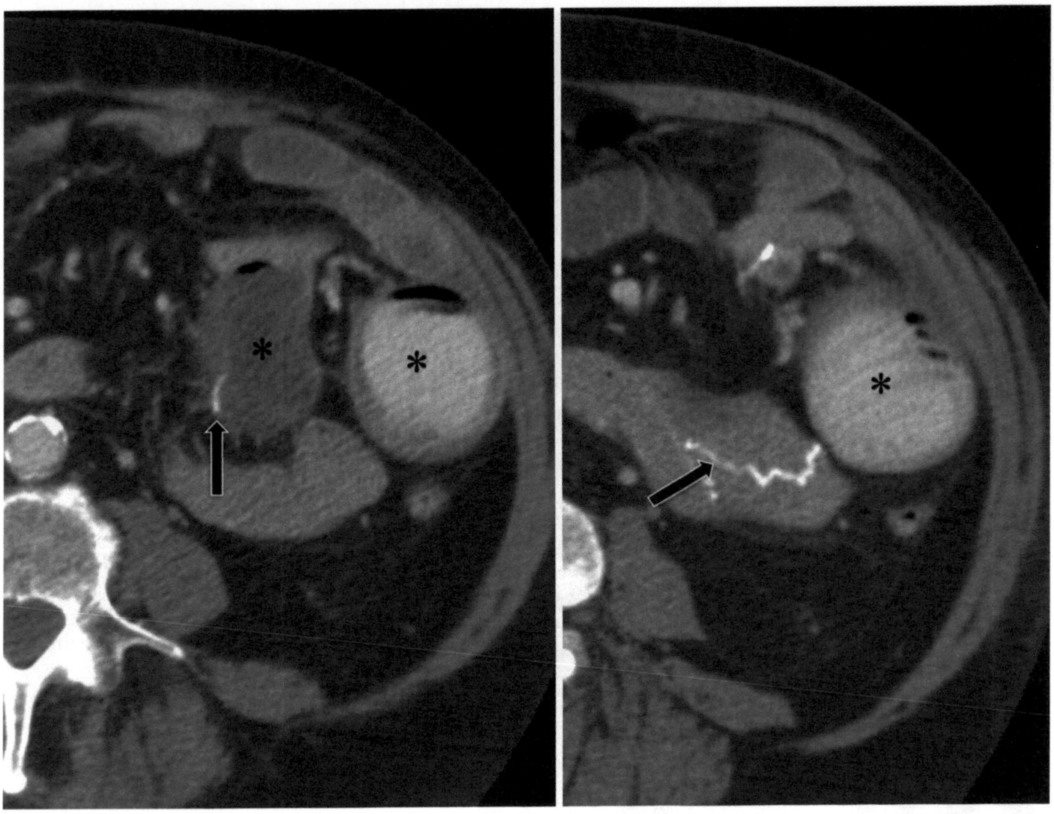

Fig. 3.64 RYGB anastomotic obstruction at the jejunojejunal anastomosis (*arrow*) with dilated contrast- and fluid-filled jejunum proximally (*asterisk*)

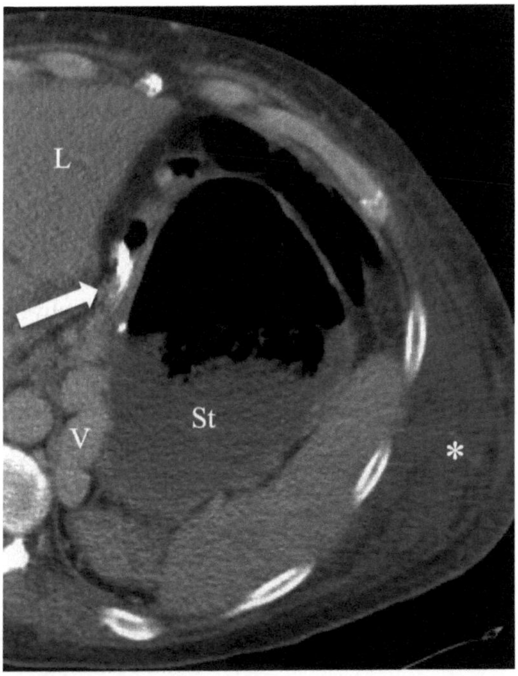

3.5.5.5 Obstruction of the Gastric Remnant and Biliopancreatic Limb

This is an uncommon complication (6% of cases) (Yu et al. 2004). Since the obstructed segment is not "in line" with the gastric pouch, patients present in a vague manner with abdominal pain, nausea, and bloating rather than vomiting. Upper GI contrast studies are normal as the obstructed stomach and small bowel are fluid filled. CT demonstrates gastric distension with the transition point indicating the etiology – gastric outlet obstruction due to peptic stricture or malignancy (Fig. 3.65), more distal jejunal obstruction due to adhesion, hernia, or anastomotic stricture (Fig. 3.66).

Fig. 3.65 RYGB excluded stomach obstruction 3 year post Roux-en-Y gastric bypass with unexplained vomiting and hypoproteinemia. The excluded stomach (*St*) is dilated due to a pyloric stricture (*not shown*). It compresses the small gastric pouch containing a nasogastric tube (*arrow*) against liver (*L*) and excluded stomach. Note edema (*asterisk*) and varices (*V*) from cirrhosis due to nonalcoholic fatty liver disease

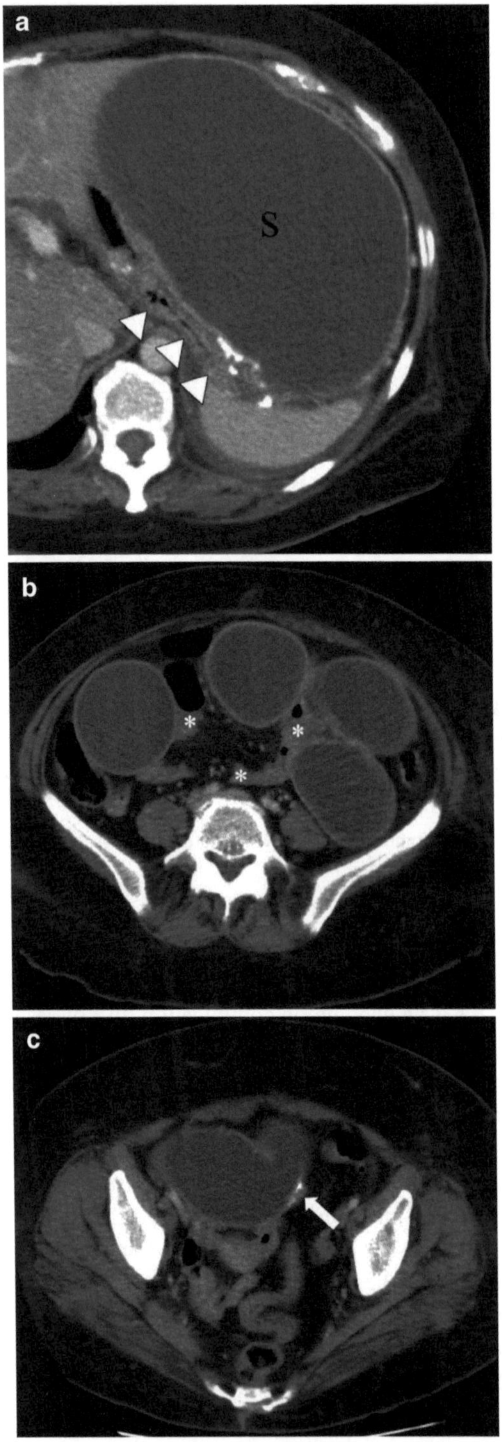

Fig. 3.66 (**a**–**c**) RYGB biliopancreatic limb obstruction. Persistent nausea after RYGB. The gastric pouch (*arrowheads*) is completely effaced by gastric dilatation (*S* stomach). The biliopancreatic limb is dilated, displacing the jejunal Roux loop (*asterisk*) due to obstruction at the jejunojejunal anastomosis (*arrow*)

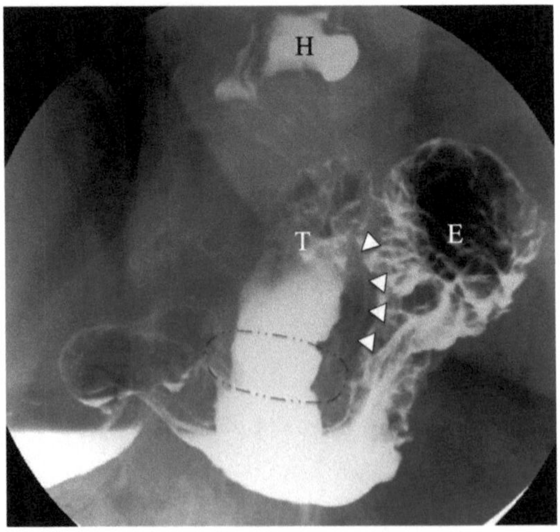

Fig. 3.67 Previous vertical banding gastrostomy with reflux symptoms. The staple line (*arrowheads*) separates the lesser curve tube (*T*) from the excluded gastric segment (*E*) with the band around the tube (*broken line*). There is no longer any restriction. Small hiatus hernia (*H*)

3.5.5.6 Lack of Restriction and Weight Gain

Unfortunately, a proportion of patients will gain weight despite surgery. This may be due to "liquid calories" overcoming the restriction, dilatation of the gastric pouch itself allowing consumption of larger meals (Fig. 3.67), lack of restriction of the gastric outflow (Fig. 3.68a), or recruitment of the blind limb of the Roux loop in RYGB to produce a sump to augment gastric volume (Fig. 3.69). Fistulation into the excluded gastric remnant is a further cause of weight gain (Figs. 3.56 and 3.57).

In cases where surgery fails to result in weight loss, revision is often required, either to add a malabsorptive component (RYGB or duodenal switch) to a restrictive procedure or alternatively to provide additional restriction (by revision of an anastomosis to make it smaller or addition of LAGB – Fig. 3.68b) or reduction in the volume of the gastric reservoir (by refashioning the gastric pouch or sleeve gastrectomy).

3.5.5.7 Complications of LAGB

Band Too Tight

Over restriction can cause vomiting, nausea, and reflux. This is indicated on contrast examinations

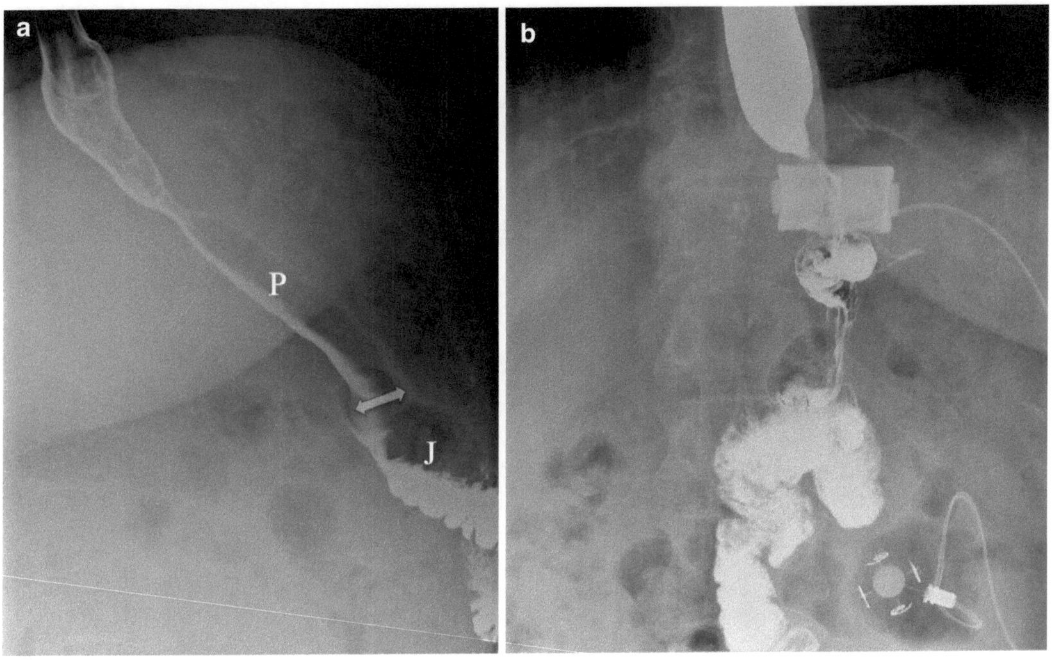

Fig. 3.68 Weight gain after RYGB. (**a**) There is no restriction between gastric pouch (*P*) and jejunum (*J*) with a wide anastomosis (*arrow*). (**b**) A gastric band has been fitted to restrict pouch outflow

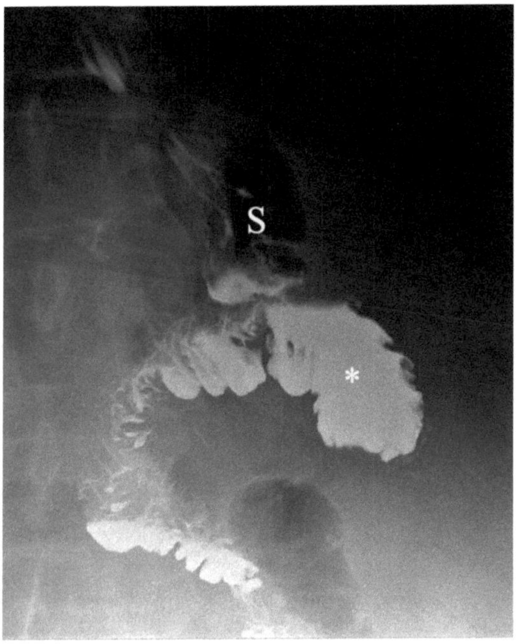

Fig. 3.69 Weight gain 1 year after RYGB. The blind limb of the Roux loop is dilated (*asterisk*) and acting as a sump to affectively increase gastric pouch volume (*S*) and reduce satiety

by dilatation of the esophagus (rather than just the small distal pouch), tertiary contractions, and in some cases atony (Fig. 3.70). It is important that restriction does not lead to chronic dilatation and secondary achalasia as this is very difficult to treat. Management is to withdraw fluid from the band reservoir. A check swallow is then performed to evaluate the adequacy of the "band tightness."

Band Migration

Migration results in the band passing inferior to the GOJ, taking up a more horizontal or vertical configuration than usual, and there is eccentric dilation of pouch proximally as the fundus and body become incorporated above it (Quigley et al. 2011). A plain film is often able to confirm the diagnosis with the balloon slipping from its usual 45° orientation (Fig. 3.71). The diagnosis can also be confirmed on contrast swallow where depending on the degree of migration, the fundus may be incorporated into the "pouch" (Fig. 3.72) or the stomach can become bizarrely dilated and distorted when migration is even more distal (Fig. 3.73). When this is observed, the band

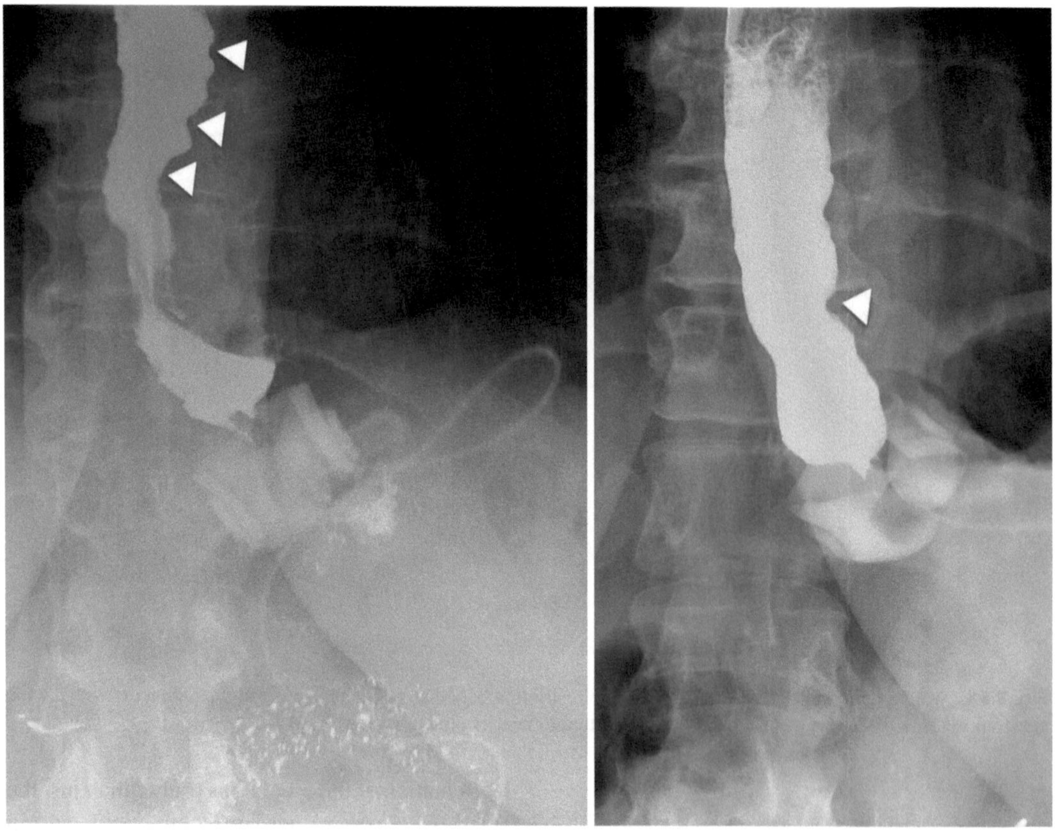

Fig. 3.70 Over restriction of gastric band inducing esophageal spasm (*arrowheads*) and stasis in the esophagus in two patients

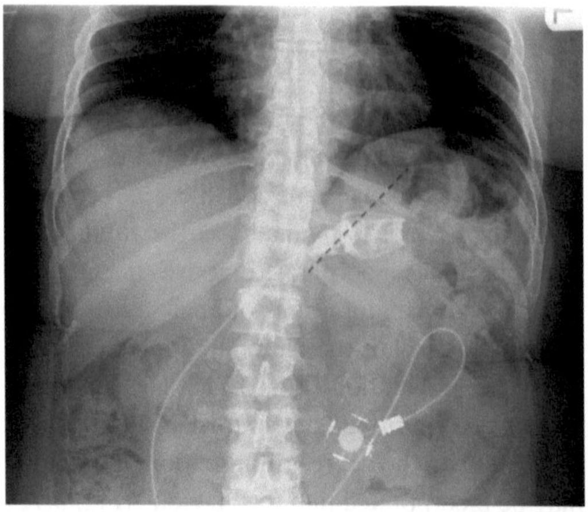

Fig. 3.71 Patient with vomiting post LAGB. Note that the band has rotated clockwise from the expected orientation (*dotted line*), raising concern for migration/displacement

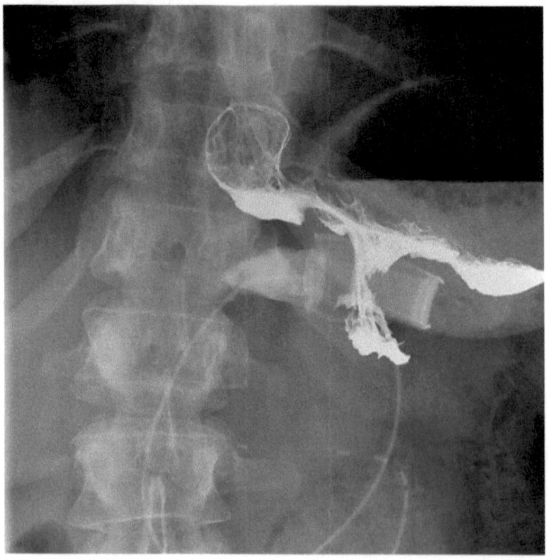

Fig. 3.72 Gastric band migration. Barium swallow shows the fundus migrated proximally through the wrap with the band constricting the mid gastric body migrated to cause annular constriction of the antrum. Urgent revision surgery was performed

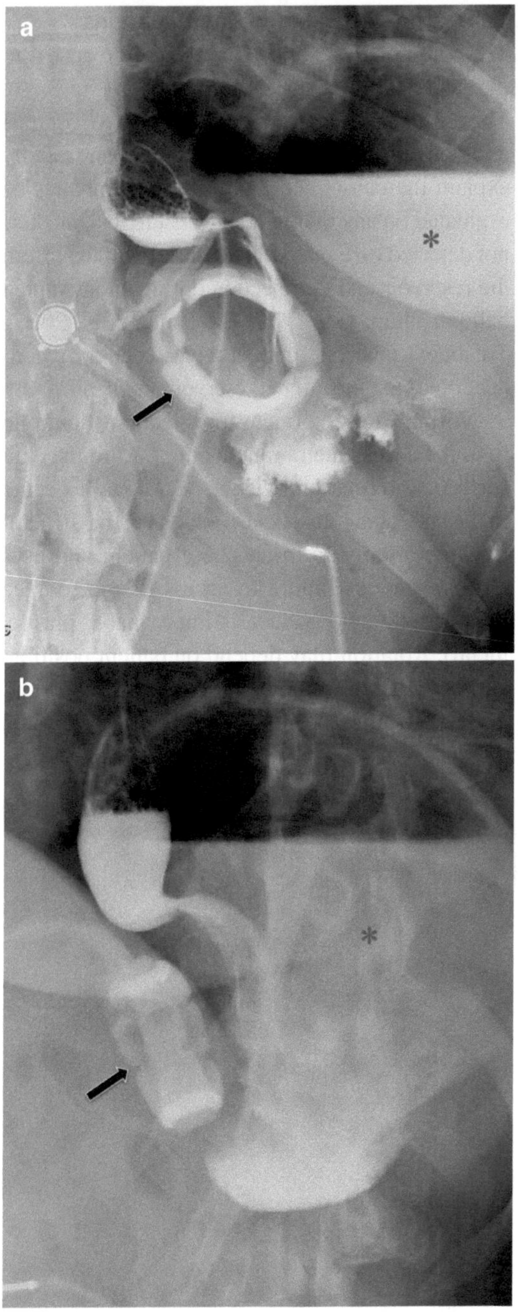

Fig. 3.73 Intractable vomiting 3 weeks after gastric band placement. (**a**) The band (*arrow*) looks normally positioned relative to the gastric cardia but is seen *en face* in the AP position, and gastric dilatation is present (*asterisk*) which should raise suspicion of migration. (**b**) In the lateral view, the band has clearly migrated to the lower body causing gross distortion of the proximal stomach

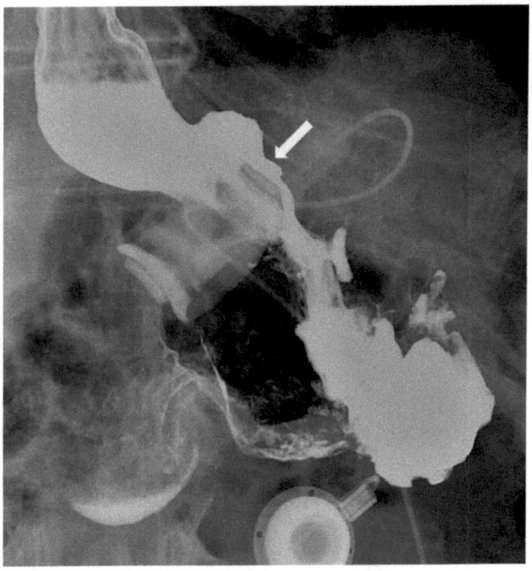

Fig. 3.74 Epigastric pain 2 years after gastric band insertion. Band erosion has occurred since the band lies in the gastric lumen (*arrow*) having eroded through the gastric wall

should be completely emptied, and the patient admitted for removal or repositioning of the balloon. Untreated migration may lead to obstruction or even gastric necrosis.

Band Erosion

This is where the gastric band erodes into the stomach through the gastric wall. This often occurs slowly over months manifesting with a lack of restriction, although in some cases erosion is heralded by severe pain. On fluoroscopy, contrast is seen within the band as well as outlining outside the band (since the tube now lies in the lumen – Fig. 3.74) (Quigley et al. 2011). CT may also indicate erosion by intraluminal location of one-half of the balloon but may be missed without adequate gastric distension or positive oral contrast.

Open Band

Rarely, the band opens due to incomplete fixation of the ring at surgery. This causes immediate release of restriction and produces a "C- or U-shaped" band rather than the usual "ring shape." Surgical revision is required to reconstitute the band (Fig. 3.75).

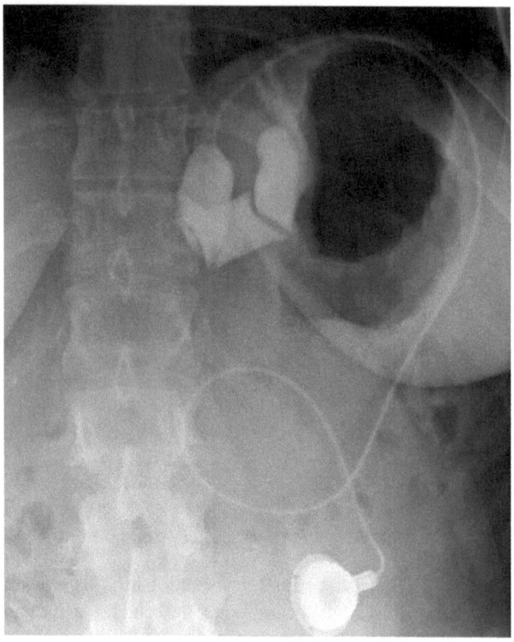

Fig. 3.75 Sudden loss of restriction after gastric band adjustment – the band is no longer in continuity and has assumed an open U shape

Tube- and Port-Related Complications

The commonest complication relating to access to the band is tube fracture or disconnection (Fig. 3.76). This results in loss of restriction due to contrast escaping from the band. Imaging can rapidly explain the cause, and the tube should always be evaluated on any radiograph to ensure it is intact. If not detected on a plain film, contrast will leak from the reservoir end on injection during an attempted balloon filling (Fig. 3.77) (Mehanna et al. 2006). Treatment involves surgical replacement or reconnection of the tube to the reservoir and band.

Normally, the port site for injection should lie with the access membrane facing toward the skin surface. Port rotation/twisting occasionally occurs in the subcutaneous pocket, which can be difficult to detect clinically in an obese patient and usually presents as failure to access the port (since the opposite side surface is impregnable plastic/metal). Rotation may depend on patient position, varying between supine and erect (Mortelé et al. 2001). The diagnosis is usually resolved with

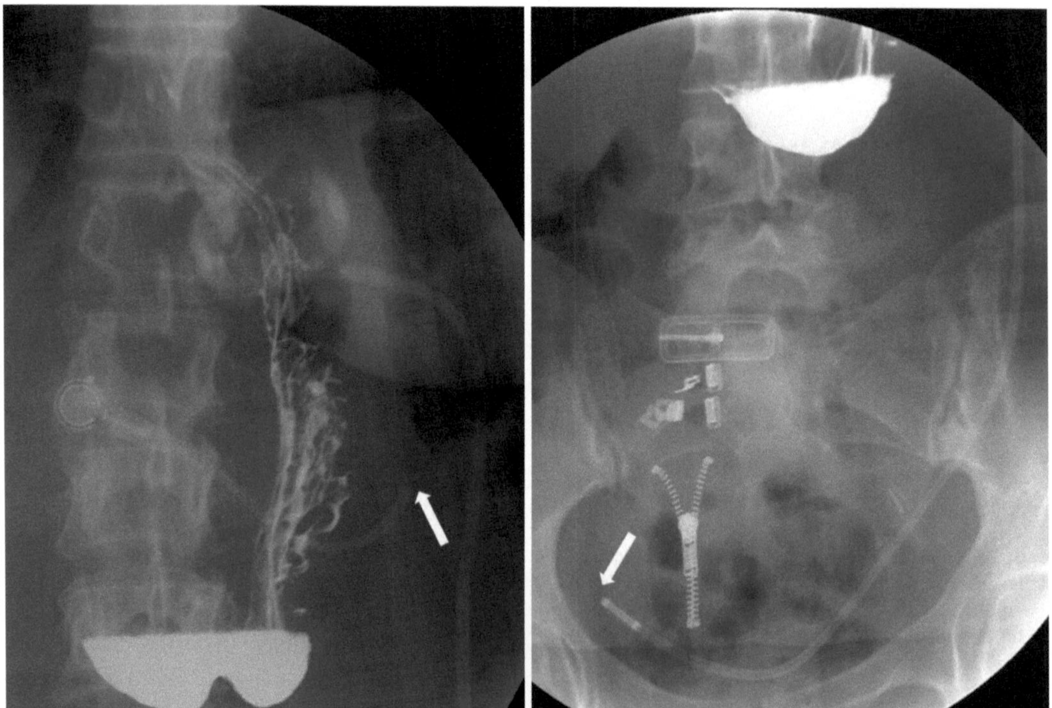

Fig. 3.76 Gastric bands in two patients with no restriction due to tube fracture (*left arrow*) and tube disconnection from the port (*right arrow*)

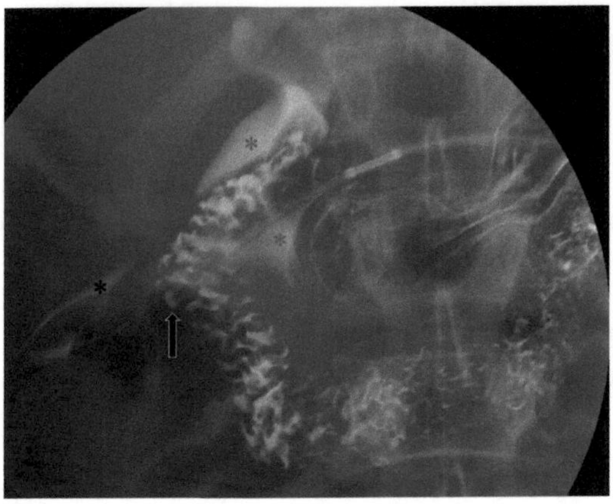

Fig. 3.77 Gastric band tube fracture not appreciated prior to filling the balloon – contrast spills into peritoneum (*asterisk*) from the fracture site (*arrow*)

imaging, as the circular port assumes either an oval or linear appearance depending on the degree of rotation (Mehanna et al. 2006). Complete rotation can be difficult to diagnose as the port retains its circular appearance. However, by screening laterally, the correct orientation of the post can quickly be determined (Mehanna et al. 2006). Some ports are made with swirled fixation anchors that are correctly oriented when the tail of the anchor is pointing in an anticlockwise direction (Figs. 3.68 and 3.71) – when abnormally rotated these anchors point clockwise (Quigley et al. 2011).

Port Site Infection

This is rare and risk is minimized by strict aseptic technique during port access to adjust the band. Imaging demonstrates fat stranding around the port, tube, or band suggesting inflammation (Mehanna et al. 2006; Blachar et al. 2007). The port and tube usually have to be removed, and the patient treated with prolonged antibiotics before a new access device is fitted.

3.6 Radiological Insertion of Gastrostomy (RIG)

3.6.1 Indications

- Temporary or permanent gastric feeding where the oral route is inadequate or contraindicated
- To "vent" the stomach for palliation of gastric outflow obstruction unresponsive to other intervention
- Gastrostomy placement where endoscopy cannot access the stomach

3.6.2 Nonradiological Techniques for Gastrostomy

Gastrostomies are created using endoscopy, surgery, or radiological placement. The radiological route is particularly useful where access to the pharynx, hypopharynx, and esophagus excludes gastric intubation by endoscopy due to stricture or other pathology. The procedure is normally performed with conscious sedation or general anesthesia.

Endoscopy is the most commonly used route: the endoscope is passed into the stomach, and a needle is then used to puncture the abdominal wall and the anterior wall of the stomach with endoscopic visualization. The correct puncture site must be checked by transillumination using the endoscope. A flexible wire is then passed through this into the stomach and grasped using endoscopic forceps and pulled back out through the mouth. The oral end of the wire is then attached to the gastrostomy tube and pulled back through the esophagus, stomach, and abdominal wall. A stiff "bumper" disc retains it (Fig. 3.78c).

Surgical gastrostomy is seldom performed and only during surgery for another reason (such as to vent the stomach), as minimally invasive techniques are usually favored as a solo procedure or feeding jejunostomy for nutrition. A needle punctures the stomach at the time of surgery and the gastrostomy placed by direct visualization.

3.6.3 Technique for RIG

These procedures are usually performed under fluoroscopic guidance. A nasogastric tube is passed prior to the procedure. This allows gastric insufflation via the tube. Sedoanesthesia is administered with appropriate monitoring of vital signs along with antispasmodic in order to maintain gastric distension (Buscopan, Boehringer

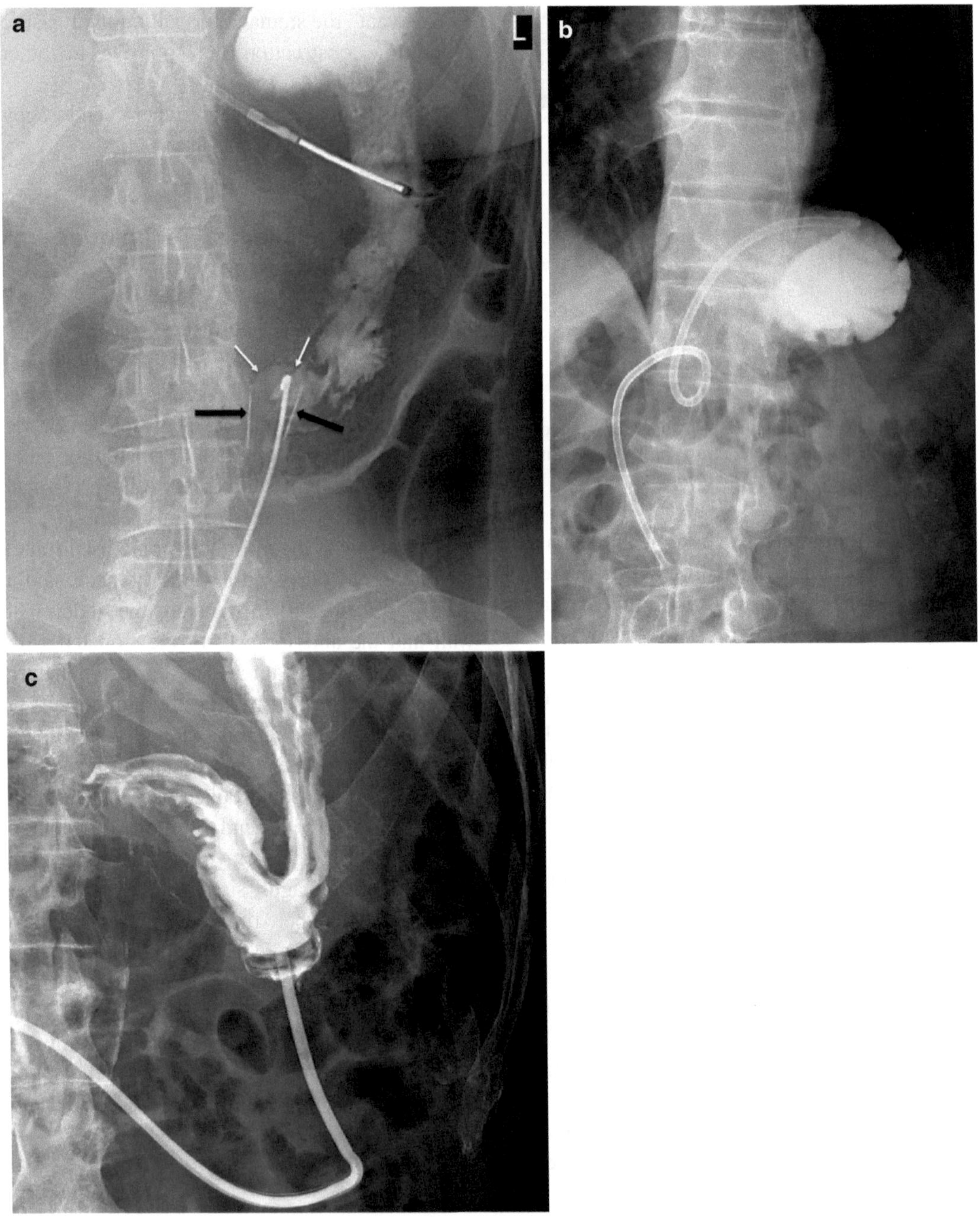

Fig. 3.78 Gastrostomy. (**a**) Radiological insertion. The nasogastric tube is placed to allow insufflation for gastric puncture. The gastrostomy puncture has been made between two gastropexy sutures in the antrum (*black arrows*). Note the water-filled gastrostomy retention balloon (*white arrows*). (**b**) A locking loop tube may be used. (**c**) Percutaneous endoscopic gastrostomy with plastic retention bumper – this is more robust than balloon retention

Ingelheim®). Using aseptic technique, the stomach is punctured, with a majority of radiologists placing 2–4 gastropexy sutures to approximate the anterior wall of the stomach to the abdominal wall. The stomach is then punctured between pexy sutures, and the track dilated over a wire to

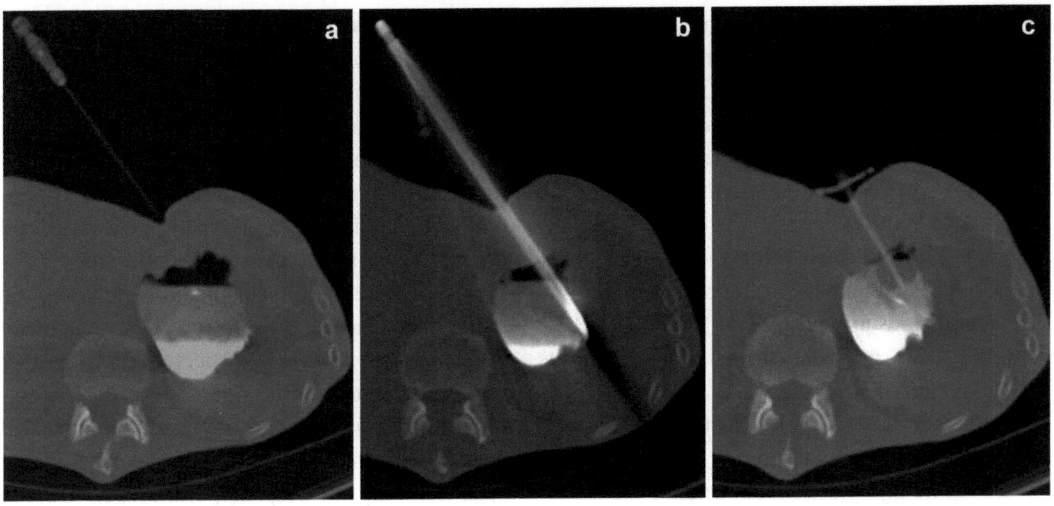

Fig. 3.79 Palliative venting gastrostomy insertion under CT guidance. "Concrete abdomen" following high-dose upper abdominal radiotherapy for lymphoma while overseas, with recurrent vomiting and no surgical access. (**a**) Gastric puncture with cannula followed by serial dilatation over wire to allow (**b**) placement of 18.5Fr peel away sheath prior to (**c**) 14Fr gastrostomy placement

allow passage of the gastrostomy. Our local practice is to dilate in order to insert an 18.5Fr peel away sheath which then allows insertion of a 14Fr balloon gastrostomy through it (Fig. 3.78a). Alternatives to using a balloon retention catheter include a locking loop catheter (Fig. 3.78b) or a small "button" gastrostomy depending on local preference.

3.6.3.1 Peroral Image-Guided Gastrostomy (PIG)

This is another less common method of imaging-guided gastrostomy placement. The stomach is insufflated with an NG tube and then punctured percutaneously in the mid body to allow a wire to pass proximally through the GOJ into the esophagus and out of the mouth. The wire is then looped around the endoscopic gastrostomy tube, which is pulled back through the esophagus, stomach, and abdominal wall (Laasch et al. 2003).

Gastrostomy may be placed using CT guidance in specific rare situations (Fig. 3.79).

3.6.4 Complications of RIG

The main complications relate to tube displacement, stoma infection, tube blockage, and postprocedure discomfort. Using the oral route for gastrostomy delivery increases infection risk. The procedure may transgress other structures, particularly the transverse colon and left lobe of liver or even lead to gastric perforation and peritonitis. Bleeding is a rare complication (Laasch et al. 2003).

3.7 Duodenal Resection and Surgery for Peptic Ulcer Disease

3.7.1 Pancreas Preserving Total Duodenectomy (PPTD) and Segmental Duodenectomy (SD)

These operations take place in subspecialist tertiary referral centers and are not commonly performed. The duodenum is normally resected as part of the Whipple procedure (Sect. 4.2.1). However, PPTD was developed to preserve the pancreas in patients with benign and premalignant disease of the duodenum and aims to reduce morbidity compared to the standard Whipple procedure. Because the pancreas remains in situ and extended lymphadenectomy is not possible, PPTD is not considered appropriate for curative resection of duodenal carcinoma. Segmental duodenectomy (SD) allows more limited resection of the duodenum either proximal (first and second part) or distal to the ampulla (third and fourth part). SD has been described particularly for removal of GIST tumors in the duodenum.

3.7.1.1 Clinical Indications

- Duodenal adenomatosis complicating familial adenomatous polyposis (FAP)
- GIST and neuroendocrine tumors of the duodenum
- Duodenal adenoma not resectable with endoscopic mucosal resection
- Duodenal injury after blunt trauma
- Duodenal benign stricture

3.7.1.2 Surgical Technique

PPTD

The jejunum is mobilized distal to the ligament of Treitz for later anastomosis. Cholecystectomy is performed, and a catheter introduced down the CBD to identify the ampulla of Vater. The duodenum is transected at the pylorus and at the ligament of Treitz and dissected free from the pancreas above and below the ampulla (Fig. 3.80a). The ampulla is then transected, and a sphincteroplasty performed to enlarge the orifice of the CBD/pancreatic duct confluence for anastomosis. The jejunum is then mobilized superiorly alongside the pancreas. Any remaining duodenal mucosa is resected from the pylorus and a pylorojejunostomy created (similar to Billroth I). The ampulla is then anastomosed to the medial wall of the jejunum (Fig. 3.80b).

A modification of the procedure involves a jejunal anastomosis to the ampulla and pylorojejunal anastomosis to the more distal jejunum (similar to Billroth II) (Fig. 3.80c).

SD

The affected duodenal segment is resected. Where the first or second part is removed, a jejunal Roux loop is formed and anastomosed to the pylorus. Where the third or fourth part is resected, an end-to-end duodenojejunostomy is fashioned. The ampulla is not disturbed (Fig. 3.81a, b).

3.7.1.3 Postoperative Imaging

Fluoroscopy allows assessment of the postoperative anastomoses and with Billroth I reconstruction can assess all anastomoses for defects. Fluoroscopy may be performed for routine assessment depending on local preference. CT is generally reserved only for evaluation of sepsis and acute pancreatitis, to plan intervention for collections or where there is suspicion of anastomotic dehiscence where a Billroth II reconstruction and duodenal stump leak are suspected. As with other pancreatic and gastric operations, the assessment should include an appraisal of abnormal fluid collections, extraluminal gas exceeding that seen normally in the postoperative period or in an unusual distribution that may indicate anastomotic leak with extraluminal positive contrast. The jejunal loop should be in continuity with no defects, and the adjacent pancreas should enhance normally (Fig. 3.82a, b). Localized peripancreatic fat stranding around the head is to be expected after dissection: more generalized pancreatic edema or altered enhancement may indicate pancreatitis.

3.7.1.4 Complications

Mortality is 1–3% with a lower postoperative blood loss compared to the Whipple procedure and no need for pancreatic replacement therapy (Müller et al. 2008). However, morbidity is still high with up to 50% cases developing postoperative complications (Al-Sarireh et al. 2008; De Castro et al. 2008). The commonest complication is a leak from the jejunoampullary anastomosis (23%) followed by the duodenojejunal anastomosis, which leaks in 8% of cases (Penninga and Svendsen 2011). Acute pancreatitis may occur as a function of ampullary edema and disruption to the main pancreatic duct. Other recognized complications include wound dehiscence and pneumonia (Al-Sarireh et al. 2008).

3.7.2 Duodenal Ulcer Surgery

Surgery continues to play an important role in management of a minority of cases with duodenal ulcer-related complications, despite advances in

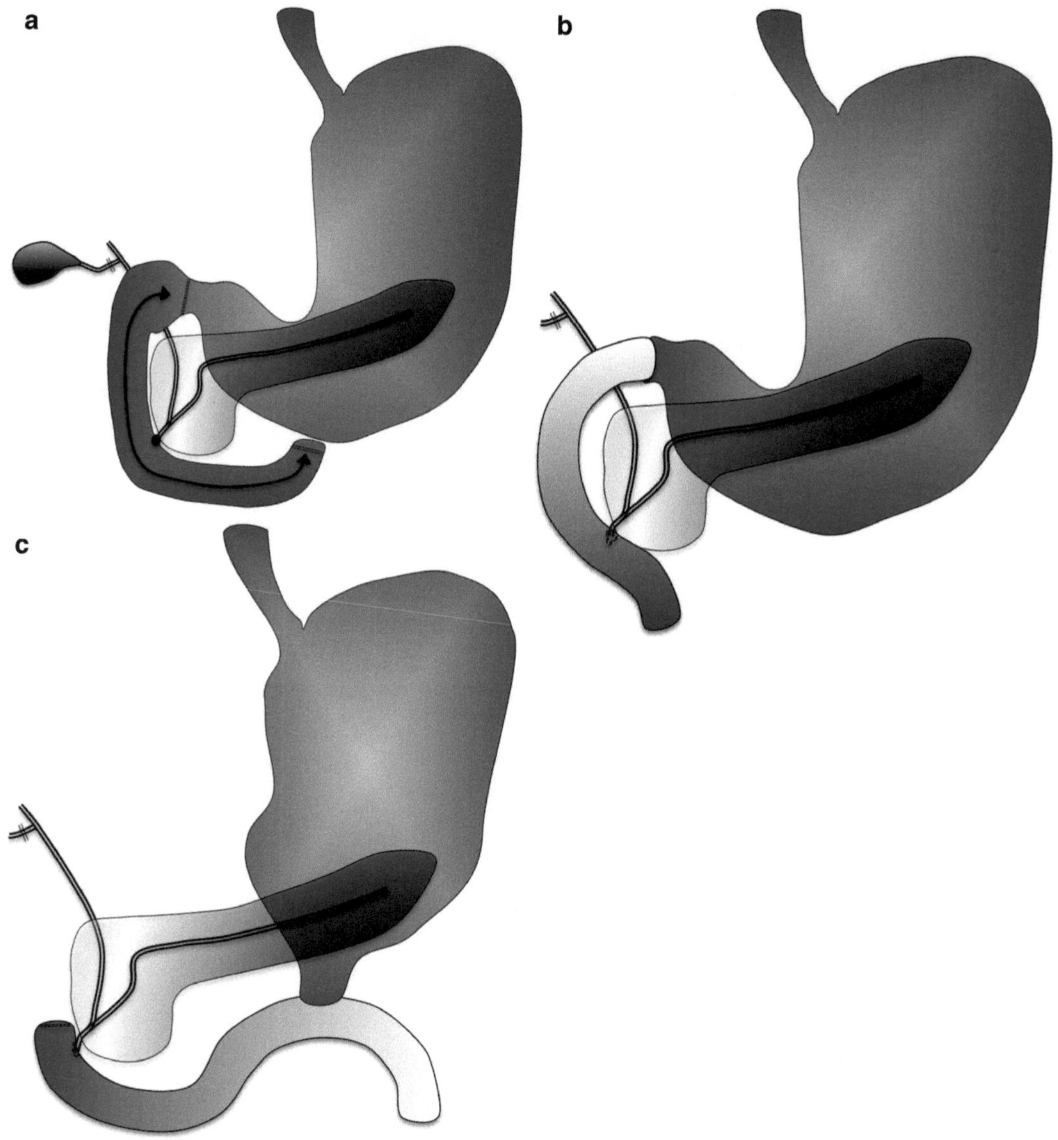

Fig. 3.80 (**a**) Pancreas preserving duodenectomy. The duodenum is transected at the proximal and distal ends and dissected from the pancreas and ampulla of Vater. Cholecystectomy is performed. (**b**) Billroth 1 anastomosis of jejunum to pylorus and to ampulla and (**c**) jejunal anastomosis to ampulla with distal gastrojejunostomy are both recognized reconstructions

both medical therapy and endoscopic techniques for treatment of bleeding. While the incidence of duodenal ulceration and ulcer-related mortality has reduced, bleeding remains the commonest presentation (73%) and perforation carries the highest mortality (Wang et al. 2010). The main indications for surgery are for uncontrolled hemorrhage refractory to endoscopic or endovascular techniques and unsealed perforation. Rebleeding after initial endoscopic treatment is most likely to occur within the first 96 h of presentation, and risk is highest where there is a visible nonbleeding vessel or adherent clot on an ulcer (Hsu et al. 1994). Duodenal ulcer perforation does not always require surgical repair, as spontaneous closure occurs in a significant proportion of cases.

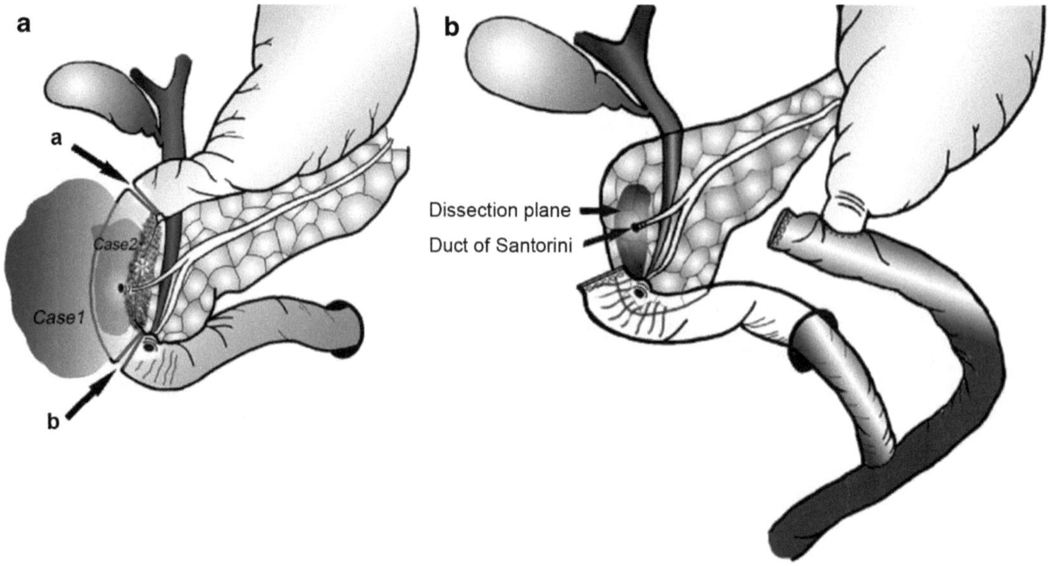

Fig. 3.81 (**a**) Segmental duodenectomy: the duodenal segment is resected between (**a**) and (**b**) sparing the adjacent pancreas and ampulla. (**b**) The stomach is subsequently anastomosed to a Roux loop

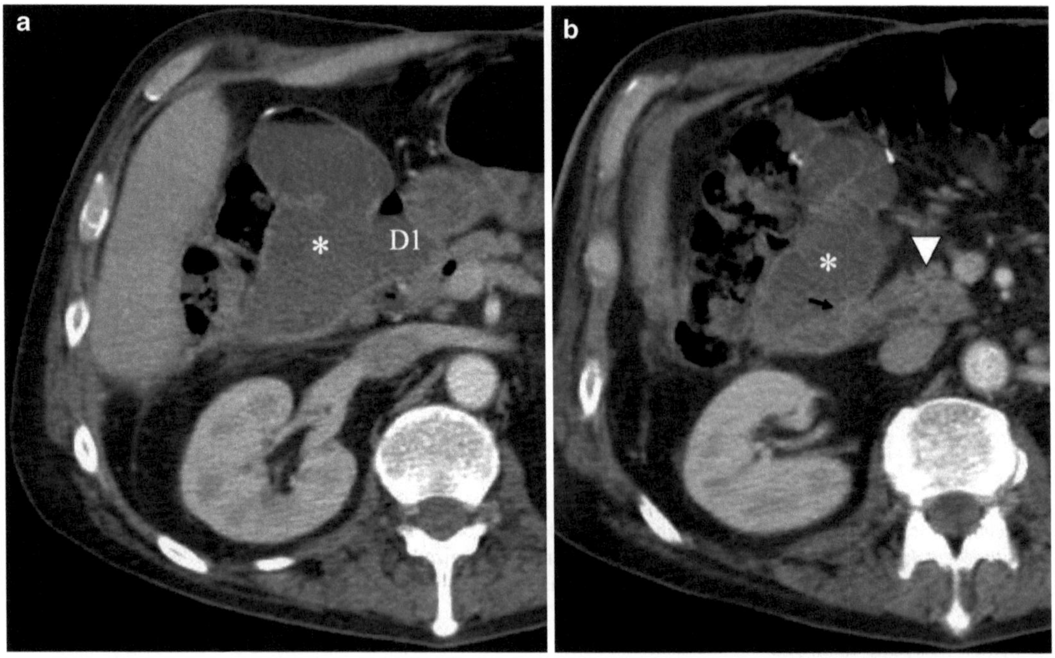

Fig. 3.82 (**a**) Pancreas preserving duodenectomy normal CT (**a, b**) Duodenectomy of second, third, and fourth part for ischemia resulting from coiling of the SMA (*not shown*) for bleeding AV malformation. CT shows the jejunal loop (*asterisk*) is anastomosed to the first part of duodenum (*D1*) and the ampulla of Vater (*black arrow*) for biliary and pancreatic drainage (*arrowhead*)

In patients with major comorbidity, the option of nonoperative management may be appropriate, since surgery itself carries a significant mortality. This may require image-guided drainage of any related collections in addition to antibiotics. Salvage surgery in a patient with ongoing leak

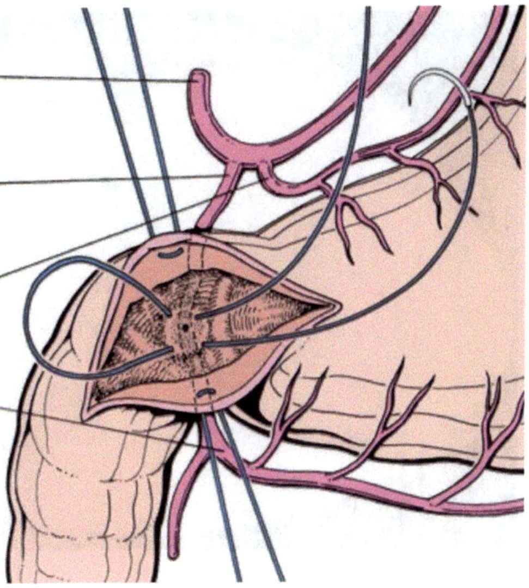

Fig. 3.83 Gastroduodenostomy and suture control of bleeding from the gastroduodenal artery. Longitudinal incision across the pylorus and proximal duodenum exposes the point of erosion into the gastroduodenal artery or branch vessel in the posterior wall of the duodenal bulb. This is best managed by undersewing the blood vessel on either side of the bleeding. The gastroduodenostomy can be closed transversely as a Heineke-Mikulicz pyloroplasty and vagotomy can also be performed

can result in increased mortality, and so radiology sometimes has a role in confirming the integrity of the duodenum with contrast studies or CT in patients where conservative management is being considered. There is little difference in the outcomes of duodenal ulcer surgery whether performed laparoscopically or open.

3.7.2.1 Surgery for Bleeding Duodenal Ulcer

The majority of cases of ulcer-related hemorrhage are managed with noninvasive techniques involving endoscopy (Anjiki et al. 2010) or angiography with embolization. A minority require surgical control (Abe et al. 2010). In this setting, the anterior wall of the first part of duodenum is opened longitudinally to allow access the posterior wall (where ulcer erosion into the gastroduodenal artery is the commonest source of bleeding). The bleeding vessel beneath the ulcer is then undersewn to prevent rebleeding. The duodenal incision then repaired (Fig. 3.83). This may be augmented with vagotomy (acid suppression) and pyloroplasty (gastric drainage).

3.7.2.2 Surgery for Perforated Duodenal Ulcer

Depending on the degree of peritoneal contamination, a range of techniques are open to the surgeon. These range from simple closure of the ulcer with an omental patch (Fig. 3.84) to antrectomy and Roux-en-Y reconstruction. Either option can be combined with a vagotomy and of course a washout of the peritoneal cavity to clear the contamination (Tsugawa et al. 2001; Jordan and Thornby 1995).

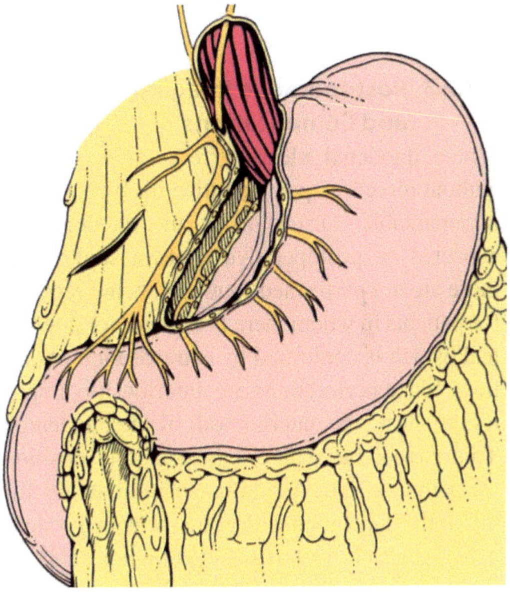

Fig. 3.84 Duodenal ulcer repair with omental patch and HSV. Perforations are patched with pedicles of greater omentum. Direct suture closure has a high risk of failure. If the patient is stable and local inflammation is not severe, a highly selective vagotomy can be performed for prevention of further episodes of ulceration

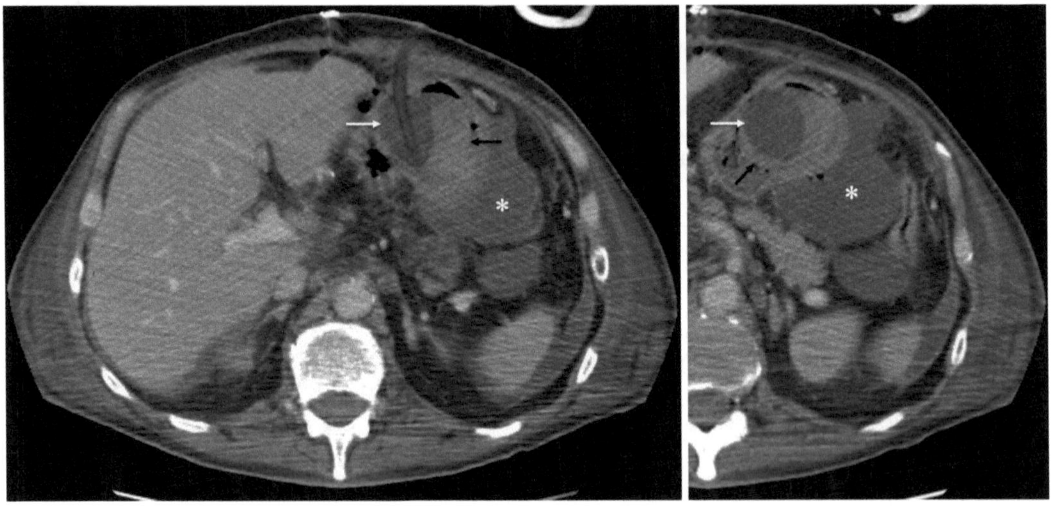

Fig. 3.85 Misplaced surgical gastrostomy for venting gastrostomy after repair of perforated duodenal ulcer with residual fluid collection adjacent to the stomach (*asterisk*). The gastrostomy balloon catheter (*white arrow*) is submucosal within the gastric wall, where this is high-density hematoma (*black arrow*)

3.7.2.3 Postoperative Imaging and Complications

Where duodenal ulcer perforation is repaired without resection, postoperative imaging is often unremarkable. Distortion of the duodenum is expected on postoperative contrast studies, but these are not performed routinely, being reserved for patients in whom there is concern for ongoing leak which is confirmed by extravasation of contrast. Since perforations are anterior, it is important to "test" the anterior wall of the duodenum. This cannot be achieved in a supine position. Therefore, a right decubitus position allows filling of the duodenum with contrast from the stomach, distension of the duodenum, and evaluation of the anterior wall. Alternatively, contrast-enhanced CT with positive oral contrast may be preferred, particularly where there is concern for undrained sepsis as well as leak, in order to plan intervention such as image-guided drainage. This may detect other unexpected complications related to the procedure (Fig. 3.85). Fluoroscopy may also be used to assess other complications including abdominal fistula (Fig. 3.86).

Likewise, repeat imaging in patients with duodenal ulcer bleeding is reserved for rebleeding or suspicion of other complications. In this setting, investigation will depend on the severity of bleeding and clinical status of the patient, with options ranging from endoscopy with hemostatic techniques, to angiography and embolization to repeat laparotomy. The choice will depend on local expertise, but endovascular techniques are attractive, particularly in patients with significant comorbidity. IV contrast-enhanced CT is only likely to be useful in the setting of ongoing bleeding where endoscopy is negative. Its role is then to search for an occult second source of hemorrhage, as rebleed of the duodenal ulcer is always the most likely cause and should be excluded in the first instance. It is essential to withhold positive oral contrast in such cases, as this will mask the site of hemorrhage.

3.7.3 Duodenal Obstruction and Palliation

3.7.3.1 Stent Versus Surgery

The duodenum and gastric outlet may become obstructed by tumors of the duodenum and antrum or by invasion from adjacent organs (particularly pancreas). While curative resection of the primary tumor is preferable (where it is not locally advanced and there is no metastatic disease), surgical bypass with gastrojejunostomy may be performed for palliation (Sect. 3.4.2.7). However, there is growing evidence for nonsurgical management of such

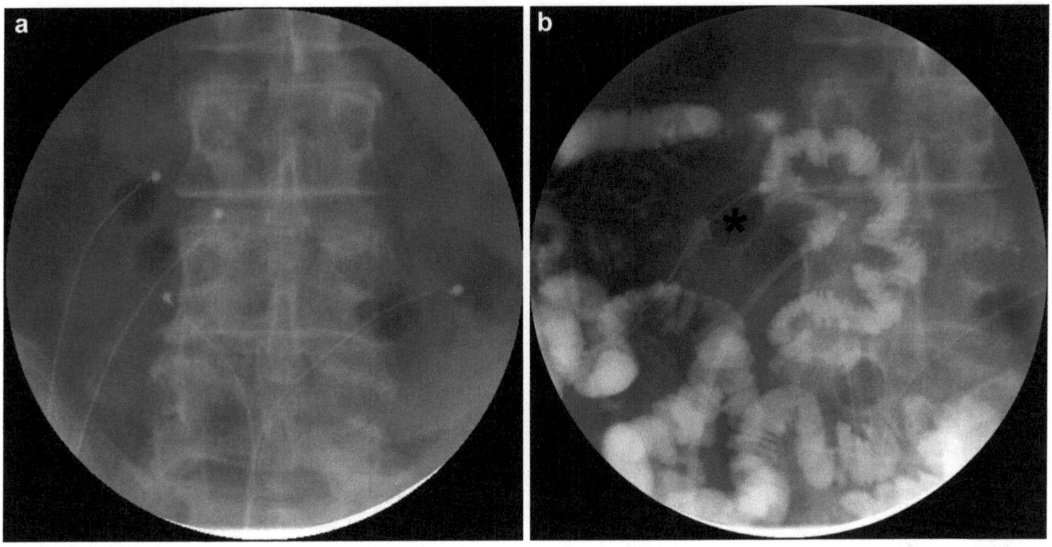

Fig. 3.86 Abdominal wall dehiscence following surgery for perforated duodenal ulcer with fistula from four sites. (**a**) Catheters have been placed in all of the cutaneous openings. (**b**) Contrast subsequently injected shows small bowel filling and no signs of distal obstruction. Management can consist of bowel rest with TPN or enteral feeding via a tube in the most distal fistula (*asterisk*)

cases with gastroduodenal stent placement. This combines a high technical success rate (>95%) with shorter hospital stay and low early complication rate (Lowe et al. 2007; Mehta et al. 2006). However, recurrent symptoms and reintervention (for stent occlusion) are more common than gastrojejunostomy, leading some authors to propose stent placement where life expectancy is short and gastrojejunostomy where life expectancy is greater than 2 months (Jeurnink et al. 2010).

Complications of stent placement mirror those in other parts of the GI tract and include migration, perforation, and occlusion (tumor ingrowth or food impaction). The incidence of such complications varies greatly between series (e.g., 8% vs. 33% for stent occlusion) (Lowe et al. 2007; Jeurnink et al. 2010), but there is little doubt that stents have an important place in the palliation of malignant gastric outlet obstruction.

3.7.3.2 Imaging

Imaging is required for stent planning and for follow-up of complications in conjunction with endoscopy. Careful planning is required particularly where there is a risk of biliary obstruction by tumor, since duodenal stent placement across the ampulla will make stent deployment across a low bile duct stricture very difficult and probably exclude endoscopic access (therefore mandating a percutaneous approach). In this case, it may be appropriate to prophylactically stent the bile duct first and then deploy a duodenal stent so that they are side by side within the duodenum.

Water-soluble contrast studies may be used to assess stent patency and check for migration where symptoms recur in order to plan reintervention (Fig. 3.87).

3.8 Teaching Points

- There are a large number of gastric reconstructions for surgery for benign and malignant indications – these share similar complications including leak, obstruction, and structure. Radiologists should be familiar with these operations to allow accurate interpretation.
- Bariatric surgery is gaining popularity, and radiologists need to be aware of the full range of operations and specific complications that may arise in this challenging patient cohort.
- Contrast studies may be required for the preoperative workup of patients to determine the form of previous surgery in patients requiring revision of bariatric, reflux, or ulcer operations where previous medical records have been lost.

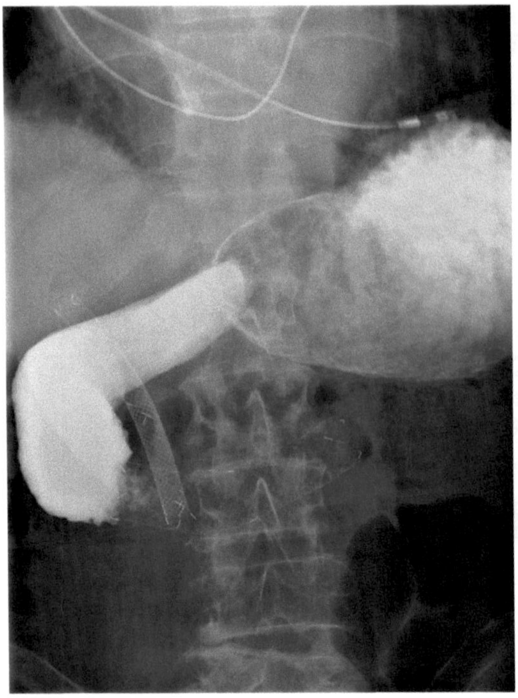

Fig. 3.87 Duodenal stent occlusion. Gradual increase in nausea 7 months following biliary and duodenal stenting for inoperable ampulla of Vater tumor due to cardiac morbidity. Despite a 20-min delay, the stomach remains distended, and no contrast passes through the duodenal stent due to tumor ingrowth at the proximal end

- Duodenal stump leak, internal hernia, and obstruction of the biliopancreatic limb are difficult to diagnose on contrast studies. CT is superior where this is clinically suspected.
- Radiological interventions to the stomach and duodenum, such as adjustment of laparoscopic gastric bands, insertion of gastrostomy or stent placement, as well as image-guided drainage, all form an essential part of modern patient management.

References

Abe N, Takeuchi H, Yanagida O, Sugiyama M, Atomi Y. Surgical indications and procedures for bleeding peptic ulcer. Dig Endosc. 2010;22 Suppl 1:S35–7.

Ahn HS, Kim JW, Yoo MW, Park do J, Lee HJ, Lee KU, Yang HK. Clinicopathological features and surgical outcomes of patients with remnant gastric cancer after a distal gastrectomy. Ann Surg Oncol. 2008;15:1632–9.

Al-Sarireh B, Ghaneh P, Gardner-Thorpe J, Raraty M, Hartley M, Sutton R, Neoptolemos JP. Complications and follow-up after pancreas-preserving total duodenectomy for duodenal polyps. Br J Surg. 2008; 95:1506–11.

Anjiki H, Kamisawa T, Sanaka M, Ishii T, Kuyama Y. Endoscopic hemostasis techniques for upper gastrointestinal hemorrhage: a review. World J Gastrointest Endosc. 2010;16(2):54–60.

Aoki M, Saka M, Morita S, Fukagawa T, Katai H. Afferent loop obstruction after distal gastrectomy with Roux-en-Y reconstruction. World J Surg. 2010;34: 2389–92.

Blachar A, Blank A, Gavert N, Metzer U, Fluser G, Abu-Abeid S. Laparoscopic adjustable gastric banding surgery for morbid obesity: imaging of normal anatomic features and postoperative gastrointestinal complications. AJR Am J Roentgenol. 2007;188:472–9.

Blachar A, Federle MP, Pealer KM, Ikramuddin S, Schauer PR. Gastrointestinal complications of laparoscopic Roux-en-Y gastric bypass surgery: clinical and imaging findings. Radiology. 2002;223:625–32.

Burhenne LJ, Fratkin LB, Flak B, Burhenne HJ. Radiology of the Angelchik prosthesis for gastroesophageal reflux. AJR Am J Roentgenol. 1984;142:507–11.

Canon CL, Morgan DE, Einstein DM, Herts BR, Hawn MT, Johnson LF. Surgical approach to gastroesophageal reflux disease: what the radiologist needs to know. Radiographics. 2005;25:1485–99.

Cleator IG, Holubitsky IB, Harrison RC. Anastomotic ulceration. Ann Surg. 1974;179:339–51.

Cuschieri A. Postvagotomy diarrhoea: is there a place for surgical management? Gut. 1990;31:245–6.

Dallemagne B, Kohnen L, Perretta S, Weerts J, Markiewicz S, Jehaes C. Laparoscopic repair of paraesophageal hernia. Long-term follow-up reveals good clinical outcome despite high radiological recurrence rate. Ann Surg. 2011;253:291–6.

de Castro SM, van Eijck CH, Rutten JP, Dejong CH, van Goor H, Busch OR, Gouma DJ. Pancreas-preserving total duodenectomy versus standard pancreatoduodenectomy for patients with familial adenomatous polyposis and polyps in the duodenum. Br J Surg. 2008;95:1380–6.

Fukagawa T, Gotoda T, Oda I, Deguchi Y, Saka M, Morita S, Katai H. Stenosis of esophago-jejuno anastomosis after gastric surgery. World J Surg. 2010;34: 1859–63.

Furnée EJ, Draaisma WA, Gooszen HG, Hazebroek EJ, Smout AJ, Broeders IA. Tailored or routine addition of an antireflux fundoplication in laparoscopic large hiatal hernia repair: a comparative cohort study. World J Surg. 2011;35:78–84.

Gayer G, Barsuk D, Hertz M, Apter S, Zissin R. CT diagnosis of afferent loop syndrome. Clin Radiol. 2002; 57:835–9.

Goh BK, Chow PK, Chok AY, Chan WH, Chung YF, Ong HS, Wong WK. Impact of the introduction of laparoscopic wedge resection as a surgical option for suspected small/medium-sized gastrointestinal

stromal tumors of the stomach on perioperative and oncologic outcomes. World J Surg. 2010;34: 1847–52.
Hainaux B, Sattari A, Coppens E, Sadeghi N, Cadière GB. Intrathoracic migration of the wrap after laparoscopic Nissen fundoplication: radiologic evaluation. AJR Am J Roentgenol. 2002;178:859–62.
Hatfield M, Shapir J. The radiologic manifestations of failed antireflux operations. AJR Am J Roentgenol. 1985;144:1209–14.
Hejazi RA, Patil H, McCallum RW. Dumping syndrome: establishing criteria for diagnosis and identifying new etiologies. Dig Dis Sci. 2010;55:117–23.
Hong X, Choi H, Loyer EM, Benjamin RS, Trent JC, Charnsangavej C. Gastrointestinal stromal tumor: role of CT in diagnosis and in response evaluation and surveillance after treatment with imatinib. Radiographics. 2006;26:481–95.
Hsu PI, Lin XZ, Chan SH, Lin CY, Chang TT, Shin JS, Hsu LY, Yang CC, Chen KW. Bleeding peptic ulcer-risk factors for rebleeding and sequential changes in endoscopic findings. Gut. 1994;35:746–9.
Jeurnink SM, Steyerberg EW, van Hooft JE, van Eijck CH, Schwartz MP, Vleggaar FP, Kuipers EJ, Siersema PD, Dutch SUSTENT Study Group. Surgical gastrojejunostomy or endoscopic stent placement for the palliation of malignant gastric outlet obstruction (SUSTENT study): a multicenter randomized trial. Gastrointest Endosc. 2010;71:490–9.
Jha S, Levine MS, Rubesin SE, Dumon K, Kochman ML, Laufer I, Williams NN. Detection of strictures on upper gastrointestinal tract radiographic examinations after laparoscopic Roux-en-Y gastric bypass surgery: importance of projection. AJR Am J Roentgenol. 2006;186:1090–3.
Johnston D, Dachtler J, Sue-Ling HM, King RF, Martin G. The Magenstrasse and Mill operation for morbid obesity. Obes Surg. 2003;13:10–6.
Jordan Jr PH, Thornby J. Perforated pyloroduodenal ulcers. Long-term results with omental patch closure and parietal cell vagotomy. Ann Surg. 1995;221:479–86.
Kim CG, Choi IJ, Lee JY, Cho SJ, Lee JH, Ryu KW, Park SR, Bae JM, Kim YW. Effective diameter of balloon dilation for benign esophagojejunal anastomotic stricture after total gastrectomy. Surg Endosc. 2009;23:1775–80.
Kim KW, Choi BI, Han JK, Kim TK, Kim AY, Lee HJ, Kim YH, Choi JI, Do KH, Kim HC, Lee MW. Postoperative anatomic and pathologic findings at CT following gastrectomy. Radiographics. 2002;22:323–36.
Kwak JM, Kim J, Suh SO. Anterograde jejunojejunal intussusception resulted in acute efferent loop syndrome after subtotal gastrectomy. World J Gastroenterol. 2010;16:3472–4.
Laasch HU, Wilbraham L, Bullen K, Marriott A, Lawrance JA, Johnson RJ, Lee SH, England RE, Gamble GE, Martin DF. Gastrostomy insertion: comparing the options – PEG, RIG or PIG? Clin Radiol. 2003;58:398–405.
Lamb PJ, Griffin SM, Chandrashekar MV, Richardson DL, Karat D, Hayes N. Prospective study of routine contrast radiology after total gastrectomy. Br J Surg. 2004;91:1015–9.
Lee HH, Hur H, Jung H, Park CH, Jeon HM, Song KY. Laparoscopic wedge resection for gastric submucosal tumors: a size-location matched case-control study. J Am Coll Surg. 2011;212:195–9.
Li XB, Lu H, Chen HM, Chen XY, Ge ZZ. Role of bile reflux and Helicobacter pylori infection on inflammation of gastric remnant after distal gastrectomy. J Dig Dis. 2008;9:208–12.
Louie BE, Blitz M, Farivar AS, Orlina J, Aye RW. Repair of symptomatic giant paraesophageal hernias in elderly (>70 years) patients results in improved quality of life. J Gastrointest Surg. 2011;15(3):389–96.
Lowe AS, Beckett CG, Jowett S, May J, Stephenson S, Scally A, Tam E, Kay CL. Self-expandable metal stent placement for the palliation of malignant gastroduodenal obstruction: experience in a large, single, UK centre. Clin Radiol. 2007;62:738–44.
Macintyre IM, Millar A, Smith AN, Small WP. Highly selective vagotomy 5–15 years on. Br J Surg. 1990;77:65.
Mehanna MJ, Birjawi G, Moukaddam HA, Khoury G, Hussein M, Al-Kutoubi A. Complications of adjustable gastric banding, a radiological pictorial review. AJR Am J Roentgenol. 2006;186:522–34.
Mehta S, Hindmarsh A, Cheong E, Cockburn J, Saada J, Tighe R, Lewis MP, Rhodes M. Prospective randomized trial of laparoscopic gastrojejunostomy versus duodenal stenting for malignant gastric outflow obstruction. Surg Endosc. 2006;20:239–42.
Mezhir JJ, Gonen M, Ammori JB, Strong VE, Brennan MF, Coit DG. Treatment and outcome of patients with gastric remnant cancer after resection for peptic ulcer disease. Ann Surg Oncol. 2011;18:670–6.
Mine S, Sano T, Tsutsumi K, Murakami Y, Ehara K, Saka M, Hara K, Fukagawa T, Udagawa H, Katai H. Large-scale investigation into dumping syndrome after gastrectomy for gastric cancer. J Am Coll Surg. 2010; 211:628–36.
Mitiek MO, Andrade RS. Giant hiatal hernia. Ann Thorac Surg. 2010;89:S2168–73.
Mortelé KJ, Pattijn P, Mollet P, Berrevoet F, Hesse U, Ceelen W, Ros PR. The Swedish laparoscopic adjustable gastric banding for morbid obesity: radiologic findings in 218 patients. AJR Am J Roentgenol. 2001; 177:77–84.
Müller MW, Dahmen R, Köninger J, Michalski CW, Hinz U, Hartel M, Kadmon M, Kleeff J, Büchler MW, Friess H. Is there an advantage in performing a pancreas-preserving total duodenectomy in duodenal adenomatosis? Am J Surg. 2008;195:741–8.
Orringer MB, Skinner DB, Belsey RHR. Long-term results of the Mark IV operation for hiatal hernia and analysis of recurrences and their treatment. J Thorac Cardiovasc Surg. 1972;63:25–31.
Pedrazzani C, Marrelli D, Rampone B, De Stefano A, Corso G, Fotia G, Pinto E, Roviello F. Postoperative complications and functional results after subtotal gastrectomy with Billroth II reconstruction for primary gastric cancer. Dig Dis Sci. 2007;52:1757–63.

Penninga L, Svendsen LB. Pancreas-preserving total duodenectomy: a 10-year experience. J Hepatobiliary Pancreat Sci. 2011;18:717–23.

Quigley S, Colledge J, Mukerjee S, Patel K. Bariatric surgery: a review of normal postoperative anatomy and complications. Clin Radiol. 2011;66(10):903–14.

Reyelt Jr WP, Anderson AA. Retrograde jejunogastric intussusception. Surg Gynecol Obstet. 1964;119:1305–11.

Scheirey CD, Scholz FJ, Shah PC, Brams DM, Wong BB, Pedrosa M. Radiology of the laparoscopic Roux-en-Y gastric bypass procedure: conceptualization and precise interpretation of results. Radiographics. 2006; 26:1355–71.

Sjöström L, Narbro K, Sjöström CD, Karason K, Larsson B, Wedel H, Swedish Obese Subjects Study, et al. Effects of bariatric surgery on mortality in Swedish obese subjects. N Engl J Med. 2007;23(357):741–52.

Smith C, Deziel DJ, Kubicka RA. Evaluation of the postoperative stomach and duodenum. Radiographics. 1994;14:67–86.

Smith C, Gardiner R, Kubicka RA, Dieschbourg JJ. Gastric restrictive surgery for obesity: early radiologic evaluation. Radiology. 1984;153:321–7.

Takahashi T, Yamashiro M, Hashimoto H, Noro T, Hino Y, Hirashima T, Kino K, Takubo K. Stomal stenosis following gastrectomy in the elderly. Nihon Ronen Igakkai Zasshi. 1992;29:758–64.

Thoeni RF, Moss AA. The radiographic appearance of complications following Nissen fundoplication. Radiology. 1979;131:17–21.

Trenkner SW. Imaging of morbid obesity procedures and their complications. Abdom Imaging. 2009;3:335–44.

Tsugawa K, Koyanagi N, Hashizume M, Tomikawa M, Akahoshi K, Ayukawa K, Wada H, Tanoue K, Sugimachi K. The therapeutic strategies in performing emergency surgery for gastroduodenal ulcer perforation in 130 patients over 70 years of age. Hepatogastroenterology. 2001;48:156–62.

Ustündag Y, Köseoglu T, Cetin F, Eroglu A, Soran A, Eskioglu E. Self-expandable metallic stent therapy of esophagojejunal stricture in a stapled anastomosis: a case report and review of the literature. Dig Surg. 2001;18:211–3.

Wang YR, Richter JE, Dempsey DT. Trends and outcomes of hospitalizations for peptic ulcer disease in the United States, 1993 to 2006. Ann Surg. 2010;251:51–8.

Watson DI. Evolution and development of surgery for large paraesophageal hiatus hernia. World J Surg. 2011;35:1436–41.

Wehrli NE, Levine MS, Rubesin SE, Katzka DA, Laufer I. Secondary achalasia and other esophageal motility disorders after laparoscopic Nissen fundoplication for gastroesophageal reflux disease. AJR Am J Roentgenol. 2007;189:1464–8.

Wiesner W, Schöb O, Hauser RS, Hauser M. Adjustable laparoscopic gastric banding in patients with morbid obesity: radiographic management, results, and postoperative complications. Radiology. 2000;216: 389–94.

Yu J, Turner MA, Cho SR, Fulcher AS, DeMaria EJ, Kellum JM, Sugerman HJ. Normal anatomy and complications after gastric bypass surgery: helical CT findings. Radiology. 2004;231:753–60.

The Pancreas

4

Krishna Menon, John Brittenden, Simon McPherson,
Nikhil M. Bhuskute, and Andrew Smith

Contents

4.1 **Introduction** 128

4.2 **Resections for Pancreatic, Duodenal, and Ampullary Tumors** 128
4.2.1 The Kausch–Whipple Procedure (PD) 128
4.2.2 Pylorus-Preserving Pancreaticoduodenectomy (PPPD) 129
4.2.3 Surgical Modifications of PD 130
4.2.4 Multivisceral Resection for Neuroendocrine Tumors (NETS) of the Pancreas 130
4.2.5 Radical Antegrade Modular Pancreatosplenectomy Surgery (RAMPS) ... 130
4.2.6 Central Pancreatectomy (Pancreas-Preserving Resections) 130

4.3 **Distal Pancreatic Operations** 131

4.4 **Operations for Chronic Pancreatitis** 131
4.4.1 Frey Procedure 132
4.4.2 Beger Procedure 132
4.4.3 Berne Procedure 133
4.4.4 Puestow Procedure 134
4.4.5 Surgical Outcomes in Chronic Pancreatitis 135
4.4.6 Imaging of Complications Following Surgery for Chronic Pancreatitis 136

4.5 **Interventions in Acute Pancreatitis** 136

4.6 **Normal Postoperative Anatomy on CT** 137
4.6.1 CT Appearances of the Anastomoses (PPPD and PD) 137
4.6.2 Postoperative Fluid/Fat Stranding 139
4.6.3 Perivascular Cuffing 139
4.6.4 Reactive Lymphadenopathy 140
4.6.5 Pneumobilia 140
4.6.6 Pancreatic Duct Dilatation 141
4.6.7 Resection Margin 141
4.6.8 Peripancreatic Inflammation 141
4.6.9 Pancreatic Atrophy 142

4.7 **Postoperative Upper GI Contrast Studies** 142

4.8 **Postoperative Complications** 142
4.8.1 Pancreatic Anastomotic Leak 142
4.8.2 Vascular Complications 144
4.8.3 Biliary Obstruction 146
4.8.4 Abscess 147
4.8.5 Acute Pancreatitis 147

4.9 **Enteric Complications** 147
4.9.1 Delayed Gastric Emptying 148
4.9.2 Gastroenterostomy Complications 148
4.9.3 Gastric Outlet and Afferent Roux Loop Obstruction 149
4.9.4 Malabsorption 149

4.10 **Tumor Recurrence** 149

4.11 **Teaching Points** 150

References 151

K. Menon, MS, FRCS
Department of Surgery, Leeds Teaching Hospitals NHS Trust, Bexley Wing, St James's University Hospital, LS9 7JT, Leeds, UK

J. Brittenden, MBChB, MRCP, FRCR (✉)
Department of Radiology, Mid Yorkshire Hospitals NHS Trust, Wakefield, UK
e-mail: john.brittenden@midyorks.nhs.uk

S. McPherson, MRCP, FRCR, BSc
Department of Radiology, Leeds General Infirmary, Leeds Teaching Hospitals NHS Trust, Leeds, UK

N.M. Bhuskute, MBBS, MS, MRCS, FRCR
Department of Radiology, Calderdale and Huddersfield NHS Foundation Trust, Huddersfield, UK

A. Smith, MBBS, DM, FRCS, BSc
Department of Surgery, Leeds Teaching Hospitals NHS Trust, Bexley Wing, St James's University Hospital, Leeds, UK

J. Brittenden, D.J.M. Tolan (eds.), *Radiology of the Post Surgical Abdomen*,
DOI 10.1007/978-1-4471-2775-8_4, © Springer-Verlag London 2012

4.1 Introduction

The complexity of pancreatic surgery along with technical variations in the types of anastomoses makes accurate understanding of normal postoperative appearances and complications imperative to avoid misdiagnosis. Mortality from surgery has significantly reduced as a result of modern interventional radiology techniques to promptly deal with complications such as hemorrhage and intra-abdominal sepsis resulting from pancreatic anastomotic leak (Zink et al. 2009). Interventional radiology is also increasingly utilized in the management of complications resulting from acute pancreatitis (Connor et al. 2005).

Pancreatic surgery is indicated in the treatment of malignancy and intractable chronic pancreatitis. Mortality rates from pancreatic cancer are dismal with pancreatic resection offering increased survival rates and the best chance of cure (Wagner et al. 2004).

The following resections are performed in the management of malignancy:

- Pancreaticoduodenectomy (PD)
- Pylorus-preserving pancreaticoduodenectomy (PPPD)
- Central pancreatectomy
- Distal pancreatectomy
- Total pancreatectomy

Surgery for chronic pancreatitis involves resection of inflamed pancreatic tissue and improvement of pancreatic ductal drainage. Procedures include:

- Puestow – pancreaticojejunostomy
- Beger – pancreatic head resection with preservation of the duodenum
- Frey – partial resection of the pancreatic head with a longitudinal pancreaticojejunostomy
- Berne – duodenum-preserving head resection

4.2 Resections for Pancreatic, Duodenal, and Ampullary Tumors

4.2.1 The Kausch-Whipple Procedure (PD)

This is indicated for benign and malignant disease involving the pancreatic head including:

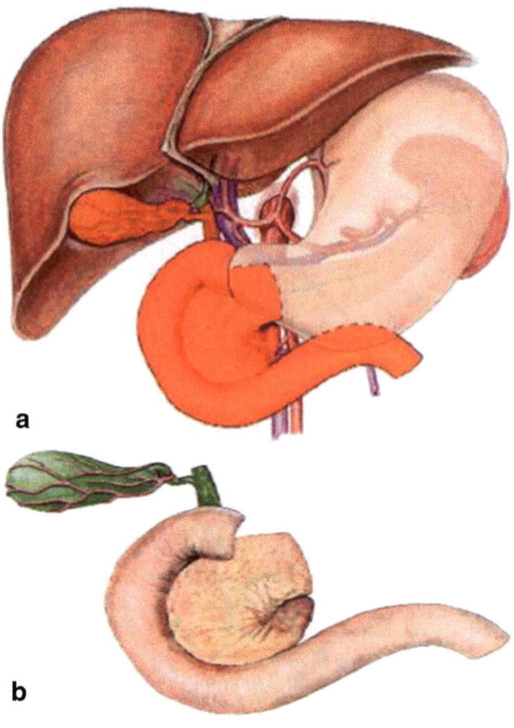

Fig. 4.1 Pancreaticoduodenectomy. (**a**) The following structures are resected (*colored orange*): (1) pancreatic head, neck, and uncinate process; (2) duodenum, pylorus, and gastric antrum; (3) gallbladder and distal common bile duct; and (4) pancreatic and peripancreatic draining lymph nodes. (**b**) Resected specimen. In a pylorus-preserving pancreaticoduodenectomy (PPPD), the gastric antrum and pylorus are preserved

- Solid pancreatic tumors (e.g., pancreatic adenocarcinoma)
- Cystic tumors (e.g., mucinous cystic neoplasms and intraductal papillary mucinous neoplasms [IPMN])
- Cholangiocarcinoma of the distal common bile duct
- Neuroendocrine carcinomas (functioning and nonfunctioning)
- Chronic pancreatitis involving the head and uncinate process
- Duodenal neoplasms
- Ampullary tumors

The most common pancreatic resection procedure is the pancreaticoduodenectomy (PD) or Kausch–Whipple procedure (pioneered by Walter Kausch and Allen Whipple) (Whipple et al. 1935).

PD involves resection of the following structures (Fig. 4.1):

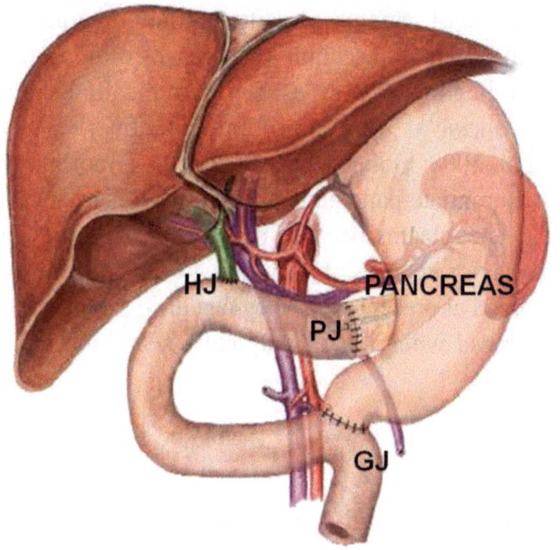

Fig. 4.2 *Line drawing* illustrating the three anastomoses used in a standard PPPD. Pancreaticojejunostomy (*PJ*), hepaticojejunostomy (*HJ*), and gastrojejunostomy (*GJ*). Note how the anastomoses are formed using a jejunal loop which is different from a Roux-en-Y small bowel loop (Fig. 4.3)

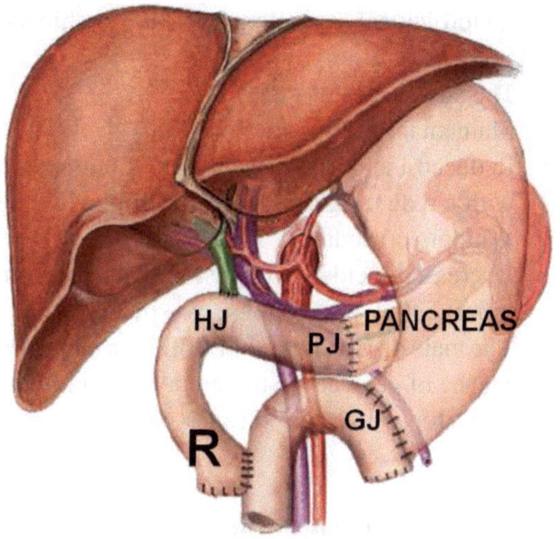

Fig. 4.3 Whipple procedure with the use of a Roux loop to fashion two of the three anastomoses. Pancreaticoduodenectomy (pylorus-resected) with use of a separate Roux-en-Y loop to fashion the pancreatic and biliary anastomoses. The gastroenterostomy is anastomosed to the proximal jejunum which is anastomosed to the Roux loop distally by a side-to-side enteroenterostomy. Pancreaticojejunostomy (*PJ*), hepaticojejunostomy (*HJ*), gastrojejunostomy (*GJ*), and Roux loop (*R*)

- Pancreatic head, neck, and uncinate process.
- Duodenum, pylorus, and gastric antrum.
- Gall bladder.
- Distal common bile duct.
- Pancreatic and peripancreatic draining lymph nodes (i.e., standard lymphadenectomy) (Pedrazzoli et al. 1998).
- Three anastomoses are formed to create drainage channels for pancreatic secretions, bile, and gastric contents in the form of pancreaticojejunostomy, hepatico/choledochojejunostomy, and gastrojejunostomy, respectively. The choledochojejunostomy is an end-to-side anastomosis. The gastrojejunostomy can be antecolic or retrocolic and is situated on the posterior wall of the stomach near the greater curve.
- The pancreatic and biliary anastomoses are hand sewn and therefore are difficult to visualize on CT. The gastrojejunostomy may be fashioned with a staple gun, and therefore, the anastomosis can be seen on CT.
- Reconstructions are fashioned on a single loop of jejunum which is positioned in the right upper quadrant. The jejunal loop is anastomosed proximally to the pancreas, then to the biliary tree, and finally to the stomach (Fig. 4.2).
- Use of a separate Roux-en-Y loop has also been practiced with the pancreatic and/or biliary anastomoses anastomosed to the Roux loop. The gastroenterostomy is anastomosed to the proximal jejunum which is anastomosed to the Roux loop distally via a side-to-side enteroenterostomy (Fig. 4.3).
- Occasionally, a stent is placed within the pancreatic duct to protect the anastomosis. This may extend from the duct through the anastomosis and out through the anterior abdominal wall. Alternatively, a short stent may be placed across the anastomosis.
- Surgical variations include anastomosis of the pancreas to the posterior wall of the stomach (pancreaticogastrostomy) (Smith et al. 2008).

4.2.2 Pylorus-Preserving Pancreaticoduodenectomy (PPPD)

This is a variation of the classic Whipple procedure in which the entire stomach is preserved and a pylorojejunal anastomosis is fashioned (Fig. 4.2).

The advantages of PPPD are:

- Maintenance of pyloric function
- Reduced incidence of weight loss (compared with a reduced gastric reservoir following the Whipple procedure)
- Decreased incidence of gastric irritation from biliary reflux (due to preserved pylorus)

The main disadvantage of PPPD is an increased incidence of delayed gastric emptying within the early postoperative period (Sect. 4.9.1).

4.2.3 Surgical Modifications of PD

Extended lymphadenectomy in conjunction with PD has been attempted to improve long-term survival in patients with pancreatic malignancy. However, studies have not demonstrated any benefit and this is now less commonly performed (Pedrazzoli et al. 1998). Isolated tumor involvement of the portal vein, portal confluence, or superior mesenteric vein is not an absolute contraindication to surgery as vascular resection and reconstruction may be performed using venous grafts (Harrison et al. 1996). Tumor involvement of venous structures is not associated with adverse outcome, but invasion into major arterial structures (e.g., the superior mesenteric artery) is a contraindication to surgery.

4.2.4 Multivisceral Resection for Neuroendocrine Tumors (NETS) of the Pancreas

Functioning NETs of the pancreas (insulinomas, gastrinomas, glucagonomas, VIPomas, somatostatinomas) can present with metastatic disease to the liver and require resection of the primary tumor (PD, distal pancreatectomy, or enucleation) as well as concomitant liver resection (either synchronously or as a staged procedure). Nonfunctioning NETs of the pancreas encompass a group of patients who often require aggressive multivisceral resection (pancreas, colon, small bowel, adrenal, liver) as they are typically locally advanced at the time of presentation (Bonney et al. 2008; Gomez et al. 2007). It is important to differentiate pancreatic NETs from other pancreatic neoplasms because despite their aggressive behavior in terms of local invasion and metastatic spread at presentation, they can have a prolonged survival when treated surgically (Fendrich et al. 2006).

4.2.5 Radical Antegrade Modular Pancreatosplenectomy Surgery (RAMPS)

RAMPS is a new technique that encompasses a more radical resection of N1 nodes and improves the posterior extent of the resection margin coupled with early rather than late control of the vasculature (Strasberg et al. 2003). RAMPS procedure can achieve negative tangential margins in a high percent of patients with resectable carcinoma of the body and tail of the pancreas.

4.2.6 Central Pancreatectomy (Pancreas-Preserving Resections)

These resections are reserved for tumors of low-grade malignant potential (mucinous cystic neoplasms, small neuroendocrine tumors, and IPMN). The operation involves removal of the central pancreas (neck and medial body) with over sewing of the medial neck margin and drainage of the remnant distal pancreas into a Roux loop (Fig. 4.4). Extended central pancreatectomy for appropriate pancreatic neoplasms is associated with less perioperative morbidity and mortality than with classic extended left or right resections (Cataldegirmen et al. 2010).

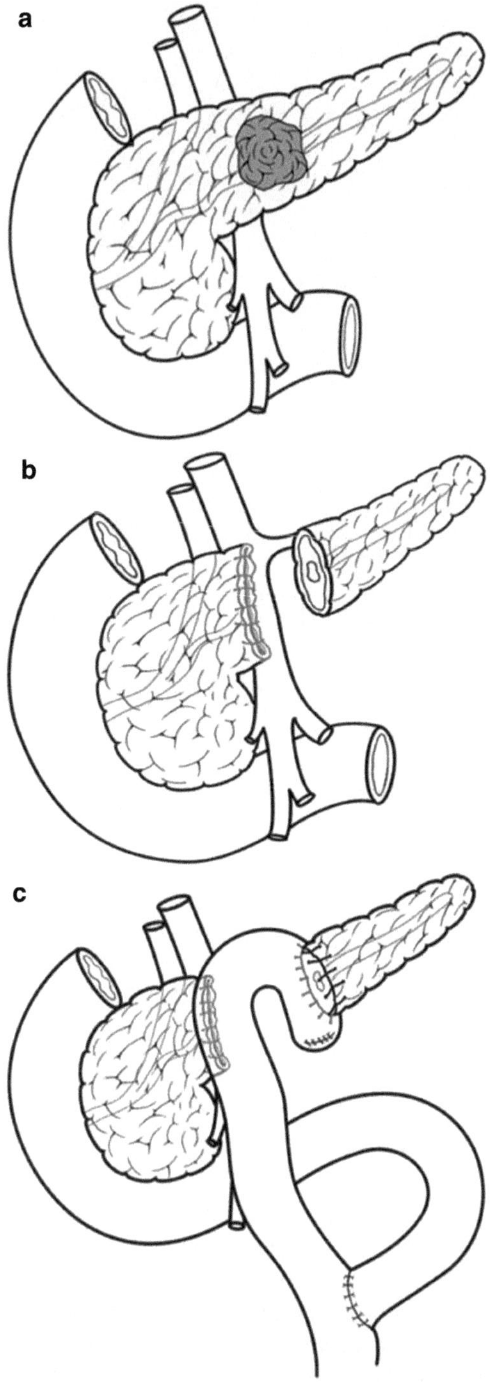

Fig. 4.4 Central pancreatectomy. (**a**) Mid pancreatic body tumor. (**b**) Removal of the central pancreas. (**c**) The distal pancreas drains into a Roux loop. The proximal pancreas is over sewn at the resection margin and drains normally into the duodenum

4.3 Distal Pancreatic Operations

Clinical indications:

- Tumors involving the body and tail of the pancreas
- Chronic pancreatitis predominantly involving the body and tail of the gland
- Pancreatic injury resulting from trauma

Distal pancreatectomy involves resection of the distal pancreas (body and tail) en bloc with the spleen and draining retroperitoneal lymph nodes (Fig. 4.5). The spleen is resected because of the intimate relationship of the pancreas with the splenic vein and artery. The operation may be performed by an open or laparoscopic approach depending on surgical preference (Fahy et al. 2002). More recently, splenic preservation has been performed, particularly for cystic tumors of the body and tail of the pancreas (Ito et al. 2010).

4.4 Operations for Chronic Pancreatitis

Chronic pancreatitis results in atrophy of the gland, strictures of the pancreatic duct, and formation of intraductal calculi that impact on exocrine function. This leads to chronic abdominal pain. Other symptoms result from endocrine and exocrine deficiencies (diabetes and malabsorption). Surgical treatment is reserved for patients with intractable symptoms. Surgical intervention reduces or resolves pain in 70% of patients and prevents further acute episodes of pancreatitis in nearly all (Sandrasegaran et al. 2005). Surgery involves resection of pancreatic tissue and/or drainage of pancreatic secretions via a pancreaticojejunostomy. The choice of surgical procedure will depend on the principle site of disease within the pancreas and on the extent of pancreatic duct dilatation. It is important to note the role of ERCP and endoscopic ultrasound-guided interventions in the management of selection of these patients.

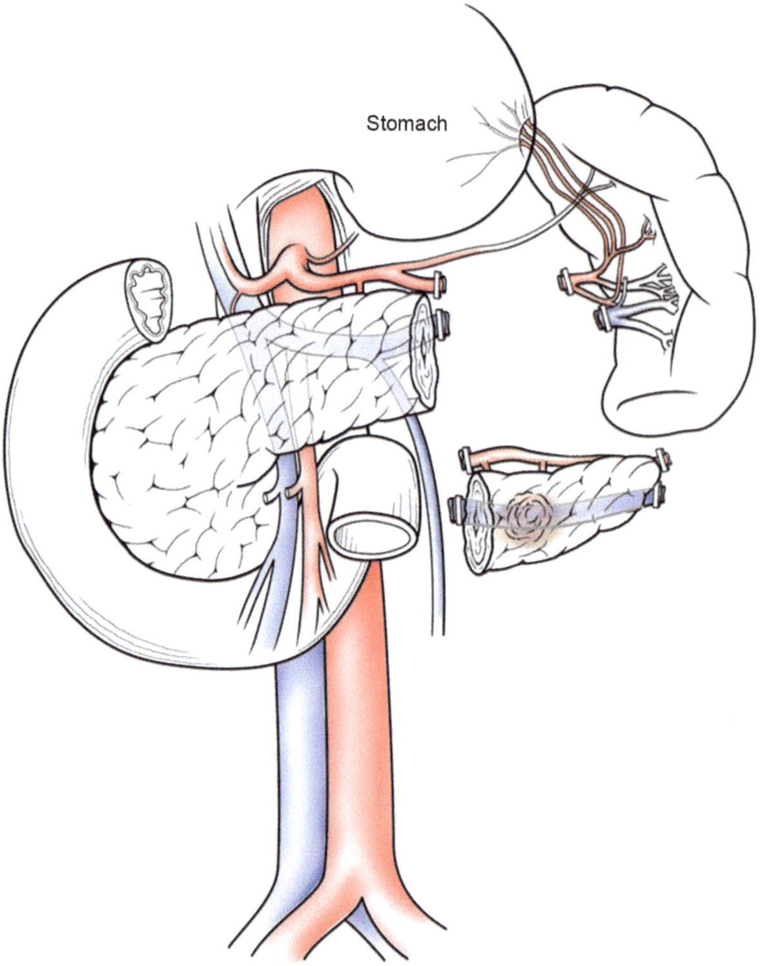

Fig. 4.5 Distal pancreatectomy. Resection of the body and tail along with the spleen and draining lymph nodes

4.4.1 Frey Procedure

The Frey procedure combines partial resection of the pancreatic head with a longitudinal pancreaticojejunostomy created via a Roux loop (Fig. 4.6). This is the preferred treatment option if chronic pancreatitis is confined to the head of the gland with upstream pancreatic duct dilatation. The presence of a duodenal or biliary stricture is a contraindication for this procedure, where a Whipple procedure would be more appropriate (Sandrasegaran et al. 2005).

4.4.2 Beger Procedure

The duodenum-preserving pancreatic head resection (DPPHR) was developed by Beger in the 1970s. The Beger procedure is a less radical surgical option compared with the Whipple procedure. It involves resection of the pancreatic head, neck, and body. A sliver of pancreatic head is left attached to the duodenum to preserve the blood supply of the latter. A pancreaticojejunostomy via a Roux loop is still required for drainage of the distal pancreas (Fig. 4.7).

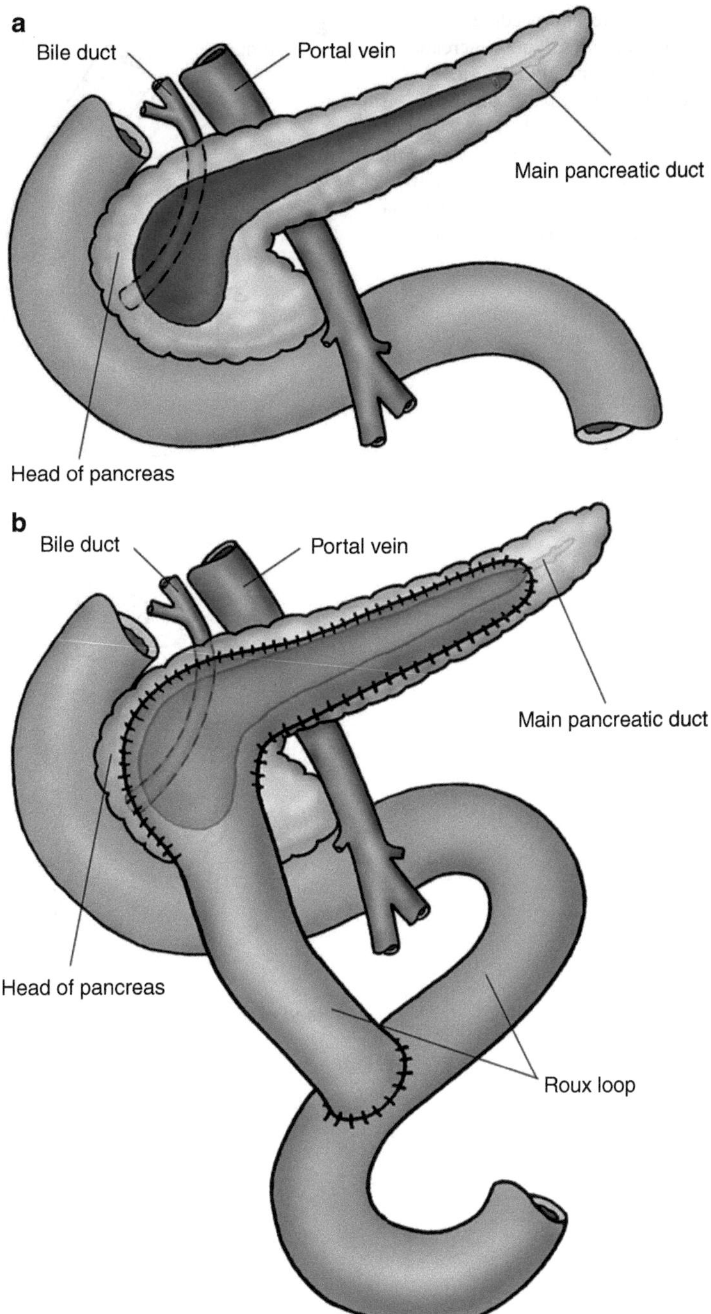

Fig. 4.6 Frey procedure. (**a**) The pancreatic head is cored out. (**b**) Pancreatic ductal drainage via a longitudinal pancreaticojejunostomy (Roux loop)

4.4.3 Berne Procedure

The Berne procedure is a modification of the Beger operation. This involves a duodenum-preserving pancreatic head resection, and a small amount of tissue within the pancreatic head is left in situ (to avoid the hazards of dissecting the pancreas from the portal vein). The cored out head is drained by a pancreaticojejunostomy fashioned from a Roux loop (Fig. 4.8) (Muller et al. 2008).

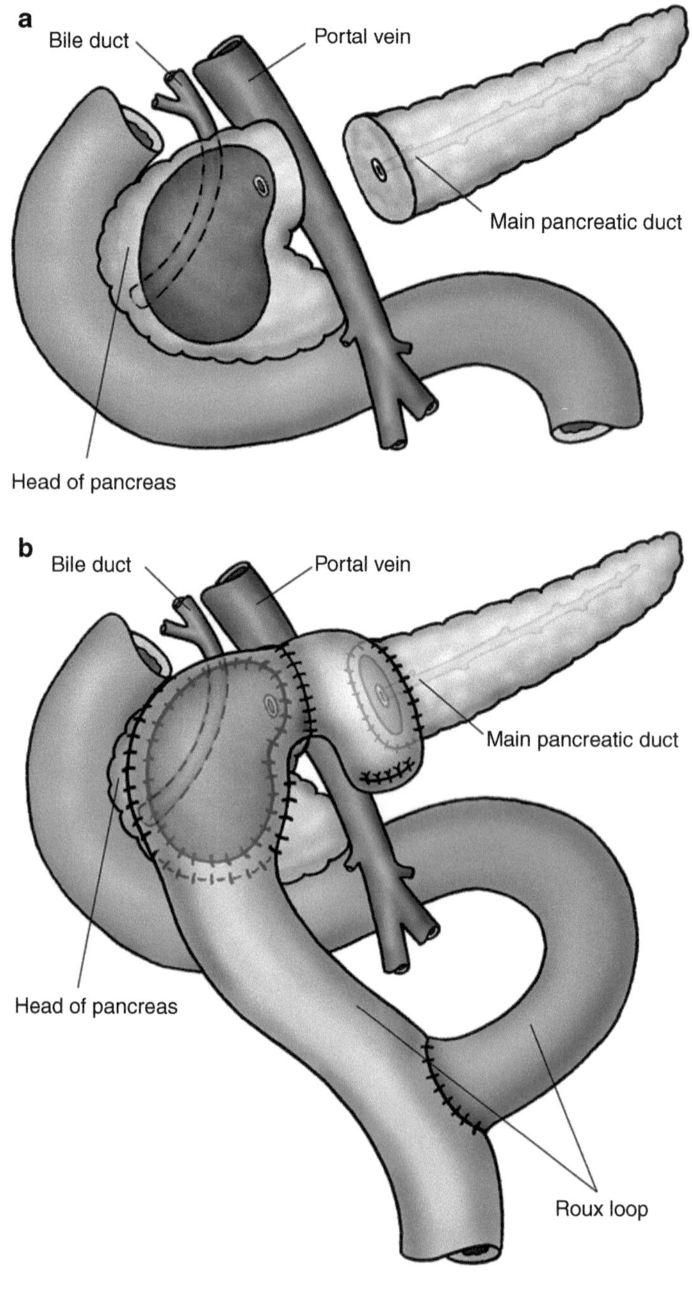

Fig. 4.7 Beger procedure. Duodenum-preserving pancreatic head resection (DPPHR). (**a**) Resection of the pancreatic head, neck, and proximal body. A sliver of pancreatic head is left to preserve the blood supply to the duodenum. (**b**) Distal pancreatic ductal drainage via a pancreaticojejunostomy (Roux loop)

4.4.4 Puestow Procedure

The Puestow procedure (lateral pancreaticojejunostomy) involves filleting of the pancreas to expose the main pancreatic duct from the neck to the tail and removal of any calculi and anastomosis of a side-to-side longitudinal pancreaticojejunostomy. This allows the main pancreatic duct to drain into a loop of jejunum. This procedure is performed on patients without significant disease involving the pancreatic head. The pancreaticojejunostomy Roux loop anastomosis is situated on the anterior surface of the pancreas. This procedure is the preferred choice if the main pancreatic duct is significantly dilated, i.e., ≥7 mm (Terrace et al. 2007). It is less commonly performed than the operations described above.

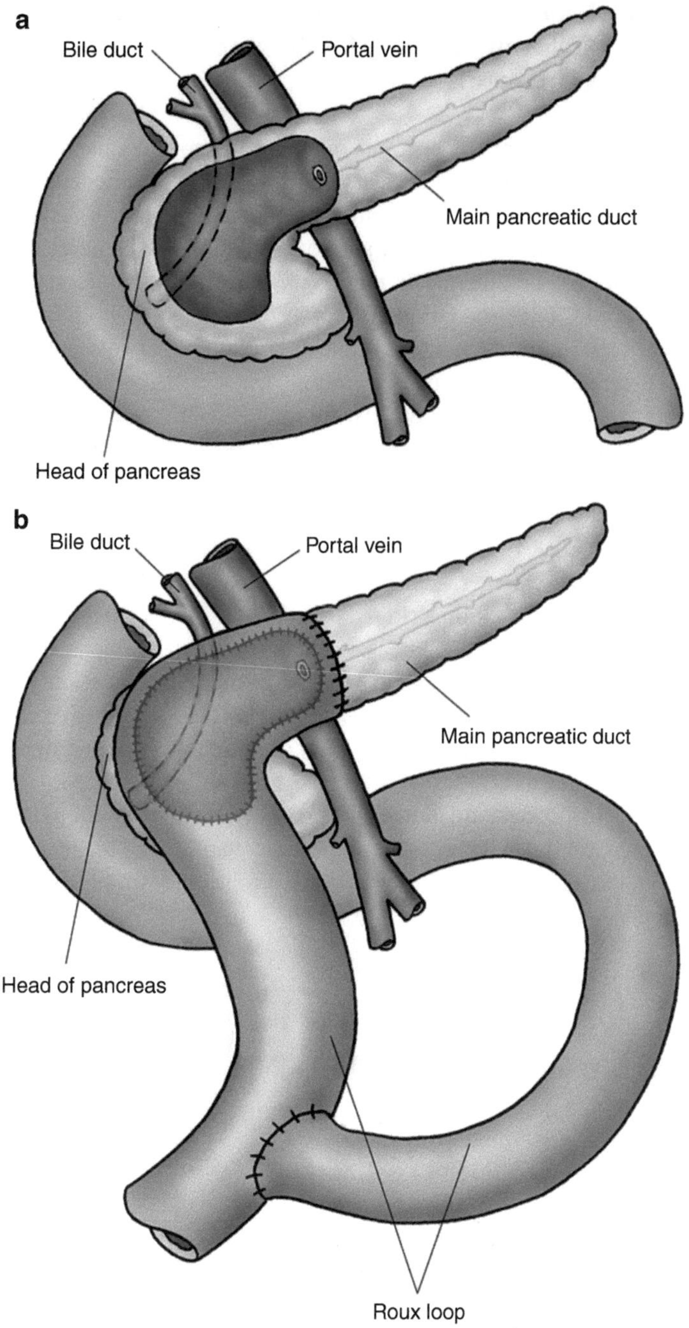

Fig. 4.8 (**a**, **b**) Berne procedure. DDPHR with preservation of a small amount of pancreatic tissue. (**b**) Pancreatic ductal drainage via a pancreaticojejunostomy (Roux loop)

4.4.5 Surgical Outcomes in Chronic Pancreatitis

Studies comparing the Beger and Frey procedures have demonstrated no statistical difference in morbidity, mortality, or endocrine/exocrine function within the two groups (Koninger et al. 2008). A prospective, randomized study to evaluate two variations of the duodenum-preserving pancreatic head resection (DPPHR), Beger procedure versus the Berne procedure, has shown that the Berne technique is technically simpler and shorter and is associated with a reduced hospital stay. Symptomatic improvement was identical in both patient groups (Strate et al. 2005).

4.4.6 Imaging of Complications Following Surgery for Chronic Pancreatitis

A detailed description of postoperative complications on CT is described in Sect. 4.8. It is important to be familiar with normal postoperative anatomy as these procedures are not commonly encountered and there are numerous potential pitfalls in CT interpretation. The procedures are illustrated in Figs. 4.5, 4.6, 4.7, and 4.8.

Potential pitfalls include:

- Puestow – the Roux loop lies within the lesser sac anterior to the pancreatic body and posterior to the stomach. It should not be misdiagnosed as an internal hernia or abdominal mass (Freed et al. 1997). In the other drainage operations (Frey, Beger, and Berne), the Roux loop lies nearer the midline (Fig. 4.9).
- Frey – the resected segment within the pancreatic head can have a cystic appearance due to the accumulation of pancreatic secretions. This should not be mistaken for a pseudocyst or neoplasm.
- Pancreatic duct dilation can persist or even increase by 1–2 mm following surgery but is not associated with an increased risk of acute pancreatitis.

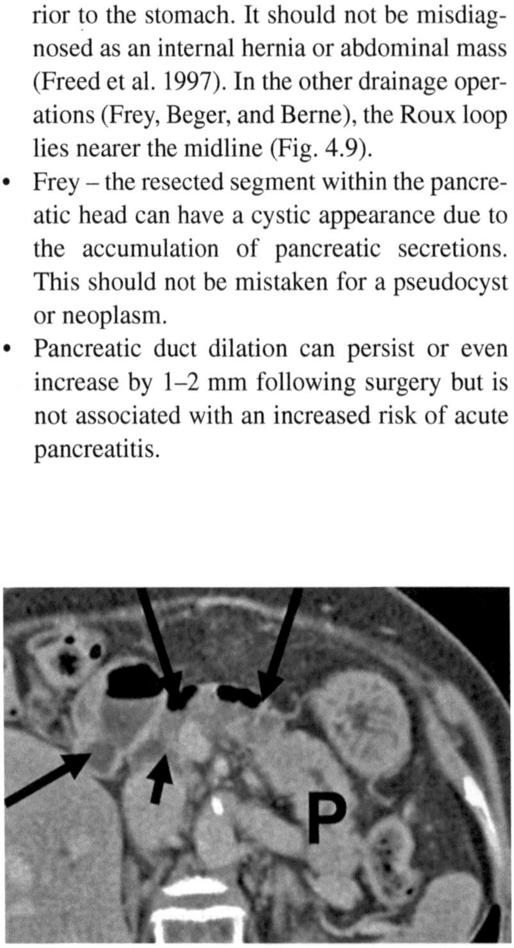

Fig. 4.9 Normal CT anatomy post Frey procedure. Curved axial reformatted CT demonstrates partial resection of the pancreatic head (*short arrow*). Pancreatic ductal drainage is facilitated by a longitudinal pancreaticojejunostomy via a Roux loop (*long arrows*). The duodenum (*black arrow*) is preserved. Residual pancreas (*P*)

4.5 Interventions in Acute Pancreatitis

The majority of patients with acute pancreatitis can be managed conservatively. In patients who clinically deteriorate or who are slow to recover, CT is performed to exclude the following complications:

- Pancreatic necrosis
- Infected fluid collections
- Pseudocyst formation
- Vascular complications

Infected pancreatic necrosis involving the body and tail of the gland can be treated with percutaneous necrosectomy. This can be performed utilizing CT guidance to place a wire within the pancreatic parenchyma (using the Seldinger technique), preferably via a retroperitoneal approach. Following serial dilatation, a 12 French drainage catheter is placed into the pancreatic bed. The surgeon then uses the drain tract to sequentially dilate and introduce a modified nephroscope to perform a necrosectomy under general anesthetic. A large diameter (>20 French) surgical drain is left in situ (Fig. 4.10). Fluid collections are common in patients with severe pancreatitis and may be located anywhere within the abdomen and not limited to the pancreas itself. The majority of collections resolve without any intervention. Suspicion of sepsis is the most common reason to request image-guided drainage. In some cases with multiple loculated collections, CT signs such as heterogeneous density, wall thickening, and enhancement may indicate an infected locule. However, aspiration and drainage of multiple collections is sometimes required.

Pleural effusions are other common sequelae of acute pancreatic inflammation (Fig. 4.11). Pleural effusions are usually reactive and are an issue when large and causing respiratory compromise. Uncommonly pleural effusions are a result of a pancreaticopleural fistula.

Pseudocysts that are infected or are large enough to cause symptoms (e.g., abdominal discomfort or gastric compression) can be drained percutaneously under image guidance or via a cystogastrostomy. This can be fashioned either surgically or endoscopically. The latter is an ideal route for draining large fluid collections within

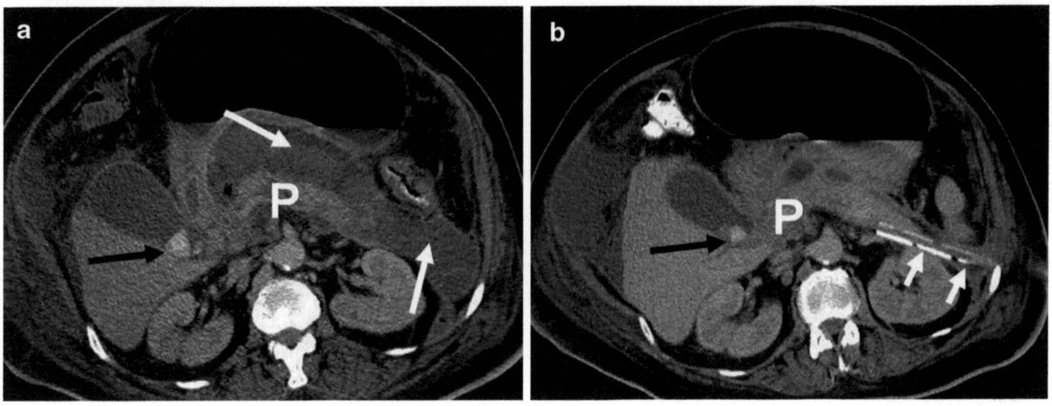

Fig. 4.10 Pancreatic necrosectomy. (**a**) Axial CT in a patient with gallstone pancreatitis who developed sepsis on day 7. There is virtually no normal enhancing pancreatic tissue within the tail of the gland with an associated well-defined peripancreatic fluid collection in keeping with pancreatic necrosis (*white arrows*). Gallstone in gallbladder neck (*black arrow*). A 12F drainage catheter was inserted via a retroperitoneal approach under CT guidance (*not shown*). (**b**) Axial CT 2 days following surgical necrosectomy (using the radiologically placed catheter as a road-map). A 22F surgical drain (*short white arrows*) has been placed in the pancreatic bed with successful drainage of the peripancreatic. Pancreas (*P*)

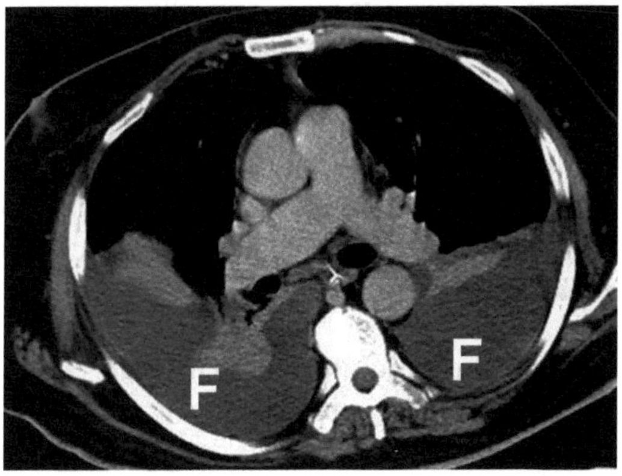

Fig. 4.11 Pleural effusions (*F*) complicating acute severe pancreatitis

the lesser sac. The posterior wall of the stomach is transilluminated, a needle puncture of the stomach is performed, and a short drainage catheter is placed over a wire through the scope into the collection. Some centers use endoscopic ultrasound for guidance rather than endoscopic visualization of the "bulge" in the gastric wall resulting from the pseudocyst. Pancreatic secretions therefore drain into the stomach in a sterile environment allowing the pancreatic duct to heal. Laparoscopic drainage of pseudocysts can be performed in certain cases not suitable for endoscopic or radiological drainage.

4.6 Normal Postoperative Anatomy on CT

CT is the most common imaging modality used in the postoperative period. Upper GI contrast studies are not as sensitive at assessing all the anastomoses and are generally reserved for the evaluation of suspected enteric complications (Sects. 4.7 and 4.9). MRI may be used if there is a history of contrast allergy.

4.6.1 CT Appearances of the Anastomoses (PPPD and PD)

Postoperative imaging involves assessment of the three surgically created anastomoses.

4.6.1.1 Pancreaticojejunostomy

This is normally positioned to the right of the residual pancreatic body and tail and is hand sewn (Figs. 4.12, 4.13, and 4.14). Oral contrast rarely refluxes into the jejunal loop which can make it difficult to visualize the anastomosis. In the immediate postoperative period, the surgical drain across the anastomosis facilitates identification. The pancreas can invaginate into the jejunal loop at the anastomotic site causing a prominent

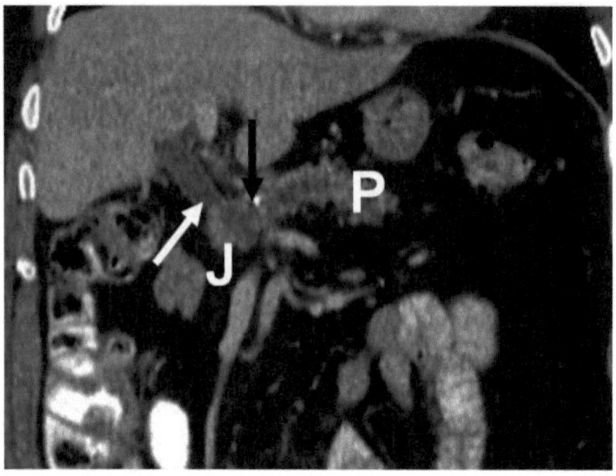

Fig. 4.12 Normal postoperative CT anatomy post Whipple procedure. Coronal CT demonstrating the jejunal loop (*J*) anastomosed to the distal common bile duct. Hepaticojejunostomy (*white arrow*) and pancreaticojejunostomy (*black arrow*). Residual pancreas (*P*). Postoperative dilatation of the pancreatic duct can be a normal finding

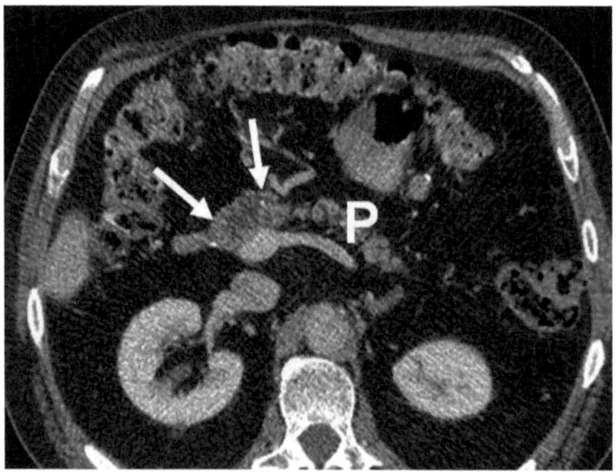

Fig. 4.13 Axial CT showing a normal pancreaticojejunostomy (*white arrows*). This can appear bulky on postoperative cross-sectional imaging and should not be misinterpreted as recurrent tumor. Pancreas (*P*)

bulge which should not be mistaken for tumor recurrence (Bluemke et al. 1997). On follow-up CT, the residual pancreas can atrophy and, therefore, the anastomosis can be hard to see.

4.6.1.2 Hepaticojejunostomy

This anastomosis is also hand sewn but can be identified at the porta hepatis (Fig. 4.15). As it is a nondependent structure, air is often seen with the jejunal loop at this site and within the intrahepatic biliary tree (particularly in the left lobe of the liver).

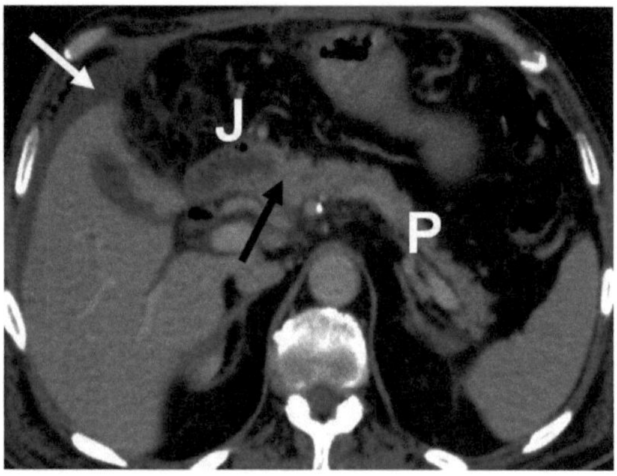

Fig. 4.14 Normal postoperative CT appearances of the pancreaticojejunostomy (*black arrow*) following PPPD. Pancreas (*P*), jejunal loop (*J*). Ascites (*white arrow*), resolved on interval imaging (see Sect. 4.6.2)

4.6.1.3 Pylorojejunostomy (in PPPD)

The pylorojejunostomy is normally positioned antecolic or in some instances retrocolic on the left side of the abdomen. It is almost always hand sewn, and therefore, the suture line is difficult to visualize on CT. It is often in the radiation port site, and therefore, the jejunal loop can appear thick walled following postoperative radiotherapy.

4.6.1.4 Gastrojejunostomy (in PD)

In patients with a gastrojejunostomy, the anastomosis is normally on the left side of the abdomen (Fig. 4.16). Surgical clips at this site and along the gastroduodenal and pancreatic artery arcades can cause artifact, obscuring the surgical bed at the site of the pancreatic head resection. If the anastomosis is performed with a stapler, then it will be identified on CT (but not if hand sewn).

The jejunal loop can have different appearances on CT depending on the presence of edema within the bowel wall (early postoperative period) and fluid and air and oral contrast within the lumen. Unopacified bowel loops, particularly in the region of the pancreaticojejunostomy and hepatico/choledochojejunostomy, can be difficult to differentiate from recurrent tumor on CT. The presence of small air bubbles and valvulae conniventes distinguishes bowel from tumor recurrence (Bluemke et al. 1997). Assessment of

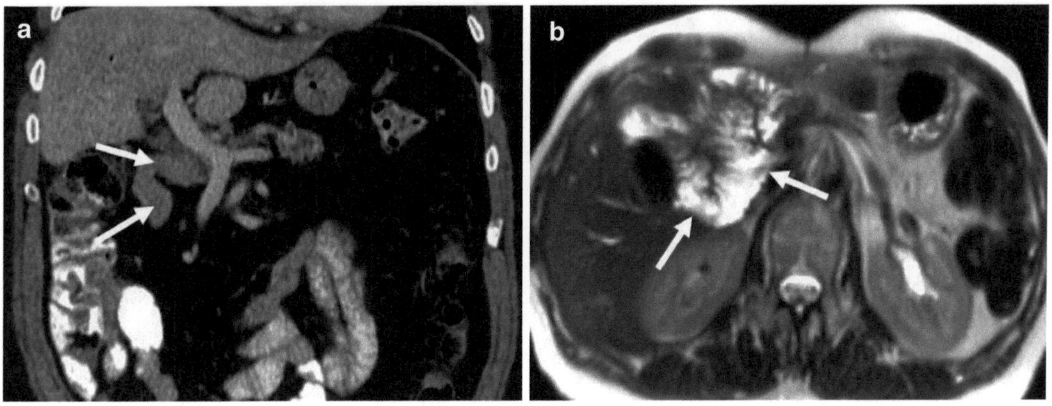

Fig. 4.15 Jejunal loop post PPPD. Appearances on (**a**) coronal CT and (**b**) axial T2WMRI show small bowel (*white arrows*) in the region of the porta hepatis which is used to create an anastomosis to the pancreas (pancreaticojejunostomy) and biliary tree (hepatico/choledochojejunostomy)

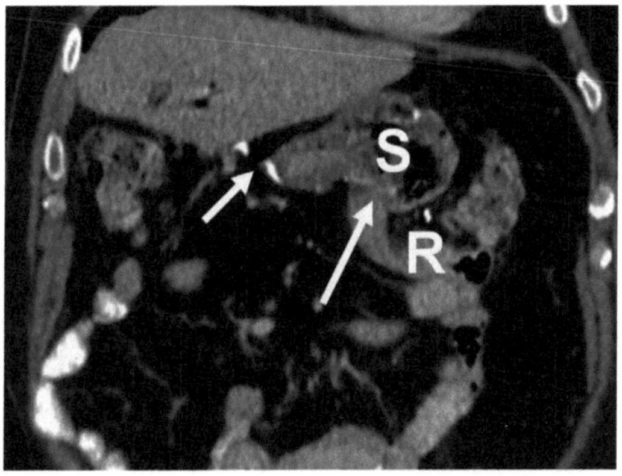

Fig. 4.16 Gastrojejunostomy. Coronal CT post Whipple procedure shows the anastomosis (*long arrow*) between the stomach and the jejunal/Roux loop (*R*). Surgical clips at the site of pyloric resection (*short arrow*).Stomach (*S*)

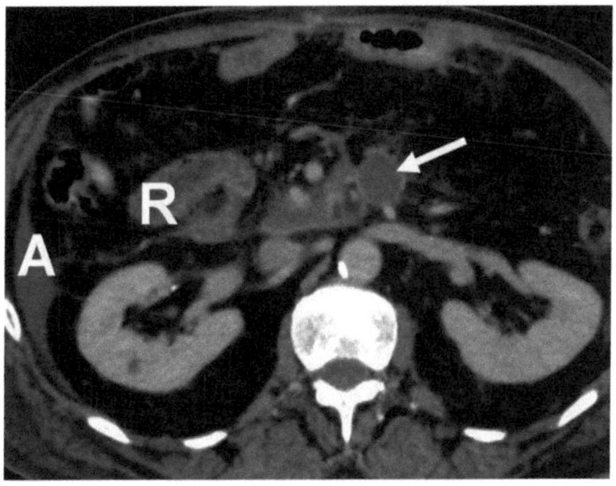

Fig. 4.17 Duodenal bed fluid collection in a pyrexial patient 6 days post PPPD. Axial CT demonstrates a small fluid collection with an enhancing rim (*arrow*). This was managed conservatively. Jejunal (Roux) loop (*R*), ascites (*A*)

coronal reformats and axial images side by side as well as previous postoperative CT imaging can assist in interpreting the tortuous course of the jejunal/Roux loop.

4.6.2 Postoperative Fluid/Fat Stranding

The most common early postoperative findings on cross-sectional imaging are stranding of the mesenteric fat and small amounts of peritoneal fluid or duodenal bed collections. The duodenal bed collections in particular can be mistaken for abscess (Fig. 4.17) formation and warrant drainage only if there are clinical signs of sepsis. Postoperative fluid and periportal hepatic edema can persist for up to 3–4 weeks after surgery.

4.6.3 Perivascular Cuffing

Perivascular cuffing on CT is a description referring to an increase in the attenuation of the intra-abdominal fat around the superior mesenteric

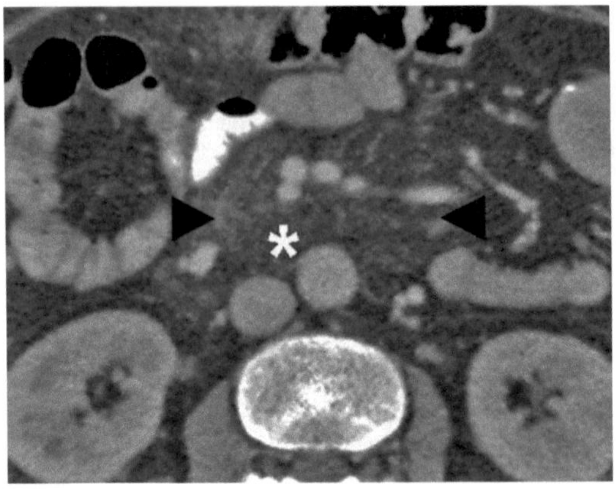

Fig. 4.18 Perivascular cuffing post PPPD for an ampullary tumor. There is subtle stranding of the abdominal fat (*asterisk*) within the surgical bed on CT. The margins of the mesenteric vascular pedicle are well defined. Lateral margins of mesenteric fat stranding (*arrowheads*). This remained unchanged on interval CT examinations. Note the difference in appearances between this benign finding and that of tumor recurrence (see Fig. 4.35)

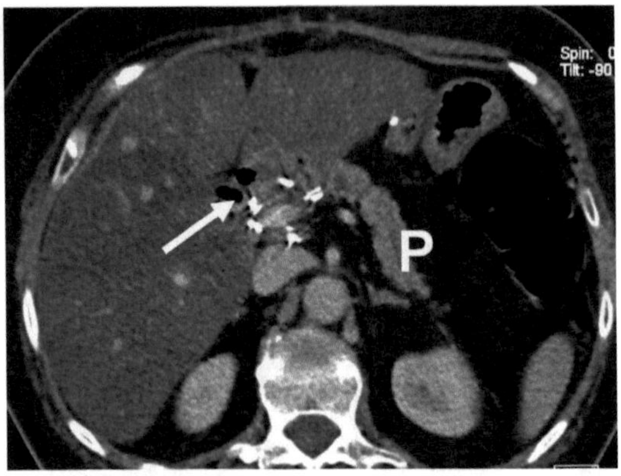

Fig. 4.19 Surgical clips post PPPD at the site of resection of the pancreatic head and draining peripancreatic lymph nodes. Pneumobilia in the CBD is a normal postoperative finding (*arrow*). Residual pancreas (*P*). Note fatty liver

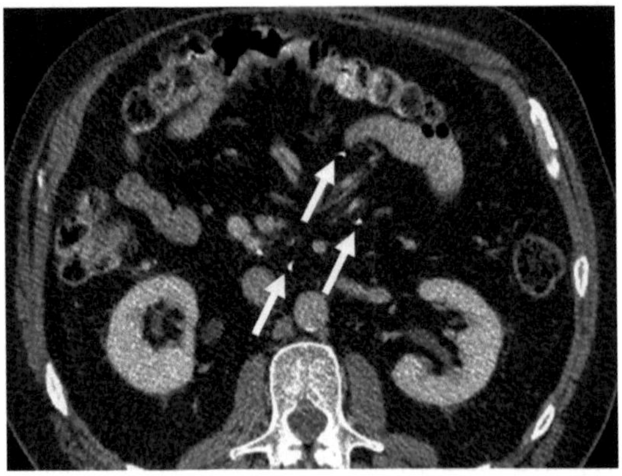

Fig. 4.20 Lymphadenectomy clips. Axial CT demonstrating surgical clips (*arrows*) at the sites of extended lymph node clearance within the retroperitoneum and small bowel mesentery

vascular pedicle (Fig. 4.18). It is due to fibrosis resulting from surgery and radiotherapy. It can also be seen around the celiac and hepatic arteries. It is commonly seen up to 6 weeks following surgery but can persist for a longer duration. It is important to distinguish perivascular cuffing from tumor recurrence, which encases the blood vessels and invades the mesenteric fat between them (Sect. 4.10, Fig. 4.35). Perivascular soft tissue associated with tumor recurrence will demonstrate an interval growth on serial CTs (Smith et al. 2008).

4.6.4 Reactive Lymphadenopathy

Reactive lymphadenopathy can be seen within the first 2–3 months following surgery. Lymph node measurements are not a reliable indicator of metastatic involvement, but reactive lymph nodes are generally less than 1 cm and regress during follow-up examinations (Scialpi et al. 2005). Lymphadenectomy clips are commonly seen along the sites of pancreatic lymph node drainage (Fig. 4.19) and occasionally at sites of extended nodal clearance within the retroperitoneum and small bowel mesentery (Fig. 4.20).

4.6.5 Pneumobilia

Pneumobilia is seen in approximately 70% of patients (Mortele et al. 2000) and is due to reflux of air into the biliary tree from the hepatico/

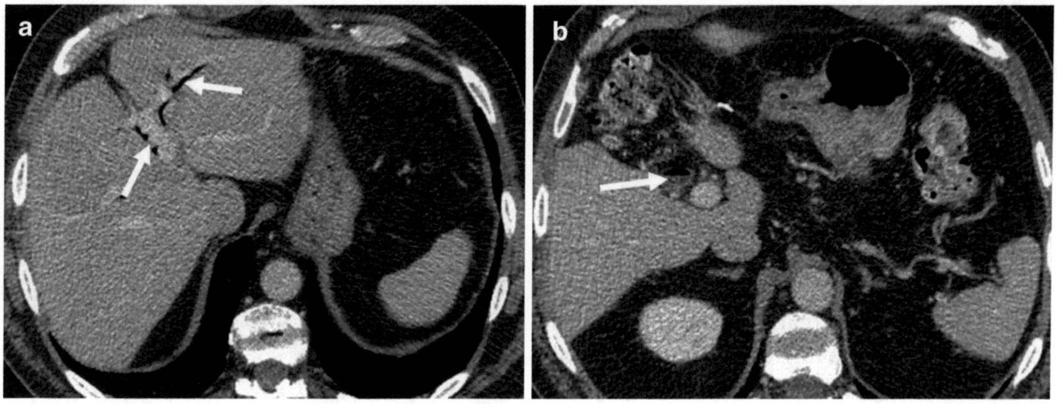

Fig. 4.21 Pneumobilia post Whipple procedure. Axial CT showing air (*arrows*) within (**a**) the left intrahepatic bile ducts and (**b**) distal common bile duct

choledochojejunostomy (Fig. 4.21). It is more prevalent within the left intrahepatic bile ducts. Mild biliary tree dilatation is also seen postoperatively.

4.6.6 Pancreatic Duct Dilatation

Pancreatic duct dilatation within 2 mm of the preoperative measurement on cross-sectional imaging is considered normal (Fig. 4.22). Dilatation of more than 2 mm should prompt a search for tumor recurrence or a stricture of the pancreatic duct at or near the anastomosis. MR using pancreatic/MRCP protocols may assist and where available the use of secretin can be useful in diagnosing strictures.

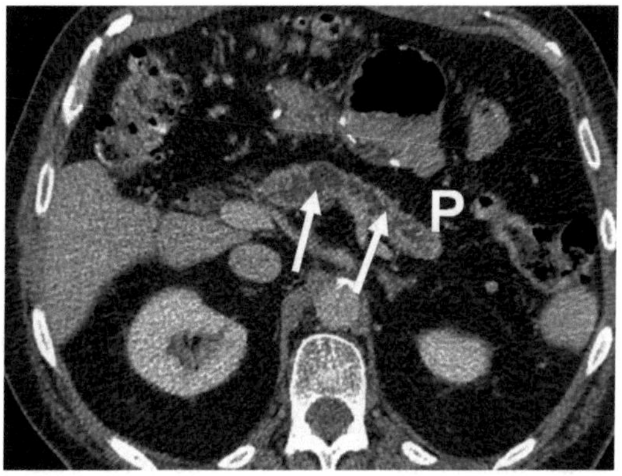

Fig. 4.22 Pancreatic duct dilatation (*arrows*) and pancreatic atrophy 2 years post PPPD. There is no evidence of tumor recurrence, and the degree of duct dilatation had not changed. Comparison with prior imaging is essential to avoid misdiagnosis. Pancreas (*P*)

4.6.7 Resection Margin

The resected edge of the residual pancreas following partial pancreatectomy can have a cystic appearance on CT within the early postoperative period. This should not be misdiagnosed as a pseudocyst or cystic tumor (particularly if the surgical resection margin was clear). The suspicion of recurrence should be raised if these appearances are new on interval imaging. Surgical clips are commonly seen at the resection margin and may cause streak artifact adjacent to the residual pancreas.

4.6.8 Peripancreatic Inflammation

Stranding within the peripancreatic soft tissues is a common CT finding within the immediate postoperative period. The appearances are similar to changes of acute pancreatitis which can also occur as a complication following pancreatic surgery. Correlation with the patient's clinical status and biochemistry are required to differentiate.

4.6.9 Pancreatic Atrophy

Although distal pancreatic atrophy can be seen on preoperative imaging due to a tumor within the proximal gland, pancreatic atrophy can also be seen on serial postoperative cross-sectional imaging (Fig. 4.22). Pancreatic atrophy can be associated with a loss of exocrine function.

4.7 Postoperative Upper GI Contrast Studies

Although CT is usually performed to evaluate normal anatomy and complications following pancreatic surgery, enteric complications can be assessed with upper GI contrast studies (Sect. 4.9). Fluoroscopic evaluation is performed early in the postoperative period using water soluble contrast media. Although there are three anastomoses, problems with delayed gastric emptying and preferential opacification of the jejunal loop distal to the pancreatic and biliary anastomoses or the efferent limb (if a Roux loop has been used) means that the pancreaticojejunostomy and hepatico/choledochojejunostomy are less commonly visualized. The pancreaticojejunostomy is the most vulnerable of the three anastomoses, and breakdown accounts for nearly 50% of deaths in the postoperative period.

Barium studies can be performed at a later date (when there is less concern regarding anastomotic integrity) to assess for gastroesophageal and jejunal biliary reflux, delayed gastric emptying, and complications resulting from adhesions (Fig. 4.23).

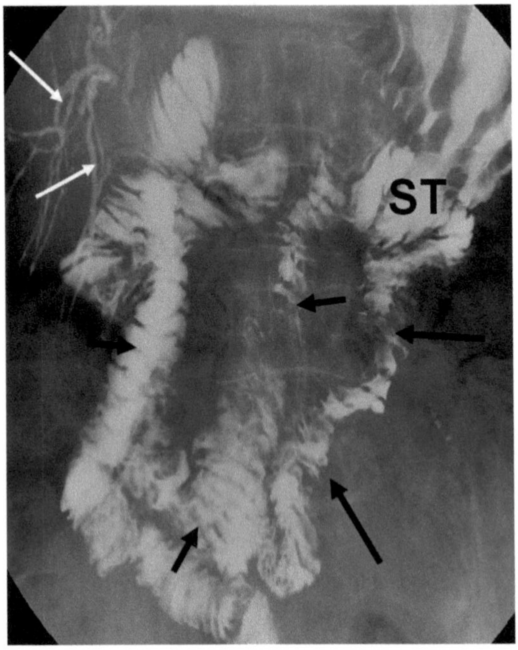

Fig. 4.23 Normal barium small bowel meal examination in a patient with intermittent vomiting 5 years post Whipple procedure. There is passage of barium into the afferent Roux loop (*short arrows*) with reflux into the biliary tree (*white arrows*) from the hepaticojejunostomy. Efferent loop (*long arrows*) and stomach (*ST*)

4.8 Postoperative Complications

4.8.1 Pancreatic Anastomotic Leak

Pancreatic anastomotic leak is the most serious postoperative complication following pancreatic surgery. The presence of pancreatic secretions within the abdominal cavity is associated with a high morbidity and mortality if not diagnosed and managed appropriately. An overall pancreatic leak rate of <10% is the acceptable standard (de Castro et al. 2005). Anastomotic leaks can cause:

- Intra-abdominal abscess
- Sepsis
- Massive hemorrhage
- Enteric fistulation

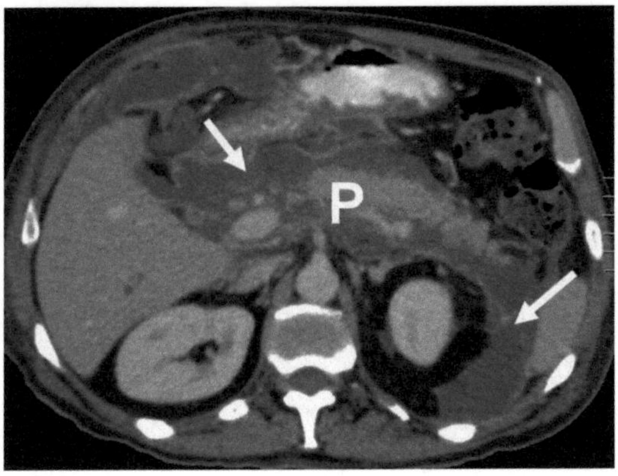

Fig. 4.24 Pancreatic anastomotic leak 5 days post PPPD. There were large volumes of amylase rich fluid within the surgical drains. Axial CT demonstrates large volume ascites within the upper abdomen (*arrows*). Pancreas (*P*). This required surgical intervention

Anastomotic leaks are multifactorial and relate to ischemia (chemotherapy, radiotherapy, sepsis, and poor nutritional status) and technical factors (quality of surgery, texture of the pancreatic remnant, and main pancreatic duct diameter) (Yang et al. 2005). Anastomotic leaks usually manifest in the first week post-surgery, and the pancreaticojejunostomy anastomosis is the most vulnerable of the three. It is usually suspected when there is a prolonged or increased output of amylase rich fluid from the intraoperatively placed drain within the pancreatic bed (Fig. 4.24). A biliary fistula from breakdown of the hepato/choledochojejunostomy will result in drainage of bile through the surgical drain (Fig. 4.25). Detection of anastomotic leaks on CT can be difficult because fluid is often seen in the region of the pancreatic bed within the postoperative period. The presence of air bubbles within the fluid is highly suggestive of anastomotic breakdown, but this can also derive from the surgical drain. If there is persisting doubt, an interval CT can be performed to evaluate any deterioration. Patients with low-output pancreatic fistulas are managed conservatively with maintenance of external drainage from the intraoperatively placed surgical drains. Complete anastomotic breakdown requires surgical intervention (Hashiomoto et al. 2007).

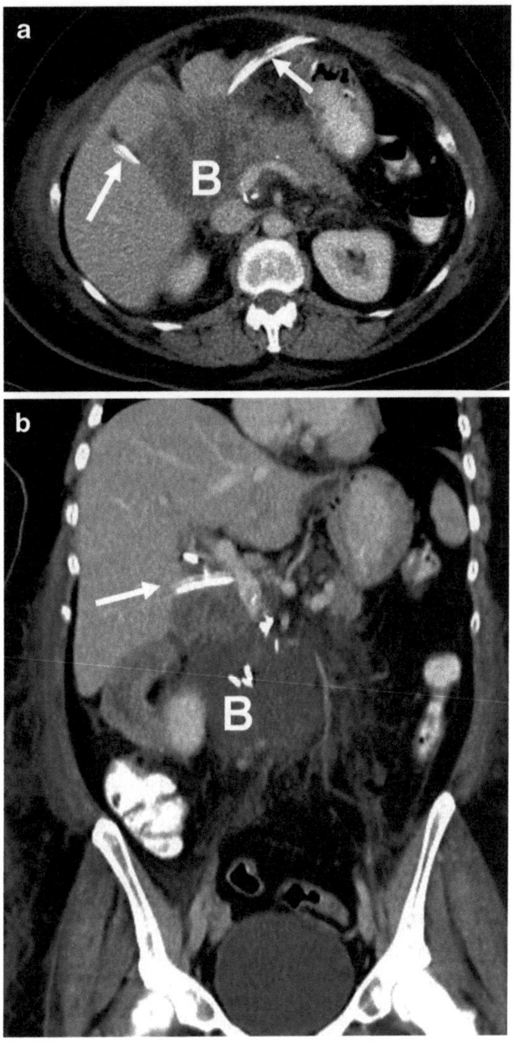

Fig. 4.25 Bile leak. (**a**) Axial and (**b**) coronal CT depicts a low attenuation collection (*B*) near the porta hepatis with intense peritoneal reaction. There was bilious material in the surgical drains (*arrows*) secondary to a biliary leak from the hepaticojejunostomy

Sepsis secondary to a pancreatic anastomotic leak can also result in the formation of gastroduodenal, hepatic, or splenic pseudoaneurysms. This is discussed in the next Sect. 4.8.2.

4.8.2 Vascular Complications

Postpancreatectomy hemorrhage (PPH) occurs in less than 10% of patients but accounts for 11–38% of deaths (Jagad et al. 2008). The International Study Group of Pancreatic Surgery classified PPH as early (≤24 h) or late (>24 h), severity (mild or severe), and location (intraluminal or extraluminal) (Wente et al. 2007). PPH into the gut (intraluminal) is manifested by hematemesis, melena, or aspiration of blood from the nasogastric tube. Extraluminal bleeding is identified in surgical drains, in abdominal wounds, or in an intraperitoneal location. Pseudo extraluminal bleeding may occur when an intraluminal hemorrhage coexists with an anastomotic dehiscence. Intraluminal hemorrhage can often be controlled by endoscopy, but extraluminal hemorrhage requires surgical or radiological intervention (Sohn et al. 2003).

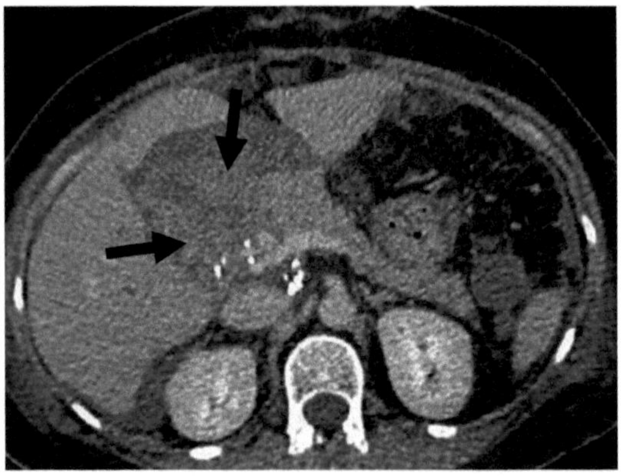

Fig. 4.26 Post operative CT (portal venous phase) in a patient post PD with bleeding into the surgical drains. There is a high density collection at the porta hepatis (*arrows*) but no active extravasation was identified on the arterial phase of imaging (*not shown*). The source of this was a suspected hepatic artery aneurysm which was identified during selective angiography and successfully stented (*not shown*)

4.8.2.1 Investigation of Vascular Complications

Exsanguinating patients require immediate laparotomy. In more stable patients, triple-phase CT (noncontrast, arterial, and portal venous phases) is the most effective technique for diagnosing the site and nature of bleeding (Smith et al. 2008) (Fig. 4.26). The unenhanced scan identifies collections and mimics of active bleeding. The arterial phase may show active bleeding and delineates the vascular anatomy. The venous phase may show slower bleeding, late filling pseudoaneurysms, or other post surgical complications. CT is most sensitive if performed at the time of active bleeding with multiplanar reformats improving the diagnostic yield and enhancing endovascular or surgical planning. The role of digital subtraction angiography (DSA) has largely changed from diagnostic to therapeutic. However, in unstable patients who are at risk from further surgery, DSA allows rapid diagnosis and intervention. A "sentinel" or "herald" bleed describes a self-limiting episode of bleeding, often from a drain. This must be investigated as it is commonly a harbinger of significant hemorrhage and a structural vascular defect should be excluded.

4.8.2.2 Radiological Management of Vascular Complications

Radiological management of PPH has increased as the endovascular armamentarium has expanded. Current commonly used techniques are embolization (coils, gelfoam, glue, or thrombin), stent grafting, intentional dissection, and percutaneous thrombin injection. Stent grafts require larger diameter access tubes (long sheaths or guiding catheters). Their insertion is not possible if the access or target vessel is small, angulated, or tortuous. Endovascular treatment is not always performed as a definitive intervention. In some cases, it will be used as a temporizing measure to control hemorrhage and allow safer surgical repair of an anastomosis. Anatomical arterial variation is common and can simplify or complicate radiological intervention.

Common scenarios include:

- Early bleeding due to failure of ligatures or arterial anastomoses. The gastroduodenal artery (GDA) stump is the first place to look. It is the commonest cause of early PPH and is often attributed to technical failure. Surgical clips next to the hepatic artery often indicate its position (Fig. 4.27). Active bleeding or a pseudoaneurysm can be treated with embolization (coils and/or glue) or stent

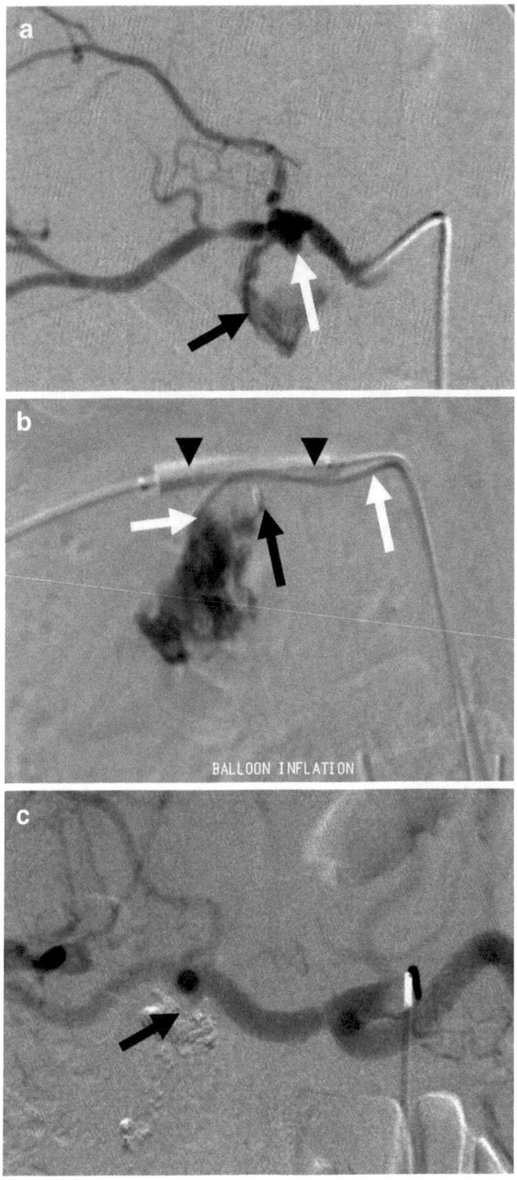

Fig. 4.27 (**a–c**) DSA of a hemodynamically unstable patient with active bleeding (*black arrow*) from the gastroduodenal artery [GDA] stump (*white arrow*) 24 h post Whipple procedure. (**b**) Balloon (*arrowheads*) inflated across the origin of the GDA after placement of a microcatheter in the GDA (*white arrows*). A surgical clip seen on this image (*black arrow*) had been used to ligate the GDA. It is not seen in (**a**) due to perfect digital subtraction. (**c**) Following injection of glue via the microcatheter, the hemorrhage has stopped (*arrow*).This is only a temporary control measure and definitive surgical care intervention is required

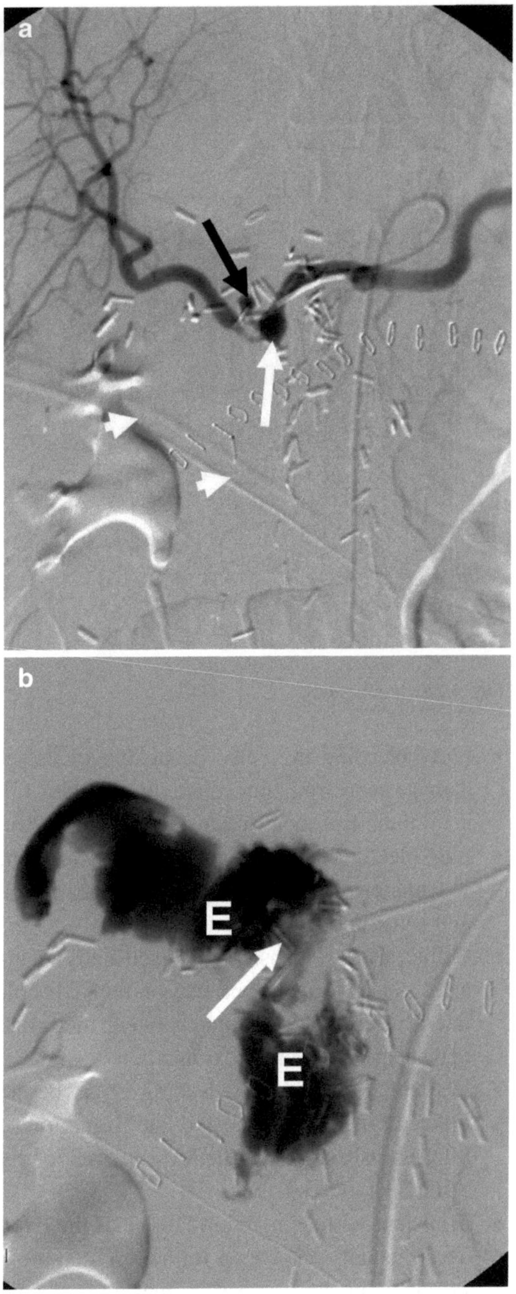

Fig. 4.28 Whipple procedure for pancreatic carcinoma with intermittent extraluminal bleeding through drain (*white arrowheads*). (**a**) No active bleeding on celiac axis run GDA stump (*white arrow*) and ligated left gastric artery (*black arrow*). (**b**) Injection with the catheter tip (*white arrow*) in the GDA stump shows active extravasation (*E*). (**c**) Following deployment of a stent graft (*white arrows*). This requires a large caliber long sheath or guiding catheter in the hepatic artery to allow deployment. It may not be possible to advance a large device into the hepatic artery. The long sheath (*black arrow*) has been withdrawn to perform angiography

grafting. Active bleeding may only be evident with injections into the GDA stump (Fig. 4.28).

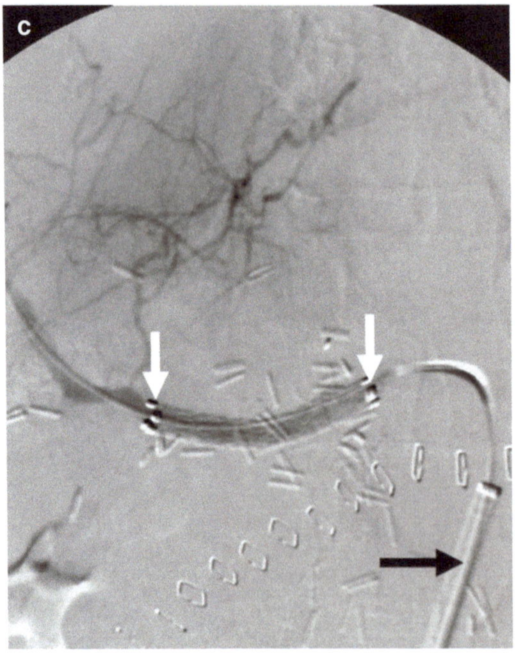

Fig. 4.28 (continued)

- Early bleeding may also occur due to vessel damage away from immediate surgical area. CT is invaluable in such circumstances (Fig. 4.29).
- Late bleeding occurs due to stress ulceration, vascular erosion secondary to pancreatic leaks, and anastomotic dehiscence (Fig. 4.30).
- Celiac artery stenosis. This is usually managed conservatively because of the rich collateral arterial blood supply between the celiac and superior mesenteric trunks.
- Hepatic arterial injury leading to ischemic injury of the biliary tree and late formation of bile duct strictures (ischemic cholangiopathy – see Sect. 6.6.5.3.1).
- Transient perfusion abnormalities of the liver. These usually resolve on follow-up imaging.
- Portal vein and superior mesenteric vein thrombosis.
- Areas of splenic infarction.

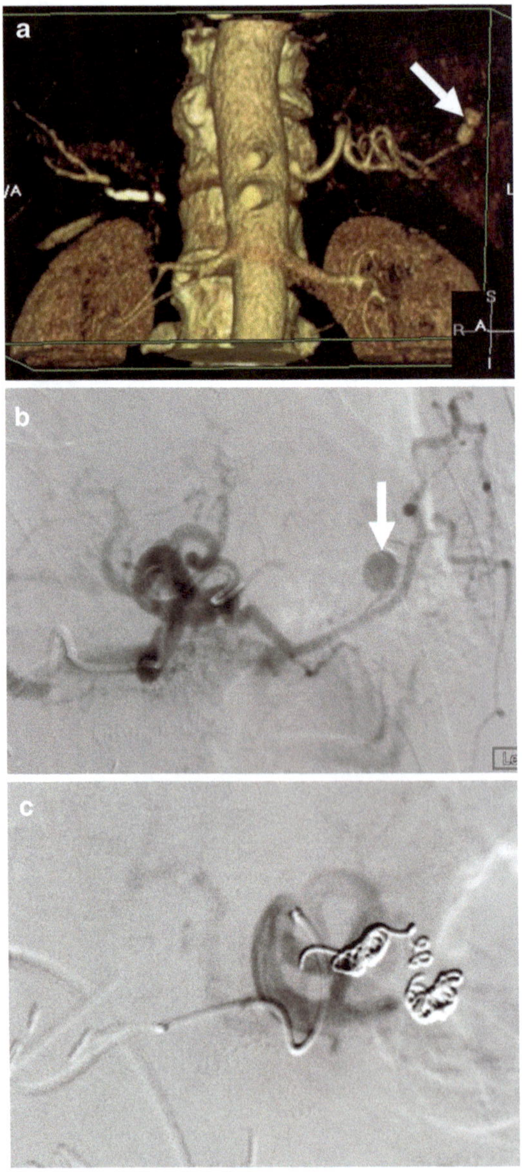

Fig. 4.29 Early hemodynamic instability postpancreatectomy. (**a**) Volume rendered coronal CT showing a pseudoaneurysm (*white arrow*) from a branch of the splenic artery. (**b**) DSA confirms a large pseudoaneurysm (*white arrow*) from a short gastric branch of the markedly tortuous splenic artery. (**c**) Following coil embolization of the short gastric artery

4.8.3 Biliary Obstruction

Biliary obstruction following pancreaticoduodenectomy can result from bile duct injury, anastomotic stricture, recurrent tumor, or biliary stones/casts. CT and MRI can be complementary in their assessment of biliary complications, but it can be difficult to differentiate benign from malignant disease particularly if there are no other features of local recurrence or metastatic disease. Because of the long jejunal or afferent loop, it is not always possible to access the

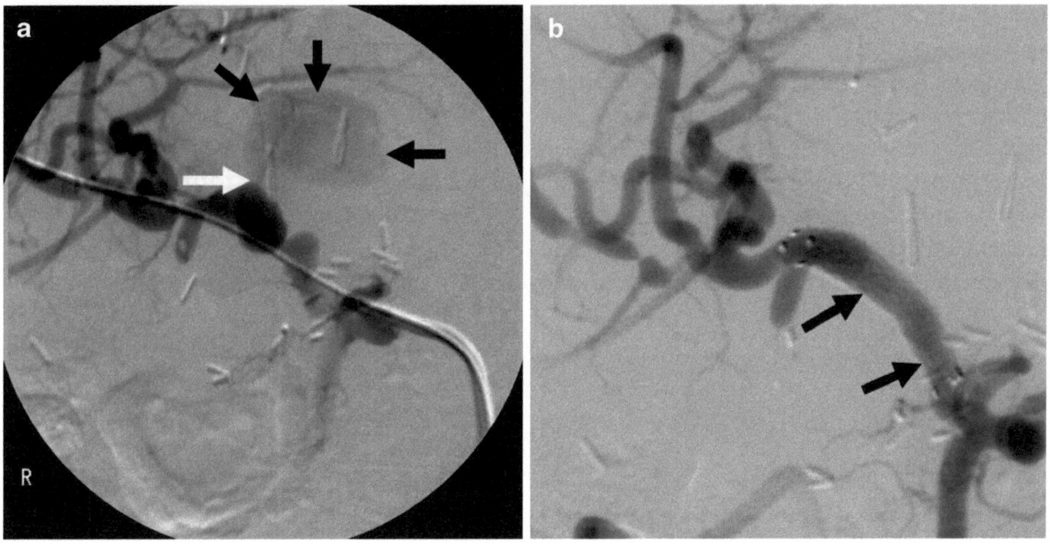

Fig. 4.30 Late rupture of the hepatic artery at 2 months. (**a**) DSA demonstrates an irregular hepatic artery with a defect (*white arrow*) and extravasation (*black arrows*). (**b**) Occlusion of the leak and remodeling of the hepatic artery following insertion of a stent graft (*black arrows*)

biliary tree by ERCP. Transhepatic techniques such as balloon dilatation of benign strictures or biliary casts and biliary drainage via stenting or catheter placement can be employed. This is discussed in the biliary chapter (Sect. 5.7.2). Biliary dilatation has been described following the Frey procedure due to ischemia of the distal common bile duct.

4.8.4 Abscess

Postoperative collections can occur at any location within the abdomen and pelvis. Common sites of abscess include the pancreatic bed, subphrenic spaces, and the pelvis (Fig. 4.31). They can be aspirated under CT or ultrasound guidance. Some surgeons will use surgical sponges (Ethicon, Livingston, UK) to achieve hemostasis. These are biodegradable hemostatic agents which may mimic an abscess due to trapped gas. This is discussed in more detail in Sect. 1.4.2.1.

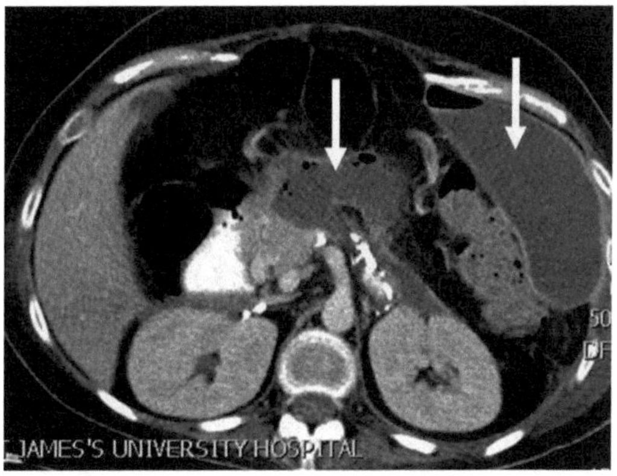

Fig. 4.31 Axial CT in a septic patient 8 days post subtotal pancreatectomy for neuroendocrine malignancy. There are rim enhancing fluid collections containing gas consistent with abscesses (*arrows*) within the surgical bed and left upper quadrant

4.8.5 Acute Pancreatitis

This occasionally occurs in the pancreatic remnant but is an infrequent complication and can only be diagnosed with clinical and biochemical correlation.

4.9 Enteric Complications

These include complications related to the gastroenterostomy and the jejunal loop.

4.9.1 Delayed Gastric Emptying

This is defined as the requirement for NG tube placement for longer than 10 days following surgery. Delayed gastric emptying is more likely to occur in patients following pyloric preserving surgery and is a common cause for prolonged hospital stay (Fig. 4.32). Patients are unable to tolerate an oral diet which is usually introduced between the fifth and seventh postoperative day. Imaging has a role to exclude a mechanical cause for obstruction (Sect. 4.9.2).

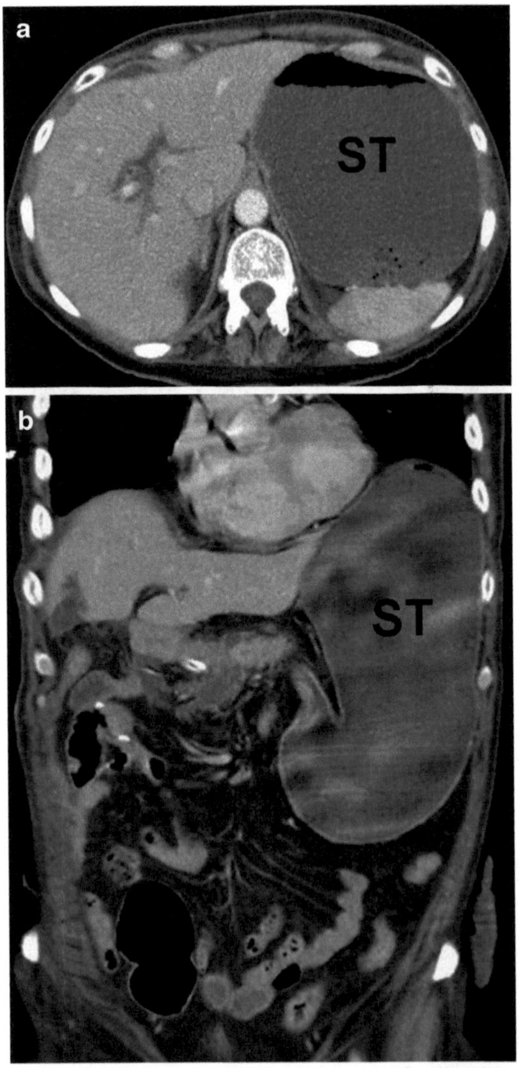

Fig. 4.32 Delayed gastric emptying in a patient 11 days post PPPD. (**a**) Axial and (**b**) coronal CT shows a severely dilated fluid filled stomach (*ST*). Endoscopy demonstrated normal appearances of the gastrojejunostomy and no obstructive mechanical cause for the dilated stomach. This was managed conservatively with nasogastric decompression

4.9.2 Gastroenterostomy Complications

Stenosis at the gastrojejunostomy site can occur at any time in the postoperative period. Upper GI contrast studies may show a delayed transit of oral contrast, but distinguishing stenosis from delayed gastric emptying can be difficult, particularly if the anastomosis is not visualized (Fig. 4.33). Endoscopy may be required to assess the caliber of the anastomosis. Ulceration within the gastric remnant or at the anastomosis does occur but is uncommon. Barium is more sensitive than gastrografin in detecting ulceration on upper GI studies but is relatively contraindicated within the early postoperative period because of the risk of anastomotic leak and subsequent barium peritonitis.

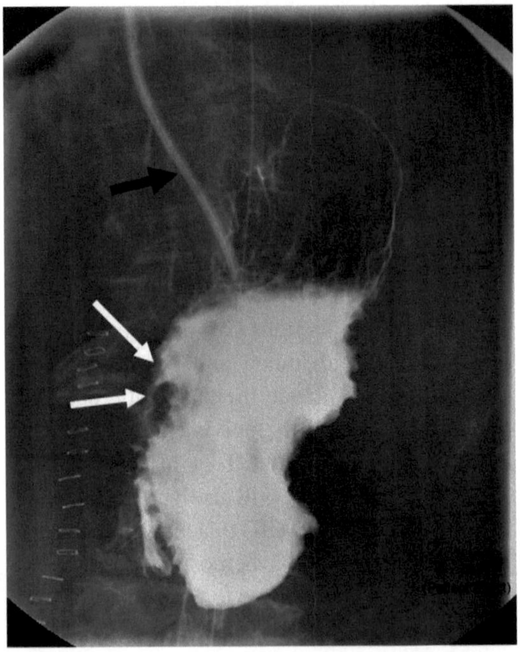

Fig. 4.33 Stomal stenosis. Oral contrast study in a patient with persistent vomiting 3 weeks post PPPD. There is ulceration (*white arrows*) at the gastrojejunostomy anastomosis. Only a small amount of contrast passes into the small bowel. NG tube (*black arrow*)

Other complications include postprandial dumping, diarrhea, dyspepsia, reflux, nausea, and vomiting. Incidences of these complications are lower in patients following pyloric preserving surgery compared with the conventional Whipple procedure (pancreaticoduodenectomy).

Dumping is a sequela of altered gastric reservoir function and abnormal postoperative gastric motor function. This is primarily a clinical diagnosis. Early dumping syndrome (30–60 min postprandial) is believed to result from accelerated gastric emptying of hyperosmolar contents into the small bowel. This causes fluid shift from the intravascular compartment into the bowel lumen, resulting in rapid small bowel distention and an increase in the frequency of bowel contractions. This results in osmotic diarrhea and vasomotor symptoms.

Late dumping occurs 1–3 h after a meal. The pathogenesis is thought to be related to the early development of reactive hyperinsulinemic hypoglycemia in response to a rapid delivery of carbohydrate high meals into the small bowel.

4.9.3 Gastric Outlet and Afferent Roux Loop Obstruction

Roux loop obstruction usually occurs early in the postoperative period. It is discussed in detail in the Roux-en-Y gastric bypass section in Chap. 3. Causative factors include edema, ulceration, or stenosis at the level of the anastomosis or internal herniation of the Roux loop through a defect within the small bowel mesentery created at the time of surgery. Chronic afferent loop syndrome results from incomplete obstruction of the jejunal lumen leading to distension with pancreatic juice and bile. The CT appearances are of a distended fluid filled small bowel loop (afferent loop) in the periportal region which is orientated transversely across the midline, adjacent to the gastroenterostomy or the jejunojejunal anastomosis (where a Roux loop is present).

Adhesions are the commonest cause of small bowel obstruction in the late postoperative period. This is discussed further in Sect. 7.2.

4.9.4 Malabsorption

Malabsorption can be caused by blind pouch or short gut syndromes. These are discussed in more detail in Sects. 7.3.4.3 and 7.3.4.8. Blind pouches usually do not form until approximately 12 weeks postsurgery. It is often the aperistaltic loop of the side-to-side distal Roux – small bowel anastomosis which starts dilating to form the blind pouch. This can lead to bacterial overgrowth which causes malabsorption. Blind pouches can be difficult to detect, but sequential upper gastrointestinal contrast studies and CT studies can assist. The blind pouch does not usually increase in size after the first year of surgery.

Excessive small bowel resection or inadvertent gastroileostomy instead of planned gastrojejunostomy can manifest as short gut syndrome. This is perhaps most easily delineated with an upper GI contrast study.

4.10 Tumor Recurrence

Tumor can recur within the pancreatic bed or at metastatic sites such as the liver, peritoneum, and lung. Patients with positive surgical margins have a higher incidence of local and systemic recurrence and a shorter disease-free survival than those with negative surgical margins. The rate of resection margin positivity (pathologically defined as R1) is usually higher in pancreatic (82%) and distal bile duct (72%) cancers but is significantly lower for ampullary tumors (25%) (Verbeke and Menon 2009). The posterior margin is most frequently involved, but margin positivity can be multifocal. The median survival of R1 pancreatic cancer patients is only 14 months.

The most common site for tumor recurrence is within the pancreatic bed (Fig. 4.34). CT assessment can be difficult in distinguishing recurrent malignancy from normal postoperative appearances (Table 4.1). Although perivascular cuffing (Sect. 4.6.3, Fig. 4.18) is a normal finding on CT in the initial postoperative period, this usually resolves (persisting in a minority). The subsequent development of fat stranding between the vascular pedicle and encasement

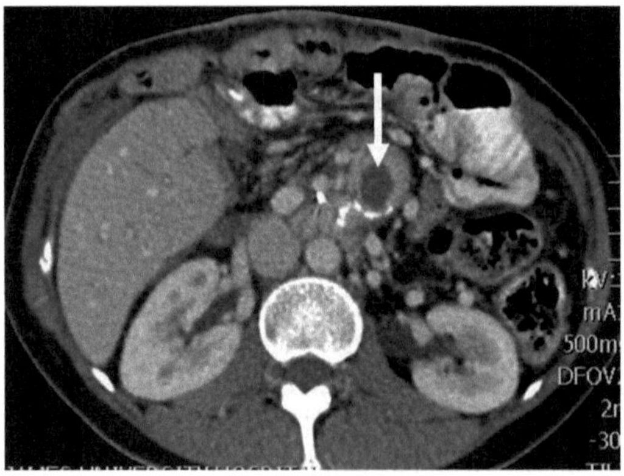

Fig. 4.34 Recurrent pancreatic malignancy (*arrow*) at the surgical resection site 15 months post PPPD for a non-functioning neuroendocrine tumor of the pancreatic head. The lesion at the staple line is cystic with an enhancing rim and should not be misinterpreted as a small bowel loop

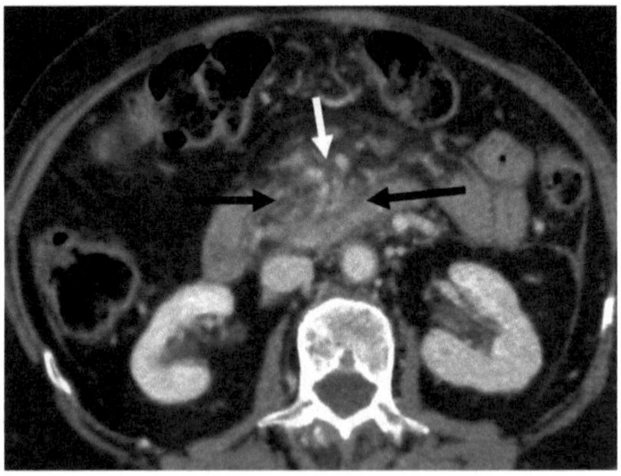

Fig. 4.35 Recurrent pancreatic malignancy within the surgical bed 18 months post PPPD for adenocarcinoma of the pancreatic head. Axial CT demonstrates ill-defined "dense" stranding within the pancreatic bed and small bowel mesentery (*black arrows*). The margins of the mesenteric vascular pedicle are indistinct indicating vascular invasion (*white arrow*). Note how the appearances differ from benign perivascular cuffing (Fig. 4.18)

Table 4.1 CT in the differentiation of normal postoperative findings and recurrent malignancy in patients following pancreaticoduodenectomy

	Normal postoperative appearances	Recurrent malignancy
Fluid collections	Located in surgical bed and Morrison pouch Resolve in 1–2 months	Ascites present after 2 months or new ascites 1 month postsurgery
Vascular soft tissue	Perivascular cuffing	Soft tissue encasing vessels
	Increased attenuation of fat along mesenteric vessels	Invasion of fat between vessels
	Usually stable	Rapid progression
	Due to postoperative fibrosis/radiotherapy	
	Can persist on follow-up CT	
Lymphadenopathy	Inflammatory response to surgery Initial size not helpful Decrease in size and number on follow-up imaging	Increase in size and number on follow-up imaging
Unopacified bowel loops	Look for small air bubbles in bowel wall	Air bubbles not a feature in recurrence

of the vessels is a strong indicator of tumor recurrence (Figs. 4.35 and 4.36). Serial CT examinations may be required to confirm this diagnosis. The development of ascites more than 30 days postsurgery has a high positive predictive value for malignancy (Mortele et al. 2000). An increase in the number and size of abdominal lymph nodes is also an indicator of recurrent disease (Fig. 4.37).

Despite adequate local control, it is important to remain vigilant for the presence of distant metastasis to the liver (Fig. 4.38) and lung.

4.11 Teaching Points

- Radiological assessment of post pancreatic surgery requires knowledge of the type of surgery performed and a sound understanding of the postoperative anatomy.
- An awareness of normal postoperative appearances and complications is essential to avoid misdiagnosis and allow prompt intervention.
- CT and upper GI fluoroscopy are the most useful tools in assessment of suspected complications.

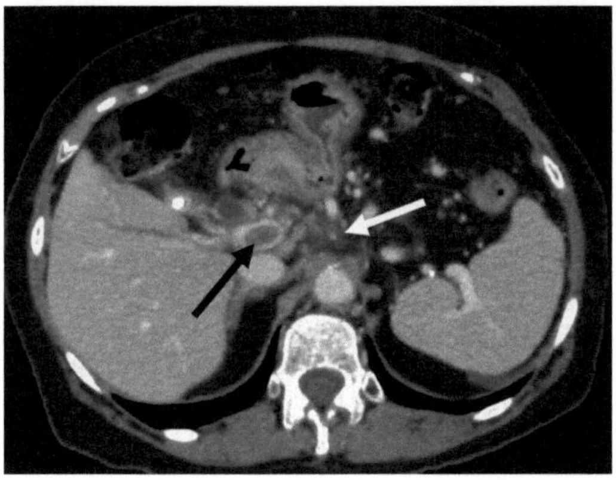

Fig. 4.36 Recurrent malignancy 12 months post pancreaticoduodenectomy. There is tumor infiltration adjacent to the celiac axis (*white arrow*) and portal vein thrombosis (*black arrow*)

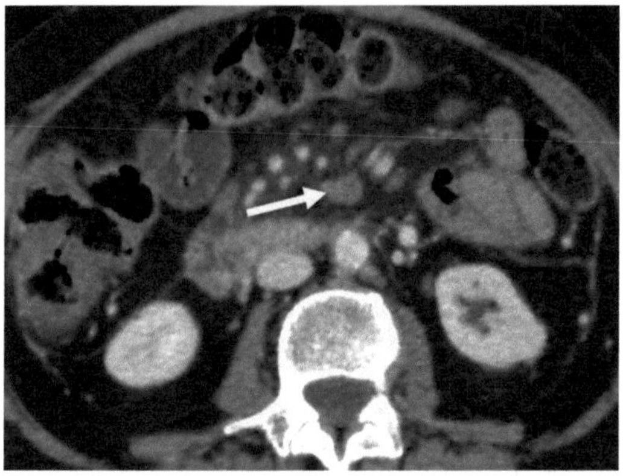

Fig. 4.37 Recurrent pancreatic malignancy with spread to local nodes. Axial CT demonstrates an enlarged mesenteric lymph node (*arrow*) which had increased in size on interval imaging

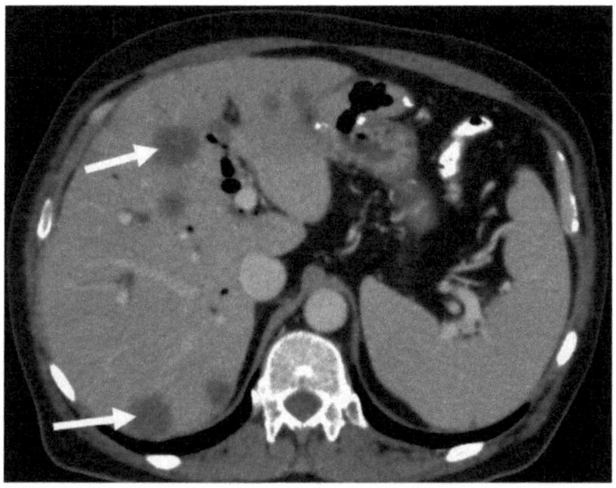

Fig. 4.38 Recurrent pancreatic malignancy. Axial CT demonstrating multiple liver metastases (*white arrows*) in a patient 18 months post Whipple procedure for pancreatic adenocarcinoma

References

Bluemke DA, Abrams RA, Yeo FE. Recurrent pancreatic adenocarcinoma: spiral CT evaluation following the Whipple procedure. Radiographics. 1997;17(2):303–13.

Bonney GK, Gomez D, Rahman SH, Verbeke CS, Prasad KR, Toogood GJ, Lodge JP, Menon KV. Results following surgical resection for malignant pancreatic neuroendocrine tumours. A single institutional experience. JOP. 2008;9(1):19–25.

Cataldegirmen G, Schneider CG, Bogoevski D, Koenig A, Kaifi JT, Bockhorn M, Deutsch LS, Vashist Y, Izbicki JR, Yekebas EF. Extended central pancreatic resection as an alternative for extended left or extended right resection for appropriate pancreatic neoplasms. Surgery. 2010;147(3):331–8.

Connor S, Raraty MG, Howes N, Evans J, Ghaneh P, Sutton R, Neoptolemos JP. Surgery in the treatment of acute pancreatitis-minimal access pancreatic necrosectomy. Scand J Surg. 2005;94(2):135–42.

De Castro SM, Busch OR, van Gulik TM, Obertop H, Gouma DJ. Incidence and management of pancreatic leakage after pancreatoduodenectomy. Br J Surg. 2005;92(9):1117–23.

Fahy BN, Frey CF, Ho HS, Beckett L, Bold RJ. Morbidity, mortality, and technical factors of distal pancreatectomy. Am J Surg. 2002;183(3):237–41.

Fendrich V, Langer P, Celik I, Bartsch DK, Zielke A, Ramaswamy A, Rothmund M. An aggressive surgical approach leads to long term survival in patients with pancreatic endocrine tumors. Ann Surg. 2006;244(6):845–51; discussion 852–3.

Freed S, Paulson E, Frederick M. Abdomen after a puestow procedure: postoperative CT appearance, complications and potential pitfalls. Radiology. 1997;203:790–4.

Gomez D, Malik HZ, Al-Mukthar A, Menon KV, Toogood GJ, Lodge JP, Prasad KR. Hepatic resection for metastatic gastrointestinal and pancreatic neuroendocrine tumours: outcome and prognostic predictors. HPB (Oxford). 2007;9(5):345–51.

Harrison LE, Klimstra DS, Brennan MF. Isolated portal vein involvement in pancreatic adenocarcinoma. A contraindication for resection? Ann Surg. 1996;224(3):342–7; discussion 347–9.

Hashimoto M, Koga M, Ishiyama K, Watarai J, Shibata S, Sato T, Yamamoto Y. CT features of pancreatic fistula after Pancreaticoduodenectomy. AJR Am J Roentgenol. 2007;188(4):W323–7.

Ito M, Horiguchi A, Asano Y, Yamamoto T, Tuda K, Morigaki S, Shimura M, Uyama I, Miyakawa S. Spleen-preserving distal pancreatectomy performed laparoscopically. Hepatogastroenterology. 2010;57(97):162–4.

Jagad RB, Koshariya M, Kawamoto J, Chude GS, Neeraj RV, Lygidakis NJ. Postoperative haemorrhage after major pancreatobiliary surgery: an update. Hepatogastroenterology. 2008;55(82–83):729–37.

Köninger J, Seiler CM, Sauerland S, Wente MN, Reidel MA, Müller MW, Friess H, Büchler MW. Duodenum-preserving pancreatic head resection-a randomized controlled trial comparing the original Beger procedure with the Berne modification (ISRCTN No. 50638764). Surgery. 2008; 143(4):490–8.

Menon KV, Gomez D, Smith AM, Anthoney A, Verbeke CS. Impact of margin status on survival following pancreatoduodenectomy for cancer: the Leeds Pathology Protocol (LEEPP). HPB (Oxford). 2009; 11(1):18–24.

Mortele KJ, Lemmerling M, Hemptinne D, De Vos M, De Bock G, Kunnen M. Postoperative findings following the Whipple procedure: determination of prevalence and morphologic abdominal CT features. Eur Radiol. 2000;10(1):123–8.

Müller MW, Friess H, Leitzbach S, Michalski CW, Berberat P, Ceyhan GO, Hinz U, Ho CK, Köninger J, Kleeff J, Büchler MW. Perioperative and follow up results after central pancreatic head resection (Berne technique) in a consecutive series of patients with chronic pancreatitis. Am J Surg. 2008;196(3):364–72.

Pedrazzoli S, DiCarlo V, Dionigi R, Mosca F, Pederzoli P, Pasquali C, Klöppel G, Dhaene K, Michelassi F. Standard versus extended lymphadenectomy associated with pancreatoduodenectomy in the surgical treatment of adenocarcinoma of the head of the pancreas: a multicenter, prospective, randomized study. Lymphadenectomy Study Group. Ann Surg. 1998; 228(4):508–17.

Sandrasegaran K, Maglinte D, Howard T, Lappas J. Surgery for chronic pancreatitis: cross sectional imaging of postoperative anatomy and complications. AJR Am J Roentgenol. 2005;184:1118–27.

Scialpi M, Scaglione M, Volterrani L, Ragozzino A, Romano S, Rotondo A. Imaging evaluation of post pancreatic surgery. Eur J Radiol. 2005;53(3):417–24.

Sohn TA, Yeo CJ, Cameron JL, Geschwind JF, Mitchell SE, Venbrux AC, Lillemoe KD. Pancreaticoduodenectomy: role of interventional radiologists in managing patients and complications. J Gastrointest Surg. 2003; 7(2):209–19.

Smith SL, Hampson F, Duxbury M, Rae DM, Sinclair MT. Computed tomography after radical pancreaticoduodenectomy (Whipple's procedure). Clin Radiol. 2008;63:921–8.

Strasberg SM, Drebin JA, Linehan D. Radical antegrade modular pancreatosplenectomy. Surgery. 2003;133(5): 521–7.

Strate T, Taherpour Z, Bloechle C, Mann O, Bruhn JP, Schneider C, Kuechler T, Yekebas E, Izbicki JR. Long-term follow-up of a randomized trial comparing the Beger and Frey procedures for patients suffering from chronic pancreatitis. Ann Surg. 2005;241(4):591–8.

Terrace JD, Paterson HM, Garden OJ, Parks RW, Madhavan KK. Results of decompression surgery for pain in chronic pancreatitis. HPB (Oxford). 2007;9(4): 308–11.

Verbeke CS, Menon KV. Redefining resection margin status in pancreatic cancer. HPB (Oxford). 2009;11(4): 282–9.

Wagner M, Redaelli C, Lietz M, Seiler CA, Friess H, Büchler MW. Curative resection is the single most important factor determining outcome in patients with pancreatic adenocarcinoma. Br J Surg. 2004;91(5):586–94.

Wente MN, et al. Postpancreatectomy hemorrhage (PPH): an International Study Group of Pancreatic Surgery (ISGPS) definition. Surgery. 2007;142(1):20–5.

Whipple AO, Parsons WB, Mullins CR. Treatment of carcinoma of the ampulla of Vater. Ann Surg. 1935; 102:763–79.

Ym Y, Tian XD, Zhuang Y. Risk factors of pancreatic leakage after pancreaticoduodenectomy. World J Gastroenterol. 2005;11(16):2456–61.

Zink SI, Soloff EV, White RR, Clary BM, Tyler DS, Pappas TN, Paulson EK. Pancreaticoduodenectomy: frequency and outcome of post-operative imaging-guided percutaneous drainage. Abdom Imaging. 2009;34(6):767–71.

The Biliary Tree

5

Vamshi P. Jagadesham, Maria Sheridan,
J. Peter A. Lodge, and John Brittenden

Contents

5.1 **Background** 153

5.2 **Laparoscopic Cholecystectomy** 154
5.2.1 Clinical Indications 154
5.2.2 Surgical Technique and Postoperative Anatomy 154
5.2.3 Modifications to Surgical Technique 154
5.2.4 Normal Radiological Appearances Following Cholecystectomy 156

5.3 **MRCP Interpretation Tips and Pitfalls** ... 157
5.3.1 MRCP Technique 157
5.3.2 Specific MRCP Pitfalls 158

5.4 **Complications of Cholecystectomy** 167
5.4.1 Bile Duct Injuries 167
5.4.2 Bile Leak 170
5.4.3 Management of Bile Leaks 174
5.4.4 Biliary Obstruction 174
5.4.5 Biliary Strictures 174
5.4.6 Retained CBD Stones 176
5.4.7 Dropped or Spilled Gallstones 177
5.4.8 Vascular Injury 179
5.4.9 Cystic Duct Stump Complications 180
5.4.10 Laparoscopic Complications 180
5.4.11 Teaching Points 180

5.5 **Mirizzi's Syndrome** 181

5.6 **Biliary Enteric Anastomoses (Hepaticojejunostomy)** 181
5.6.1 Clinical Indications 181
5.6.2 Surgical Technique and Postoperative Anatomy 181
5.6.3 Modifications to Surgical Technique 181

5.7 **Complications of Biliary Enteric Anastomoses** 182
5.7.1 Anastomotic Leak 182
5.7.2 Anastomotic Stricture 183
5.7.3 Nonanastomotic Stricture 184
5.7.4 Stone Formation 184

5.8 **Teaching Points** 184

References 185

V.P. Jagadesham, BSc (Hons), MBChB (Hons), MRCS, MD
Department of Surgery, Yorkshire and Humber Deanery, Leeds, UK

M. Sheridan, MBChB, MRCP, FRCR
Department of Radiology, Leeds Teaching Hospitals NHS Trust, Leeds, UK

J.P.A. Lodge, MD, FRCS
Department of Surgery, Leeds Teaching Hospitals NHS Trust, Leeds, UK

J. Brittenden, MBChB, MRCP, FRCR (✉)
Department of Radiology, Mid Yorkshire Hospitals NHS Trust, Wakefield, UK
e-mail: john.brittenden@midyorks.nhs.uk

5.1 Background

Approximately 50,000 cholecystectomies are performed annually in the UK for symptomatic gallstone disease. The majority of cases are performed laparoscopically (Gurusamy et al. 2010) with benefits of reduced morbidity and postoperative stay and improved cosmetic results compared with an open procedure. The timing of cholecystectomy following an acute episode of cholecystitis is debated with differing opinions on the optimal timing of the procedure.

J. Brittenden, D.J.M. Tolan (eds.), *Radiology of the Post Surgical Abdomen*,
DOI 10.1007/978-1-4471-2775-8_5, © Springer-Verlag London 2012

Some advocate early removal of the gallbladder, while others wait for the inflammation to resolve and operate approximately 6 weeks later.

Inadequate identification of the surgical anatomy increases the risk of common bile duct (CBD) injury during laparoscopic cholecystectomy. If magnetic resonance cholangiopancreatography (MRCP) has been performed prior to surgery to assess for intraductal stones, the radiologist should be vigilant for variations of ductal anatomy, which increase the risk of surgical complications, e.g., low insertion of the cystic duct into the common bile duct. The surgeon occasionally performs intraoperative cholangiography if there is doubt regarding biliary tree anatomy. Where there is continuing concern regarding accurate anatomical identification, the procedure will be converted from a laparoscopic to open cholecystectomy.

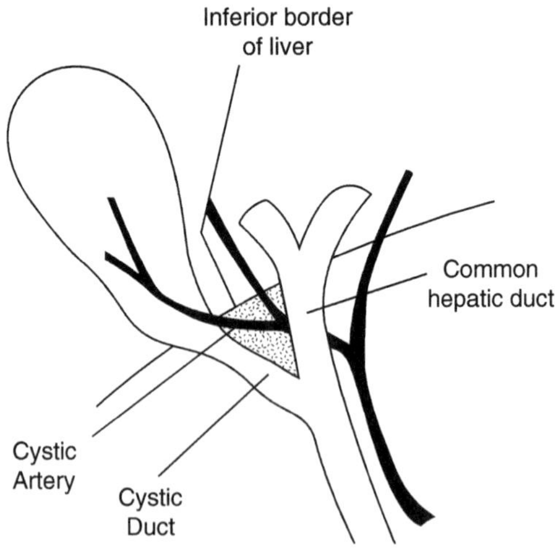

Fig. 5.1 Calot's triangle (*shaded area*). This is demarcated by the inferior border of the liver, the common hepatic duct, and the cystic duct. It contains the cystic artery (a branch of the right hepatic artery)

5.2 Laparoscopic Cholecystectomy

5.2.1 Clinical Indications

- Symptomatic cholelithiasis – biliary colic, cholecystitis
- Gallstone pancreatitis
- Gallbladder dysfunction/nonfunctioning gallbladder
- Large gallbladder polyps (>1 cm)

5.2.2 Surgical Technique and Postoperative Anatomy

- Single-port laparoscopic cholecystectomy is now possible using modified instruments.
- Following induction of a pneumoperitoneum with carbon dioxide via a periumbilical incision, the gallbladder is visualized to assess whether laparoscopic cholecystectomy is feasible.
- The primary trocar and laparoscope are placed through the umbilical incision.
- Two or three other port sites are used to assist. The epigastric port is the main operative port with accessory right midclavicular and right anterior axillary line ports used for retraction.
- Dissection of Calot's triangle is performed via a retrograde dissection. The boundaries of Calot's triangle include the inferior border of the liver, the common hepatic duct, and the cystic duct (Fig. 5.1). It contains the cystic artery and lymph nodes. Accurate identification and dissection of this area is integral to performing an uncomplicated cholecystectomy.
- Cystic artery and duct are clipped (titanium or plastic clips) and divided between clips (Fig. 5.2).
- Gallbladder is dissected from the liver bed and removed via laparoscopic port.
- Surgical drain may be positioned in the gallbladder fossa.

5.2.3 Modifications to Surgical Technique

- If the cystic duct is too dilated to safely apply clips, an extracorporeal absorbable suture is tied and placed around the duct.

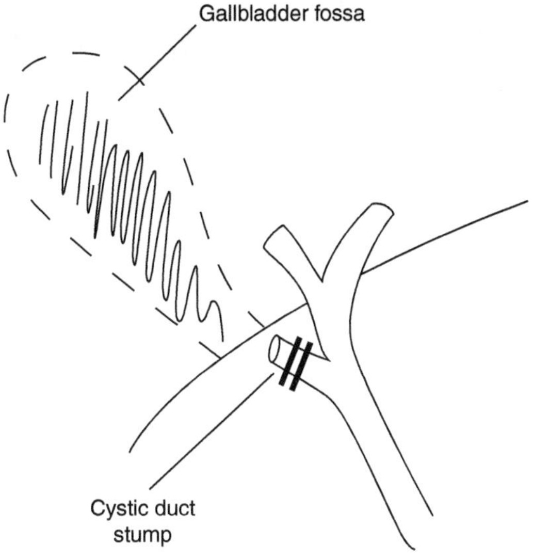

Fig. 5.2 Normal postoperative appearances following cholecystectomy. The cystic duct has been clipped close to the insertion with the common hepatic duct

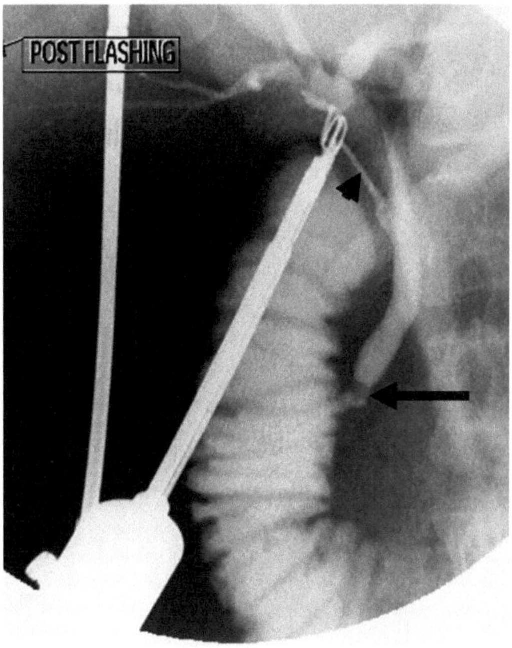

Fig. 5.3 Intraoperative cholangiogram (IOC). The cystic duct has been cannulated (*arrowhead*), and injected iodinated contrast outlines a small calculus in the distal CBD (*arrow*)

- Fundus-first cholecystectomy – is performed when dissection in Calot's triangle may be deemed difficult (e.g., chronic cholecystitis).
- Conversion to open cholecystectomy via a right subcostal (Kocher's) or upper midline incision.
- Subtotal cholecystectomy (laparoscopic/open) – if dense adhesions are present in Calot's triangle, which preclude safe dissection, a subtotal cholecystectomy can be performed. The gallbladder is dissected from the liver bed (fundus first) and incised at the level of Hartmann's pouch. The neck of the residual gallbladder may be sutured, and a drain is left in the gallbladder fossa to monitor bile drainage. A persistent bile leak is managed with ERCP and placement of a temporary plastic stent within the CBD to facilitate distal biliary drainage.
- Intraoperative cholangiography (IOC) – IOC is performed by some surgeons to outline the anatomy of the biliary tree (to prevent ligation of structures other than the cystic duct) and to identify stones in the bile ducts (Fig. 5.3). Its role, however, is controversial, and there is a wide variation of surgical practice. Some advocate IOC in all patients undergoing laparoscopic cholecystectomy, while others only use it in selective cases, i.e., patients at risk of bile duct injury due to aberrant ductal anatomy or if bile duct stones are suspected. Studies have shown that despite the use of IOC during laparoscopic cholecystectomy, bile duct injuries were not recognized at the time of surgery in a large proportion of patients (Slater et al. 2002).
- Laparoscopic/open bile duct exploration – if the choledochotomy is not primarily closed, a T-tube is placed and removed after 10–14 days following a T-tube cholangiogram (Fig. 5.4).
- Cholecystostomy – this is usually performed in patients with acute cholecystitis not responding to antibiotics or if there is empyema of the gallbladder. Cholecystostomy can be carried out under ultrasound or CT (Fig. 5.5) guidance preferably by a transhepatic approach (to prevent a bile leak into the abdomen). During a difficult laparoscopic cholecystectomy where conversion to an open procedure is not likely to be successful, a surgical drain can be inserted directly into the gallbladder.

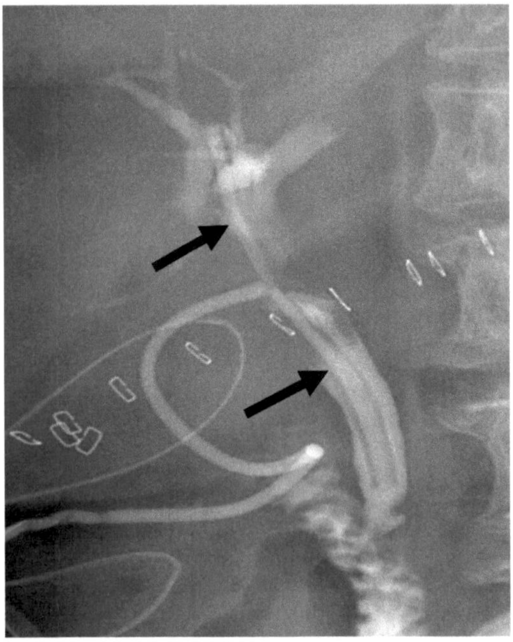

Fig. 5.4 Normal T-tube cholangiogram performed 10 days after an open cholecystectomy in which there were concerns regarding CBD stones. Contrast outlines the biliary tree and duodenum with no evidence of obstruction or intraductal calculi. Proximal and distal limbs of the T-tube (*arrows*)

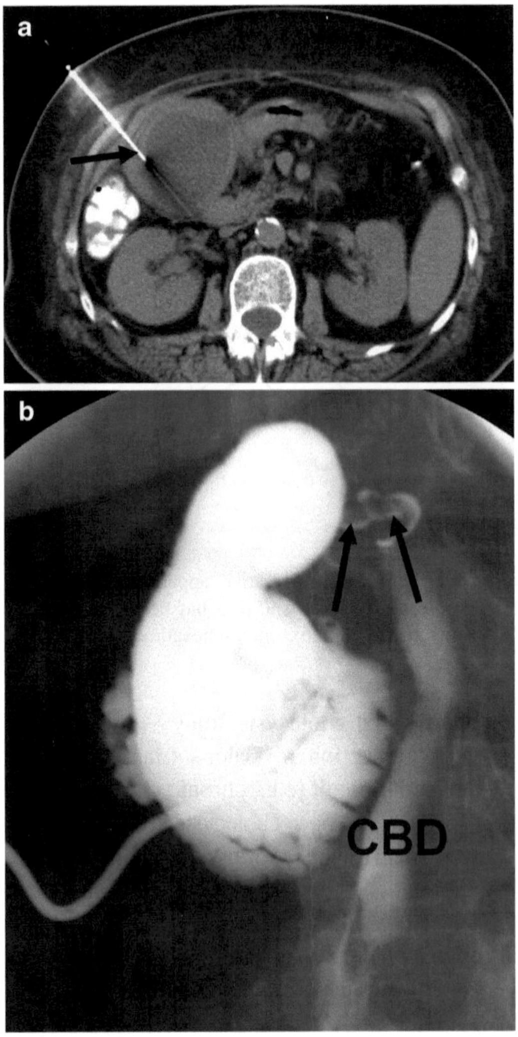

Fig. 5.5 Cholecystostomy in a patient with an empyema of the gallbladder. (**a**) Axial CT showing a Longdwell needle within a distended thick-walled gallbladder (*arrow*). Pus was aspirated, and a 10F locking-loop pigtail catheter was inserted. (**b**) Cholecystogram (4 days later when the patient had clinically improved) shows a thick-walled fissured gallbladder with filling defects within the cystic duct secondary to gallstones (*arrows*). Some contrast does enter the common bile duct (*CBD*)

5.2.4 Normal Radiological Appearances Following Cholecystectomy

Imaging is usually only requested following suspected complications after laparoscopic cholecystectomy (Thurley and Dhingsa 2008). Ultrasound, MRCP, and CT may be requested depending on local availability and expertise.

5.2.4.1 Postoperative Fluid

It is common to see a small amount of fluid in the gallbladder fossa 3–5 days postcholecystectomy. This fluid is secondary to small collections of bile or blood. One of the possible causes for a small bile leak is injury to persistent congenital connections that connect the gallbladder directly to the right lobe of the liver (ducts of Luschka). These fluid collections in an uncomplicated cholecystectomy should have no distinct or well-demarcated borders on CT (Quinn et al. 1992). Other common findings include small amounts of free pelvic fluid and some increased density of the fat at the laparoscopic port sites (Moran et al. 1994). As always, correlation between the presence of these findings and the clinical status of the patient is advised.

5.2.4.2 Biliary Dilatation

The diameter of the CBD may increase postcholecystectomy, with a maximal diameter of 13 mm recognized (Feng and Song 1995). When biliary dilatation is identified on postoperative imaging, correlation with preoperative imaging and current clinical features and biochemistry is advised. Biliary dilatation can be seen following sphincterotomy and may persist in patients with CBD stones despite treatment.

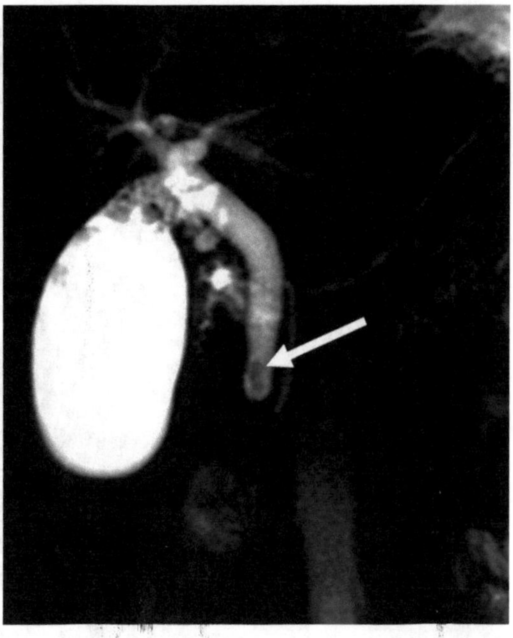

Fig. 5.6 Single-shot FSE MRCP sequence obtained in a 4-s breath hold shows a mildly dilated CBD with the stones at the lower end (*arrow*)

5.3 MRCP Interpretation Tips and Pitfalls

In our institution, MRCP is the most common modality requested in the postoperative period to investigate suspected complications following biliary surgery. If tolerated, MRCP provides information on ductal anatomy and the presence of intraductal stones or strictures and can detect fluid collections in the gallbladder fossa and upper abdomen. It is however associated with pitfalls in interpretation both in the pre- and postoperative settings, and the radiologist should be familiar with these.

5.3.1 MRCP Technique

Magnetic resonance cholangiopancreatography (MRCP) is an effective noninvasive imaging technique for demonstration of disorders of the bile and pancreatic ducts. MRCP uses heavily T2-weighted fast spin-echo (FSE) sequences in which slowly moving or stationary fluid has very high signal intensity. The signal from the background tissue is suppressed because of the shorter T2 relaxation time, resulting in an image that looks like a conventional cholangiogram or pancreatogram. While MRCP is robust and reproducible, attention needs to be given to the clinical question to ensure that the correct technique is employed.

The FSE sequence allows cholangiographic images to be obtained in a short breath hold. The rapid acquisition of the image also reduces motion artifact from peristalsis. Both single-slice thick slab and multislice images can be generated.

Single-slice fast spin-echo technique produces a thick slab (30–80 mm) in less than 5 s (Fig. 5.6). Single-shot FSE sequences with partial Fourier techniques, e.g., half-Fourier acquisition single-shot fast spin-echo (HASTE), are extremely useful for producing high-resolution images and demonstration of fine structures (Fig. 5.7). Techniques such as HASTE produce up to eleven 2–4-mm slices in a 20-s breath hold. HASTE imaging is usually performed in both the axial plane and the optimal coronal or coronal oblique plane, which will be chosen on the basis of the FSE images.

More recently, it has been possible to perform high-resolution 3D MRCP, which has the advantage of an increase in the signal-to-noise ratio for a given TE or a lower repetition time for the same signal-to-noise ratio. Contiguous sections can then be reconstructed in any plane

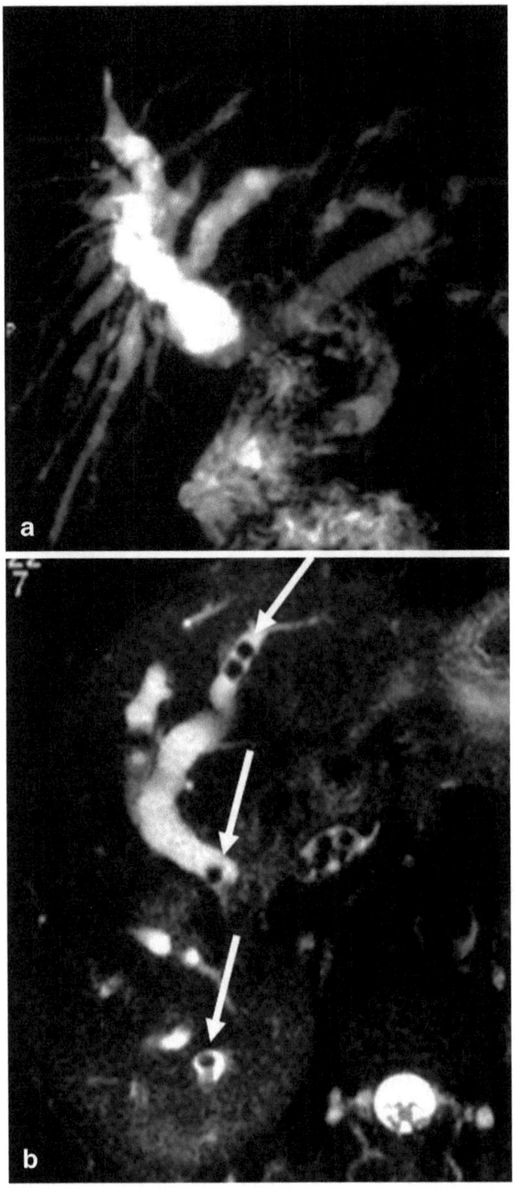

Fig. 5.7 (**a**) Single-shot FSE thick slab shows multiple stones in a dilated common bile duct. (**b**) HASTE images, however, show detail of the intrahepatic ductal stones much more clearly (*arrows*)

to produce a maximum intensity projection (MIP) image. It is essential however that the source images are reviewed as some detail can be overlooked on the MIP images (Fig. 5.8). 3D MRCP does not require breath holding, but the patient must breathe regularly. Irregular excursions of the diaphragm reduce image quality considerably. Any degree of patient movement also causes significant image degradation (Fig. 5.9).

Pitfalls in the interpretation of MRCP imaging may be divided into those related to inappropriate or inadequate technique, misinterpretation (particularly when the patient has had previous intervention), and finally where pathology is arising outside the ducts. In these cases, it might then be necessary to add in conventional liver or pancreatic sequences.

In our department, basic MRCP protocol includes an overall view of the anatomy of both the ducts and the soft tissues in the upper abdomen using a steady-state precession technique (true FISP, BFFE, or FIESTA). This technique produces an excellent anatomical overview and is particularly useful for demonstration of vessels (Fig. 5.10). It also allows a single slice to be obtained in less than a second and therefore can give extremely helpful information in patients who are uncooperative (Fig. 5.11). It is usually recommended that patients fast for approximately 4 h prior to the examination to prevent fluid in the stomach and duodenum, causing difficulty with interpretation. Fasting, however, is not essential in most cases. A negative oral contrast agent can be used such as iron oxide or pineapple juice if luminal fluid is thought to be problematic.

The true FISP sequences can be used effectively to allow accurate positioning for the FSE images (Fig. 5.12). It is essential that an appropriate slice thickness is chosen. This may be particularly important when looking for small stones or detail of short strictures (Fig. 5.13).

5.3.2 Specific MRCP Pitfalls

5.3.2.1 Vascular Compression

The most common site of vascular compression is at the hilum of the liver where the right hepatic

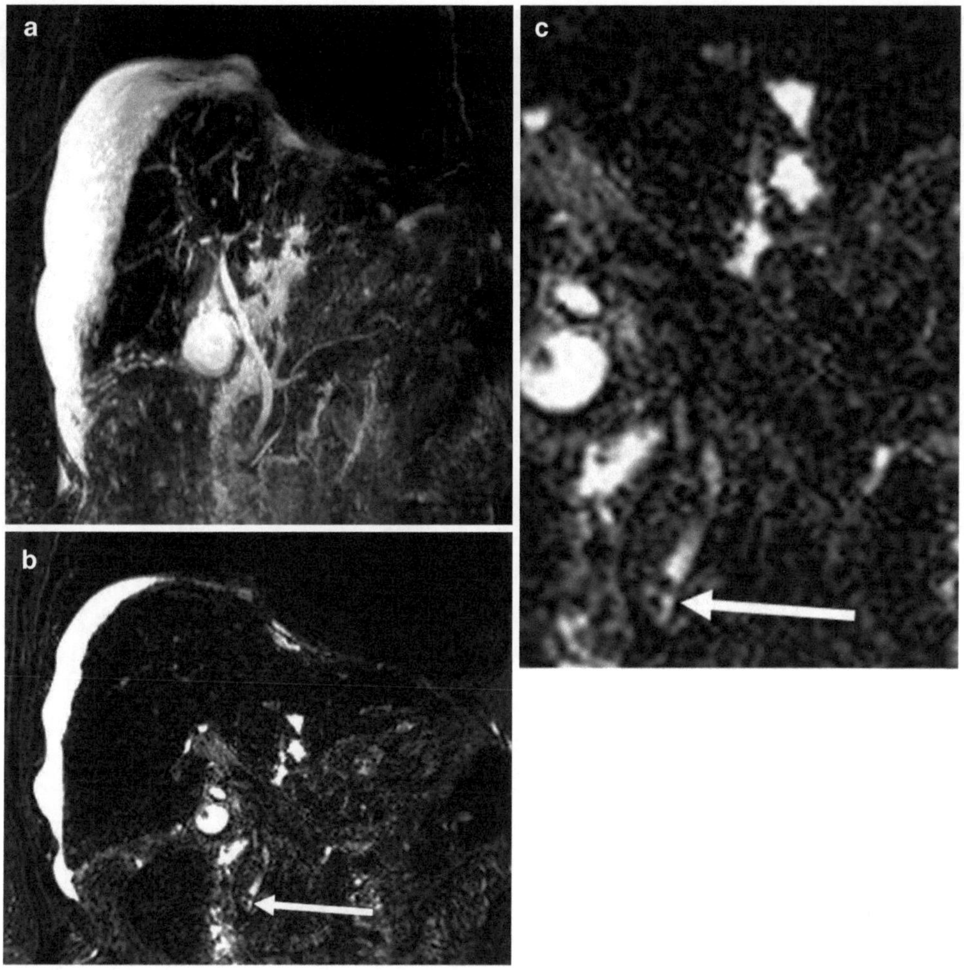

Fig. 5.8 (**a**) 3D MRCP MIP image in a patient with sclerosing cholangitis, end-stage liver disease, and ascites. The source images (**b** and **c**), however, show stones at the distal end of the bile duct (*arrows*), which were the cause of the patient's recent deterioration

artery crosses the common hepatic duct just below the hilum. This can be easily misinterpreted as a short hilar stricture (Fig. 5.14). Where there is doubt, gadolinium-enhanced imaging may clarify (particularly if it has been performed in a similar plane to the MRCP image). In a standard MRCP examination, dynamic imaging is not generally performed. Vessels, however, are well seen on true FISP images, and review of the FISP sequence may allow correct interpretation. At the lower end of the bile duct, the gastroduodenal artery can cause a filling defect most frequently seen on axial imaging behind the bile duct, and this can be misinterpreted as a small distal stone. Again, review of true FISP images is helpful.

5.3.2.2 Flow Artifact

In standard HASTE images, there may be a filling defect lying centrally in the distal CBD (Fig. 5.15). This is usually about 1–2 mm in diameter and generally only occurs in the axial plane. This is thought to represent a flow artifact. This artifact may be particularly problematic

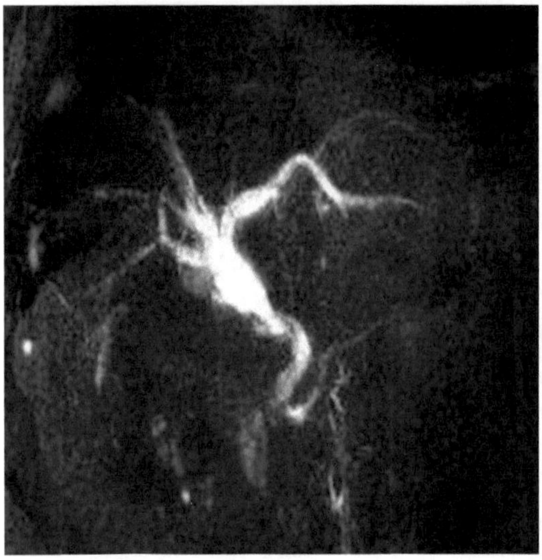

Fig. 5.9 3D MRCP degraded by movement artifact. Detail of structures is extremely poor

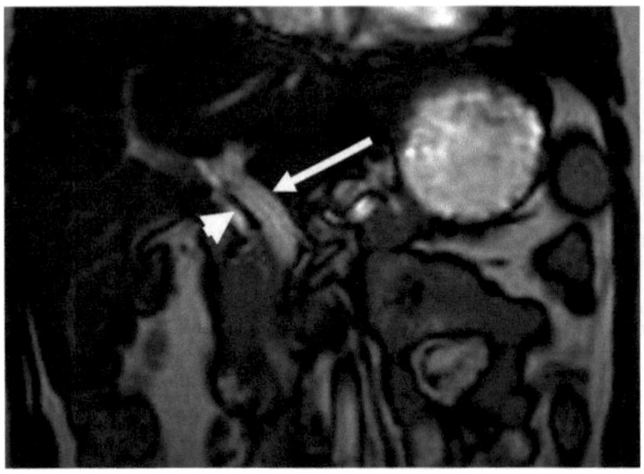

Fig. 5.10 True FISP sequence demonstrating vessels and overall anatomy. Portal vein (*arrow*), CBD (*arrowhead*)

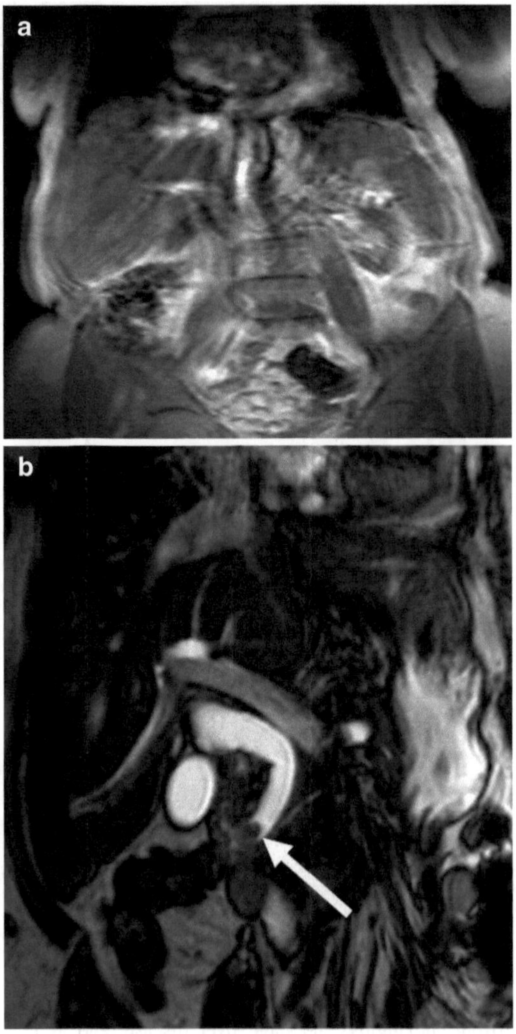

Fig. 5.11 (**a**) Localizer image in a patient who is having difficulty with breath holding in which there is considerable movement artifact. (**b**) True FISP image obtained in less than a second, demonstrating a stone at the lower end of the bile duct (*arrow*)

around the cystic duct insertion where flow dynamics may be more complex.

5.3.2.3 Pseudocalculus

The normal sphincter of Oddi complex can look like a filling defect at the lower end of the bile duct. This occurs when there is a relative degree of spasm. Repeated imaging over a period of time should demonstrate relaxation of the sphincter. Because the 3D sequence is acquired over several minutes, the sphincter is less likely to be closed throughout this time, and therefore this artifact is rarely a problem with this sequence (Fig. 5.16).

5.3.2.4 Air in the Bile Ducts (Pneumobilia)

This most frequently occurs following an endoscopic sphincterotomy, surgical sphincteroplasty, or formation of a biliary enteric anastomosis. On axial imaging, the distinction may be relatively straightforward; air accumulates in the

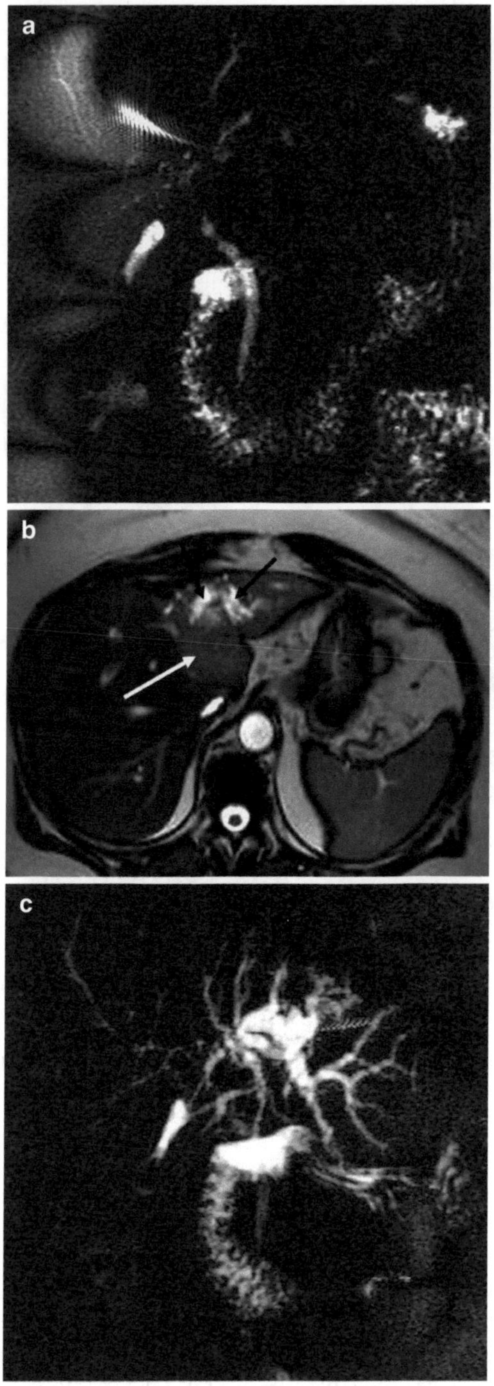

Fig. 5.12 (**a**) Single-shot FSE showing the extrahepatic bile duct but very poor detail of the intrahepatic ducts. Review of the true FISP imaging in (**b**) shows that the left lobe ducts are crowded (*black arrows*) and there is left lobe atrophy (*white arrow*). (**c**) Repositioning of the acquisition slab results in much better detail of the intrahepatic biliary tree

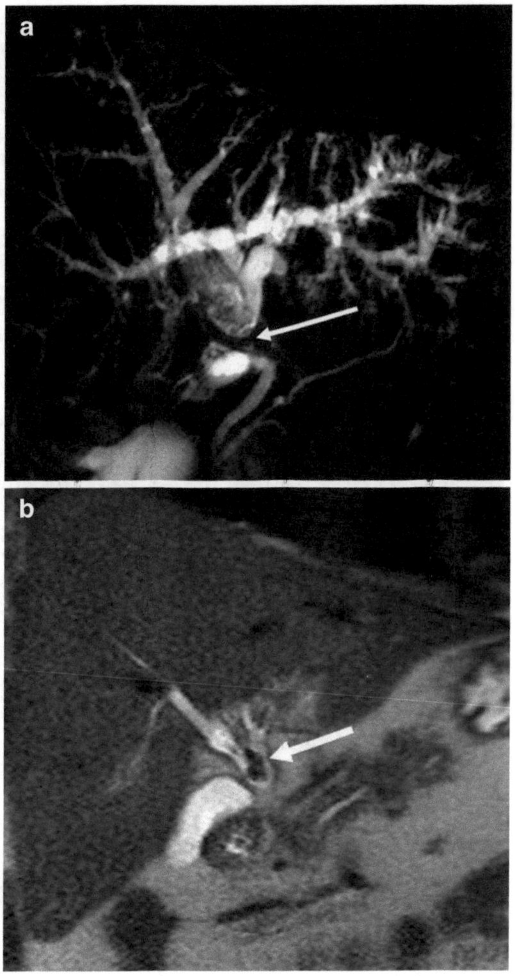

Fig. 5.13 Patient referred for MRCP with a suspected cholangiocarcinoma. (**a**) Thick slab FSE shows obstruction of the common bile duct. 4-mm HASTE images were performed but did not demonstrate the nature of the obstruction (*not shown*). (**b**) 2-mm slices were performed, and they clearly demonstrate that the obstruction is due to stone disease (*arrow*). In some patients, stones in the gall bladder and bile ducts are high signal on T1 images

least dependent part of the bile ducts, usually the left-sided intrahepatic ducts. Air is usually seen lying anteriorly in a dilated bile duct forming an air-fluid level. This can be extremely difficult to appreciate on coronal or coronal oblique images, where it can be misinterpreted as a stricture or stones (Figs. 5.17 and 5.18). In the axial plane, stones generally lie posteriorly in a bile duct as they are heavier than bile.

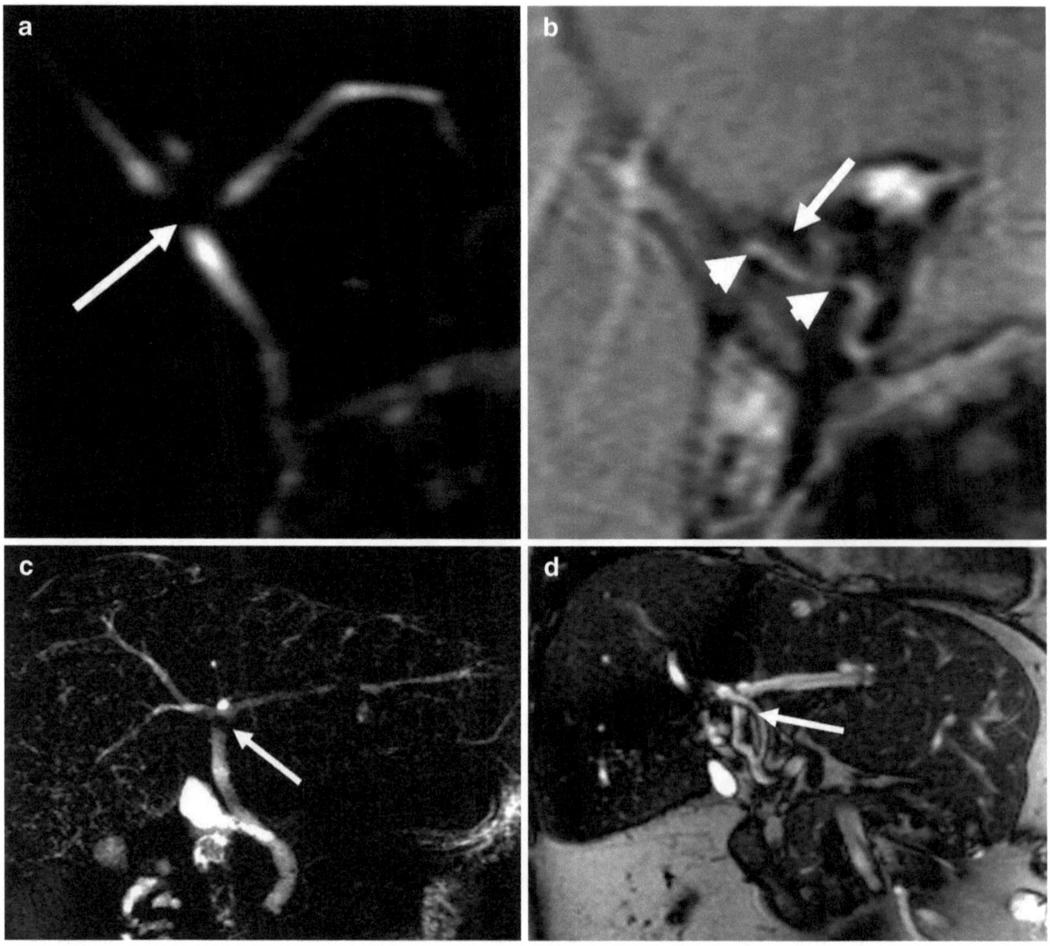

Fig. 5.14 Vascular compression in two patients. (**a**) Shows an apparent stricture at the hilum of the liver (*arrow*). (**b**) Gadolinium-enhanced image in a right coronal oblique projection showing the hepatic artery (*arrowheads*) crossing the bile duct at the same level. The "stricture" (*arrow*) is a pulsation artifact. (**c**) There is an oblique filling defect (*arrow*) at the proximal common hepatic duct with no dilatation proximal to this. (**d**) True FISP image from the same patient demonstrates the right hepatic artery (*arrow*) crossing the bile duct at this level

5.3.2.5 Stents, Clips, and Drains

While drains, clips, and stents are relatively easy to see on CT examinations, they can be very difficult to appreciate on standard MRCP sequences. A tubular structure containing high signal fluid with low signal edges should raise the possibility of a drain. A tubular structure containing either fluid or air within the bile duct should raise the possibility of a plastic stent (Fig. 5.19). One of the advantages of MRCP sequences is that they are relatively insensitive to susceptibility artifact from metal clips and stents. However, there may be small areas of artifact, and this should be considered where there is an apparent defect in a bile duct. The metallic nature of the abnormality may be appreciated on the true FISP sequence, and if that does not help, then in- and opposed-phase T1-weighted images can verify a metallic artifact

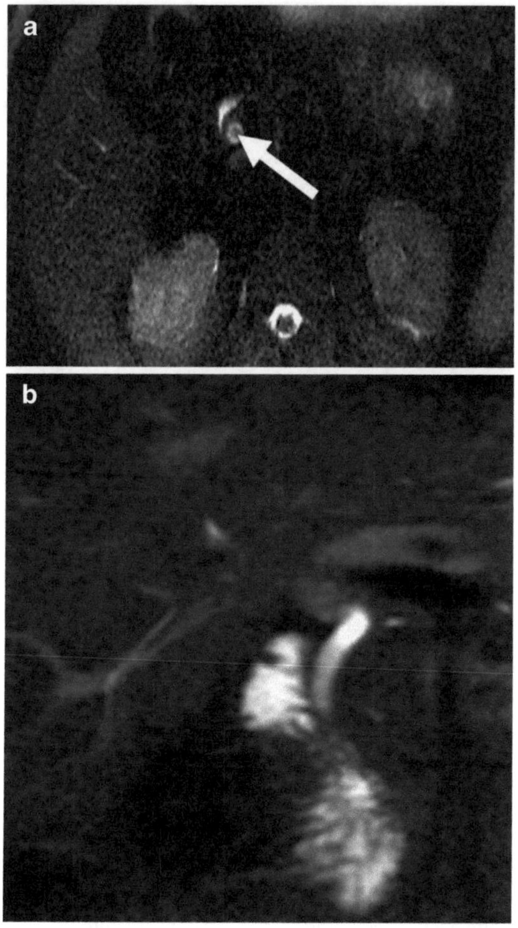

Fig. 5.15 Flow artifact. (**a**) Axial HASTE image with an apparent filling defect in the center of the distal bile duct (*arrow*). This is not seen on the coronal HASTE image (**b**) and represents a flow artifact. These are most frequently seen below the level of the cystic duct insertion

(Fig. 5.20). The degree of signal dropout due to clips is greatest on the T1 in-phase sequences compared with the opposed-phase sequences (due to the longer echo time and therefore increased susceptibility artifact).

5.3.2.6 Pathology Originating Outside the Ducts

While MRCP sequences are designed to look specifically at the ductal system and signal from the

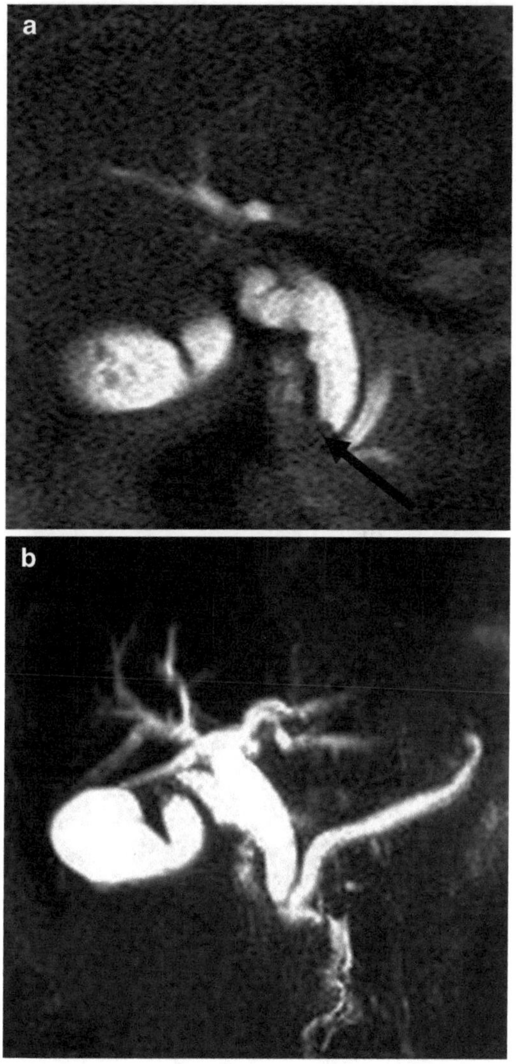

Fig. 5.16 Pseudocalculus. (**a**) This is due to contraction of the sphincter of Oddi at the distal end of the duct on the HASTE sequences (*arrow*). (**b**) The 3D sequence shows a normal distal duct. During this prolonged acquisition sequence, the sphincter relaxes

surrounding soft tissues is suppressed, useful information can nevertheless be detected. Normal vessels are seen as areas of flow artifact, but thrombosed vessels will be seen as areas of relatively high signal rather than a flow void (Fig. 5.21).

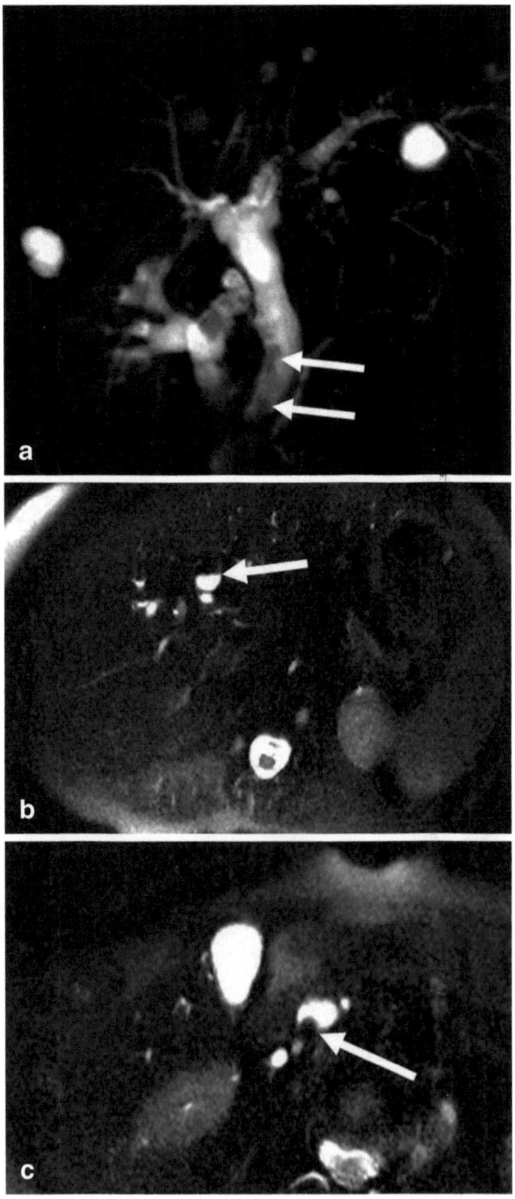

Fig. 5.17 Pneumobilia and ductal stones in a patient with a previous sphincterotomy for CBD stones. (**a**) Coronal thick slab FSE image with multiple filling defects in the distal bile duct (*arrows*). Differentiating stones from air can be difficult on coronal sequences. (**b**) Axial HASTE shows an air-fluid level in the proximal common bile duct secondary to pneumobilia (*arrow*). (**c**) A stone is seen lying posteriorly in the distal common bile duct (*arrow*)

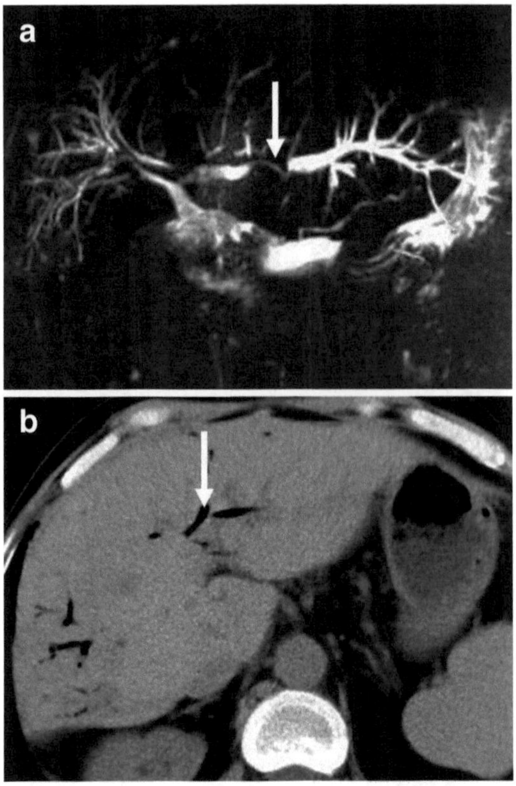

Fig. 5.18 Pneumobilia. (**a**) An apparent left hepatic duct stricture (*arrow*) is seen on the thick slab FSE image with mildly dilated left-sided intrahepatic ducts. Review of the CT (**b**) scan shows that there is air (*arrow*) in the intrahepatic ducts, accounting for the apparent stricture

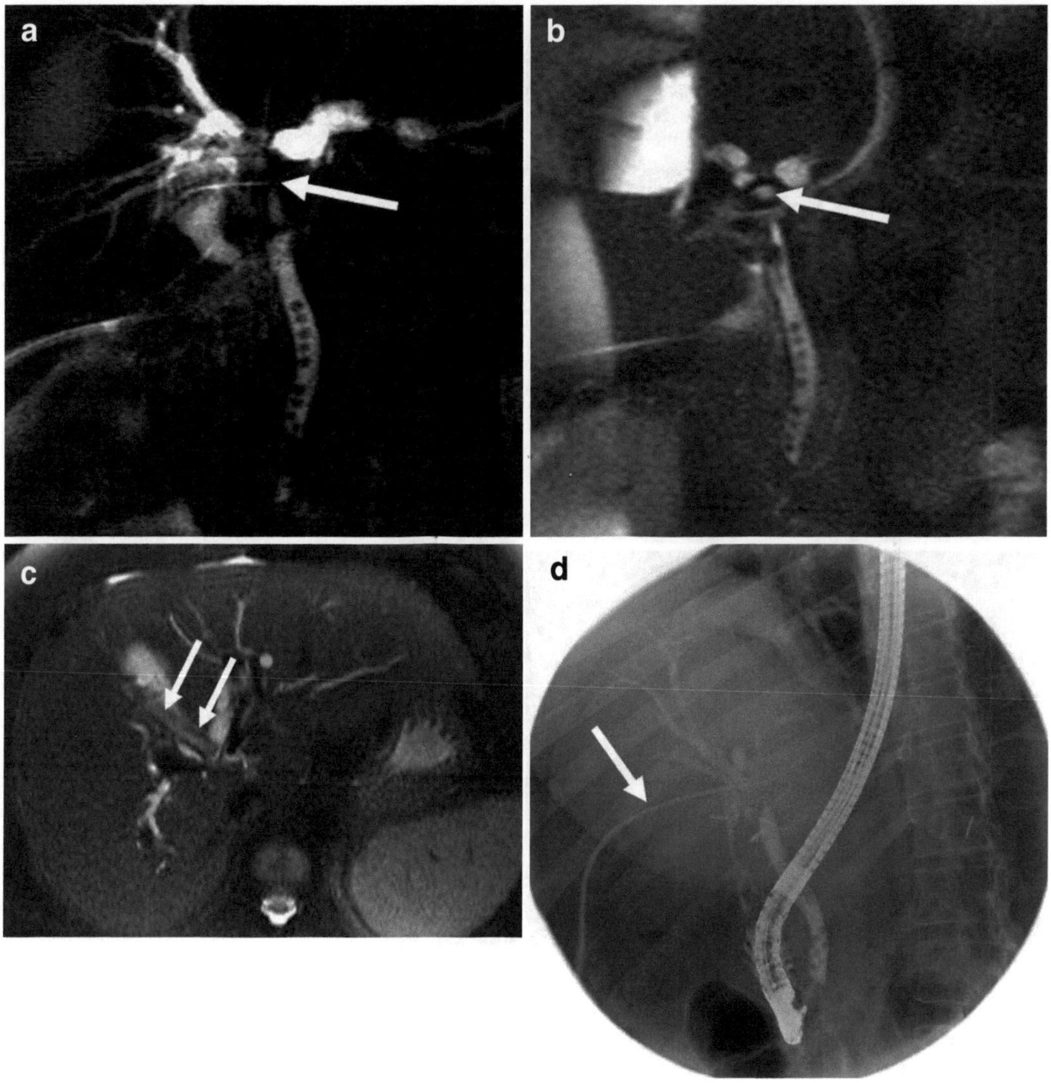

Fig. 5.19 (**a**) Axial thick slab FSE image with stones in the distal bile duct. The intrahepatic ducts are dilated, and there is a signal void at the hilum of the liver (*arrow*). (**b**) HASTE image in a coronal plane with an area of signal void at the hilum surrounding an area of higher signal intensity (*arrow*). On the axial images (**c**), this represents a tubular structure (*arrows*) which was lying very close to the hilum of the liver and potentially obstructing the ducts. This represents a surgical drain. (**d**) The position of the drain (*arrow*) is confirmed on the ERCP

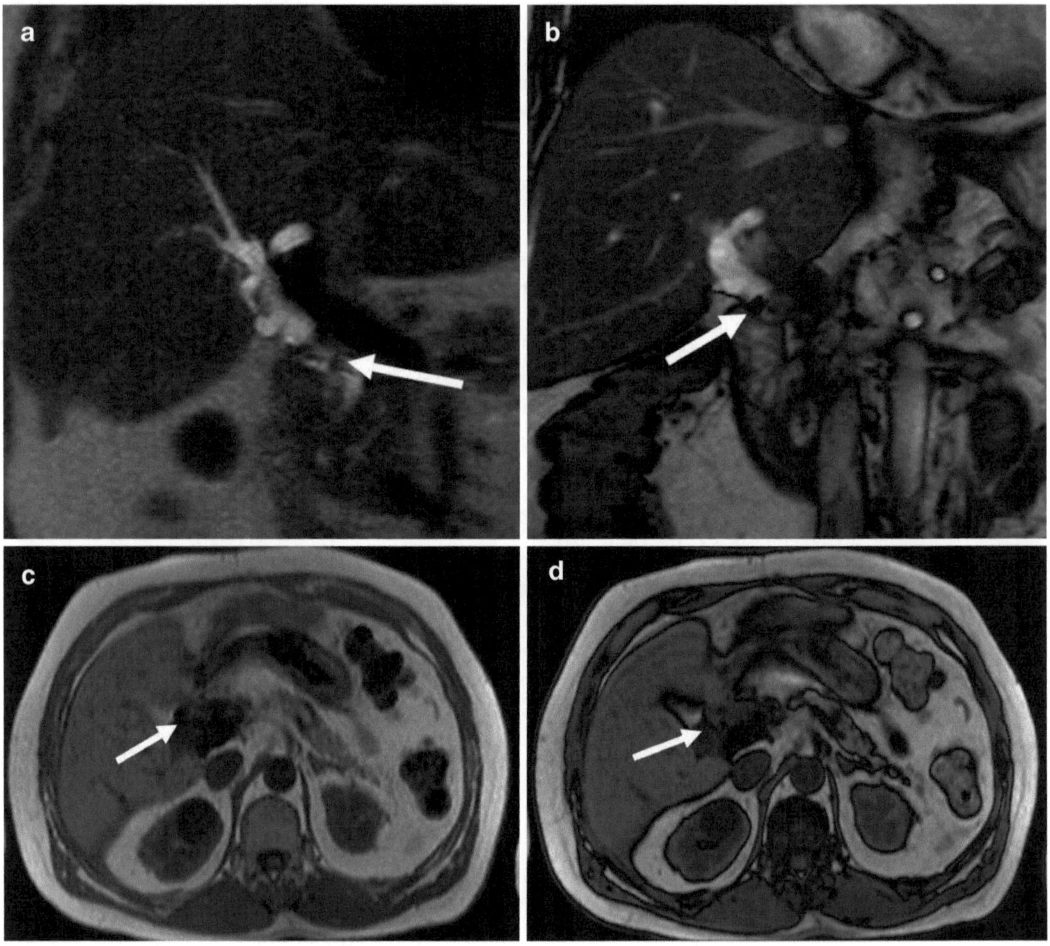

Fig. 5.20 Surgical clips. (**a**) Thin slice HASTE image with an apparent filling defect on the lateral margin of the bile duct at the level of the cystic duct (*arrow*). This is very linear and it was thought may represent metallic clips from the recent laparoscopic cholecystectomy. The metallic nature is evident on the true FISP image (**b**) where there is marked signal dropout (*arrow*). This is confirmed on the in-phase (**c**) and opposed-phase (**d**) T1-weighted images where the artefact (*arrow*) is more obvious on the in-phase than the opposed-phase (because of the longer TE and greater susceptibility artifact)

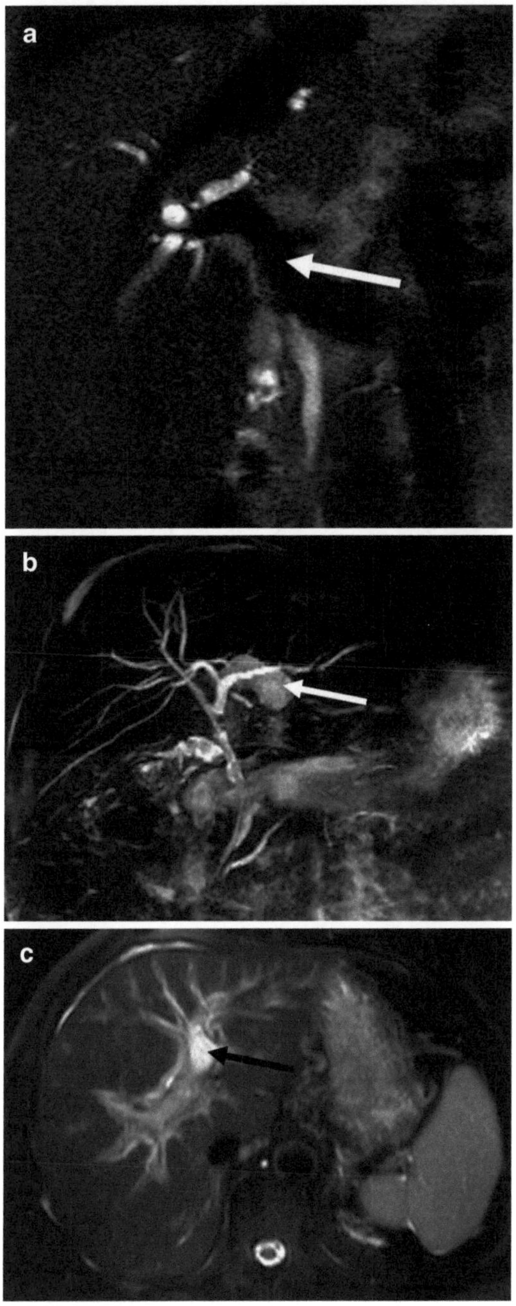

Fig. 5.21 Thrombosed vessels. (**a**) Coronal thin slice HASTE image with a normal caliber common bile duct and the normal portal vein is seen as a signal void (*arrow*). (**b**) Coronal 3D MRCP image, showing additional high signal in the left lobe of the liver (*arrow*). On the axial HASTE images (**c**), this is shown to be a thrombosed left portal vein (*arrow*). Note the varying signal intensity within the portal vein, indicating thrombus of different ages

5.4 Complications of Cholecystectomy

Although solitary complications do occur, complex multiple complications do frequently coexist. The following will be discussed:

- Bile duct injury – leaks, strictures, transection/ligation
- Biliary obstruction – retained gallstones, misplaced surgical clips, and diathermy injury
- Dropped gallstones
- Vascular complications
- Laparoscopic complications

5.4.1 Bile Duct Injuries

Bile duct injuries are rare (0.3–0.7%) but are more common following laparoscopic cholecystectomy for acute cholecystitis and biliary pancreatitis, where inflammation prevents adequate identification of biliary anatomy. Injury is also associated with anatomical anomalies of the biliary tree (Christensesn et al. 1992). The most common examples include (Fig. 5.22):

- Short or long cystic duct
- Long cystic duct winding round the hepatic duct
- Cystic duct arising from right hepatic duct
- Aberrant right hepatic duct
- Accessory hepatic duct draining into the gallbladder

The biliary tree can also be injured secondary to inadvertent ligation, laceration, resection, or thermal injury. Bile duct injury can potentially cause a biliary leak, obstruction, or delayed stricture formation.

A high index of suspicion must be observed in all patients postcholecystectomy who present with the following symptoms: abdominal pain, (obstructive) jaundice, pyrexia, tachycardia, and sepsis as these are clinical hallmarks of potential postoperative biliary complications. In the presence of a bile leak, patients may develop a localized bilioma or biliary peritonitis.

Bile duct injuries are classified according to Strasberg's classification (Fig. 5.23), which are

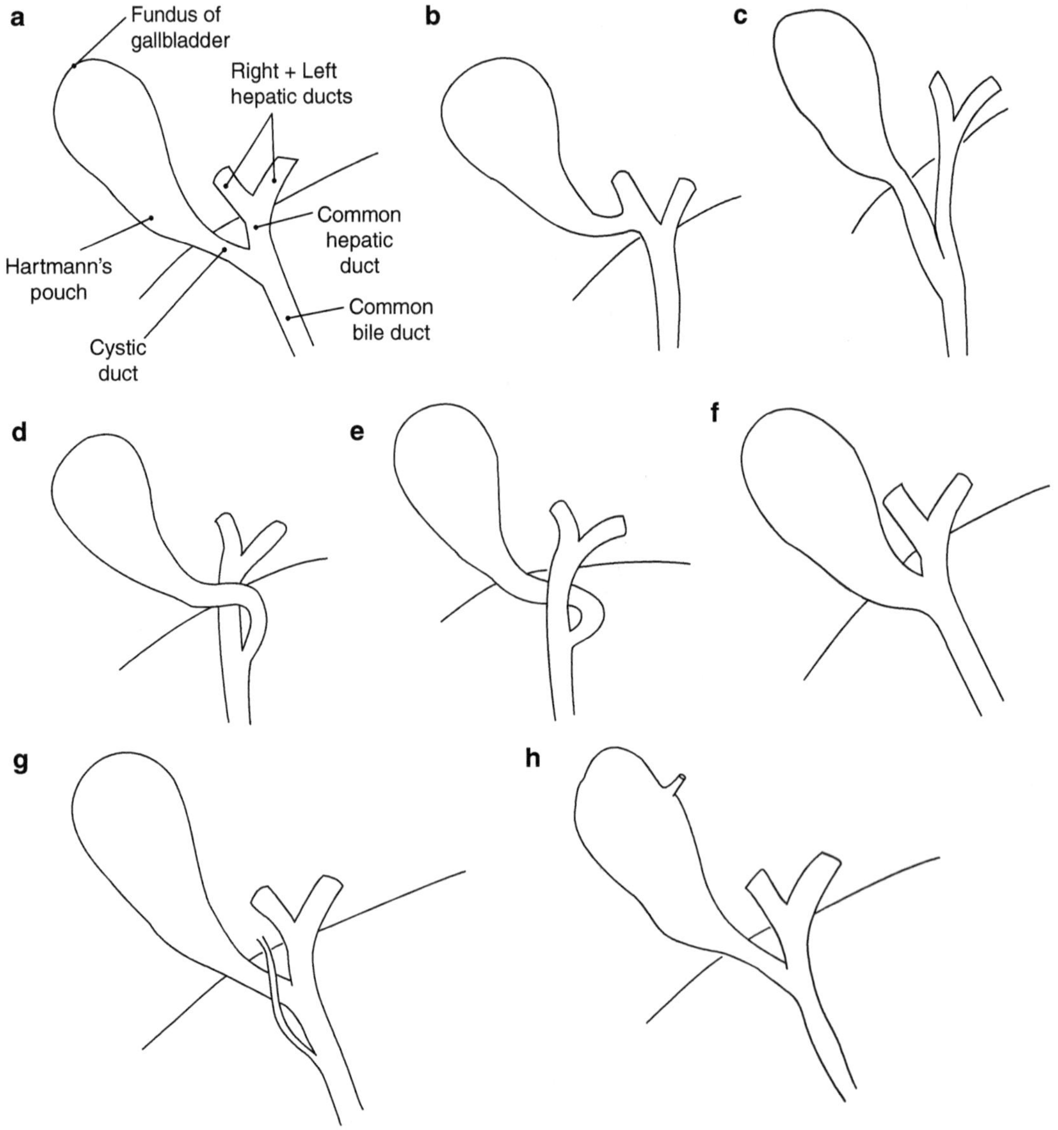

Fig. 5.22 (**a**, **b**) Biliary anatomy and common variants. (**a**) Normal biliary anatomy. (**b**) Cystic duct arising from right hepatic duct. (**c**) Long cystic duct running parallel in proximity to the common hepatic duct with low insertion into the common bile duct. (**d**) Long cystic duct winding anterior to the common hepatic duct. (**e**) Long cystic duct winding posterior to common hepatic duct. (**f**) Short cystic duct. (**g**) Accessory hepatic duct draining into the common bile duct. (**h**) Accessory hepatic duct draining into the gallbladder

categorized from A to E and according to location, mechanism of injury, and the continuity of the biliary system (Strasberg et al. 1995). Type E injuries involve the main biliary ducts and are further subdivided (E1–E5) based on Bismuth's classification (Fig. 5.24) (Bismuth and Majno 2001). In the presence of a bile leak, the biliary tree is rarely dilated on imaging. The management of bile duct injuries depends very much on the location and extent of injury. For example, proximal biliary tree injuries involving the confluence of the main ducts are technically more difficult to manage than those that involve the distal CBD. Where bile duct injury is recognized at the time of surgery, immediate remedial action is taken, whereas a delayed presentation will

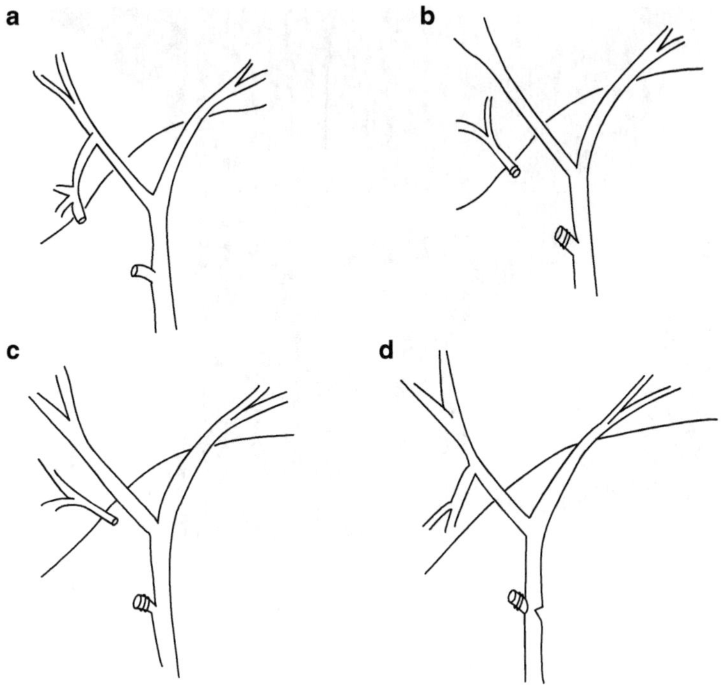

Fig. 5.23 Strasberg classification of bile duct injuries. (**a**) Bile leak from the cystic duct or liver bed. (**b**) Occlusion of part of the biliary tree, typically an aberrant segmental or sectoral duct. (**c**) Bile leak from an aberrant segmental or sectoral duct. (**d**) Partial lateral injury to the extrahepatic bile duct

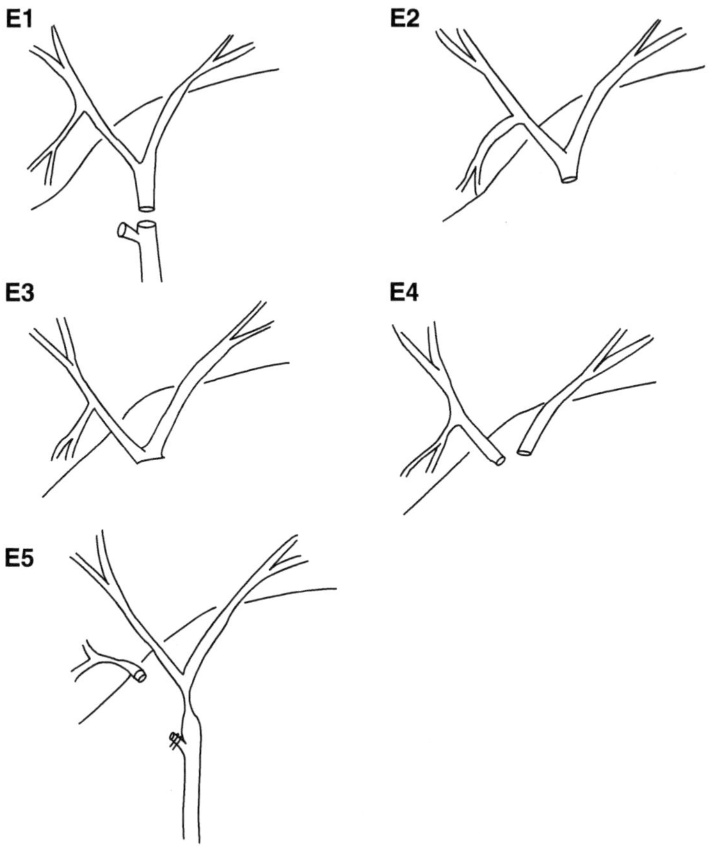

Fig. 5.24 Bismuth subclassification of main bile duct injury. (*E1*) Circumferential injury to the common hepatic duct with a residual stump >2 cm in length. (*E2*) Circumferential injury to the common hepatic duct with a residual stump <2 cm in length. (*E3*) Hilar injury at the confluence with preservation of hepatic duct continuity. (*E4*) Hilar injury at the confluence with loss of hepatic duct continuity. (*E5*) Involvement of an aberrant right sectoral hepatic duct alone with or without concomitant stricture of the common hepatic duct

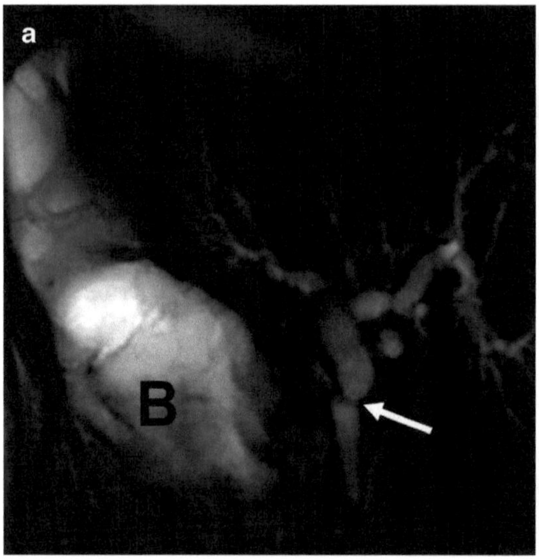

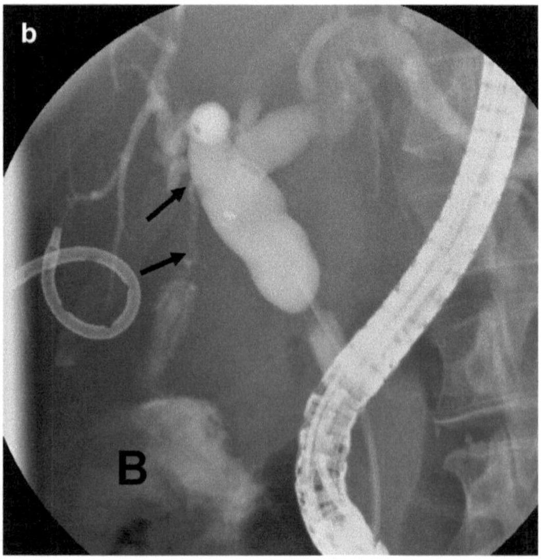

Fig. 5.25 Bile leak and CBD injury following complicated cholecystectomy in which tumor was unexpectedly encountered arising from the gallbladder fundus. (**a**) Thick slab coronal T2W MRCP shows a large bile leak (*B*) within the right upper quadrant. There is an abrupt "cutoff" of the CBD possibly due to a clamping injury (*white arrow*). The bile leak was drained under ultrasound guidance. (**b**) At ERCP, the short CBD stricture was traversed with a guidewire. Injection of contrast through a catheter confirms the bile leak from a sectoral duct (*black arrows*) communicating with the collection (*B*). Note the pigtail drainage catheter. An 8F plastic stent was placed within the CBD to facilitate bile drainage (*not shown*)

require a delay for peritoneal contamination/sepsis to abate. This invariably needs imaging to confirm the diagnosis and direct intervention.

5.4.2 Bile Leak

A leak from the cystic duct stump is the most common cause of a postoperative bile leak. It occurs when surgical clips become dislodged or do not encompass the entire cystic duct. Bile leaks from the cystic duct are more pronounced in the presence of distal obstruction secondary to a retained CBD calculus because of obstruction to the distal flow of bile. Bile leaks can also occur from the gallbladder fossa when the plane of dissection within the liver bed is too deep and segmental biliary radicles are injured. Such an injury is more likely to occur with an intrahepatic gallbladder or an adherent gallbladder following chronic cholecystitis (Hoeffel et al. 2006). Incomplete resection of the gallbladder can also lead to a sustained bile leak.

The most common sites of bile collections are in the gallbladder fossa and the subhepatic and the right subphrenic spaces (Fig. 5.25). Free intraperitoneal fluid may also be seen, although this is a nonspecific finding in a postoperative patient. When the collections are well demarcated and have a defined wall, these are defined as biliomas and can occur in an intra- or extrahepatic location (Fig. 5.26). Free leakage of the bile into the peritoneal cavity can produce biliary peritonitis.

5.4.2.1 Imaging of Suspected Bile Leaks

Although repeat laparoscopy can be used to identify bile leaks, ultrasound, MRCP, CT, and nuclear imaging (HIDA) are noninvasive modalities that are more commonly utilized. The preferred choice of imaging will depend on local availability and expertise. CT is better at demonstrating the full extent of the leak within the peritoneal cavity (Fig. 5.27). If fluid is detected around the liver or gallbladder on postoperative imaging, diagnostic aspiration can be performed using CT or ultrasound guidance. The content of the aspirate,

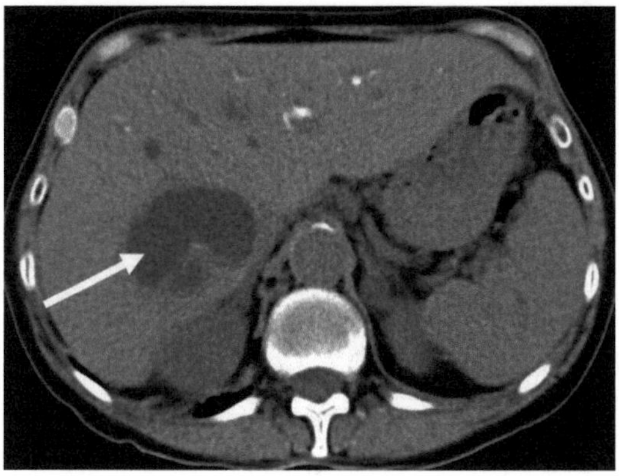

Fig. 5.26 Liver bilioma. Axial CT cholangiogram in a patient with a history of complicated cholecystectomy shows a well-demarcated bilioma (*arrow*). There was biliary obstruction secondary to CBD stones (*not shown*)

e.g., serous, bilious, hemorrhagic, or purulent, will determine subsequent intervention (Fig. 5.28). Percutaneous radiological guided drainage can be performed at the same time in most cases of localized bile leaks. MRCP is a useful adjunct as it demonstrates the residual biliary tree anatomy (if reconstruction is necessitated) and identifies the presence of retained CBD calculi. These studies, however, only provide indirect evidence of a bile leak (e.g., free fluid or collection). Dynamic studies which provide direct evidence of a bile leak are discussed below (Sect. 5.4.2.2). The exclusion of biliary dilatation is important to allow differentiation of a leak from duct ligation/stricture, as management pathways are different.

5.4.2.2 Dynamic Studies Used to Diagnose Bile Leaks

HIDA

Radionuclide scanning with technetium-labeled HIDA is widely available and advantageous in patients who cannot tolerate MRCP (Fig. 5.29). The addition of hybrid SPECT-CT imaging allows accurate anatomical cross-sectional correlation with the radioisotope study. Following a 4-h fast, 150 MBq (scaled down for children) of Tc-99 m mebrofenin (2,2′-[[2-[(3-bromo-2,4,6-trimethylphenyl)-amino]-2-oxoethyl] imino]) (Bracco Diagnostics, Princeton, NJ) or other IDA derivative is administered intravenously. Images are acquired at 1 and 2 min, then at 5-min intervals to 45 min. Anterior or right anterior oblique views are taken to include the liver and duodenum. Additional views are obtained as needed to tailor the study to the individual postoperative anatomy of the individual patient. Later acquisitions (up to 24 h) are obtained as required to show the onward drainage of bile, to show minor leaks or fistulae,

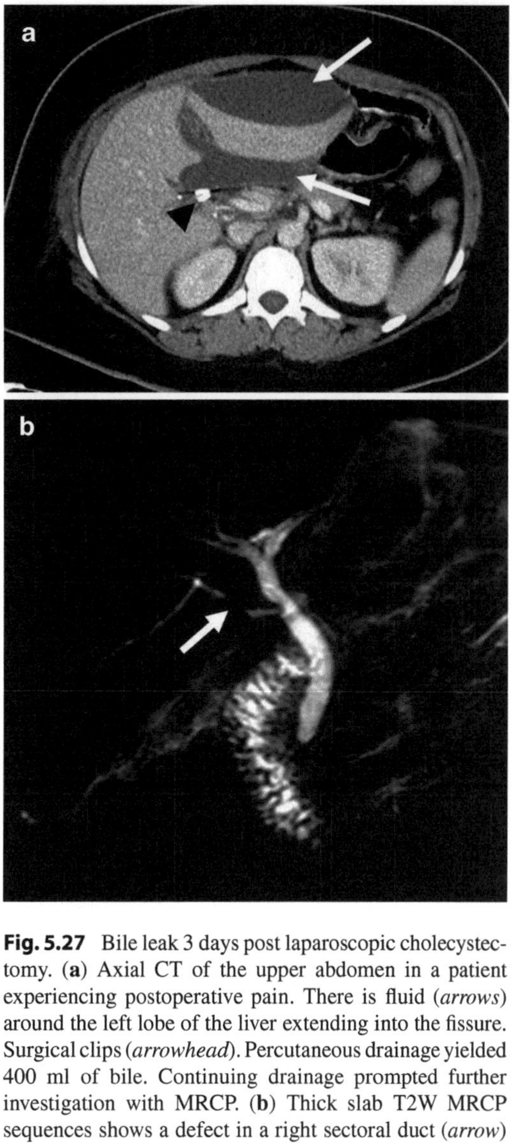

Fig. 5.27 Bile leak 3 days post laparoscopic cholecystectomy. (**a**) Axial CT of the upper abdomen in a patient experiencing postoperative pain. There is fluid (*arrows*) around the left lobe of the liver extending into the fissure. Surgical clips (*arrowhead*). Percutaneous drainage yielded 400 ml of bile. Continuing drainage prompted further investigation with MRCP. (**b**) Thick slab T2W MRCP sequences shows a defect in a right sectoral duct (*arrow*) consistent with transection. This drains directly into the common hepatic duct and was the source of the bile leak but had been mistaken for the cystic duct. Review of the pre operative MRCP did confirm aberrant ductal anatomy but this was not reported. It is important to highlight any anatomical ductal variants on preoperative MRCP

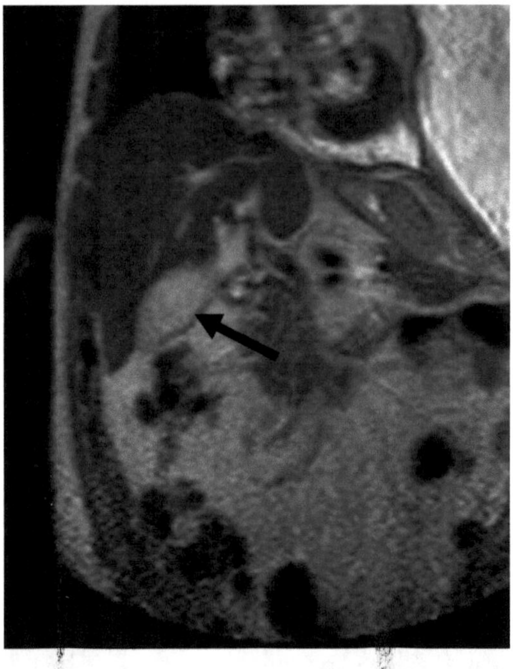

Fig. 5.28 Postoperative hematoma. Coronal T2W MRCP in a patient who had a recent cholecystectomy shows a high signal small hematoma in the gall bladder bed (*arrow*)

and to show delayed excretion of tracer in cases of reduced liver function. Drainage catheters and bags should be included in the field of view.

Contrast-Enhanced MRCP

Contrast-enhanced MRCP utilizes agents which are primarily excreted via the biliary tree (Hoeffel et al. 2006). Examples include mangafodipir trisodium [Teslascan; Nycomed Amersham Imaging, Oslo, Norway] or Primovist (Bayer Schering Pharma). The dynamic excretion of these contrast agents provides anatomical and functional information on the postoperative biliary tree, e.g., confirming a bile leak and identifying the source of the leak (Fig. 5.30). Limitations include the assessment of the peripheral intrahepatic bile ducts and opacification of the biliary tree in the presence of biliary obstruction.

CT Cholangiography

The site of a bile leak can be identified with CT cholangiography (although the required contrast agent Biliscopin [Bayer Schering Pharma AG] is

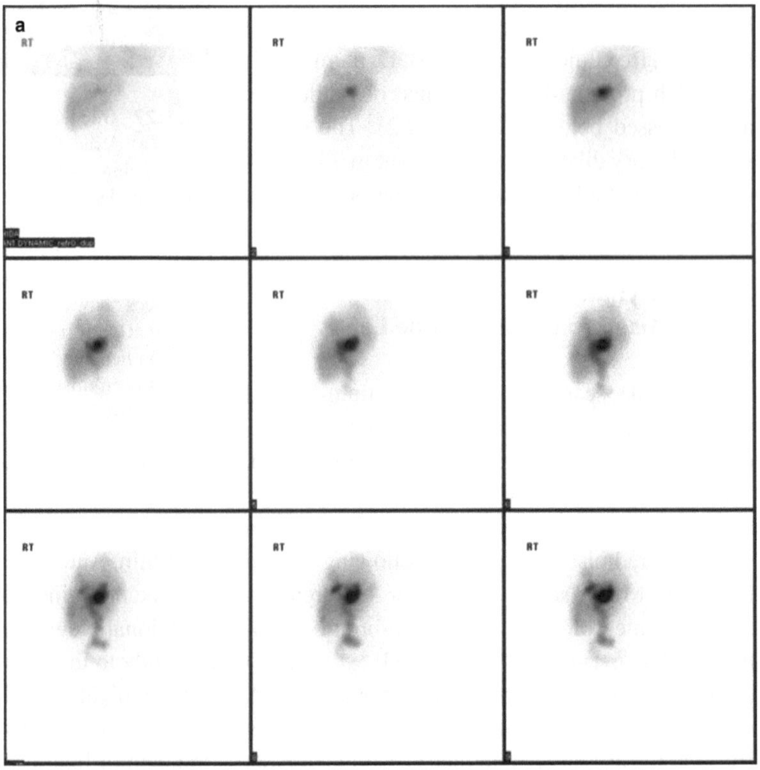

Fig. 5.29 Tc-99 m HIDA scintigraphy in the investigation of suspected bile leak. (**a**) Sequential planar images from the dynamic acquisition showing pooling of the leak. (**b**) Overview from SPECT-CT which localizes this to a collection adjacent to the surface of the liver (Courtesy of Dr. Andrew Scarsbrook, Leeds TH NHS Trust)

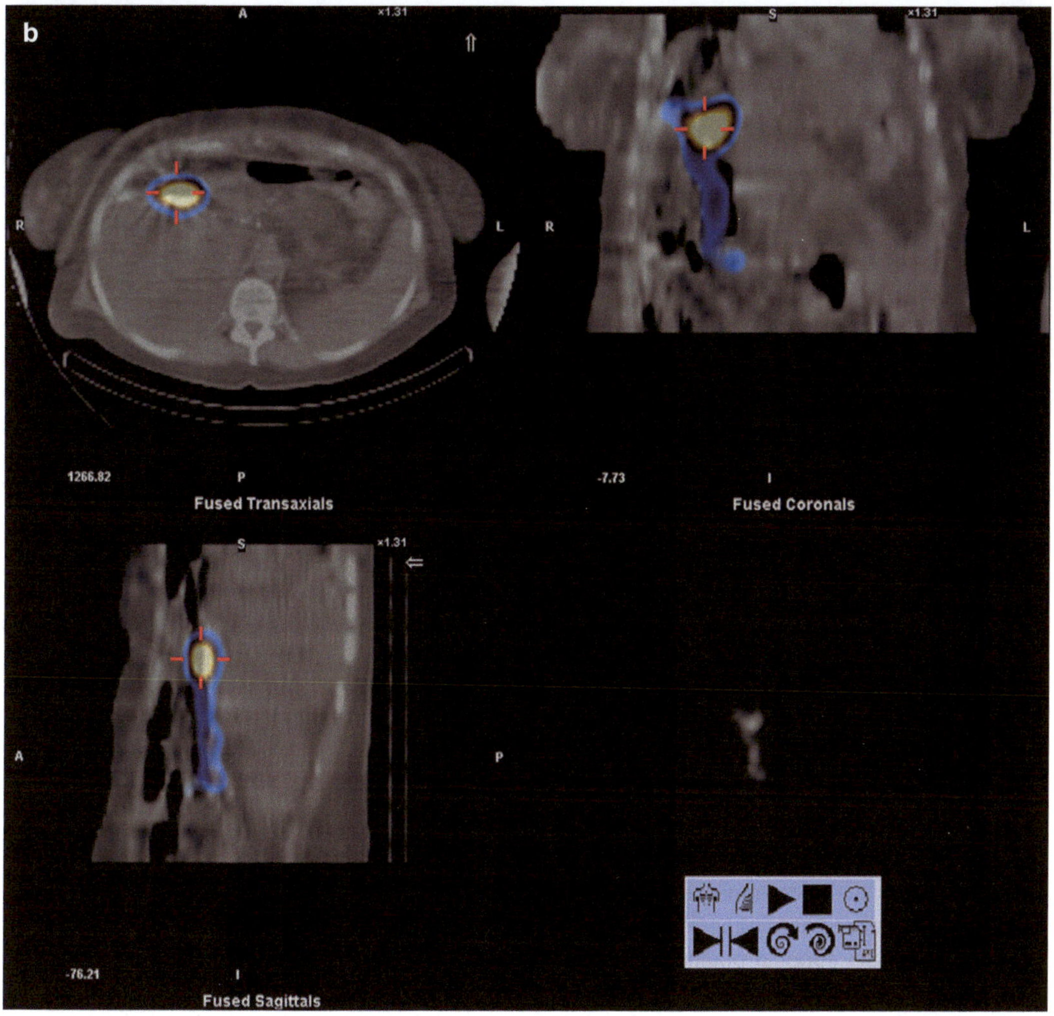

Fig. 5.29 (continued)

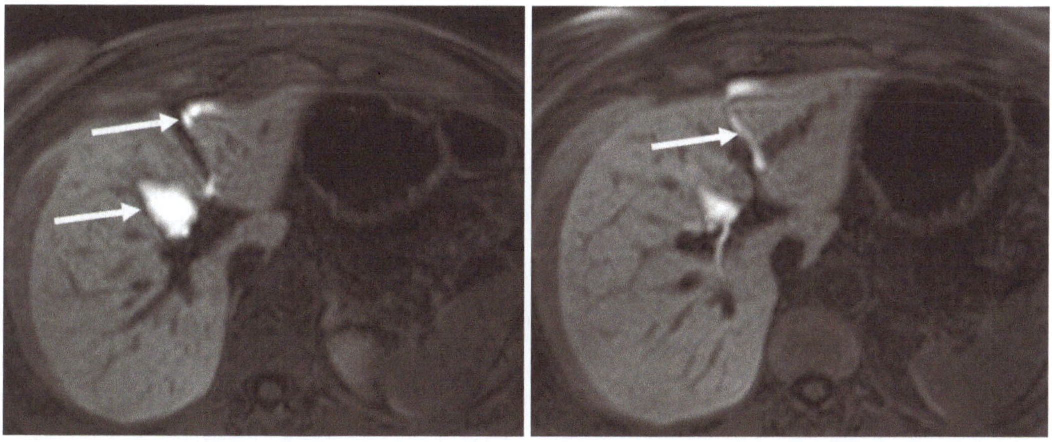

Fig. 5.30 Contrast-enhanced MRCP using mangafodipir trisodium (Teslascan; Nycomed Amersham Imaging, Oslo, Norway) in a patient with a suspected bile leak post laparoscopic cholecystectomy. There is extravasation of contrast from the biliary tree into a small collection at the porta and adjacent to the edge of the left lobe of the liver (*arrows*)

being withdrawn in Europe). CT cholangiography is performed following infusion of 100 ml of Biliscopin over 30–40 min. The upper abdomen is scanned during a single breath hold with MDCT, and axial, sagittal, and coronal oblique reformatted images are viewed on the CT workstation. Reduced opacification of the biliary tree occurs if the infusion is delivered too quickly or if the patient has a high serum bilirubin level (>100 mmol/l). As with contrast-enhanced MRCP, the peripheral intrahepatic ducts are usually inadequately opacified.

5.4.3 Management of Bile Leaks

Bile leaks are commonly managed with endoscopic retrograde cholangiopancreatography (ERCP) and the placement of a plastic biliary stent (Fig. 5.31). The stent is typically required to hold open the sphincter of Oddi and therefore reduce the transpapillary pressure gradient. This facilitates distal drainage of bile and reduces the amount of proximal extravasation. However, if there has been a major injury to the common hepatic or common bile duct (or particularly where the duct has been transected), ERCP or MRCP can confirm the diagnosis and level of injury. This allows surgical planning for biliary reconstruction. Surgical repair is generally reserved for ductal injuries close to or involving the confluence of the main bile ducts with fashioning of a biliary enteric anastomosis (hepaticojejunostomy) (Lefebvre-Chartrand et al. 1994). Primary duct-to-duct repair is however associated with a high incidence of postoperative stricture formation, so hepaticojejunostomy is favored in experienced centers. In some instances, the site of leak from the common bile duct can be crossed and a temporary plastic stent be inserted. Any associated bile collections can be managed with percutaneous image-guided drainage.

5.4.4 Biliary Obstruction

Biliary obstruction can be complete or segmental and occurs either as a result of inadvertent ligation of the common, aberrant, or intrahepatic bile ducts at cholecystectomy (Fig. 5.32) or from the passage of a calculus into the CBD. Patients present with progressive postoperative obstructive jaundice. The consequences of ligation of an aberrant duct will depend on the volume of the liver parenchyma drained by the duct. Focal intrahepatic biliary dilatation often accompanies this scenario.

Ultrasound and MRCP are the usually first-line investigations to define duct dilatation and exclude choledocholithiasis. With MRCP, in particular, the transition at the point of duct ligation can be identified. This is most common at the level of the common hepatic duct. ERCP is useful in confirming the diagnosis, with PTC reserved for rare cases to either treat biliary sepsis or confirm biliary anatomy where a complex injury is suspected. Iatrogenic bile duct injury is not usually appreciated at the time of cholecystectomy. Surgical repair is required in the form of a biliary enteric anastomosis, i.e., choledocho- or hepaticojejunostomy (Sect. 5.6).

5.4.5 Biliary Strictures

Biliary strictures occur when the cystic duct is clipped in close proximity to its junction with the common hepatic duct or, where a portion of the wall of the common hepatic duct is inadvertently ligated. Thermal injury secondary to overzealous use of diathermy in Calot's triangle may also lead to bile duct injury and subsequent stricture formation.

The diagnosis of a biliary stricture is usually confirmed by MRCP or ERCP following the demonstration of intra- and extrahepatic biliary dilatation on ultrasound. ERCP alone may fail to optimally demonstrate the site of injury due to the difficulty in opacifying the biliary tree proximal to a "tight" stricture. MRCP, however, does not rely on contrast opacification of the biliary system. The stricture may appear as a signal void or discontinuity of a bile duct segment on the axial and coronal sequences with biliary dilation proximal to the point of narrowing (Fig. 5.33). PTC is now less commonly utilized to delineate the biliary tree in this situation.

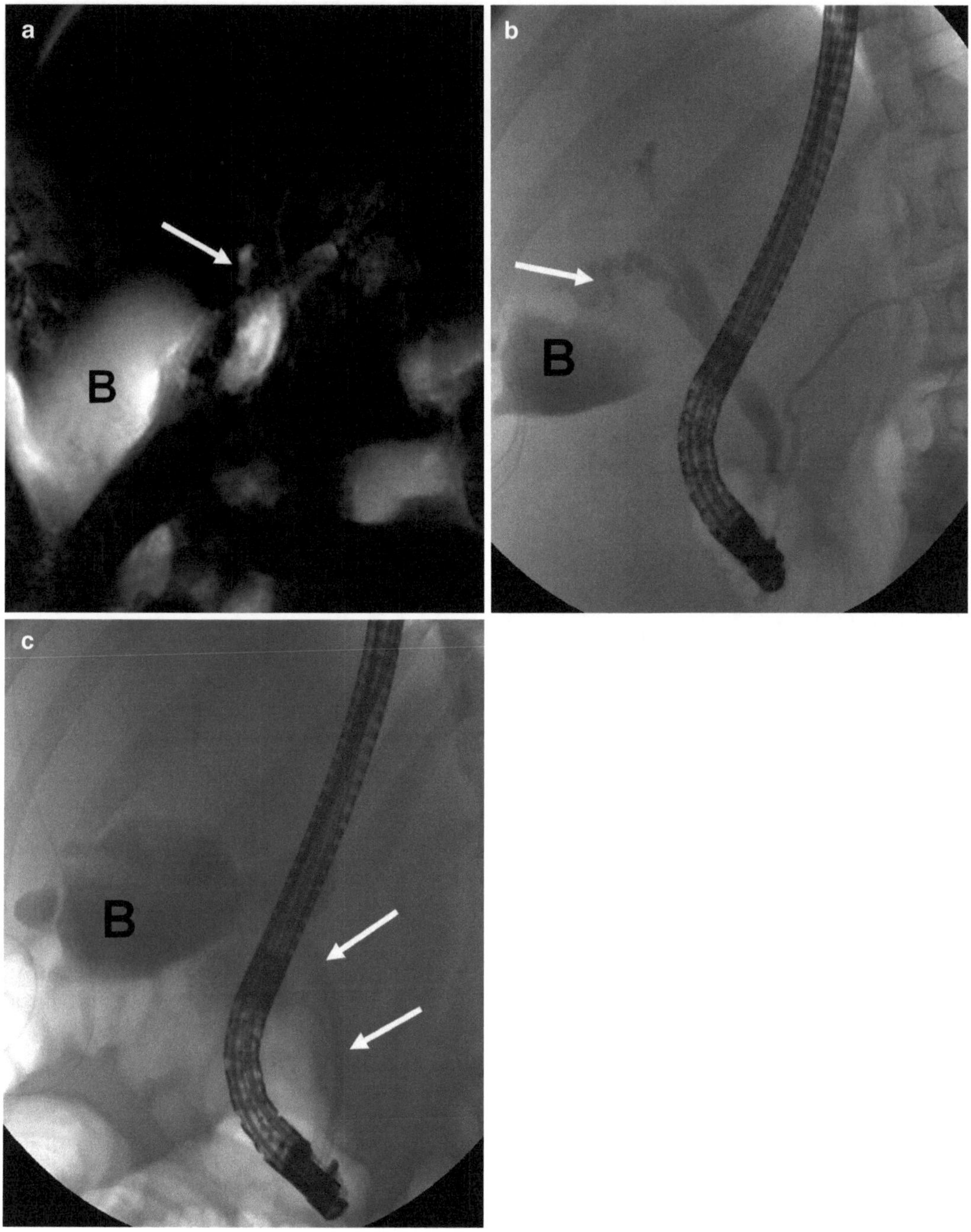

Fig. 5.31 Cystic duct leak postcholecystectomy. (**a**) Thick slab coronal T2W MRCP image shows a fluid collection in the region of the gallbladder fossa (*B*) with indirect evidence to suggest that the leak is originating from the cystic duct (*arrow*). It also confirms a normal caliber biliary tree and the absence of duct dilatation, stones, or strictures. (**b**) ERCP confirms direct evidence of a leak from the cystic duct (*arrow*). (**c**) A plastic biliary stent (*arrows*) was placed to improve distal biliary drainage

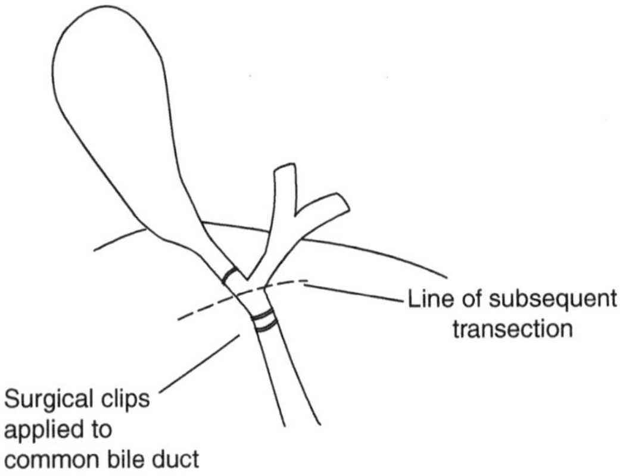

Fig. 5.32 Classic bile duct injury. Excessive caudal traction of Hartmann's pouch results in misinterpretation of biliary anatomy and clipping of the common bile duct. *Dotted line* indicates line of division

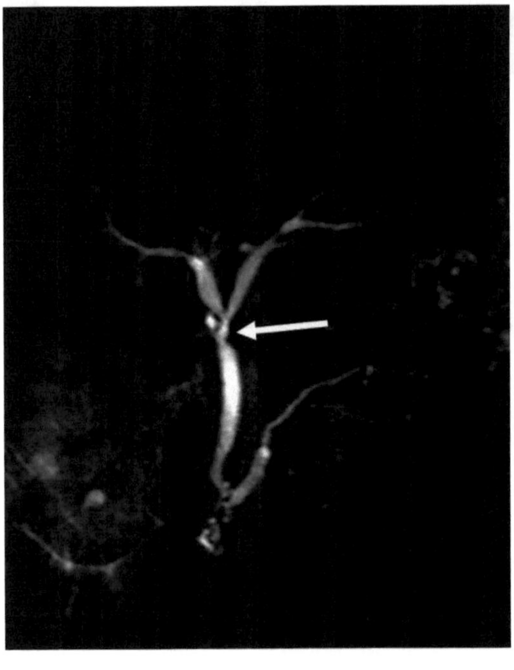

Fig. 5.33 Bile duct injury and subsequent stricture 6 months post laparoscopic cholecystectomy. Thick slab coronal T2W MRCP demonstrates a stricture (*arrow*) of the common hepatic duct with moderate dilatation of the right and left hepatic ducts

5.4.6 Retained CBD Stones

Patients with CBD stones diagnosed preoperatively are usually managed with ERCP or occasionally perioperatively using a choledochoscope which is used to explore and clear the bile duct. In the postoperative period when retained CBD stones are suspected, an ultrasound may demonstrate biliary dilatation or the presence of CBD stones. Where ultrasound is equivocal, MRCP is the modality of choice and is now routinely performed for this indication both pre- and postoperatively (Fig. 5.34).

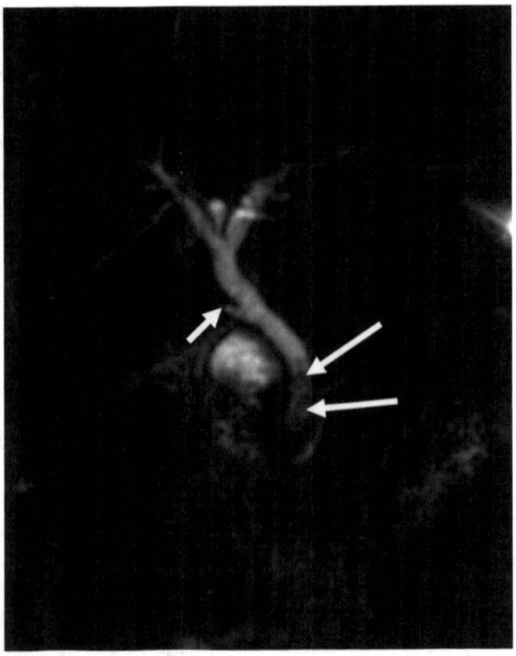

Fig. 5.34 Common bile duct stones. Thick slab coronal T2W MRCP in a patient presenting with obstructive jaundice 9 months postcholecystectomy shows multiple CBD calculi (*arrows*). Cystic duct stump (*short arrow*). A sphincterotomy and stone extraction was subsequently performed

Choledocholithiasis may occur during cholecystectomy if stones are accidentally milked into biliary tree at the time of surgery and not recognized. Calculi may also remain in the cystic duct remnant or in the intra- or extrahepatic bile ducts (Fig. 5.35). Primary duct stones can also form within the CBD de novo (Fig. 5.36). Following a cholecystectomy, 2–5% of patients will develop symptoms secondary to choledocholithiasis (Hoeffel et al. 2006).

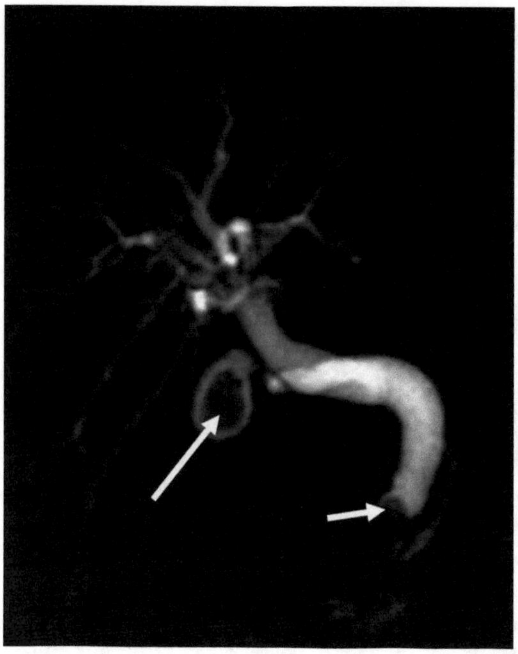

Fig. 5.35 Subtotal cholecystectomy and residual intraductal calculi. Partially resected gallbladder despite conversion from laparoscopic to open cholecystectomy (limited visualization due to adhesions). Coronal thick slab MRCP demonstrates a stone in Hartmann's pouch (*long arrow*) and in the distal CBD (*short arrow*)

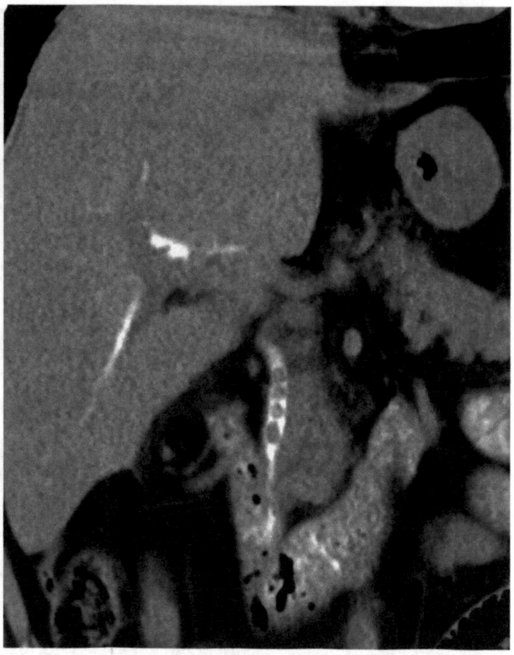

Fig. 5.36 CT cholangiogram in a patient with deranged liver function tests 2 years postcholecystectomy, unable to have an MRCP because of a cardiac pacemaker. Ultrasound demonstrated mild intrahepatic biliary tree dilatation, but there were poor views of the common bile duct. Coronal reformatted CT shows multiple CBD calculi

5.4.6.1 Management of Choledocholithiasis

The management of CBD stones is variable and is dictated largely by the available resources, time of presentation, and local expertise. Current techniques include:

- ERCP with sphincterotomy and extraction of stones
- Laparoscopic transcystic CBD exploration or choledochotomy with extraction of stones
- Open choledochotomy +/– choledochoscopy and extraction of stones
- Laser and ultrasound lithotripsy (Fig. 5.37)

ERCP offers the advantage of minimizing the risk of complications from future choledocholithiasis when sphincterotomy is performed prior to stone extraction. Furthermore, ERCP does not require an incision of the CBD, which may be complicated by future stricture formation. However, ERCP is not without risks which include pancreatitis, cholangitis, and duodenal perforation. Multiple large calculi may be present, and the choice of whether to opt for ERCP or laparoscopic duct exploration may be influenced by the overall stone burden, size of stones, as well as anatomical factors limiting access to the ampulla (e.g., presence of a biliary enteric anastomosis, gastrojejunostomy, or a large periampullary duodenal diverticulum). If ERCP or laparoscopic techniques fail, an open approach is the last resort.

5.4.7 Dropped or Spilled Gallstones

Spillage of gallstones occurs secondary to inadvertent entry into the gallbladder during dissection or at the time of gallbladder extraction

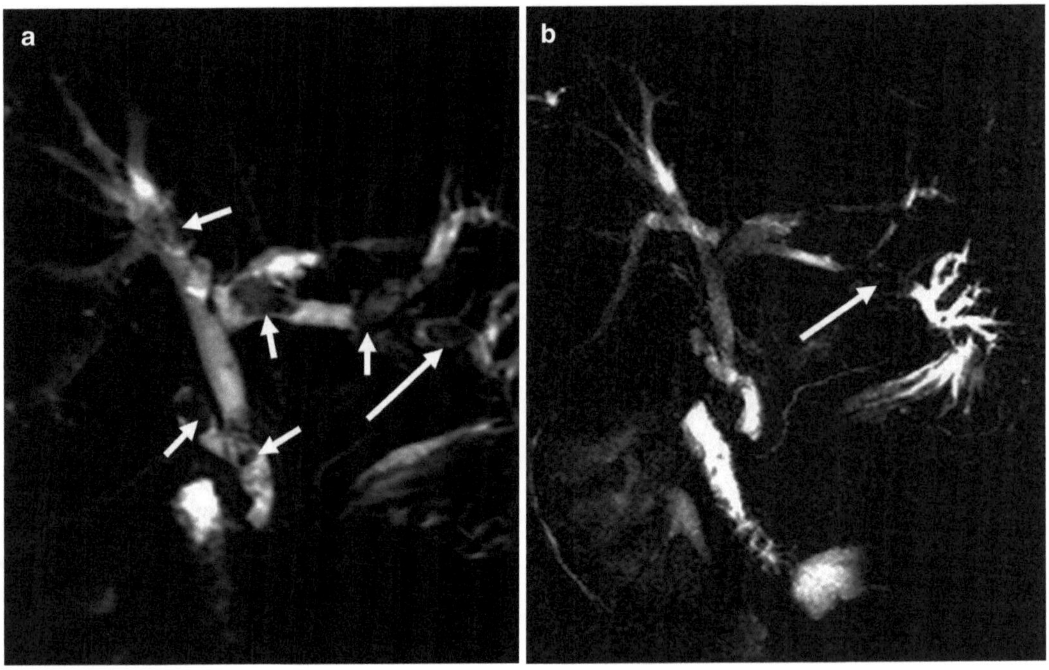

Fig. 5.37 (**a**, **b**) Multiple biliary tree stones post laparoscopic cholecystectomy. Despite attempted clearance with ERCP stone extraction and sphincterotomy, multiple stones (*short arrows*) remain in the cystic duct, CBD, and intrahepatic biliary tree. A T-tube was left in situ. The stones were successfully lasered using a 10F ureteroscope via following dilatation of the T-tube tract (under general anesthetic). (**b**) Postprocedure MRCP demonstrates successful removal of most of the stones. There is some mild bile duct stricturing within the left lobe and some dilatation upstream of a stone that was too peripheral to reach via the ureteroscope (*long arrow*)

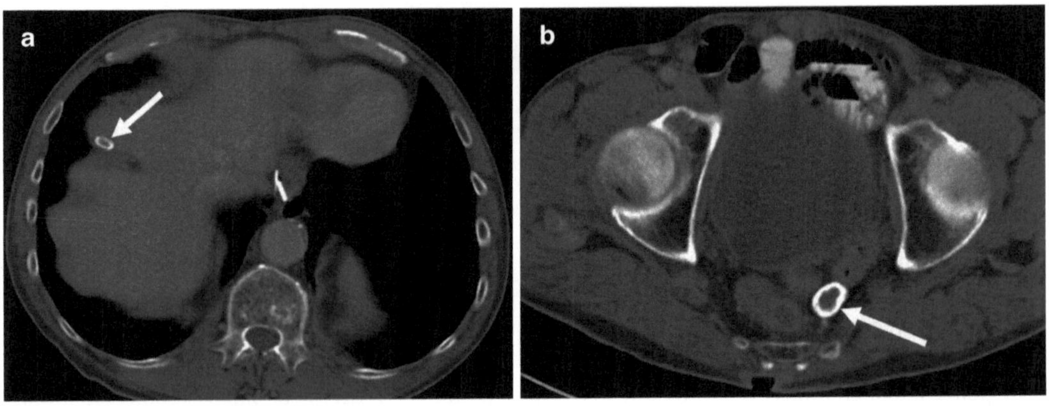

Fig. 5.38 (**a**, **b**) CT examinations in two different cases of dropped stones (*arrows*) post laparoscopic cholecystectomy

through the port site. The reported incidence is variable, ranging from 0.1% to 20%. The majority of "dropped" gallstones are sited within the right upper quadrant, but they may migrate to dependent areas (right paracolic gutter or pelvis) (Fig. 5.38). Although most "dropped" gallstones do not cause further problems, a small proportion cause significant complications since they incite a local foreign body reaction (Thurley and Dhingsa 2008).

Abscess formation is the most common complication resulting from "dropped" stones and may develop months following cholecystectomy (Fig. 5.39). The diagnosis is suggested by the presence of abdominal abscess in a postcholecystectomy patient without another obvious source (e.g., appendix, colonic diverticulitis). This can be a difficult diagnosis to make since the majority of calculi are radiolucent on CT. Fistula or sinus formation may also occur either eroding to the overlying skin surface or migrating to the pleural cavity and the lungs, resulting in the formation of an empyema or, more rarely, expectoration of calculi (cholelithoptysis). These complications can largely be prevented by giving antibiotics in the postoperative period to prevent abscess formation.

5.4.8 Vascular Injury

Peri- or postoperative hemorrhage is usually caused by injury to the vessels during trocar insertion (Shamiyeh and Wayand 2004). This occurs in the surgical bed or the abdominal wall and is usually easily diagnosed on noncontrast CT and ultrasound as high attenuation/heterogeneous fluid collections, respectively. Ongoing active bleeding is best demonstrated on CT after intravenous contrast administration with a combination of arterial and portal venous phase imaging.

During operative dissection of Calot's triangle, the right hepatic artery is the most common vessel to be injured followed by the portal vein (Thurley and Dhingsa 2008). Hepatic artery ligation is not always recognized at the time of operation and may lead to the development of an ischemic cholangiopathy, with most patients presenting months after surgery with jaundice. MRCP may show irregular ductal dilatation and stenosis. Postoperative bleeding occurs commonly from the liver bed or rarely from the cystic artery when the clip(s) have been displaced from cystic artery stump. Failure to identify aberrant or coaxial vessels can also lead to delayed postoperative bleeding. In this situation, endovascular therapies can be very effective. Portal vein injury, a rare and life-threatening complication, requires acute surgical repair to achieve hemostasis.

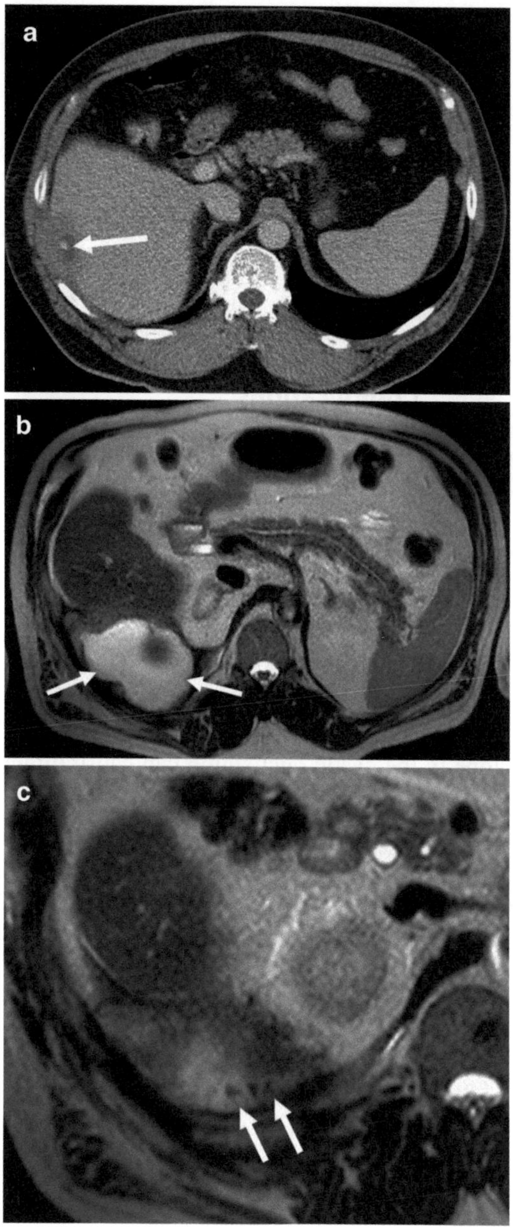

Fig. 5.39 Two cases of dropped stones and associated sepsis. (**a**) Case 1. Axial CT of a patient with right upper quadrant pain postcholecystectomy demonstrates a dropped stone and an associated small perihepatic abscess (*arrow*). (**b**, **c**) Case 2. Axial T2W MRI of a patient with a recurrent right perihepatic abscess (*arrows*) treated with percutaneous drainages 2 years postcholecystectomy. (**c**) Within the most caudal aspect of the collection, there are small gallstones (*arrows*) (magnified image)

Intra-abdominal hematoma may form following postoperative bleeding and carries a small risk of infection. Where there are clinical features of sepsis, image-guided drainage can be offered, although most uncomplicated hematomas resolve spontaneously with time. Routine aspiration of sterile hematomas is not appropriate due to the risk of introducing infection.

5.4.9 Cystic Duct Stump Complications

A cystic duct stump or remnant of 1–2 cm is usually left at surgery, although stumps up to 6 cm in length may be seen. A longer stump may be left after cholecystectomy when a long, parallel cystic duct or low medial insertion is present.

Retained calculi are the most common complication to affect the cystic stump (Fig. 5.40), with longer stumps at particular risk. A large stone in the cystic duct stump can cause direct compression or edema of the common hepatic duct (Mirizzi's syndrome type I). Rarely, the stone may erode through the cystic duct wall into the common hepatic duct (Mirizzi's syndrome type II). A "re-formed" gallbladder may be seen due to bulbous dilatation of the proximal portion of a very long cystic duct remnant, which is prone to stasis and stone disease. The stump may occasionally become distended with mucus forming a mucocele, leading to impingement on the common hepatic duct (Hoeffel et al. 2006).

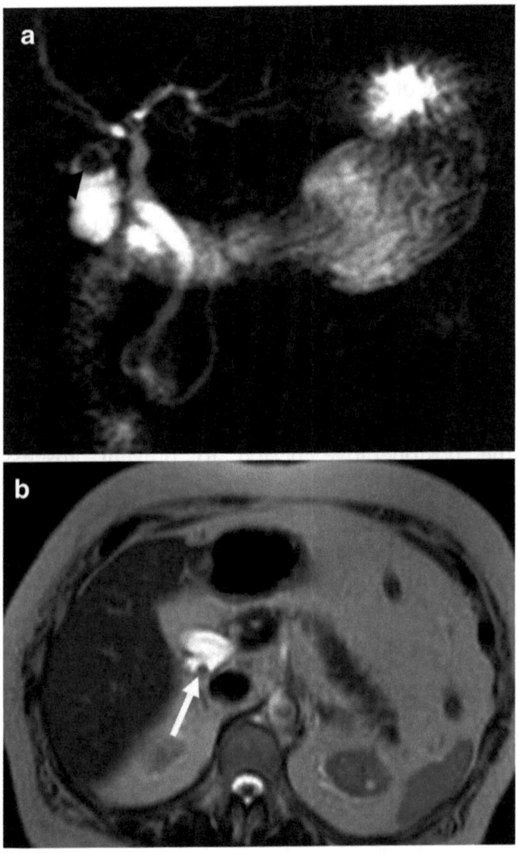

Fig. 5.40 Two cases of cystic duct stones postcholecystectomy. (**a**) Coronal thick slab MRCP image demonstrates a small filling defect (*arrow*) within the cystic duct stump consistent with a retained stone. (**b**) Axial T2W MRI showing a small calculus (*arrow*) within a short cystic duct stump

5.4.10 Laparoscopic Complications

These include:

- Abdominal wall and omental bleeding
- Abdominal and retroperitoneal vascular injury
- Gastrointestinal perforation
- Bladder perforation
- Solid organ injury
- Port site hernia

They are discussed in more detail in Sect. 1.7.

5.4.11 Teaching Points

- Complications following cholecystectomy require multimodality imaging.
- Biliary leaks and obstruction are the most common postoperative complications.
- Management of bile duct injury and leaks is complex.
- Where conservative management fails in the treatment of bile leaks and postoperative strictures, surgery is advocated (fashioning a biliary enteric anastomosis).
- MRCP in the pre- and postoperative setting of biliary disease is associated with numerous pitfalls with which the radiologist should be aware.

5.5 Mirizzi's Syndrome

Although Mirizzi's syndrome is a not a postoperative complication, it can cause confusion on preoperative imaging. The diagnosis of Mirizzi's syndrome may be made incidentally during laparoscopic cholecystectomy (usually necessitating open conversion). Preoperative diagnosis is made more complex by the fact that imaging findings can be difficult to differentiate from a primary cholangiocarcinoma due to the presence of an inflammatory mass at the porta hepatis.

It is a rare complication of cholelithiasis (<0.5%) and is due to an extrahepatic biliary stricture usually in the absence of CBD stones. Mirizzi's syndrome type I is defined as extrinsic compression (direct pressure or edema) of the common hepatic duct secondary to a gallstone in the cystic duct or Hartmann's pouch. Type II is associated with the presence of a fistula secondary to erosion of the aforementioned gallstone into the common hepatic duct. Patients commonly present with abdominal pain, pyrexia, and tachycardia and sometimes deranged liver function tests.

The surgical management of Mirizzi's syndrome is complex, and although laparoscopic approaches have been reported, it is generally safer to perform open surgery for both types I and II. Intraoperative cholangiography may be required to assess biliary anatomy with a focus on the extrahepatic stricture. Bile duct exploration may be necessitated with the subsequent insertion of a T-tube. In type II, the defect in the common hepatic duct may be primarily closed over a T-tube or, if significant, may require formation of a hepaticojejunostomy to restore biliary continuity. Type I may also require a biliary enteric anastomosis if the stricture is significant enough to compromise biliary continuity.

5.6 Biliary Enteric Anastomoses (Hepaticojejunostomy)

5.6.1 Clinical Indications

- Component of pancreaticoduodenectomy
- Liver resection for malignancy (cholangiocarcinoma, hepatocellular carcinoma, colorectal liver metastases)
- Liver transplantation when duct-to-duct reconstruction is either not possible or undesirable (e.g., PSC)
- Bile duct injury
- Biliary strictures (fibrosis, sclerosing cholangitis)
- Hepatolithiasis (intrahepatic gallstone disease)
- Choledochal cyst resection
- Gallbladder carcinoma infiltrating the CBD

5.6.2 Surgical Technique and Postoperative Anatomy

- Depending on the indication, prior to a hepaticojejunostomy (HJ), patients may require assessment of the biliary tree anatomy with MRCP, ERCP, or percutaneous transhepatic cholangiography.
- An HJ can be performed either laparoscopically or via an open approach, although the latter is generally favored.
- HJs are performed with a Roux-en-Y configuration. Following division of a proximal loop of jejunum ~50 cm from the duodenojejunal flexure, the distal limb (Roux limb) is brought up (retro- or anterocolic) to be anastomosed to the common hepatic duct to perform an end-to-side or side-to-side anastomosis (Fig. 5.41). The proximal limb is reanastomosed to the Roux limb ~50 cm usually with a side-to-side anastomosis (to minimize the risk of enteric reflux and damage to the biliary tree) from the terminal end (of the Roux limb) to complete the Roux-en-Y configuration.

5.6.3 Modifications to Surgical Technique

- If the jejunal loop cannot be directly anastomosed to the common hepatic duct, an anastomosis to the left or right hepatic ducts, or intrahepatic ducts can be performed.
- If there is an adequate length of healthy proximal common bile duct, then surgeons may opt to perform a choledochojejunostomy (end-to-side anastomosis).
- Choledochoduodenostomy is an alternative anastomosis whereby the supraduodenal

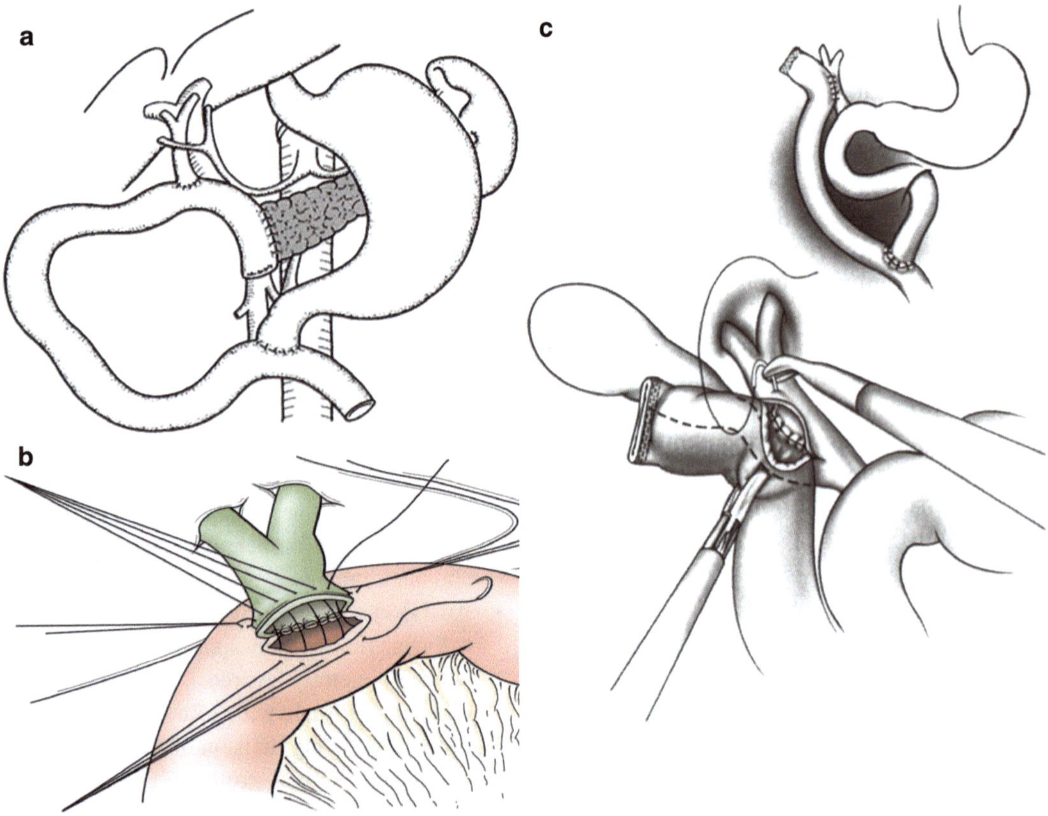

Fig. 5.41 Roux-en-Y hepaticojejunostomy. (**a**, **b**) Example of an end-to-side biliary enteric anastomosis following a pylorus-preserving duodenectomy. (**c**) Side-to-side biliary enteric anastomosis

CBD is anastomosed to the first part of the duodenum. Today, this approach is rarely used to achieve biliary drainage, but it offers the option of postoperative access to the biliary system via endoscopy.

- Cholangiocarcinoma of the mid- and distal CBD requires either a radical bile duct resection or a pancreaticoduodenectomy (Sect. 4.2). Bile duct resection plus partial hepatectomy may be necessary for hilar cholangiocarcinoma. Biliary continuity is then restored with an HJ.
- Gallbladder cancer may be diagnosed on preoperative imaging, at the time of cholecystectomy, or on histological analysis following a routine cholecystectomy. Depending on the stage of the tumor, surgical management may include a combination of cholecystectomy with lymphadenectomy, wedge resection of the gallbladder bed, bile duct resection, resection of segments IV and V, or extensive partial hepatectomy.
- Cholecystojejunal bypass is an uncommon operation that may be performed as a palliative procedure to relieve biliary obstruction due to pancreatic head malignancy. It is usually reserved for patients with no duodenal access for ERCP and hepatic metastasis precluding PTC biliary drainage. The gallbladder is anastomosed to a jejunal loop (Fig. 5.42).

5.7 Complications of Biliary Enteric Anastomoses

5.7.1 Anastomotic Leak

The incidence of an anastomotic leak following an HJ is variable and very much dependent

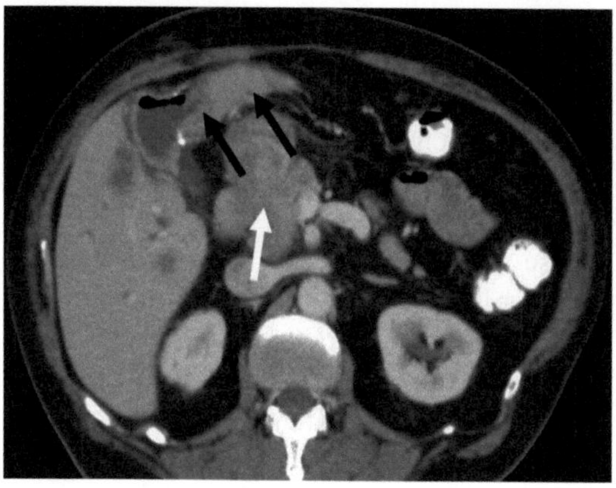

Fig. 5.42 Cholecystojejunal bypass in a patient with biliary obstruction secondary to inoperable pancreatic cancer (*white arrow*). Stenting via ERCP was unsuccessful, and the number of liver metastases precluded PTC. A Roux loop of jejunum has been anastomosed to the gallbladder (*black arrows*)

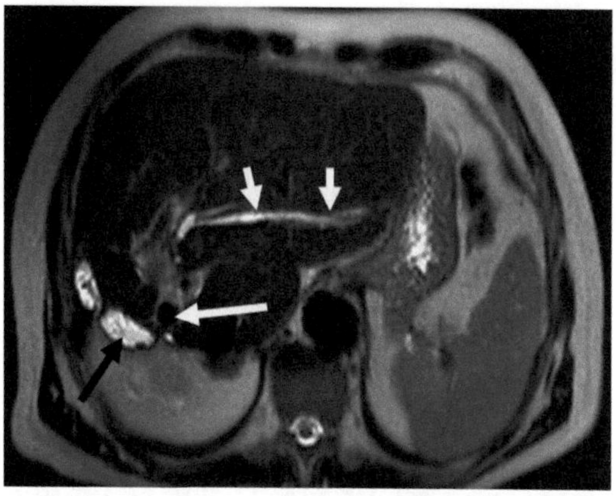

Fig. 5.43 Benign biliary enteric anastomotic stricture and intraductal stone disease 2 years post extended right hepatectomy and hepaticojejunostomy (HJ) for liver metastases from a colorectal primary tumor. Axial T2W MRCP shows compensatory hypertrophy of the left lobe of the liver and dilatation of the intrahepatic biliary tree (*short white arrows*). Intraductal calculus (*long white arrow*). The HJ was refashioned, and the stone was removed at laparotomy. Jejunal Roux loop (*black arrow*)

on the indication for the index procedure. An anastomotic leak is suggested by the presence of bile in abdominal drains. Confirmation of a suspected leak requires either a US or CT to demonstrate a collection in the region of the perihepatic anastomosis. Management of an anastomotic leak is dependent on the clinical status of the patient. Conservative management with the preservation of intra-abdominal drains may be used until the bile leak has resolved. Alternatively, percutaneous transhepatic approaches with drainage and stent placement may be used (due to the inaccessibility of the biliary system to ERCP). In rare circumstances, surgical exploration is necessitated and involves drainage with or without a redo HJ procedure.

5.7.2 Anastomotic Stricture

The incidence of anastomotic stricture involving biliary enteric anastomoses is in the region of 4–10% (Selvakumar et al. 2008) and occurs late in the postoperative period (several months to years). It is due to postoperative fibrosis. Patients who develop an anastomotic stricture may present with obstructive jaundice or cholangitis (Fig. 5.43). Ultrasound or MRCP may demonstrate the presence of biliary tree dilatation. ERCP is generally not possible due to inaccessibility via the endoscopic approach, although the presence of a gastric access loop (blind end of Roux loop anastomosed to gastric antrum) may make such an approach feasible. Anastomotic stricture can less commonly be due to recurrent malignancy and should be suspected if liver resection has been previously performed for primary liver tumors or colorectal liver metastases (Fig. 5.44).

Revision surgery is complex and associated with significant morbidity and further stricture formation. Hence, percutaneous transhepatic balloon dilatation with or without stent insertion is the preferred primary management strategy. Failure to achieve adequate biliary drainage or recurrent episodes of obstructive jaundice with cholangitis may ultimately require revisional surgery. This is fraught with difficulty but is required to prevent long-term complications of HJ strictures, i.e., hepatic atrophy and secondary biliary cirrhosis, that may require liver transplantation.

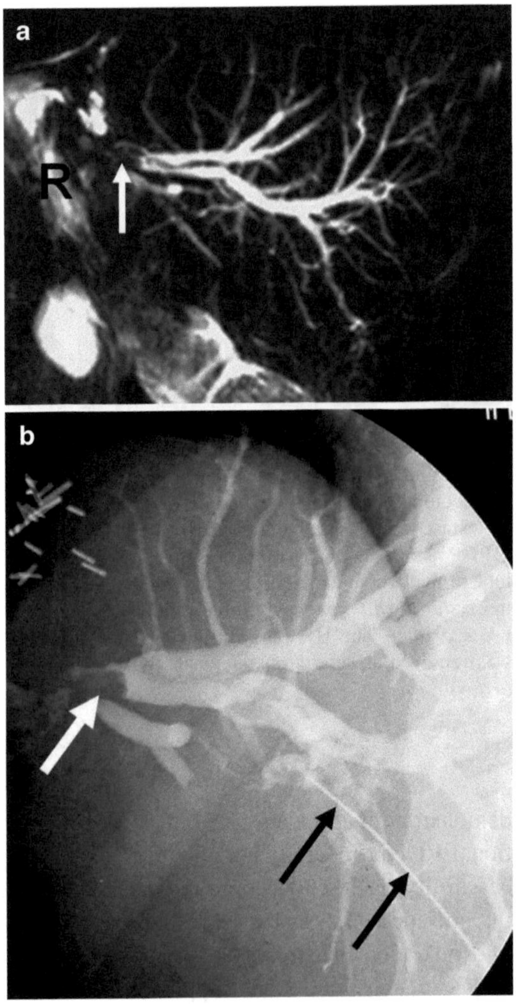

Fig. 5.44 Malignant biliary enteric anastomotic stricture following right trisectionectomy for colorectal liver metastases. (**a**) Coronal oblique thick slab T2W MRCP and (**b**) cholangiogram via a left lobe bile duct puncture (*black arrows*) show a filling defect (*white arrow*) proximal to the hepaticojejunostomy (*R*) and biliary dilatation. CT (*not shown*) confirmed recurrent disease

5.7.3 Nonanastomotic Stricture

Nonanastomotic strictures involving biliary enteric anastomoses are usually the result of an ischemic process and not related to iatrogenic bile duct injury. They are more common in patients who have an HJ in association with liver transplantation. Thrombosis of the hepatic artery (blood supply to the biliary tree) is the most common cause. Other causes, particularly in the setting of liver transplantation, include:

- Transplant rejection
- Prolonged preservation time
- Cholangitis
- Use of DCD (donation after cardiac death) donor liver

Nonanastomotic strictures are usually central and involve the main ducts close to the hilum (Hoeffel et al. 2006). They are usually longer in length than anastomotic strictures. If biliary necrosis also occurs, e.g., in the presence of hepatic arterial occlusion, bile leaks may be seen on imaging. Management is difficult and includes dilatation, stenting, surgical revision, or retransplantation.

5.7.4 Stone Formation

This is typically a consequence of biliary stasis from stricture but may occur de novo. Sludge or bile casts in the region of the anastomosis can be managed percutaneously with balloon dilatation (Fig. 5.45). However, the management of intraductal calculi is difficult and may require surgical removal and revision of the anastomosis.

5.8 Teaching Points

- Biliary enteric anastomosis entails fashioning a small bowel Roux loop to the extrahepatic biliary tree (hepatico- or choledochojejunostomy).
- It is a component of numerous abdominal operations, e.g., pancreaticoduodenectomy, liver resection, and transplantation, and in the treatment of bile duct injury from cholecystectomy.
- Most common complications are anastomotic strictures and stone formation.

Acknowledgments We would like to thank Dr. Daniel Madigan (Consultant GI and Interventional Radiologist, Royal Adelaide Hospital, South Australia) for his help with the chapter and his kind permission for the use of many of the images.

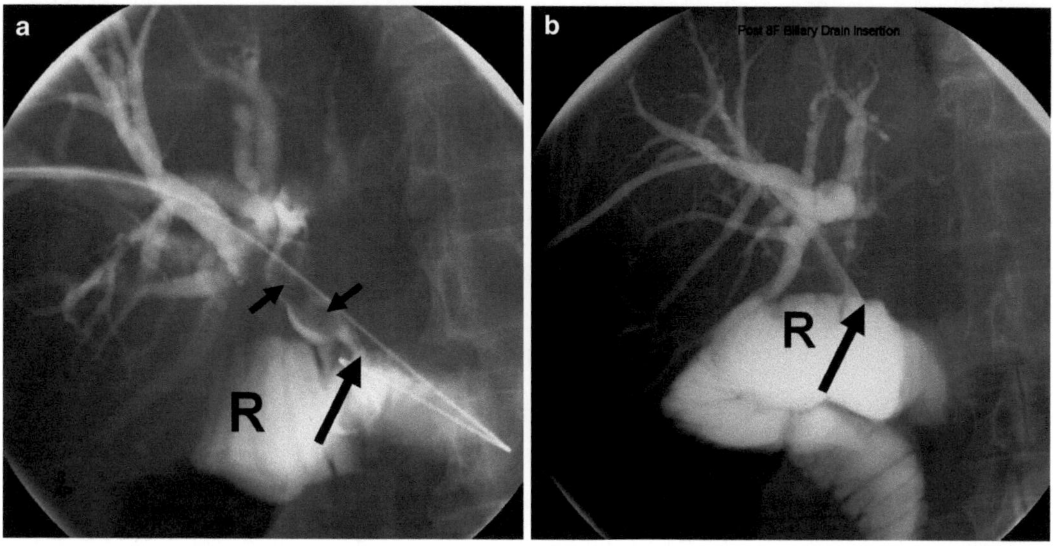

Fig. 5.45 Biliary obstruction in a patient 3 years post pancreaticoduodenectomy for ampullary carcinoma. MRCP (*not shown*) demonstrated filling defects within the common hepatic duct proximal to the hepaticojejunostomy. These were thought to represent biliary casts/sludge in association with an anastomotic stricture. PTC and cholangiogram. (**a**) Confirms filling defects (*small arrows*). Roux loop (*R*), hepaticojejunostomy (*arrow*). A wire has been placed within the Roux loop and the bile casts/sludge angioplastied with an 8-mm balloon. Temporary external drainage achieved (**b**) with an 8F locking-loop pigtail catheter

References

Bismuth H, Majno PE. Biliary strictures: classification based on the principles of surgical treatment. World J Surg. 2001;25(10):1241–4.

Christensesn RA, van Sonnenberg E, Nemcek AA, D'Agostino HB. Inadvertent ligation of the aberrant right hepatic duct at cholecystectomy: radiologic diagnosis and therapy. Radiology. 1992;183:549–53.

Feng B, Song Q. Does the common bile duct dilate after cholecystectomy? Sonographic evaluation in 234 patients. AJR Am J Roentgenol. 1995;183:1559–66.

Gurusamy K, Samraj K, Gluud C, Wilson E, Davidson BR. Meta-analysis of randomized controlled trials on the safety and effectiveness of early versus delayed laparoscopic cholecystectomy for acute cholecystitis. Br J Surg. 2010;97(2):141–50.

Hoeffel C, Azizi L, Lewin M, Laurent V, Aube' C, Arrive' L, Tubiana J-M. Normal and pathologic features of the post operative biliary tract at 3D MR Cholangiopancreatography and MR imaging. Radiographics. 2006;26:1603–20.

Lefebvre-Chartrand C, Dufresne M-P, Lafortune M, Lapointe R, Dagenais M, Roy A. Iatrogenic injury to the bile duct: a working classification for radiologists. Radiology. 1994;193:523–6.

Moran J, Del Grosso E, Wills JS, Hagy JA, Baker R. Laparoscopic cholecystectomy: imaging of complications and normal postoperative CT appearance. Abdom Imaging. 1994;19:143–6.

Quinn SF, Sangster W, Standage B, Schuman E, Gross G. Biliary complications related to laparoscopic cholecystectomies: Radiologic diagnosis and management. Surg Laparosc Endosc Percutan Tech. 1992;2(4):279–86.

Selvakumar E, Rajendren S, Balachandar TG, Kannan DG, Jeswanth S, Ravichandran P, Surendran R. Long term outcome of gastric access loop in hepaticojejunostomy. Hepatobiliary Pancreat Dis Int. 2008;7(2):152–5.

Shamiyeh A, Wayand W. Laparoscopic cholecystectomy: early and late complications and their treatment. Langenbecks Arch Surg. 2004;389:164–71.

Slater K, Strong RW, Wall DR, Lynch SV. Iatrogenic bile duct injury: the scourge of laparoscopic cholecystectomy. ANZ J Surg. 2002;72:83–8.

Strasberg SM, Hertl M, Soper NJ. An analysis of the problem of biliary injury during laparoscopic cholecystectomy. J Am Coll Surg. 1995;180(1):101–25.

Thurley PD, Dhingsa R. Laparoscopic cholecystectomy: post operative imaging. AJR Am J Roentgenol. 2008;191:794–801.

The Liver

6

J. Ashley Guthrie, Hajamohideen M. Salahudeen, and J. Peter A. Lodge

Contents

6.1 **Introduction** 187

6.2 **Normal Liver Anatomy** 188

6.3 **Liver Resection and Metastasectomy** 190
6.3.1 Clinical Indications 190
6.3.2 Surgical Technique and Postoperative Anatomy 190
6.3.3 Modifications of Surgical Technique 192
6.3.4 Normal Postoperative Imaging 194
6.3.5 Postoperative Complications 196
6.3.6 Imaging Recurrent Disease 200
6.3.7 Teaching Points 202

6.4 **Radiofrequency Ablation (RFA)** 202
6.4.1 Introduction 202
6.4.2 Clinical Indications 204
6.4.3 RFA Technique 204
6.4.4 Modifications to RFA Technique 205
6.4.5 Imaging Post-RFA 205
6.4.6 Post-RFA Complications 205
6.4.7 Recurrent Disease 207
6.4.8 Teaching Points (RFA) 208

6.5 **Transcatheter Arterial Chemoembolization (TACE)** 209
6.5.1 Introduction 209
6.5.2 Clinical Indications 209
6.5.3 TACE Technique 209
6.5.4 Imaging Post-TACE 210
6.5.5 Post-TACE Complications 211
6.5.6 Imaging of Recurrent Malignancy Post-TACE 212
6.5.7 Teaching Points (TACE) 214

6.6 **Orthotopic Liver Transplantation** 214
6.6.1 Introduction 214
6.6.2 Surgical Technique 214
6.6.3 Modifications of Surgical Technique 215
6.6.4 Normal Postoperative Imaging 216
6.6.5 Postoperative Complications 218
6.6.6 Teaching Points 224

References 224

J.A. Guthrie, BA, MB, BChir, MRCP, FRCR (✉)
Department of Radiology, Leeds Teaching Hospitals NHS Trust, Leeds, UK
e-mail: ashley.guthrie@leedsth.nhs.uk

H.M. Salahudeen, MBBS, MD, MRCP, FRCR
Department of Radiology, Calderdale and Huddersfield NHS Foundation Trust, Huddersfield, UK

J.P.A. Lodge, MD, FRCS
Department of Surgery,
Leeds Teaching Hospitals NHS Trust, Leeds, UK

6.1 Introduction

The first reported liver resections were performed following trauma in 1716 by Berta and for malignancy by Langenbuch in 1888. However, the first anatomic resection for malignancy was only performed in 1952 by Lortat-Jacob (1952). The techniques for anatomic resection have developed since then with a major contribution by Bismuth (1982). Couinaud's excellent description of the segmental anatomy of the liver has lead to a better understanding of the segmental functional anatomic planes now utilized in liver

J. Brittenden, D.J.M. Tolan (eds.), *Radiology of the Post Surgical Abdomen*,
DOI 10.1007/978-1-4471-2775-8_6, © Springer-Verlag London 2012

resection and is discussed in Sect. 6.2. Liver resection or hepatectomy is now widely practiced in specialized centers to treat various benign and malignant conditions.

The only potentially curative option for primary and metastatic liver tumors is surgical resection, with expected 5-year survival rates of 25–35% for hepatocellular carcinoma (HCC) and 30–40% for colorectal metastases (Fong et al. 1997; Nagorney et al. 1989). The commonest indication for liver resection in the West is colorectal metastasis confined to the liver. HCC is the fifth most common cancer worldwide and accounts for 80–90% of primary liver tumors. In untreated cases, the prognosis is poor with a median survival of 6–9 months in early stage tumors and only 1–2 months in advanced disease. With advances in imaging techniques and earlier detection because of surveillance programs, an increasing number of patients are now considered suitable for surgical treatment. Surgical resection is the treatment of choice in noncirrhotic individuals. In cirrhotic patients with HCC, there are numerous clinical and biochemical parameters which determine treatment options. Surgery is the preferred option if there is sufficient functional hepatic reserve within the residual liver to tolerate this. Radiofrequency ablation can be utilized if the tumors are small and if the patient is not deemed suitable for resection. Liver transplant may be offered to patients with a limited burden of malignant disease. The usual criteria for transplantation are a maximum of three HCCs not greater than 3 cm in diameter or a single HCC less than 5 cm (Milan criteria), without any evidence of microvascular invasion or metastases.

Background knowledge of the resection planes and postoperative imaging anatomy is essential to detect postoperative complications and recurrence. Cross-sectional imaging plays a major role in the assessment of postoperative complications. The preoperative workup usually consists of CT of the chest, abdomen, and pelvis and MR of the liver. FDG-PET CT is increasingly being used to identify extrahepatic disease prior to resection for colorectal metastases. The preoperative imaging provides an essential baseline when assessing the findings on postoperative imaging.

6.2 Normal Liver Anatomy

The liver was initially divided into left and right lobes along the line of the umbilical fissure at the insertion of the falciform ligament. When divided on this basis, the left lobe is much smaller than the right. Cantlie divided the liver into functional left and right lobes on the basis of the vascular inflow. The line of division is often referred to as Cantlie's line; this describes the plane running from the inferior vena cava superiorly to the gallbladder fossa inferiorly and contains the middle hepatic vein and the point of bifurcation of the portal vein into left and right main branches. Current surgical anatomic concepts were advanced by Claude Couinaud, who extended the functional divisions further and divided the liver into eight segments each described by the hepatic and portal venous supply relationships (Couinaud 1957, 1999). Each segment has an independent vascular inflow, outflow, and biliary drainage (Figs. 6.1 and 6.2).

Using Couinaud's classification, the left and right lobes are divided, as described by Cantlie. The right lobe is divided into four functional components by the right hepatic and right main branch of the portal vein. Segment 5 is inferior to the right portal vein and anteromedial to the right

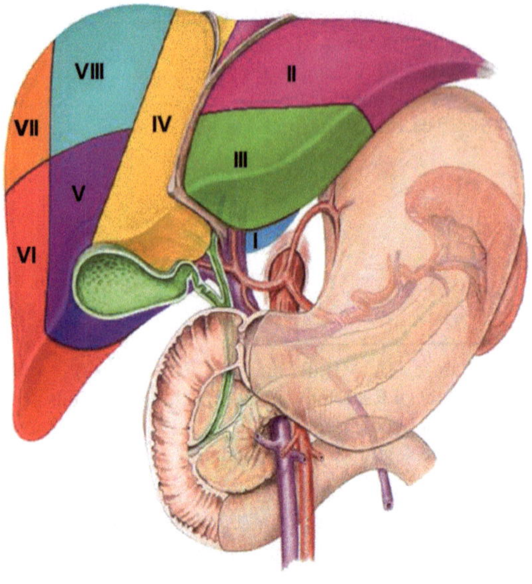

Fig. 6.1 Drawing depicting Couinaud's classification of segmental liver anatomy

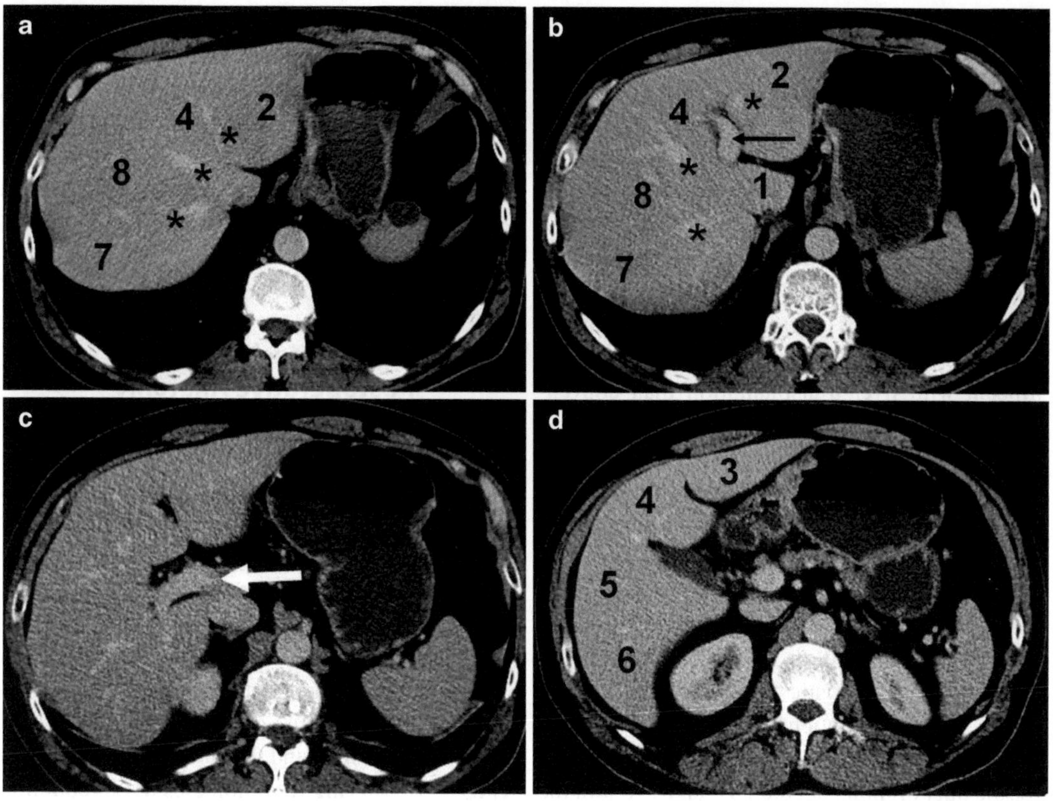

Fig. 6.2 CT illustration of segmental liver anatomy. (**a**) Cranial to the main portal vein. (**b**) At the level of left portal vein (*arrow*). (**c**) At the level of the main portal vein (*arrow*). (**d**) Caudal to the main portal vein. Hepatic veins (*asterisks*)

hepatic vein, and segment 6 is inferior to the right portal vein but posterolateral to the right hepatic vein. Segment 7 is above the right portal vein and posterolateral to the right hepatic vein, and segment 8 is above the right portal vein and anteromedial to the right hepatic vein. The central component of the left lobe is segment 4 (formerly referred to as the quadrate lobe) and is bounded by the umbilical fissure and Cantlie's line. The left lateral segments, i.e., segments 2 and 3, are located to the left of the falciform ligament with segment 2 above the left portal vein and segment 3 below. Segment 1 (caudate lobe) is functionally separate from the rest of the liver and is located posterior to the porta, predominantly to the right of the cava and bounded on the left by the ligamentum venosus.

The liver has two sources of inflow of blood; between one third and a quarter of the blood supply to the normal liver is from the hepatic artery with the majority being derived from the portal vein. There are many anatomic variations of the hepatic arterial supply (classified by Mitchel):

- The commonest anatomic arrangement is for all to be derived from the coeliac axis via the common hepatic artery, but this only occurs in approximately 55% of patients.
- The right hepatic artery arises from the superior mesenteric artery in approximately 11% of patients, with an additional (accessory) right hepatic artery in 7%.
- In 10% of patients, the left hepatic artery supply arises from the left gastric artery.
- In 8%, there is an additional accessory left hepatic artery arising from the same vessel (Catalano et al. 2008).
- There are additional rarer variants.

The hepatic artery supplying segment 4 variably arises from the left or right hepatic artery or at the bifurcation between the two. This becomes significant if a potential liver donor has a segment 4 artery arising from the right hepatic artery when a right lobe graft is planned, as this may compromise the arterial supply of this segment.

The main nonarterial inflow is from the portal vein, with variable additional input from aberrant right gastric and parabiliary veins (Matsui et al. 1997). There are variations in the morphology of the branch pattern of the portal vein such as an absent main right portal vein trunk, or an H-shaped bifurcation; these tend to be more significant with liver transplantation than conventional liver resections.

The hepatic venous drainage is classically via the left and middle hepatic veins (which join immediately proximal to the inferior cava) and a right hepatic vein. The pattern of branching within the liver, and dependent territories, is more variable with the drainage of segments 5 and/or 8 into either the right or middle hepatic veins. Accessory right hepatic veins are also present within 30–50% of patients.

The classic biliary anatomic arrangement is for the duct draining segments 6 and 7 to join the duct draining segments 5 and 8 to form the right main duct, with tributaries from segments 2–4 fusing to form the left main duct. Segment 1 may drain into the left or the right systems. The left and right ducts join to form the common hepatic duct and the cystic duct draining the gallbladder fuses with the common hepatic duct to form the common bile duct. This arrangement is present in approximately 58% of patients. The commonest variants are for the right posterior duct to join the left main duct or the left and right bifurcation to form a trifurcation. These are discussed further in Sect. 5.4.1.

6.3 Liver Resection and Metastasectomy

6.3.1 Clinical Indications

- Colorectal metastasis (most common indication for liver resection)
- Hepatocellular carcinoma (without liver decompensation)
- Cholangiocarcinoma
- Neuroendocrine metastasis
- Selected cases of genitourinary, breast, gastric, sarcoma, and melanoma metastases (i.e., localized disease confined to the liver after a long disease-free interval)
- Benign hepatic neoplasm, e.g., hepatic adenoma
- Benign biliary disease
- Traumatic laceration

6.3.2 Surgical Technique and Postoperative Anatomy

Liver resections can be broadly divided into anatomical or nonanatomical. Anatomical resections involve removing contiguous functional liver units or segments which may extend beyond one lobe. Nonanatomical resections are smaller local wedge resections performed to remove a focal liver lesion with a small cuff of adjacent liver. There are numerous combinations of liver resections that are possible depending upon the location, number, size, and distribution of the lesions (Fig. 6.3). Varying terminologies are in common use, but an attempt at standardization was defined by the Brisbane 2000 Terminology of Hepatic Anatomy and Resection. This proposed dividing the liver into four sections, namely, the right anterior section (segments 5 and 8), right posterior section (segments 6 and 7), left medial section (segment 4), and left lateral section (segments 2 and 3). The corresponding terminologies used for removal of these sections are given below (Figs. 6.4, 6.5, 6.6, 6.7, and 6.8):

- Right hepatectomy or right hemihepatectomy – resection of segments 5, 6, 7, and 8
- Extended right hepatectomy (right trisectionectomy) – right hepatectomy and resection of segment 4
- Left lateral hepatectomy (left lateral sectionectomy) – resection of segments 2 and 3
- Left hepatectomy – resection of segments 2, 3, and 4
- Extended left hepatectomy or extended left hemihepatectomy left hemihepatectomy also includes resection of segments 5 and 8
- Central hepatectomy – resection of segments 4, 5, and 8
- Right posterior sectionectomy – resection of segments 6 and 7

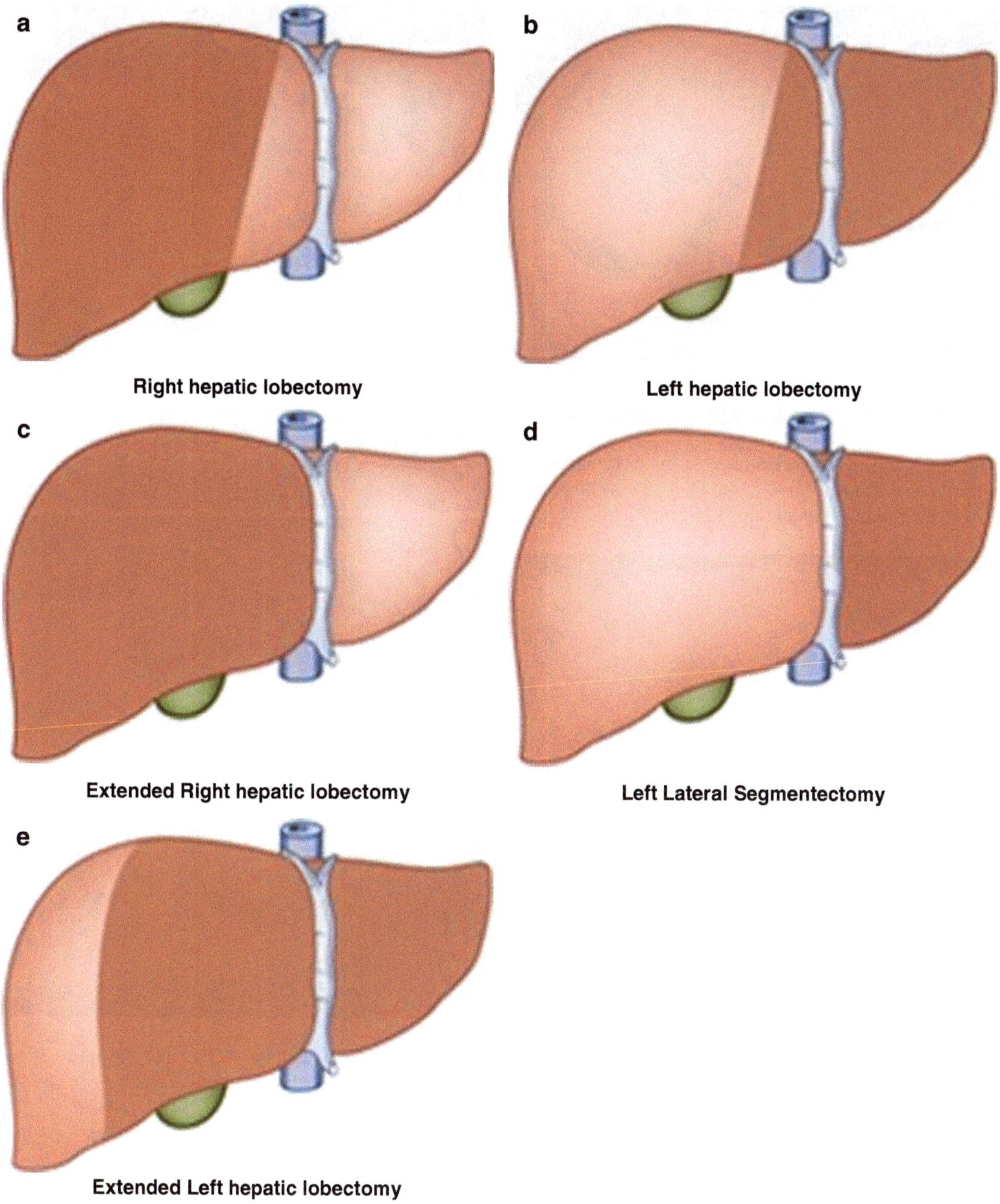

Fig. 6.3 Illustration of some of the commonly performed anatomic segmental liver resections. The resected liver is represented by the darker colour. (**a**) Right hepatectomy (removal of segments 5, 6, 7, and 8). (**b**) Left hepatectomy (removal of segments 2, 3, and 4). (**c**) Extended right hepatectomy/trisectionectomy (right hepatectomy + removal of segment 4). (**d**) Left lateral hepatectomy (removal of segments 2 and 3). (**e**) Extended left hepatectomy/trisectionectomy (left hepatectomy + removal of segments 5 and 8). Other resections (*not shown*) include central hepatectomy (removal of segments 4, 5, and 8), right inferior hepatectomy (removal of segments 5 and 6), and right superior hepatectomy (removal of segments 7 and 8)

- Right inferior hepatectomy – resection of segments 5 and 6
- Right superior hepatectomy – resection of segments 7 and 8
- Caudatectomy – resection of segment 1 (this may be used in combination with the above operations, i.e., radical excision of hilar cholangiocarcinoma)

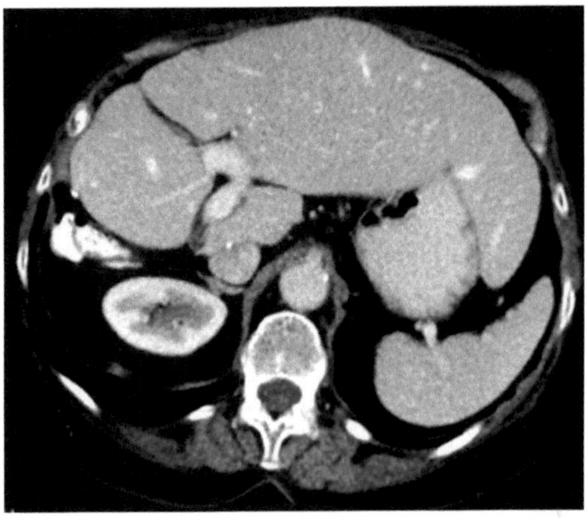

Fig. 6.4 Axial CT 3 months post right hepatectomy (resection of segments 5, 6, 7, and 8). There is compensatory hypertrophy of the left lobe segments

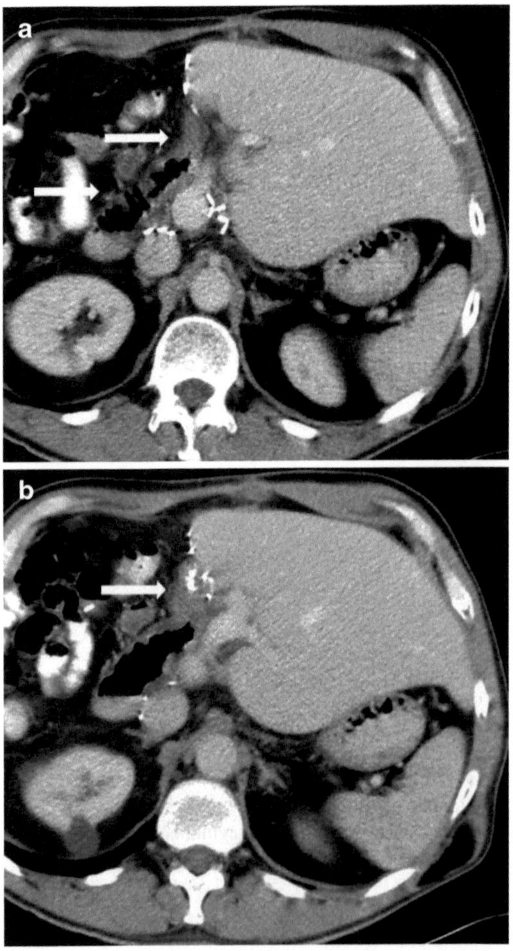

Fig. 6.5 (**a**, **b**) Extended right hepatectomy (right hepatectomy and resection of segment 4) and caudectomy. Axial CT shows the biliary-enteric anastomosis and Roux loop (*arrow*)

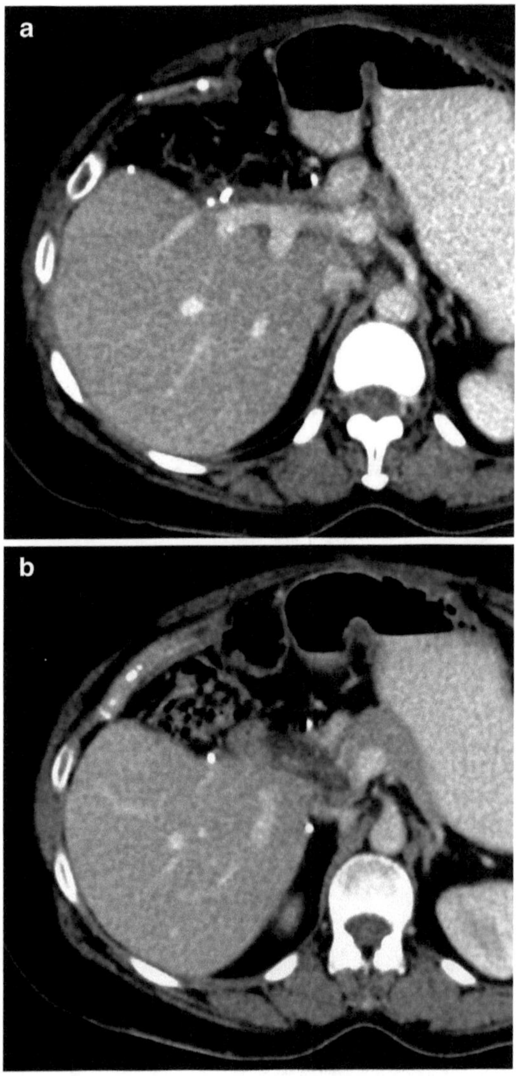

Fig. 6.6 Left hepatectomy. CT at (**a**) the level of the portal vein and (**b**) below the hilum showing resection of segments 2, 3, and 4

6.3.3 Modifications of Surgical Technique

- The extremes of liver resection are becoming more divergent. There is a progressive tendency to perform more limited resections for a given burden of disease so as to preserve as much liver parenchyma as possible, whereas at the other end of the spectrum, patients are undergoing resections with a greater number and volume or wider distribution of disease using combinations

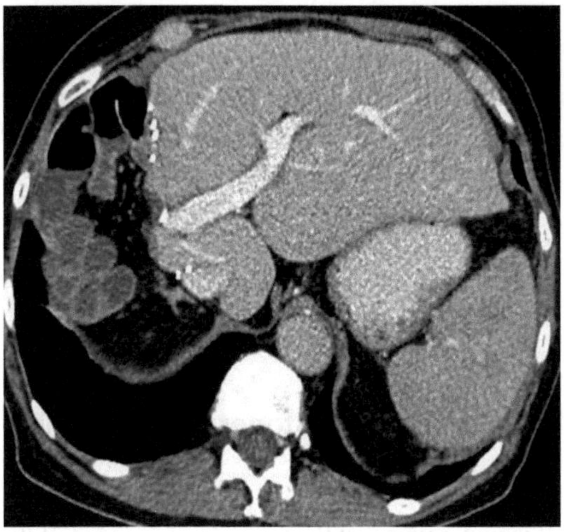

Fig. 6.7 Extended right hepatectomy (right hepatectomy and resection of segment 4). The caudate lobe is also retained

of resections or other therapeutic techniques, e.g., radiofrequency ablation (RFA) and transcatheter arterial chemoebolization (TACE).

- Nonanatomic wedge resection is increasingly used for small superficial lesions (Fig. 6.9), but for deeper lesions, formal segmental resection is more commonly required. The advantages of wedge resection over segmental resection include conservation of the liver parenchyma and function, less hemorrhage and sepsis, and therefore a shorter hospital stay. It is essential that an adequate resection margin (Liau et al. 2004) is still obtained.
- Nonanatomic wedge resections may be used in combination with conventional segmental resections when there is bilateral disease.
- Sufficient hepatic parenchyma to support life must be retained. If the proposed residual segments are too small, embolization or ligation of the portal vein branches that supply the liver to be removed may be performed to induce hypertrophy in the segments to be retained. This may be performed as part of a two-stage operative procedure if there is bilateral disease, or as an interventional radiological technique (Fig. 6.10).
- Chemotherapy may be given prior to liver surgery either to reduce the volume of metastases to enable resection in otherwise inoperable cases or as adjuvant therapy after the colonic

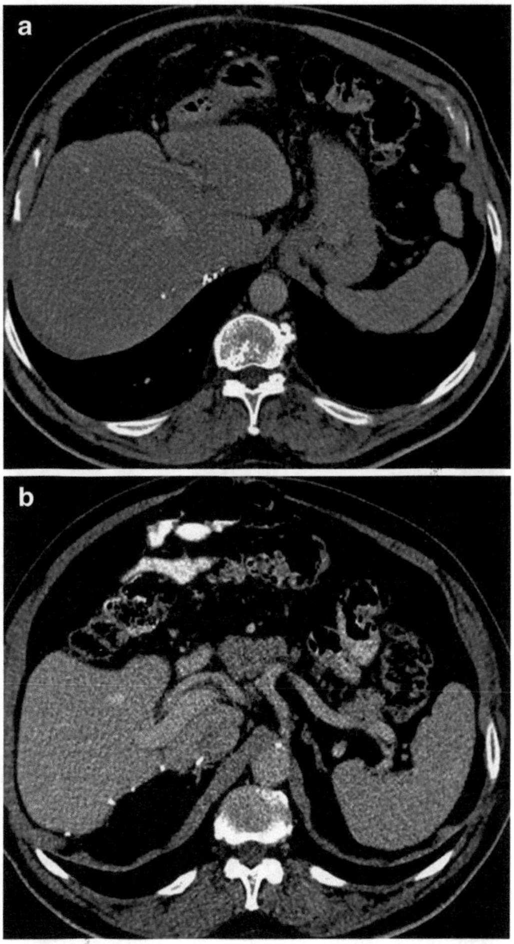

Fig. 6.8 (**a**, **b**) CT on a patient with a colonic tumor and liver metastasis following combined right hemicolectomy and right posterior sectionectomy (removal of segments 6 and 7)

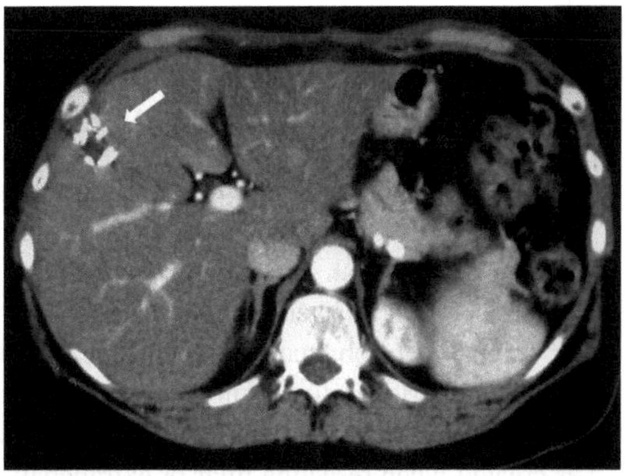

Fig. 6.9 Metastasectomy (*arrow*). CT demonstrating a "chip shot" from the right lobe of the liver

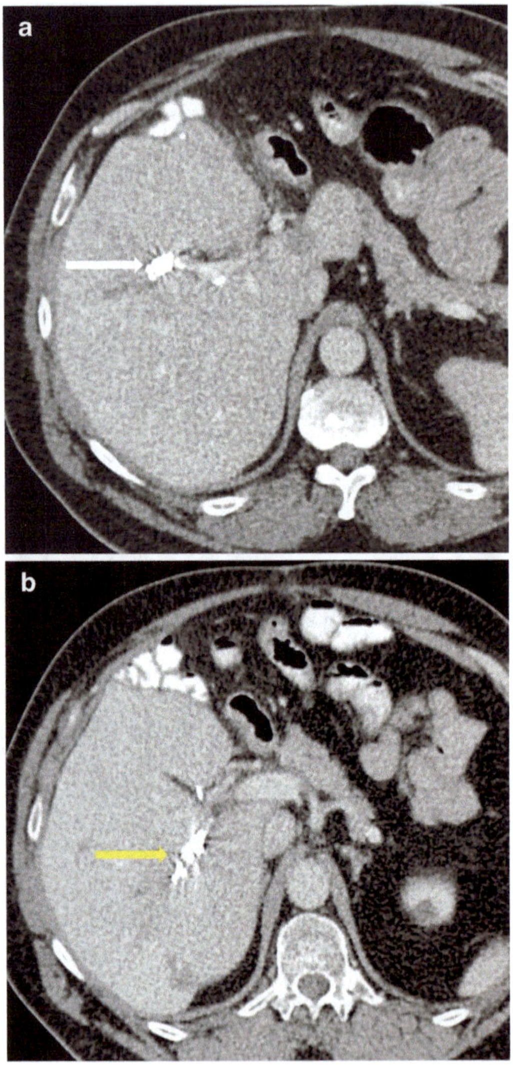

Fig. 6.10 (**a**, **b**) Interim CT in a patient with bilateral colorectal liver metastases. Following a left lateral sectionectomy (resection of segments II and III), the anterior (*white arrow*) and posterior divisions (*yellow arrow*) of the right portal vein have been embolized to promote hypertrophy of segment IV prior to a right hemihepatectomy

primary has been resected (if the primary has adverse histological features putting the patient at high risk of systemic recurrence). This can result in liver injury (steatohepatitis or sinusoidal obstructive syndrome) and increased perioperative complications.

- A biliary-enteric anastomosis (i.e., Roux-en-Y) is created when resecting hilar or extrahepatic cholangiocarcinomas or if there is other significant extrahepatic biliary pathology.
- Some patients might have additional local ablation treatments such as radiofrequency ablation performed at the time of a surgical resection.
- With limited synchronous colorectal metastatic disease, the liver resection may be performed at the time of the primary colonic resection.
- During major resections, the gallbladder is usually removed as an opportunistic procedure to prevent future problems with cholelithiasis.

6.3.4 Normal Postoperative Imaging

6.3.4.1 CT

It is imperative that the radiologist is aware of the indication for surgery and the nature of the surgical procedure. Other considerations include the presence of preexisting benign lesions in the residual liver and any additional treatments performed, e.g., local ablative treatments. The radiological question to be addressed will depend on the temporal relationship to the surgery. Imaging in the early postoperative period is only performed if there are clinical features of an early complication. The first planned follow-up CT is usually performed between 3 and 6 months postoperatively. This is performed to identify occult metastases not seen on preoperative imaging, new primary lesions within the liver, or new extrahepatic metastases. The nature of the original disease will have a bearing on the sites at high risk of further disease.

6.3.4.2 CT in the Early Postoperative Period

Abdominal drains are left in situ after major resections and usually removed at around the fifth postoperative day if the drainage fluid is serous and not blood or bile stained. It is common to see small low attenuation fluid collections at the resection site due to transient accumulation of blood and bile. These collections are confined to the limits of resection margin, conform to the shape of that margin and adjacent anatomic compartment, and usually regress over time (Figs. 6.11 and 6.12).

Extraluminal gas accumulation while usually resolving within 10 days can rarely persist up to 2 months postoperatively even in uncomplicated

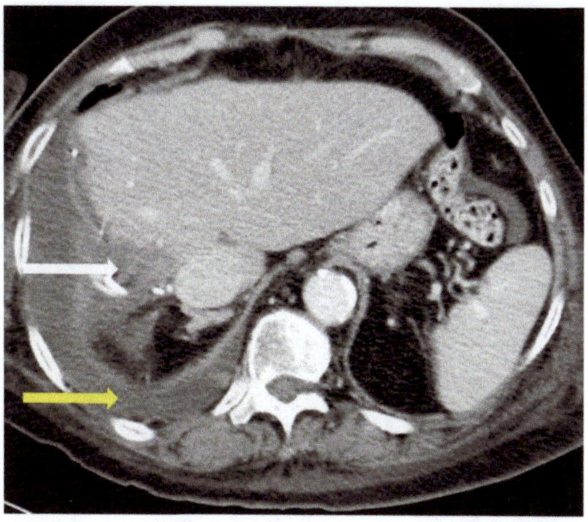

Fig. 6.11 Fluid collection adjacent to the resection margin post-right hepatectomy (*white arrow*). Right pleural effusion (*yellow arrow*)

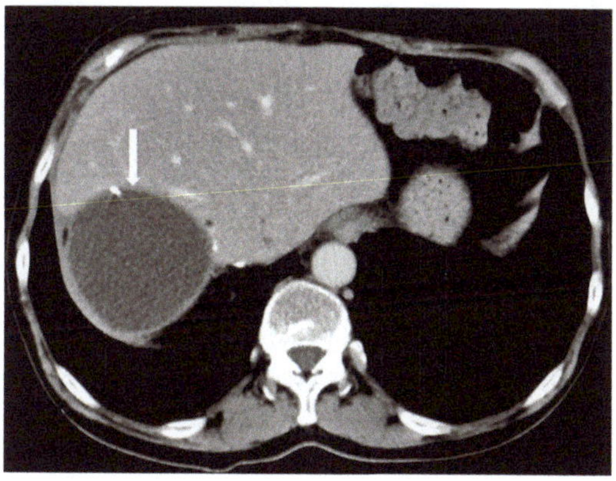

Fig. 6.12 Organized postoperative fluid collection posterior to the resection site on axial CT (*arrow*)

cases. Correlation with the clinical condition of the patient is therefore required to exclude the possibility of localized sepsis, anastomotic leak, or perforation.

Sympathetic pleural effusions are common after liver surgery, particularly on the right. These may require draining if they become symptomatic.

Artificial hemostatic agents such as those made from oxidized regenerated cellulose (Surgicel – Ethicon, Gargrave, UK) are used to control intraoperative bleeding (Fig. 6.13) (see Sect. 1.4.2.1). Small gas bubbles may be seen in association with fluid at the metastasectomy site in the immediate postoperative period in such cases without implying infection. Over time, these collections resolve spontaneously. In the past, some surgeons

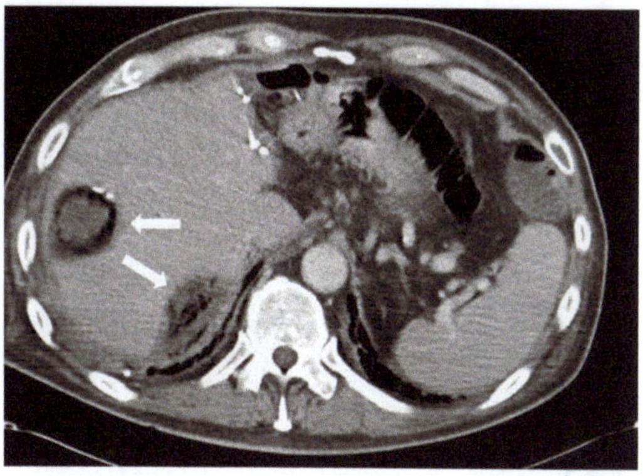

Fig. 6.13 Surgicel – Ethicon, Gargrave, UK. Early postoperative CT following left lateral sectionectomy with segment VII and VIII metastasectomies. The metastasectomy sites (*arrows*) are packed with oxidized regenerated cellulose with small bubbles of gas present at the interface with the liver

used to sew an omental patch to the resection margin, and this appeared as an area of low attenuation on CT. Between this patch and the resection margin, a small collection of fluid can be seen in the early postoperative period.

6.3.4.3 CT in the Late Postoperative Period

Following major liver resection, the remnant liver undergoes regeneration (Fig. 6.14). It occurs most rapidly in the first week following surgery, and it can reach up to 70% of the total preoperative volume. Thereafter, the remnant liver continues to regenerate to reach up to 85% of preoperative volume by the end of the first year. However, regeneration may be slower in the presence of cirrhosis, and this is potentially a contributing factor to poorer outcomes. Preexisting benign lesions such as cysts and hemangiomas in the remnant liver may change in configuration due to parenchymal hypertrophy.

Following partial hepatectomy, the anatomical relationship of the upper abdomen undergoes rearrangement. The right kidney and bowel fills the liver bed following right hepatectomy; transverse colon and stomach fills the space after left hepatectomy. Local ablative treatment sites and Roux loops can be misinterpreted on postoperative imaging if not considered by the radiologist.

The size of the spleen may increase following major resection presumably as a consequence of

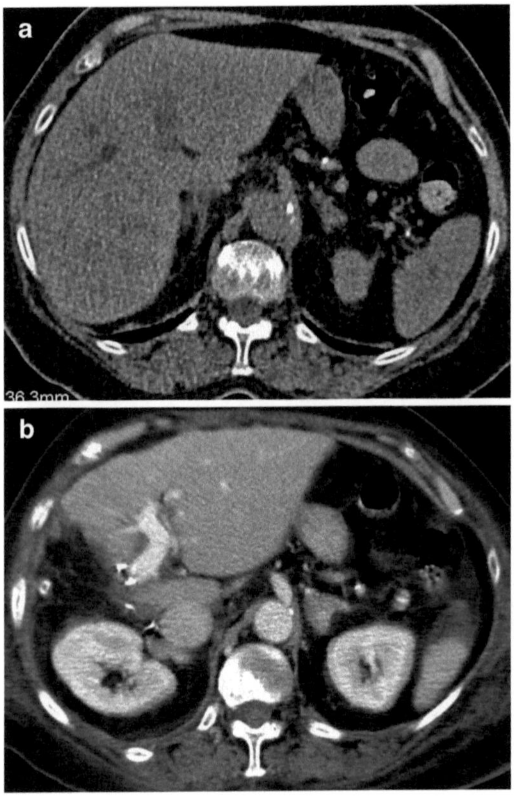

Fig. 6.14 Liver regeneration following right hepatectomy. The volume of the left lobe has increased by approximately one third between (**a**) a preoperative noncontrast CT and (**b**) a postcontrast CT 9 days postresection

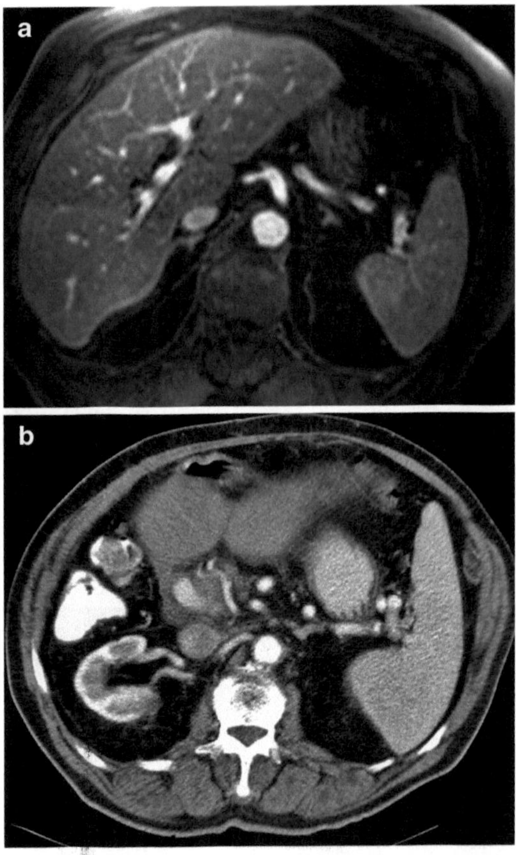

Fig. 6.15 Splenic hypertrophy following right hepatectomy. (**a**) Normal sized spleen on preoperative MRI. (**b**) On postoperative CT, the spleen has enlarged to 17 cm

altered portal venous dynamics, although varices are not usually seen (Fig. 6.15). Oxaliplatin is frequently used either pre- or post liver resection for colorectal metastases, and an increase in spleen size has been observed in some patients with liver injury caused by chemotherapy, particularly sinusoidal obstructive syndrome related to oxaliplatin treatment (Overman et al. 2010).

6.3.4.4 MRI

MRI is mainly used as a problem solver to supplement CT or ultrasound findings when recurrence is suspected within the remnant liver or if biliary complications are suspected. MR is also used when re-resection is planned for recurrent disease.

At the site of liver resection, a small area of high signal intensity on T2-weighted images is to be expected in the early postoperative period, and this may persist for months. The signal intensity on both T1 and T2 will depend on the relative contribution of serous fluid, bile, hematoma, or surgically applied hemostatic agents. In the early postoperative period, it may be difficult to differentiate this from residual or recurrent tumor. Extracellular contrast agents (gadolinium chelates) are helpful. Surgical clips cause susceptibility and therefore usually appear darker and larger on sequences sensitive to susceptibility; for this reason, clips appear darker upon in phase chemical shift T1 images than opposed phase T1 at 1.5T (Sect. 5.3.2.5).

6.3.5 Postoperative Complications

In series published in the 1970s, mortality for liver resection was approximately 20%. With current practice, overall mortality is low with perioperative morbidity rates of 15–35% (Simmonds et al.

2006; Farid et al. 2010). If less than 3 segments are resected mortality in major units is less than 1% whereas if 6 segments are resected this may reach 7.8% (Jarnagin et al. 2002). The major cause of mortality apart from a cardiac event is sepsis, multiorgan failure, and hemorrhage (Farid et al. 2010). Many of these are interrelated as poor hepatic reserve may lead to hemorrhage and subsequent increased risk of sepsis which can create a positive feedback loop with the sepsis causing further liver function impairment and renal failure.

6.3.5.1 Sepsis

The most common indication for imaging in the early postoperative period (ultrasound or CT) is in septic patients to exclude an intra-abdominal collection. As described above, fluid adjacent to the liver edge is a normal postoperative finding. Hematoma, perihepatic abscess, or biloma usually do not confine to the resection margin or fill an anatomic shape (Letourneau et al. 1988). Hematoma in the early stages has a relatively high attenuation particularly within the center of the collection. The presence of gas suggests infection (Fig. 6.16), and image-guided percutaneous aspiration is often required for confirmation.

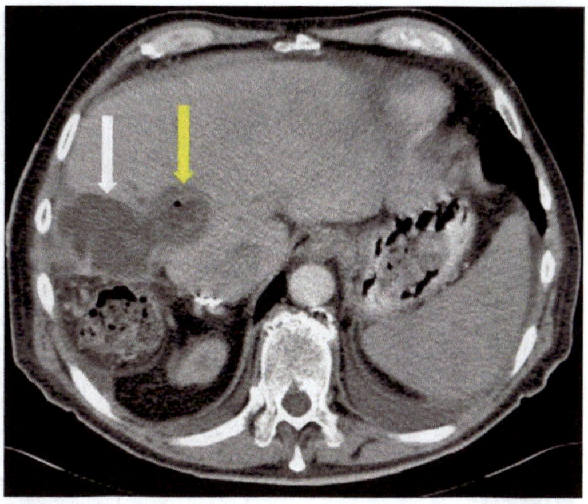

Fig. 6.16 Infected postoperative fluid collection. Axial CT shows an infected fluid collection adjacent to the resection margin (*white arrow*) which has penetrated the liver capsule forming a liver abscess (*yellow arrow*). A tiny gas locule is present within the liver collection

6.3.5.2 Biliary Complications

The main biliary complications associated with liver resection are bile leaks and biliary obstruction. Although the reported complication rate is 3–4%, they are associated with a high incidence of liver failure. Clinical presentation includes intra-abdominal sepsis, biliary peritonitis, and jaundice.

Bile Leak

The common sites of bile leaks include the hepatic duct stump of the resected lobe, the biliary-enteric anastomosis, common hepatic ducts, and T-tube insertion sites (Lo et al. 1998). Bile in postoperative surgical drains should prompt urgent investigation with direct cholangiography if a T-tube is present, or more usually MRCP, scintigraphy (Fig. 6.17), PTC, or ERCP or in order to establish the site and nature of the leak (Sect. 5.4.2.1). There is often little to see on US and CT if the drain is effective at preventing fluid accumulation. The majority of cases can be managed conservatively with percutaneous drainage

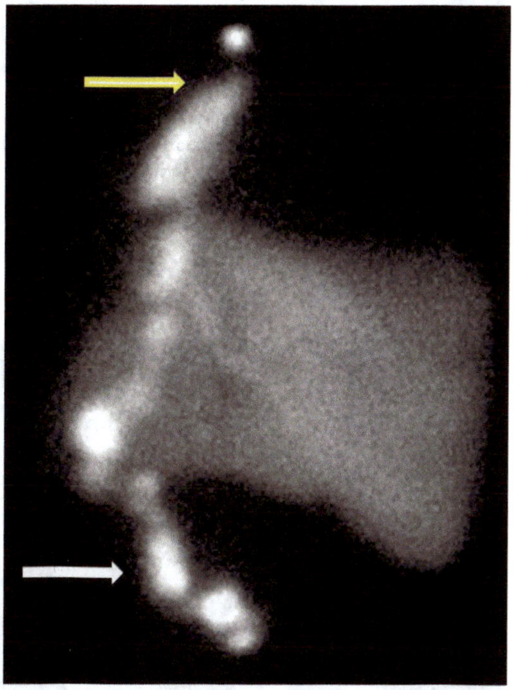

Fig. 6.17 Bile leak and subsequent biliary-bronchial fistula. A 35-min anterior planar image from a technetium-99 m mebrofenin scintigram in a patient who had previously undergone a right trisectionectomy for liver metastasis. The bile drainage inferiorly (*white arrow*) is into a Roux loop and superiorly (*yellow arrow*) into the bronchial tree (Courtesy Dr. Andrew Scarsbrook Leeds TH NHS Trust)

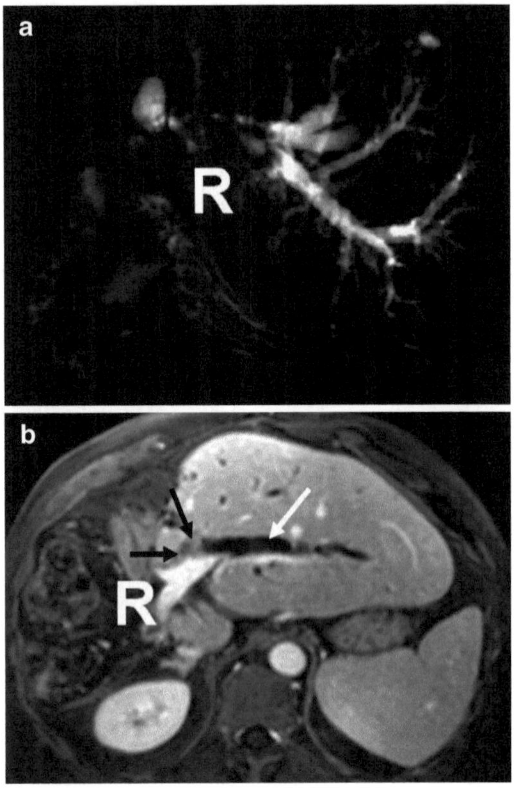

Fig. 6.18 Recurrent malignant anastomotic biliary obstruction following right hepatectomy for colorectal metastases. (**a**) MRCP MIP images show dilatation of the left biliary tree proximal to the biliary-enteric anastomosis (*R*). (**b**) Axial postgadolinium fat-suppressed T1 image demonstrates biliary dilatation (*white arrow*) due to tumor recurrence (*black arrows*)

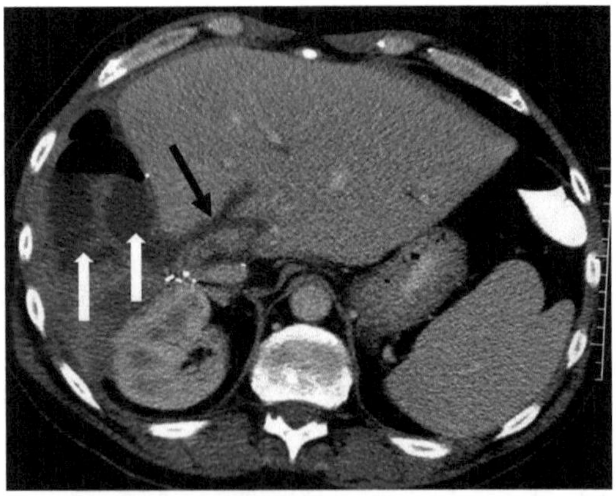

Fig. 6.19 Roux loop obstruction post-liver resection. Mildly dilated fluid-filled Roux loop on axial CT suggestive of obstruction (*white arrows*) with dilatation of the biliary tree (*black arrow*). There are some ill-defined postoperative inflammatory changes within the surgical bed adjacent to the right kidney

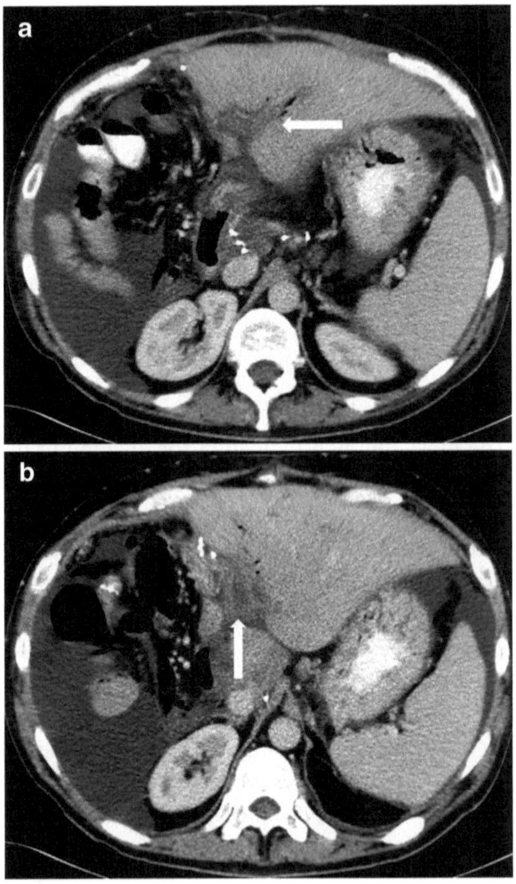

Fig. 6.20 (**a**, **b**) Portal venous thrombosis post liver resection. Axial CT shows nonenhancement of the left portal vein (*arrow*) indicating venous thrombosis. There is a reduction in perfusion of the residual left lobe of the liver. Pneumobilia and moderate volume of ascites are noted

and stenting via either an endoscopic or transhepatic approach. Surgery is reserved for cases that have been unsuccessfully managed by stenting but is associated with a high complication rate, e.g., subsequent development of bile duct strictures. This is also discussed in Sect. 5.4.3.

Biliary Obstruction

Biliary obstruction can be due to postoperative fibrosis or recurrent malignancy (Fig. 6.18) at the biliary-enteric anastomosis. Obstruction of the Roux loop can also occur (Fig. 6.19).

6.3.5.3 Ascites

Ascites occurs more commonly in postoperative patients with documented cirrhosis than in patients with normal liver function (Pol et al. 1999).

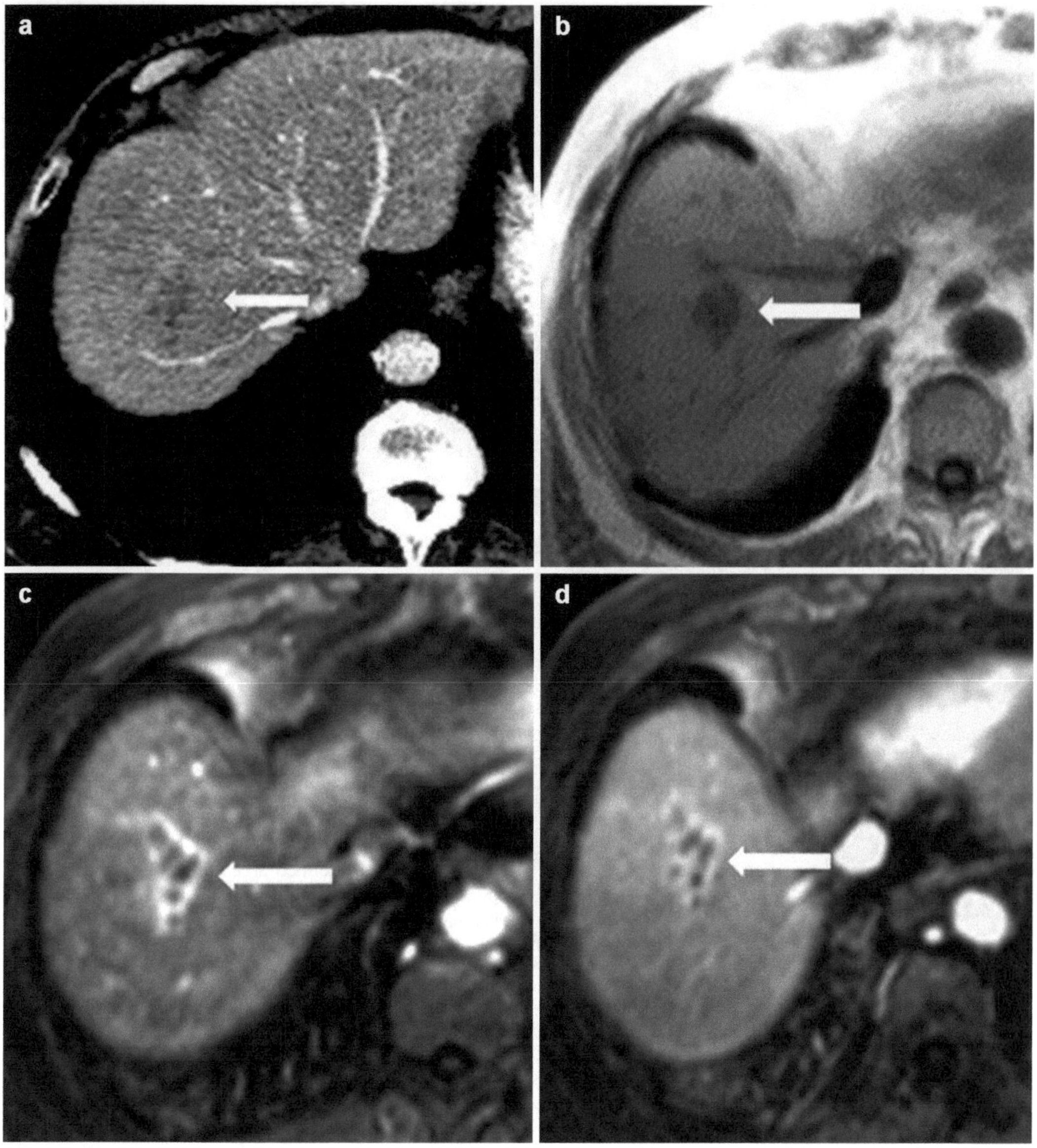

Fig. 6.21 Branch portal vein thrombosis posthepatectomy. (**a**) A poorly defined hypodense lesion on axial CT (*arrow*) was worrisome for a new metastasis. (**b–d**) Further characterization of the "lesion" with MRI demonstrates (**b**) low signal on axial in phase T1W gradient echo sequences. (**c**, **d**) Arterial and portal venous phase postgadolinium shows a lack of central enhancement (*arrows*) with confirmed thrombosed portal venous branches (Images used with permission)

6.3.5.4 Vascular Complications

Vascular complications include thrombosis of the portal (Figs. 6.20 and 6.21) and hepatic venous (Figs. 6.22 and 6.23) circulation. It is an uncommon complication but should be considered in the early postoperative period in patients who develop a transient deterioration in liver function. Doppler ultrasound of the liver is a sensitive in detection of venous thrombosis, but the diagnosis can also be made with contrast-enhanced CT and MRI. Vascular thrombosis is usually self-limiting owing to the formation of collateral vessels. After multiple or complex resections, the hepatic venous outflow may fibrose to cause the remnant liver to become congested. In these patients, the enhancement pattern of the liver resembles Budd-Chiari syndrome.

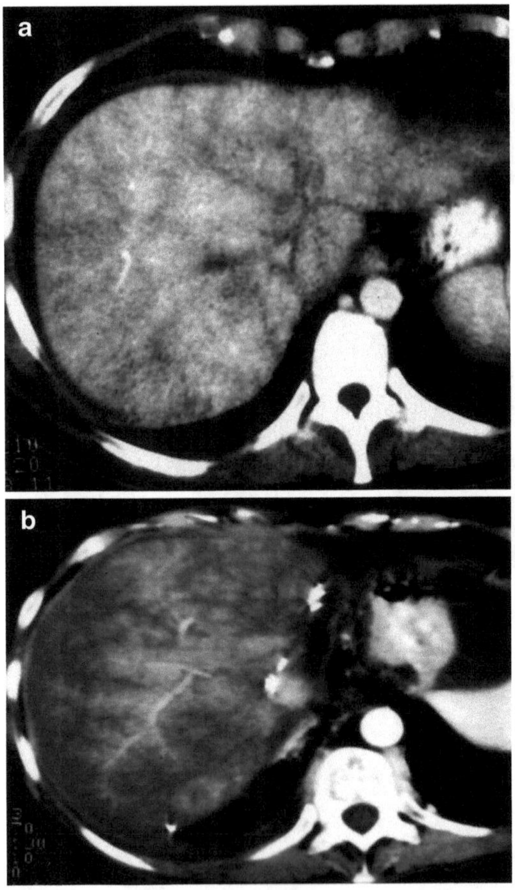

Fig. 6.22 (**a**, **b**) Budd-Chiari syndrome post liver resection. Axial CT demonstrates patchy enhancement of the remnant liver and lack of enhancement of the hepatic veins

6.3.6 Imaging Recurrent Disease

After resection of colorectal liver metastasis, serum CEA (carcinoembryonic antigen) measurements are routinely measured combined with clinical assessment and regular CT of the chest, abdomen, and pelvis. Different units perform this at differing intervals. The CEA level should return to normal if the surgery is successful. If the CEA remains persistently elevated postoperatively or begins to rise after normalization, a CT should be performed, and if negative, a PET-CT, to look for any treatable sites of disease.

Major liver resections are associated with a massive increase in cytokine production which apart from having a regenerative effect on the liver may serve to promote the growth of occult metastases. The liver is the commonest site of

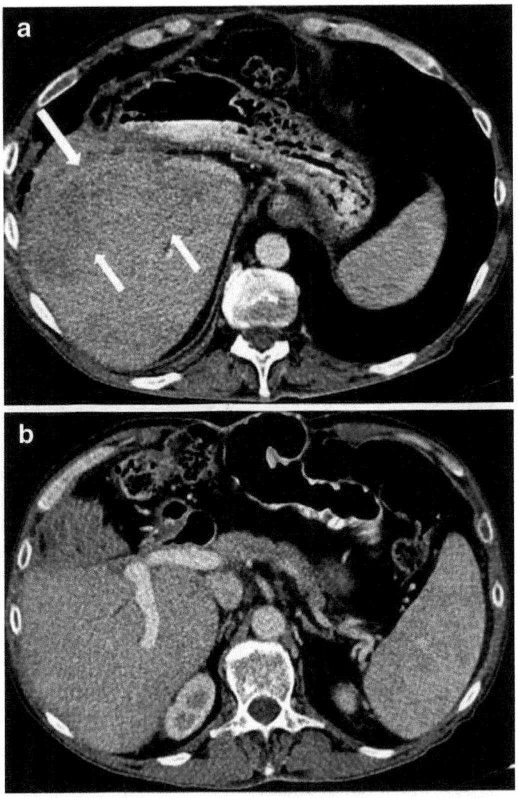

Fig. 6.23 Hepatic venous compromise following left trisectionectomy for cholangiocarcinoma on axial CT. (**a**) There is a poorly defined area of low attenuation in the anterosuperior aspect of the remnant liver (*arrows*). (**b**) The portal vein branches are patent

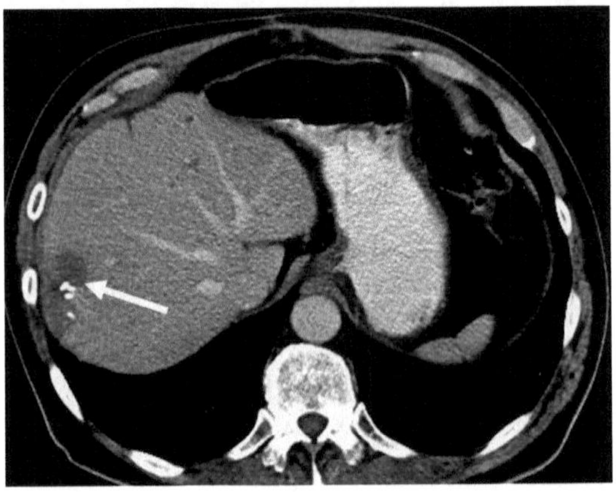

Fig. 6.24 Local recurrence at the site of a previous metastasectomy. An ill-defined area of low attenuation (*arrow*) at the site of surgical resection (staples) indicates local recurrence

recurrence (Fig. 6.24) (occurring in nearly 50%) following colorectal metastases resection, but patients may be suitable for further resection.

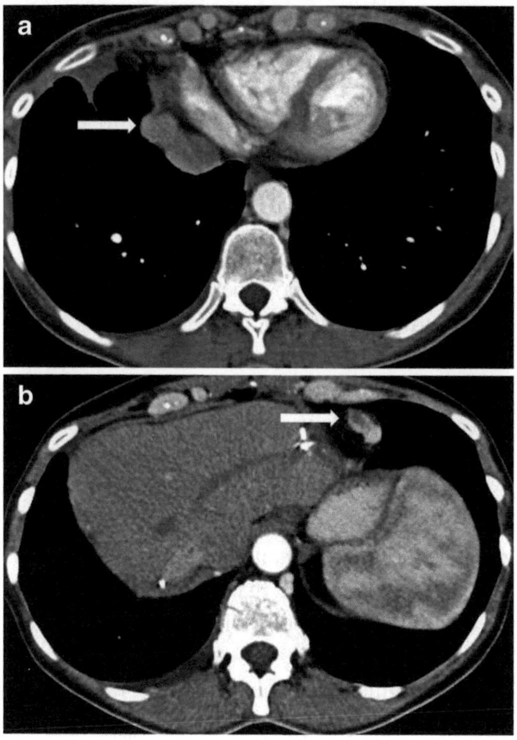

Fig. 6.25 Supradiaphragmatic nodal recurrence of a carcinoid tumor 6 months post right hemicolectomy and bilateral liver resection. (**a**) Enlarged lymph node (*arrow*) anterior to the IVC and (**b**) a further node adjacent to the left lobe of liver are shown (*arrow*)

The next commonest site of recurrence is the lung (reported in 25%), followed by other intra-abdominal sites (Fig. 6.25).

Presurgical imaging is invaluable in the assessment of focal abnormalities detected on follow-up imaging. It should be appreciated that the axis of the liver may change post resection and this will have a bearing on the location of preexisting liver lesions. The presence of surgical clips helps to identify sites of metastasectomy and nonanatomic wedge resection. However, if surgical clips were not used, it may not be so obvious. Beware of low attenuation tissue which projects into the liver beyond surgical clips as this should raise suspicion for locally recurrent disease. The risk of recurrence at a resection margin is higher at a metastasectomy site than an anatomic segmental resection margin, as the margins are usually greater with the latter. New segmental or subsegmental biliary dilatation is highly suggestive of an underlying liver metastasis even if a metastasis is not identified.

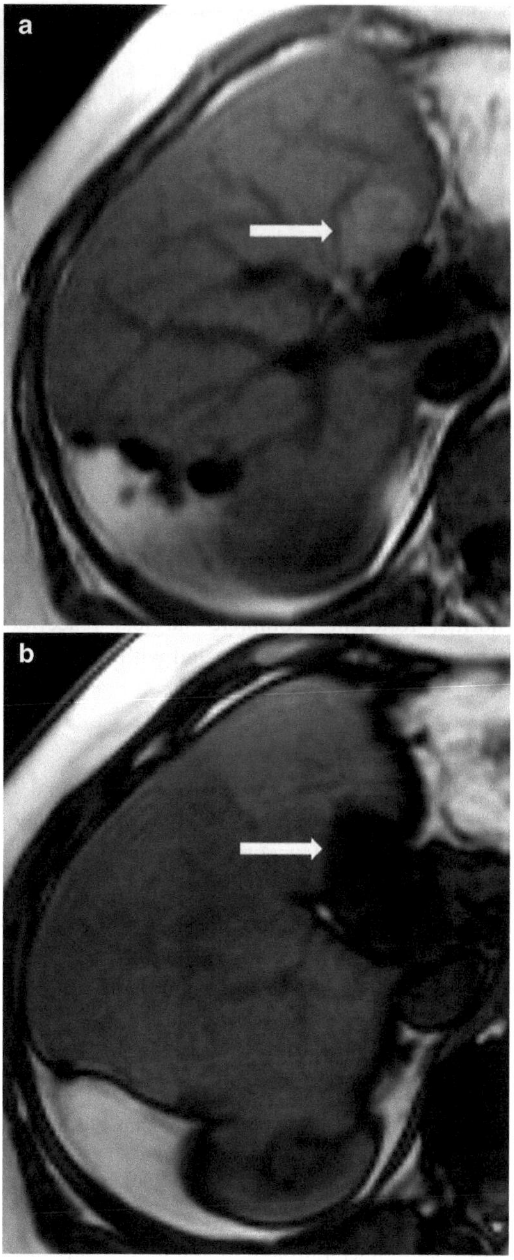

Fig. 6.26 Focal fatty infiltration following liver resection. (**a**) In and (**b**) opposed phase axial T1W gradient MRI images show an area of signal drop out on the opposed phase image in keeping with focal fatty infiltration (*arrow*). Lack of enhancement on dynamic postgadolinium T1W fat-suppressed images (*not shown*) confirms benign disease

Fatty livers may obscure recurrent tumors, and occasionally altered liver perfusion effects may result in focal fat deposition mimicking recurrent disease (Figs. 6.26 and 6.27).

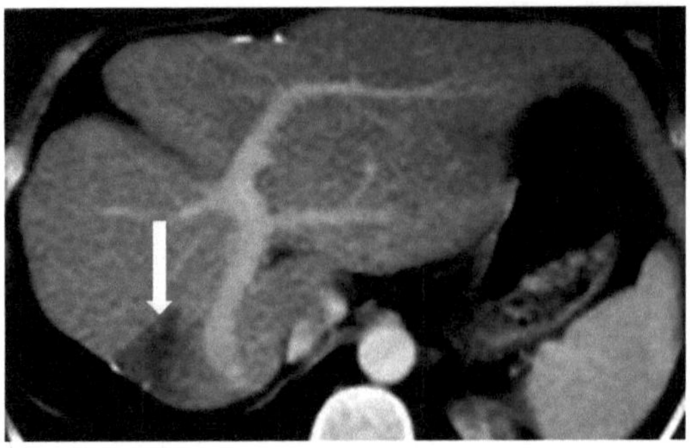

Fig. 6.27 Focal fatty infiltration at the resection site following right hepatectomy. Clear resection margin on initial follow-up CT (*not shown*). Six months later, there is a new hypodense area at the resection site posteriorly (*arrow*). Confirmed as focal fat on MRI (*not shown*)

If the AFP (alpha-fetoprotein) level is elevated before surgery, for HCC, it should return back to normal following complete surgical resection. Recurrence should be suspected with rising AFP levels (Fig. 6.28).

6.3.6.1 CT

For the detection of recurrence, it is crucial to scan patients at the appropriate vascular phase depending on the tumor histology:

- Portal venous phase examination of the liver alone would be sufficient in cases of colorectal metastasis and cholangiocarcinoma. Metastatic lesions are hypovascular and have a low attenuation.
- Dual phase (arterial and portal venous phase) examination is appropriate for hypervascular tumors such as hepatocellular carcinoma and neuroendocrine metastases.

6.3.6.2 MRI

Pre- and postcontrast imaging is indicated. Collections at resection margins may have a complex signal in the early postoperative period; this should not be misinterpreted as residual tumor. The signal intensity of metastases should be similar to that of the original resected metastasis, and early enhancement following gadolinium at the interface between the tumor and the liver is a helpful sign, whereas with collections, this is either absent or if a fibrous wall has formed progressively accumulates contrast (Robinson and Ward 2006).

6.3.7 Teaching Points

- Knowledge of segmental liver anatomy and types of resection are important to interpret postoperative liver appearances.
- Following major resection, the remnant liver undergoes hypertrophy, which can alter the configuration of preexisting benign lesions.
- In the immediate postoperative period, imaging in particular with CT helps to identify complications and direct appropriate treatment.
- Depending on tumor histology, CT scanning at the appropriate vascular phase is imperative.
- Low attenuation on CT at a resection site should be expected and not misinterpreted as tumor recurrence.
- Tissue of lower attenuation than normal liver parenchyma on CT that projects into the liver beyond surgical clips is likely to represent recurrent disease.
- New segmental or subsegmental biliary dilatation is highly suggestive of recurrent disease.

6.4 Radiofrequency Ablation (RFA)

6.4.1 Introduction

RFA involves delivery of high-frequency alternating current to the tissues via a needle electrode. Heat is created around the tip of the electrode that exceeds 60–100°C as a result of agitation of the ions in the tissue. This leads to localized thermal coagulation necrosis and protein denaturation. The first proposal to destroy small malignant liver tumors using a modified radiofrequency technique was made in early 1990s. Since then, there have been several modifications in the needle probe design and method of delivering the RF current. The technique itself has undergone further refinements with an improved overall success rate. Although there are several thermal ablation techniques (i.e., cryoablation, microwave, laser, and high-intensity focused sonography) are available used to treat liver tumors, radiofrequency ablation (RFA) is currently the most widely practiced technique. RFA is considered to be a safe,

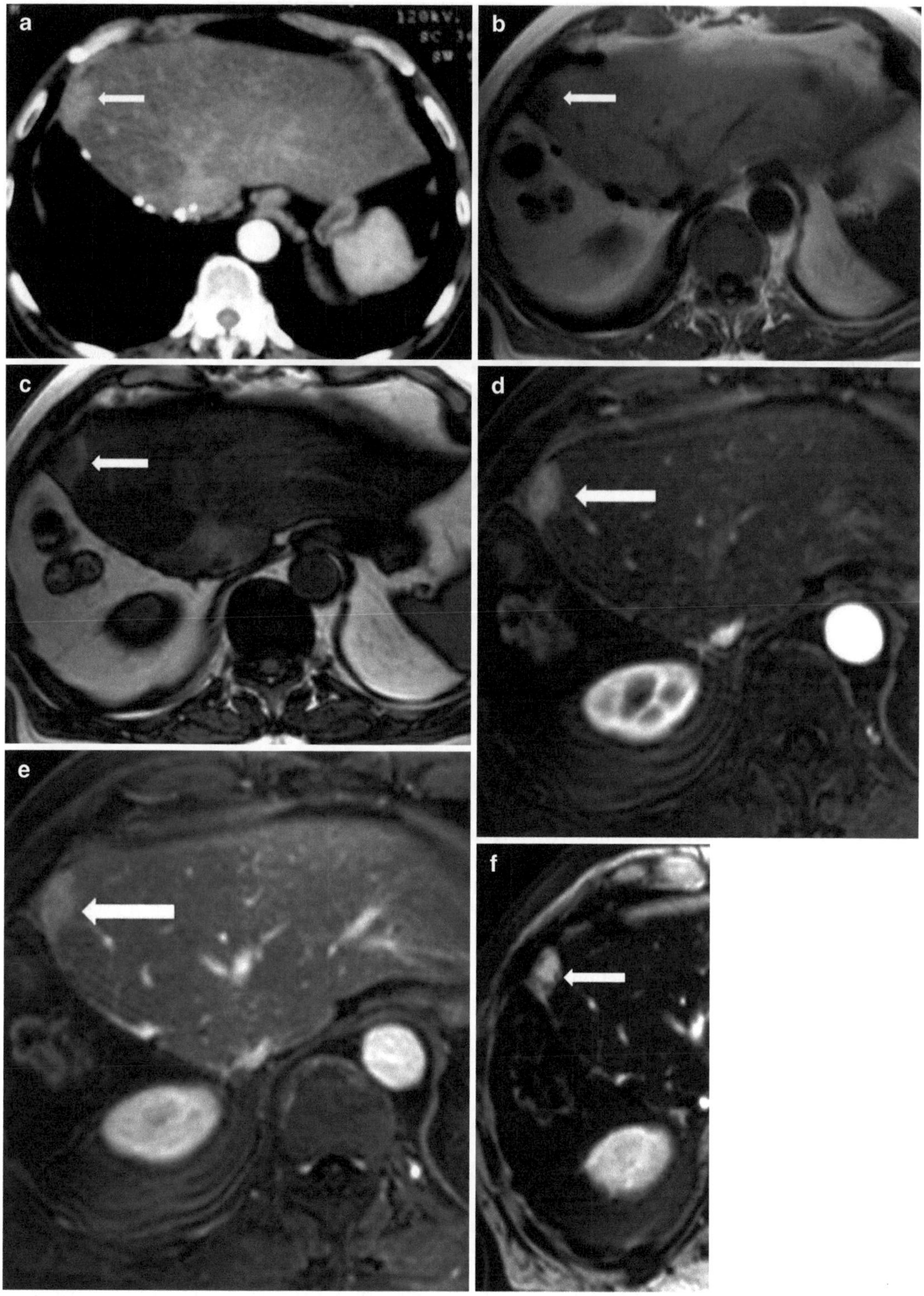

Fig. 6.28 HCC recurrence at resection margin site in a patient with a rising alpha-fetoprotein (AFP). (**a**) Small hyperdense lesion at the resection site on axial CT (*arrow*). Focal fatty sparing in a fatty liver and tumor recurrence were considered. (**b**) In and (**c**) opposed phase axial T1W gradient MRI images demonstrate diffuse signal loss within the liver consistent with a fatty liver. The lesion is, however, more prominent on the opposed signal sequence confirming it does not contain fat (*arrow*). (**d, e**) Dynamic postgadolinium fat-suppressed T1 images show (**d**) early arterial phase enhancement and (**e**) some washout in the equilibrium phase. (**f**) Lack of superparamagnetic iron oxide (SPIO) uptake by the lesion confirms recurrent HCC (*arrow*)

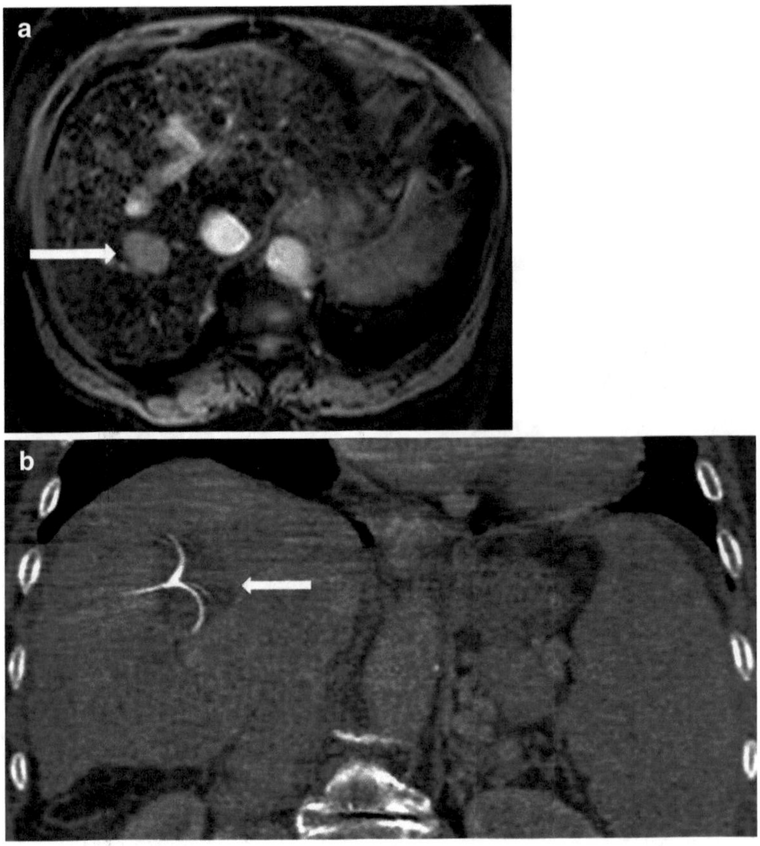

Fig. 6.29 CT-guided RFA in the treatment of HCC. (**a**) MRI following SPIO (superparamagnetic iron oxide) confirms liver cirrhosis and a lack of SPIO (iron) uptake within a lesion consistent with HCC (*arrow*). (**b**) Unenhanced coronal CT images obtained during initial RFA treatment. There is good positioning of the needle (LeVeen RFA needle-4 cm) centered on the lesion and satisfactory deployment of the electrode arms (*arrow*)

well-tolerated, and an effective treatment procedure for unresectable hepatic malignancies less than 3.0 cm in diameter, although can be used for larger tumors.

Only 5–15% of newly diagnosed HCC or colorectal cancer liver metastasis patients are eligible for a potentially curative resection, and there is a role for local ablative treatments in prolonging the survival of selected patients unable to tolerate surgery or as a bridge to transplantation.

6.4.2 Clinical Indications

- Small volume but nonresectable HCC
- Either as a definitive treatment, in combination with transarterial chemoembolization (TACE), or as a bridge to transplantation in patients with limited disease awaiting liver transplant
- Colorectal liver metastases
- Neuroendocrine metastases – to reduce tumor bulk and hormone secretion
- Other liver metastases (rare)

6.4.3 RFA Technique

- An RF needle electrode is introduced into the lesion percutaneously or laparoscopically using ultrasound as guidance or by an open (laparotomy) method.
- A typical RF needle electrode has a long insulated cannula containing a number of electrode arms. Once the needle is satisfactorily positioned within the lesion, the individual electrode arms are deployed which takes the shape of a hook or a tine.
- The electrode is then attached to an RF generator, and two dispersive electrodes (return or grounding pads) are placed on the patient, one on each thigh.

- RF energy is then applied using an established treatment algorithm. A single ablation lasts between 8 and 20 min.

6.4.4 Modifications to RFA Technique

- CT or MR can also be used as a guide to place the needle (Fig. 6.29).
- A laparoscopic approach which has advantages and disadvantages. The peritoneal cavity can be inspected to exclude extrahepatic disease, and better resolution can be achieved with laparoscopic ultrasound.
- Multiple overlapping ablations might be required to treat large lesions, or, alternatively, a newer generation probe which covers a larger area can be used.
- Treatments may have to be repeated to ensure adequate response.

There are several advantageous to the percutaneous approach. It is the least invasive, may be performed with conscious sedation, and repeated as necessary to treat recurrent tumor. It is also associated with minimal morbidity (McGhana and Dodd 2001). The main advantage of ultrasound-guided RFA over CT and MRI is its real-time capabilities, vascular assessment, availability, speed, and low cost. The primary disadvantage is its limited ability to assess the effectiveness of an ablation due to the echogenic response seen immediately following treatment.

6.4.5 Imaging Post-RFA

Imaging is vital to assess the completeness of the ablation and to detect any complications in the early stages posttreatment. Given its easy accessibility, a contrast-enhanced CT is more commonly performed, although MR is also equally accurate.

6.4.5.1 Ultrasound

Ultrasound has a limited role in the assessment of treated lesions because necrotic and viable tumor can have similar echogenic appearances on posttreatment scans. However, contrast-enhanced ultrasound using agents such as SonoVue (Bracco Diagnostics) can be used as an imaging tool in assessing for tumor recurrence (Fig. 6.30).

6.4.5.2 CT

In the first few days following ablation, the treated lesion appears low in attenuation on CT. The overall size of the lesion is larger than the original tumor owing to tumor necrosis, although it is expected to gradually decrease over a period of time. The ablated lesion may also contain gas, but this usually disappears within the early posttreatment period provided there is no clinical evidence of superadded infection.

Within the first month following RFA, peripheral rim enhancement reflecting reactive inflammatory tissue and hyperemia is commonly seen. This rim is of uniform thickness unlike recurrence (Lim et al. 2001).

Distal to the lesion within the liver parenchyma, a wedge-like area of enhancement can be seen. This is thought to represent iatrogenic arteriovenous shunting (Fig. 6.31).

6.4.5.3 MRI

As with CT, most ablated lesions appear larger than the pretreatment lesion. Frequently, it produces high signal on unenhanced T1-weighted images owing to hemorrhage or proteinaceous material. On T2-weighted sequences, ablated lesions can appear low in signal due to the dehydrating effects of thermal treatment (Dromain et al. 2002). Marked T2 hyperintensity, however, implies a biloma or liquefactive necrosis.

6.4.6 Post-RFA Complications

Complications are usually related to either placement of the needle electrode or resultant thermal injury (Rhim et al. 2004).

6.4.6.1 Vascular Complications and Bleeding

Vascular injury (0.6–1.6%) is due to inadvertent traversing of vessels by the RFA electrode or

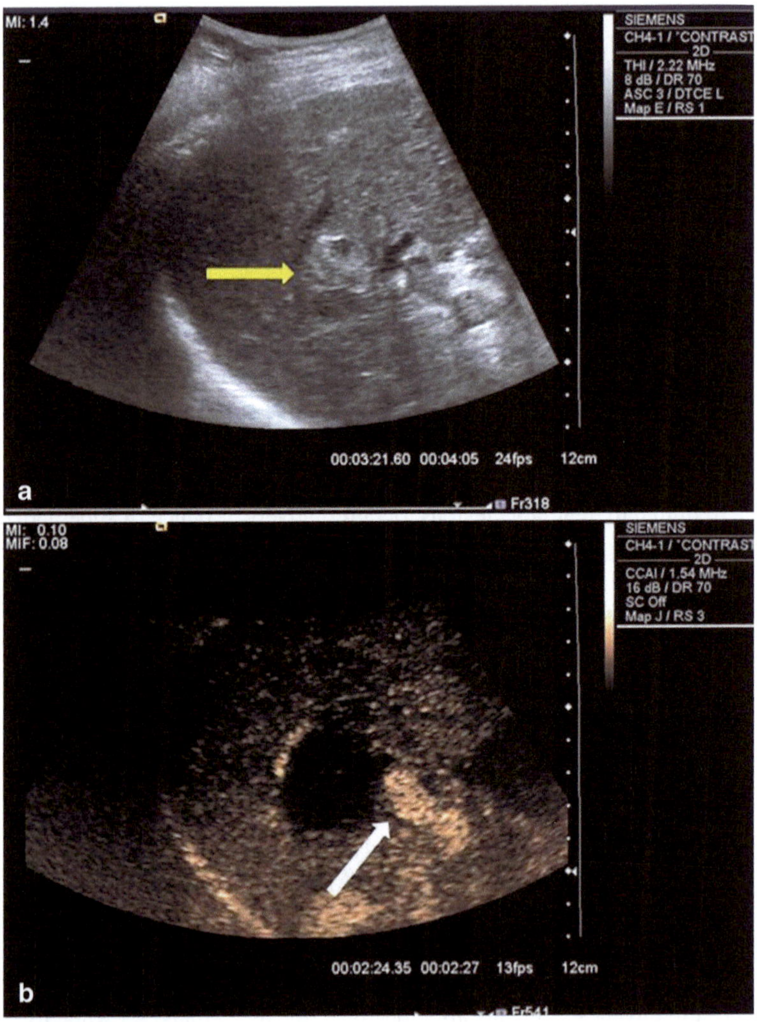

Fig. 6.30 Contrast ultrasound assessment post-RFA for HCC. (**a**) Pretreatment ultrasound shows an HCC within the right lobe of the liver (*yellow arrow*). (**b**) Contrast ultrasound assessment 1 month post treatment (SonoVue – Bracco Diagnostics) shows the treated lesion is predominantly echo-poor but there is a small enhancing nodule posteriorly suggestive of viable tumor (*white arrow*). This was retreated with RFA (Courtesy Dr. TzeWah, Leeds Teaching Hospitals NHS Trust)

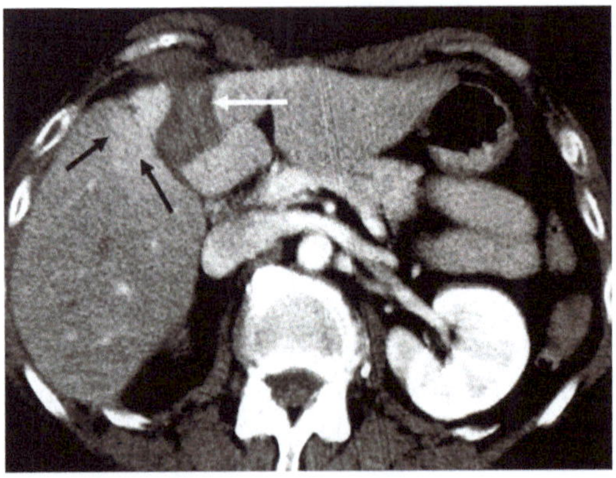

Fig. 6.31 Normal CT appearances post RFA. Day 30 posttreatment of a solitary colorectal metastasis in segment 4. Axial CT demonstrates a well-defined zone of ablation with clear nonenhancing margins (*white arrow*). There is adjacent increased perfusion which is uniform (*black arrows*)

thermal injury sustained during the procedure. Arterial bleeding, venous thrombosis, pseudoaneurysm, and arteriovenous fistula are other recognized vascular complications. Patients usually present a few hours posttreatment with pain and/or bleeding. Patients with underlying cirrhosis are at increased risk of bleeding from the ablation site. Dual phase CT (noncontrast and postcontrast [portal phase]) is usually performed. A subcapsular hematoma is identified as an area of crescentic or biconvex high attenuation along the hepatic surface and/or extending into the adjacent extraperitoneal space.

A filling defect within the portal vein on contrast-enhanced CT indicates venous thrombosis. Portal venous thrombosis can also be implied indirectly if there is segmental enhancement of the liver parenchyma in the arterial phase distal to the site of thrombosis. Hepatic infarction manifests as a well-defined wedge-shaped area of low attenuation that extends to the liver surface.

6.4.6.2 Damage to Adjacent Structures

Thermal damage to adjacent structures such as the biliary system or bowel can result in cholecystitis, bile duct strictures (1.0%), and bowel perforation (0.5%), respectively. The colon is at increased risk of perforation compared with the stomach or small bowel owing to its close proximity to the liver. Infusion of dextrose into the abdomen during RFA can be utilized to separate bowel from the adjacent liver and reduce the likelihood of thermal of injury (Akahane et al. 2005).

6.4.6.3 Thoracic Complications

Pleural complications (pneumothorax, pleural effusion, and hemothorax) or diaphragmatic injury can occur if the lesion is located close to the diaphragm.

6.4.6.4 Skin Burns

These occur at the grounding pad sites but are rare (<2%).

6.4.6.5 Postablation Syndrome

Postablation syndrome is characterized by a low-grade pyrexia, malaise, and myalgia and occurs in up to one third of patients undergoing RFA (Wah et al. 2005). It is managed conservatively with analgesia.

6.4.6.6 Abscess

A persistent fever should alert to the possibility of abscess formation which usually develops 2–8 weeks after the procedure. Diabetes and preexisting biliary-enteric anastomoses are recognized risk factors. Clinical correlation is required when gas is seen within the treated lesion on follow-up CT as this can be a normal finding.

6.4.6.7 Tumor Seeding

Tumor seeding of the needle tract, pleura, or peritoneum has been reported to occur 3–12 months after the procedure. Aggressive tumors, subcapsular location, and high levels of alpha-fetoprotein have been associated with this complication.

6.4.7 Recurrent Disease

The assessment of treatment efficacy following RFA and detection of early recurrence is best achieved by cross-sectional imaging modalities such as CT or MRI.

6.4.7.1 CT

Contrast-enhanced multiphasic helical CT acquisition during arterial, portal venous, and equilibrium phase is usually required for lesion characterization. For assessment of treatment efficacy, a scan at 1 month posttreatment followed by three monthly scans thereafter is recommended.

Two reliable imaging features of complete ablation are the size and margin characteristics. In the initial period, successful ablation is represented by an ovoid or round area of homogenous low attenuation which should be centered on and larger than the original lesion. Lack of contrast enhancement indicates necrosis. A smooth sharply demarcated margin best appreciated following intravenous contrast defines the interface between necrotic tissue and surrounding normal liver (Choi et al. 2001).

During the first month of treatment, not infrequently, a peripheral reactive enhancing rim can be seen which should not be misinterpreted as residual tumor. An iso- or hyperattenuating peripheral rim during portal venous and equilibrium phases indicates reactive change, whereas if it appears low in attenuation in the equilibrium phase, tumor recurrence should be suspected.

Early detection of residual or locally recurrent HCC following ablation can facilitate successful retreatment. On the other hand, if detected late, the tumor may be more difficult to treat due to a combination of size and unfavorable geometry.

Absence of tumor recurrence at the margin of ablated HCC lesion at 12 months is a good indicator of adequate treatment response.

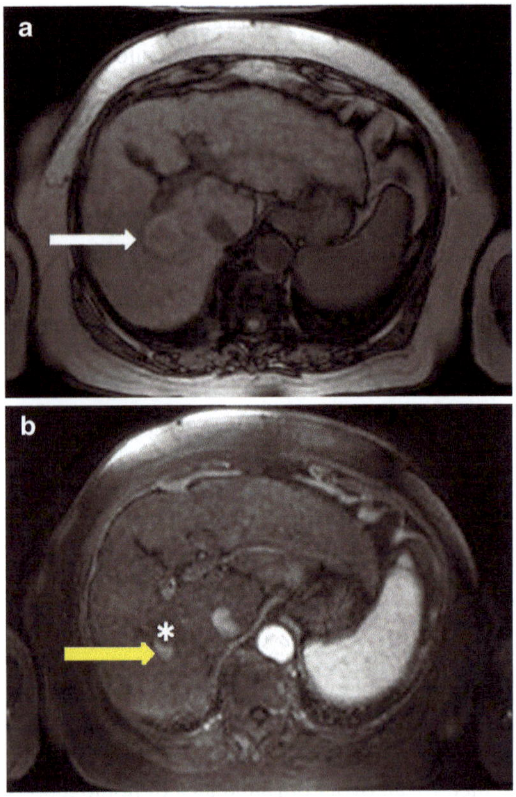

Fig. 6.32 Early tumor recurrence 2 months post RFA. (**a**) Axial T1W GRE opposed phase image shows mixed high mixed signal indicating hemorrhage and central necrosis (*white arrow*). (**b**) Axial T1W fat-suppressed arterial phase postgadolinium shows the lesion is mostly avascular (*white asterisk*) but there is a small nodular area of enhancement posteriorly (*yellow arrow*)

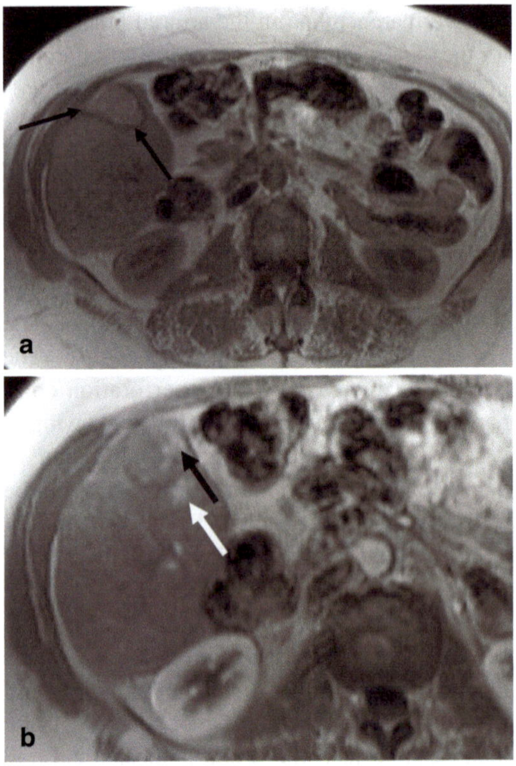

Fig. 6.33 Tumor recurrence in another patient post RFA for a solitary HCC in segment 5. (**a**) Axial T1W MRI at 1 month shows high signal within the zone of ablation (due to hemorrhage/proteinaceous material) and a low-signal margin (*black arrows*) consistent with successful ablation. There was no enhancement following gadolinium (*not shown*). (**b**) Axial T1W (magnified image) post-contrast at 3 months shows areas of enhancement at the margin of the lesion (*black arrow*) secondary to recurrent HCC with a satellite lesion posteriorly (*white arrow*). This was treated with further RFA

6.4.7.2 MRI

The signal intensity on the unenhanced T1- and T2-weighted sequences can be variable due to uneven evolution of the necrotic area and, therefore, contrast is essential to differentiate this from recurrence. The ablated tumor is characterized by low signal on T2-weighted sequences, but viable tumor produces moderate high signal intensity. Contrast enhancement is also specific for residual viable tumor (Lim et al. 2006) (Figs. 6.32 and 6.33). Features of successful treatment 2 months following the treatment include uniform hypointensity on T2-weighted sequence and nonenhancement of the RF-treated area on contrast-enhanced T1-weighted images.

6.4.8 Teaching Points (RFA)

- RF ablation is widely used to treat nonresectable HCC and colorectal metastases.
- Careful patient selection and planning helps to reduce potential complications.
- Complications can be related to needle placement or the thermal effects of ablation.
- Most complications are detected by contrast-enhanced CT in the immediate posttreatment period.
- Knowledge of the expected evolution and the pattern of an ablated lesion is required to avoid misinterpretation.

- Early detection of residual tumor or early recurrence is crucial in facilitating further ablative treatments.

6.5 Transcatheter Arterial Chemoembolization (TACE)

6.5.1 Introduction

Dr. R. Yamada, a Japanese radiologist, was the first to use transcatheter arterial chemoembolization (TACE) to treat patients with unresectable HCC (Yamada et al. 1983). Since then, TACE has been widely used to treat malignant liver lesions. The principles of TACE are to deliver chemotherapeutic agents directly to the lesion and embolize its principle arterial supply, i.e., branches of the hepatic artery. The advantages of TACE over standard chemotherapeutic agents are that direct injection into the arterial supply of the liver can produce tumor ischemia and attain higher concentrations than peripherally administered intravenous agents. Furthermore, higher intracellular drug concentration helps to overcome drug resistance and reduce systemic toxicity (Brown et al. 2006).

HCC is the most common and one of the most fatal malignancies of the liver. Surgical resection and transplantation offers the only possibility of a cure, but only a small proportion of patients are suitable for surgery. Underlying cirrhosis in 70–80% of patients with or without hepatic dysfunction and the angioinvasive nature of the lesion are the main reasons that preclude surgery. The median survival is 4–6 months for patients with unresectable tumors.

TACE plays an important role in the treatment of HCCs which are otherwise considered inoperable. Most HCCs are supplied exclusively by the hepatic artery. Meta-analysis of randomized controlled trials in 1,605 patients showed significant reduction in the overall 2-year mortality following chemoembolization of unresectable HCCs (Camma et al. 2002). The degree of lesion hypervascularity on preprocedure CT has been shown to predict prognosis and response to treatment in one study (Katyal et al. 2000). Even large tumors are routinely treated by repeated courses of chemoembolization spread over a period of several months, to reduce tumor vascularity. The major contraindications are main branch portal venous occlusion, usually by tumor, when concomitant hepatic arterial obstruction can lead to hepatic ischemia and decompensation, and poor liver functional reserve (Kokudo and Makuuchi 2004).

Chemoembolization can be technically challenging with great potential to cause complications. For the procedure to be safe and effective, it is important to understand the vascular anatomy of the upper abdomen and identify the presence or absence of extrahepatic collaterals and nontarget arteries. Radiologists should also be familiar with the imaging appearances following chemoembolization that do not necessarily alter patient management or affect prognosis but might concern the inexperienced.

6.5.2 Clinical Indications

- Unresectable HCC – most common and widely performed
- Bridge to transplantation in patients with resectable HCC to prevent tumor progression
- Neoadjuvant/adjuvant treatment to downsize a previously inoperable tumor
- Combined therapy with RFA in large tumors
- Metastases (mainly palliative) – colorectal metastases, metastatic neuroendocrine tumors, and metastatic sarcoma

6.5.3 TACE Technique

- The hepatic artery is selectively catheterized via a femoral artery puncture.
- Simultaneous embolization of the nutrient hepatic artery with a concentrated dose of chemotherapeutic drugs (cisplatin, doxorubicin, fluorodeoxyuridine, or mitomycin suspended in ethiodized oil) and embolization particles (gelatine foam) (Fig. 6.34).
- Alternative chemotherapy preparations include drug-eluting beads (DC beads–Biocompatibles International plc (BTG), Surrey, UK),

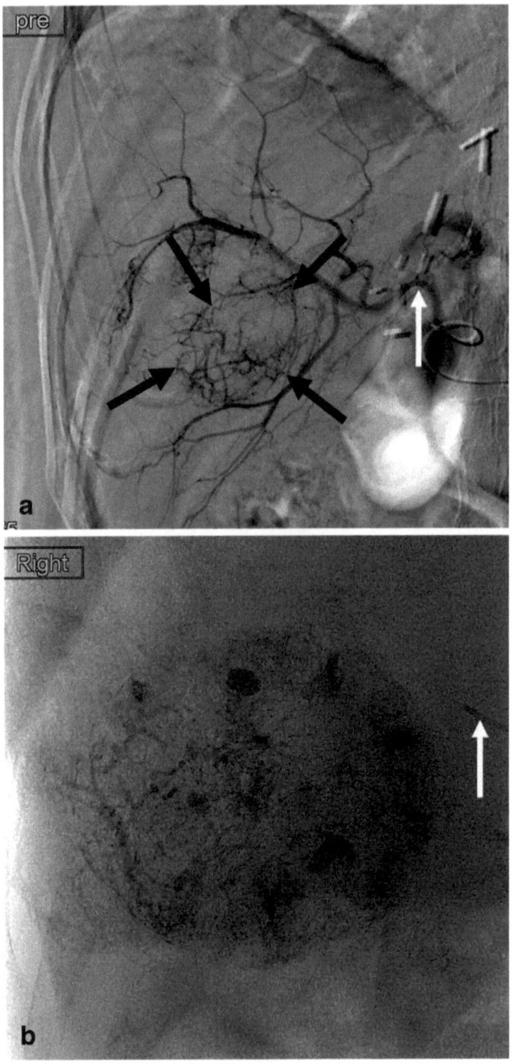

Fig. 6.34 (**a**) Angiogram demonstrating the tumor circulation of an HCC within the right lobe of the liver (*black arrows*). Angiographic catheter is positioned within the common hepatic artery (*white arrow*). (**b**) Retained lipiodol within the tumor at the end of the procedure (note the selective catheter has been advanced into a feeding hepatic segmental artery – *arrow*)

which are commercially produced and enable more accurate dosing of chemotherapeutic agents (lipiodol is not present in these preparations).

- Selective internal radiation therapy (SIRT) is a further variation in technique. Yttrium-90, a pure beta emitter, is bonded to microspheresis and delivered angiographically via the hepatic artery. The technique is more involved than other TACE techniques, and in order to ensure the agent is not delivered elsewhere, potential sources of collateral flow such as the gastroduodenal artery are occluded.

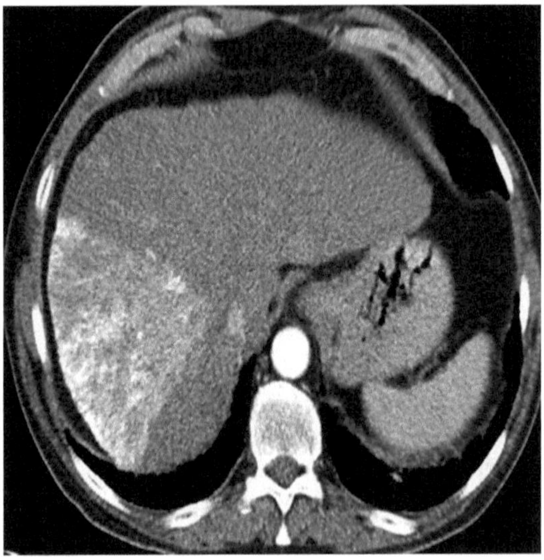

Fig. 6.35 CT within the first few days post TACE. The lipiodol has not yet been cleared from a segmental distribution within the right lobe of the liver

6.5.4 Imaging Post-TACE

The purpose of imaging follow-up with either CT or MRI is to assess the distribution, pattern and resorption of ethiodized oil, the size and morphology of tumor, overall liver size and to look for new lesions or metastasis.

6.5.4.1 CT

CT is used to assess therapeutic response and detection of any associated complications. During the initial few weeks of treatment, the lesion appears high in attenuation with resultant artifacts due to the presence of ethiodized oil, and as a consequence, characterization at this stage is not possible. Therapeutic response is therefore better assessed after few weeks when the iodized oil has cleared from the tumor (Fig. 6.35).

6.5.4.2 MRI

Dynamic MRI has specific advantages over CT because iodized oil has no paramagnetic effect and has little influence on signal characteristics. However, it is better to perform MRI after the first week post-TACE as the high concentration of oil can produce high signal on T1-weighted sequences. The signal characteristics are variable due to a combination of hemorrhage, liquifaction and necrosis and should always be assessed with contrast agents. Diffusion weighted imaging alone is also unreliable in assessing response.

Imaging characteristics of tumor recurrence on CT and MRI are discussed in Sect. 6.5.6.

6.5.5 Post-TACE Complications

Complications following TACE can be divided into those affecting the target organ (liver) or nontarget areas.

6.5.5.1 Target Organ Complications

- Hematoma – at the vascular access sites (usually resolves within a few weeks).
- Chemical arteritis – involving small vessels supplying the bile ducts can cause bile duct necrosis (12.5%). This can lead to biloma formation and bile duct strictures.
- Liver abscess (Fig. 6.36) – increased risk in patients with biliary-enteric anastomoses due to possible combined effect of biliary tree contamination and bile duct injuries (Kim et al. 2001). Normally occurs between the second and fourth week post-TACE.
- Postembolization syndrome – manifests by transient nausea, vomiting, fever, and abdominal pain. This occurs in the initial few days, whereas a liver abscess tends to occur 2–4 weeks following embolization.
- Rupture of the liver – this is a potential but uncommon complication if the liver capsule is breached before embolization or if the tumor is near to the capsular surface.
- Hepatic parenchymal atrophy – this is caused by ischemic injury to the liver parenchyma, especially in patients with decreased portal venous perfusion caused by thrombosis.
- Following SIRT radiation hepatitis may rarely occur.

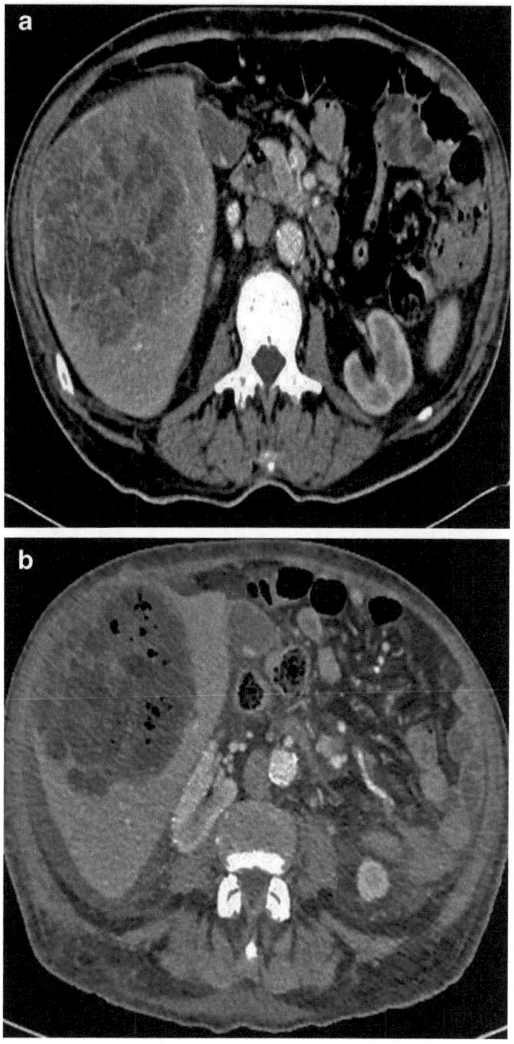

Fig. 6.36 Liver abscess post TACE. (**a**) CT of a large HCC with typical "mosaic" morphology within segments 5 and 6. (**b**) Post-TACE treatment arterial phase CT performed for pyrexia and pain shows reduced vascularity but confirms a large abscess containing gas

6.5.5.2 Nontarget Organ Complications

- Extrahepatic uptake – chemoembolization material can be deposited in extrahepatic sites such as the lung, stomach, pancreas, duodenum, gallbladder, diaphragm, and spleen. Fortunately, the amount deposited is only small and is usually insignificant (Gates et al. 1999).
- Lung or pleural uptake – occurs commonly (up to 25%) and it can be bilateral. There may be secondary inflammatory changes, and large amounts can cause pulmonary infarction.

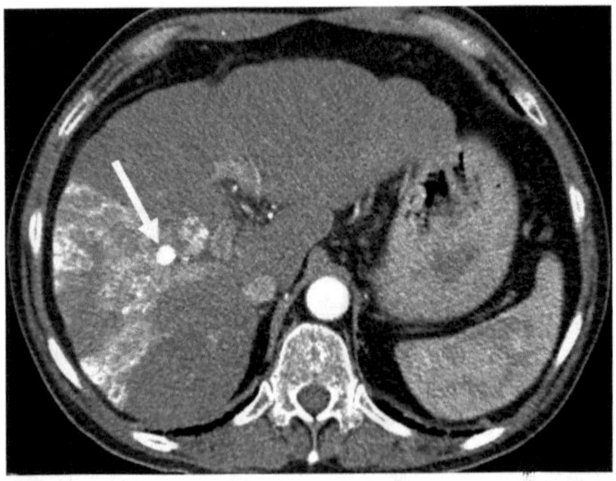

Fig. 6.37 CT in the assessment of therapeutic response post TACE. Axial CT (arterial phase) post TACE shows homogenous uptake of lipiodol within the lesion (*arrow*) with good uptake around the tumor

- Diaphragmatic weakness – secondary to inadvertent phrenic artery embolization.
- Pleural effusion and ascites have been reported.
- Duodenal or pancreatic injury – can occur due to reflux of small quantities of embolization material into the coeliac artery (despite selective catheterization).
- Gastric deposition – is characteristically found in the mucosal lining (1%) resulting in peptic ulceration.
- Gallbladder wall deposition – this is not uncommon (14%) but again is not associated with any adverse outcome. Cases of emphysematous cholecystitis and gallbladder infarction have been reported in the literature.
- Splenic infarction – due to reflux of chemoembolization material into the splenic artery.

6.5.6 Imaging of Recurrent Malignancy Post-TACE

Tumor marker levels are routinely checked before and after chemoembolization.

6.5.6.1 CT

CT is frequently used to assess the therapeutic response of HCC to chemoembolization. The amount of iodized oil accumulation within the lesion has been shown to correlate with necrosis. The therapeutic effect can be assessed by looking at the pattern and distribution of iodized oil.

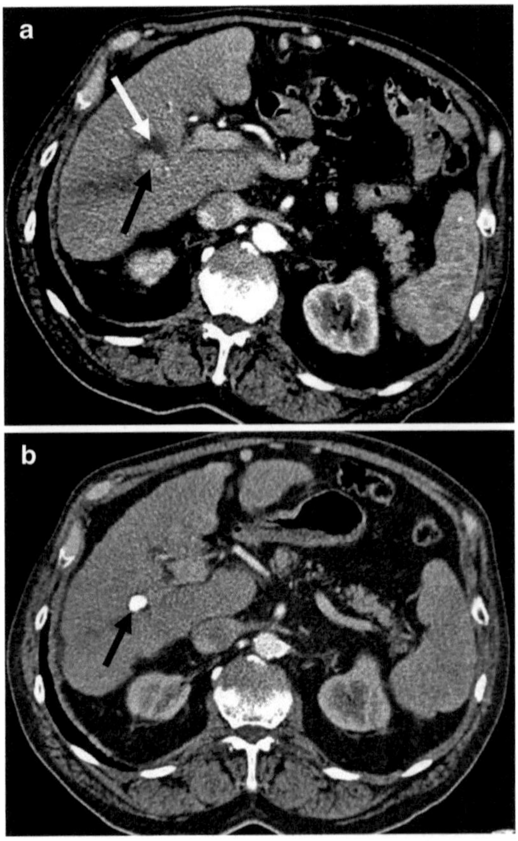

Fig. 6.38 HCC treated with RFA and TACE. (**a**) CT (arterial phase) 3 months post RFA for an HCC shows a hypervascular nodule (*black arrow*) at the edge of the ablation site (*white arrow*) in keeping within tumor recurrence within the right lobe of the liver. This was treated with TACE. (**b**) A subsequent CT demonstrates good uniform uptake of lipiodol (*black arrow*)

Classification of the degree of accumulation of iodized oil within the lesion has been described (Nishimine et al. 1994) but in practice is not widely used. This can range from homogenous, partial to faint or no uptake (Figs. 6.37, 6.38, 6.39, and 6.40). The presence of a focal defect or washout of iodized oil within the contrast-enhanced lesion suggests viable tumor. It should be appreciated that there is no lipiodol when DC beads (or SIRT) are used and assessment is made on the basis of enhancement and tumor size (Fig. 6.41).

6.5.6.2 MRI

Evaluation of contrast enhancement, which is a feature of viable tumor on CT, can be challenging

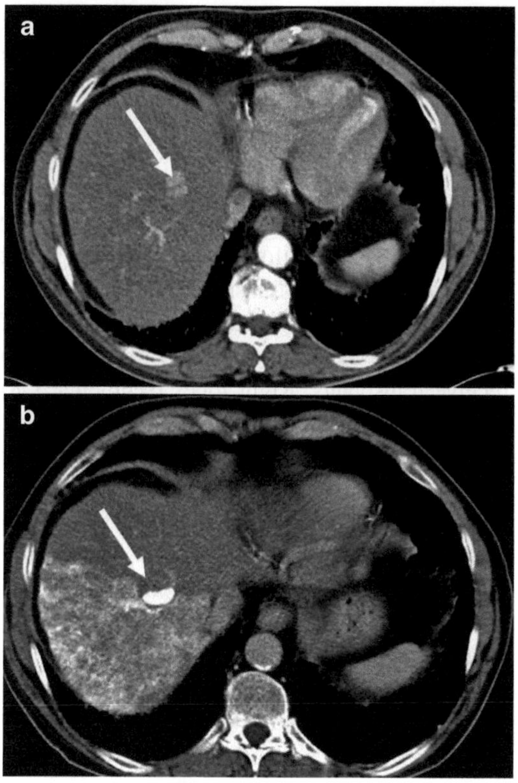

Fig. 6.39 CT in the assessment of therapeutic response post-TACE. (**a**) Pretreatment axial CT (arterial phase) shows a small HCC within segment 8 (*arrow*). (**b**) Post-TACE treatment demonstrates only partial uptake of lipiodol indicating viable tumor (*arrow*)

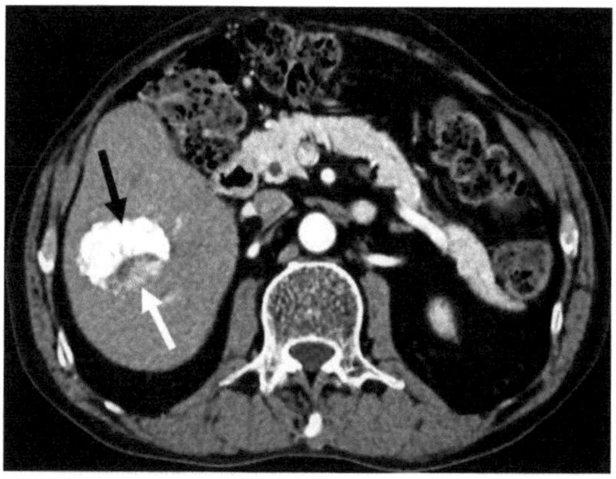

Fig. 6.40 Arterial phase CT 3 months post TACE with dense lipiodol uptake within the majority of an HCC located in segments 5 and 6 (*black arrow*). There is no uptake within the arterialized posterior-medial component (*white arrow*) in keeping with viable tumor

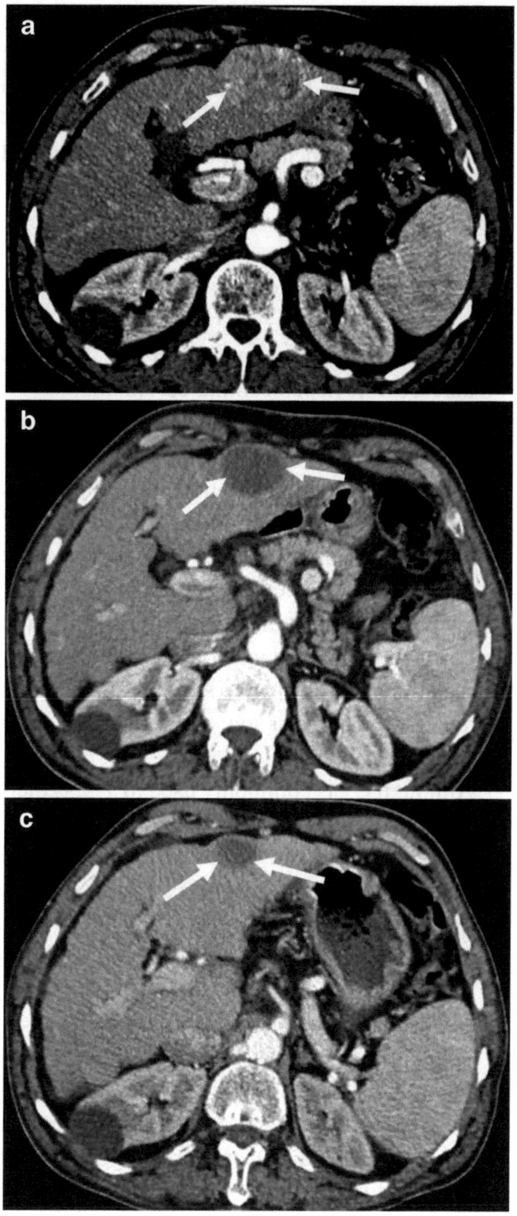

Fig. 6.41 HCC treatment with DC beads (drug-eluting beads). (**a**) Pretreatment arterial phase CT of an HCC within the left lobe of the liver (*arrows*). Posttreatment with DC beads shows the tumor to be avascular with a progressive reduction in size on CT at (**b**) 2 months and (**c**) 6 months. Note that lipiodol is not present in this preparation

due to the beam hardening effect of high-density iodized oil. In this respect, MRI is advantageous as the signal intensity is not influenced by the iodized oil. Although contrast resolution is good with MRI, small residual tumor in the capsule of the lesion can be difficult to detect as the capsule appears as a hyperintense ring on both early and late dynamic enhancement. T2 hypointensity represents tumor necrosis, whereas hyperintensity corresponds to residual tumor or hemorrhage. Viable tumor demonstrates enhancement on postcontrast-enhanced T1-weighted sequences (Lim et al. 2006).

6.5.7 Teaching Points (TACE)

- The most common indication for TACE is unresectable hepatocellular carcinoma.
- Knowledge of the vascular anatomy including any variants is crucial to avoid complications.
- Knowledge of the embolization technique is important as there is no lipiodol when DC beads are used and assessment is made on the basis of enhancement and tumor size.
- Complications are mainly due to deposition of chemoembolization material in various organs including extrahepatic sites, although the amount deposited is low and frequently clinically insignificant.
- Although CT is commonly used to assess therapeutic response, when there is dense accumulation of lipiodol, beam hardening effect of high attenuation iodized oil can preclude adequate assessment.
- TACE and RFA can be used in combination to treat HCC.
- MRI has a distinct advantage over CT in evaluating tumor response as the signal intensity is not affected by iodized oil.
- T2 hyperintensity and contrast enhancement on T1-weighted images are suggestive of residual tumor.

6.6 Orthotopic Liver Transplantation

6.6.1 Introduction

Starzl and colleagues pioneered the technique of human whole liver transplantation in 1963 (Starzl et al. 1963). Over the years with improvement in surgical and organ preservation techniques and better immunosuppression, liver transplantation has been accepted as a successful form of treatment for end-stage liver disease.

With the incidence of cirrhosis increasing and conventional sources of grafts reducing, there is presently a shortage of cadaveric donors. Newer techniques have therefore evolved such as living donor and split liver transplantation and the use of organs from non-heartbeating donors, all of which allow increased numbers of patients to receive transplants. Right lobes (segments 5–8) are most commonly implanted in adults and left lateral segments in children. In case of larger recipients, extended right lobes or trisections (segments 4–8) are used (Seamen 2001).

Maintaining grafts particularly in the early postoperative period requires a multidisciplinary approach with contributions from surgeons, physicians, intensivists, and radiologists. One of the most serious complications is acute graft rejection which occurs in 10–30%. of patients, but most cases are successfully managed with modifying immunosuppression. The diagnosis of rejection is established with graft biopsy and histology (Nghiem 1998). The primary role of imaging is to exclude other complications following transplantation which can mimic the clinical signs and symptoms and biochemical profile of rejection. The radiology of liver transplantation is complex and diverse, and most radiologists will only encounter a few cases during their lifetime. It is important to note that many of the complications are medical and are managed by hepatologists. This section will provide a brief overview of the operative technique and the main complications which the radiologist will be asked to image.

6.6.2 Surgical Technique

Removal of the diseased liver (hepatectomy) and replacing it with a healthy liver in exactly the same location (implantation) is referred to as orthotopic liver transplantation (OLT). Commonly, cadaveric donors are used (Fig. 6.42):

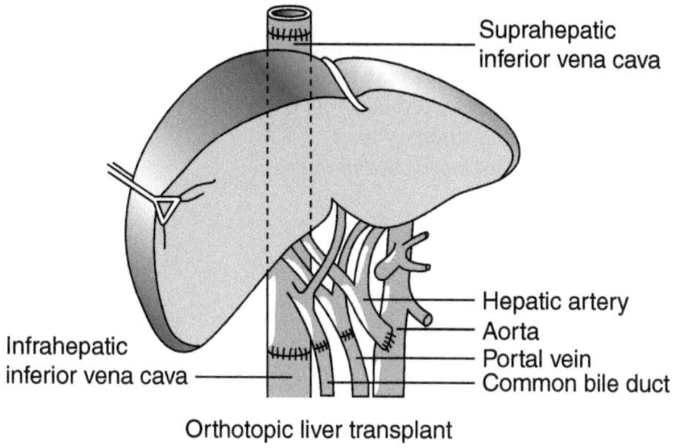

Fig. 6.42 Line drawing of orthotopic liver transplantation (OLT)

- The recipient's hepatic artery, portal vein, and common hepatic duct are ligated close to the liver.
- The inferior vena cava may be resected leaving upper and lower caval cuffs.
- The implantation of the donor liver cava can be performed using by standard or piggyback techniques.
- The standard technique involves anastomosis of the suprahepatic followed by the infrahepatic vena cava (Fig. 6.43a).
- With the piggyback technique, a common venous cuff is formed from three main hepatic veins which is then anastomosed to the donor suprahepatic cava. The donor's infrahepatic cava is stapled or tied (Fig. 6.43b).
- The hepatic artery is anastomosed in an end-to-end fashion.
- A donor to recipient bile duct to bile duct reconstruction if the recipient bile duct is normal. If the recipient CBD is diseased (e.g., primary sclerosing cholangitis), a biliary-enteric anastomosis is formed (Roux-en-Y jejunal loop).

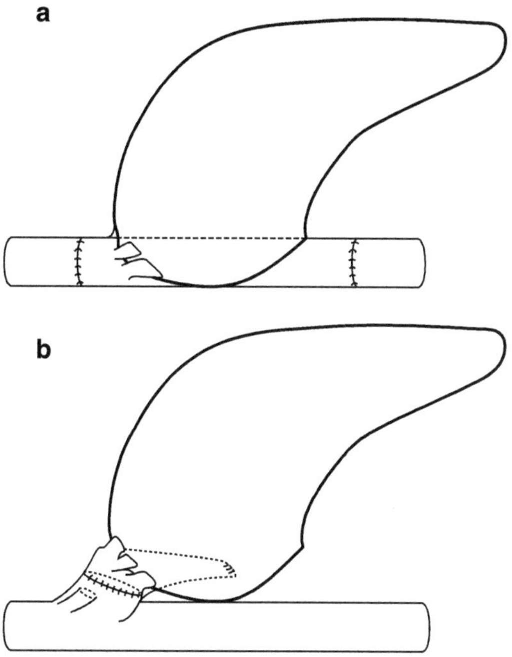

Fig. 6.43 (**a**) Conventional liver transplantation technique with end-to-end anastomosis of the donor and recipient vena cava. (**b**) Piggyback technique in which the donor suprahepatic vena cava is anastomosed to the joint ostium of the recipient hepatic veins

6.6.3 Modifications of Surgical Technique

Split liver transplantation. The donor liver is transected into two through the falciform ligament or main portal fissure. Typically, the left lobe is given to a child and the extended right or right lobe to an adult:

- Living-donor liver transplantation. A further form of split liver graft with the donor hepatic vein anastomosed to inferior vena cava. A detailed presurgical anatomic assessment is made of the potential donors' liver to identify any vascular or biliary variants that may compromise the graft. In addition, a volumetric assessment is made to enable a judgment as to

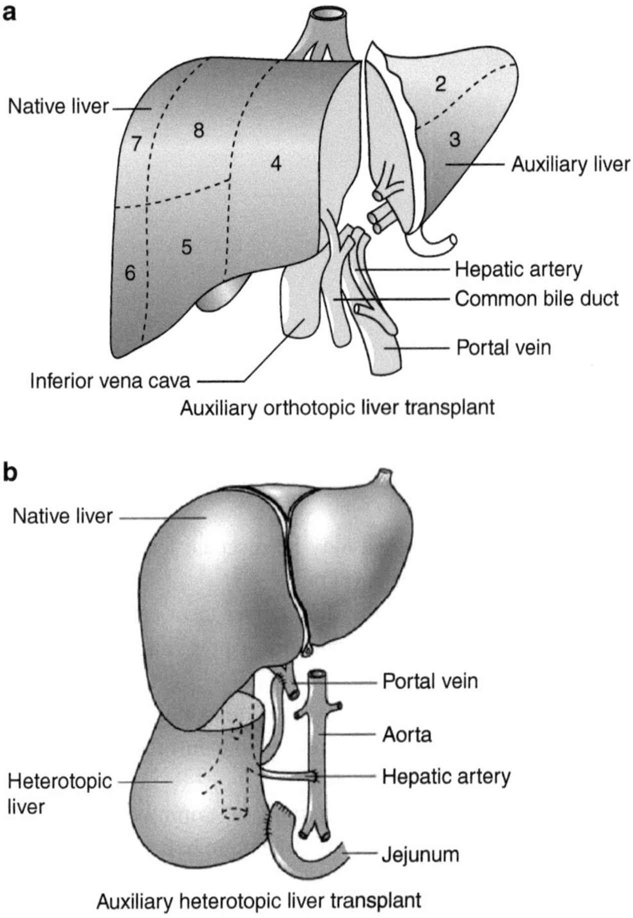

Fig. 6.44 Line drawing of (**a**) standard auxiliary liver transplantation, the left native left lateral segment may be resected (as illustrated) or preserved (see Fig. 6.45) and (**b**) heterotopic auxiliary liver transplantation (*not performed in our institution*)

whether the liver can be split with adequate tissue to support both the recipient and donor. The right lobe is usually donated in adults; alternatively, if a child is to be the recipient, the left lateral segment is donated. The recipient must have favorable anatomy as there is no scope to use iliac vein grafts to supplement vascular deficiencies.

- Livers have classically been harvested from donors fulfilling the criteria for brain stem death. Due to the shortage of such organs, non-heart-beating donors are now being used in many centers. This results in a greater ischemic time for the organ and increases the risk of ischemic biliopathy (Sect. 6.6.5.3).
- Auxiliary liver transplantation (Fig. 6.44). If the patient has acute fulminant hepatic failure and the liver is expected to recover, e.g., following paracetamol overdose, transplantation may be used to enable the native liver to recover, and immunosuppression is withdrawn. In this situation, only part of the native liver is resected, usually the right lobe and the graft inserted in the created space in the right upper quadrant (Fig. 6.45).

6.6.4 Normal Postoperative Imaging

Ultrasound and CT are the most commonly used imaging modalities in the postoperative period following OLT. Ultrasound is routinely requested to assess the patency of the vessels within the donor liver. Knowledge of the type of transplant, nature of the surgical technique, and appreciation of the vascular and biliary anastomoses is crucial for interpretation of post surgical anatomy and complications.

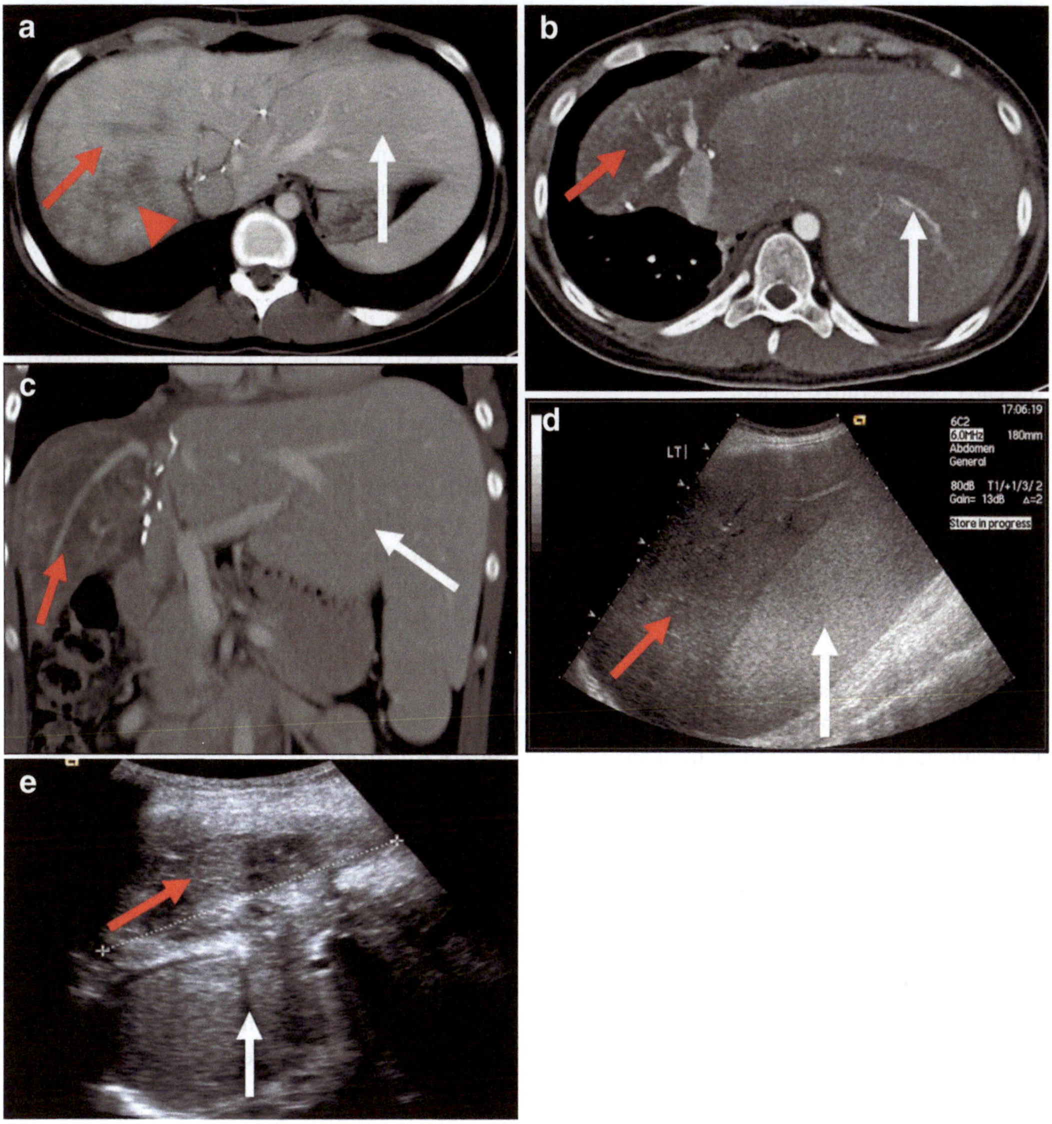

Fig. 6.45 Auxiliary liver transplantation for acute liver failure secondary to paracetamol overdose. (**a**) Axial CT shows heterogeneous attenuation of the diseased native liver (*red arrow*). Healthy left lateral graft (*white arrow*). Thrombosis within right posterior portal vein branch (*red arrowhead*). Follow up CT's, (**b**) axial and (**c**) coronal images demonstrate progressive hypertrophy of the transplanted left lobe segments (*white arrow*) and progressive volume loss within the diseased native liver (*red arrow*). Ultrasound images of the same patient show a coarse echotexture within the native liver (*red arrow*) and more echogenic transplant liver. (**e**) Follow up ultrasound at 1 year demonstrating that the native liver remains diseased with further volume loss

6.6.4.1 Ultrasound Appearances

Hepatic Artery Anastomosis

The normal hepatic artery waveform shows rapid systolic upstroke and a continuous diastolic blood flow. The resistive index of a normal hepatic artery is 0.5–0.8, the higher end of the range typically occurring in the immediate postoperative period. The normal acceleration time (from end diastole to the first systolic peak) is less than 0.08 s. Both main branches and the anastomotic site should be evaluated as a normal waveform at the porta does not exclude hepatic arterial thrombosis.

Portal Vein Anastomosis

The normal portal vein in a liver graft has a regular contour with smooth walls and an anechoic lumen. A mild reduction in vessel caliber at the anastomotic site can be expected. The Doppler waveform is monophasic and varies with respiration with a hepatopetal direction (toward the liver). Turbulent flow may be a normal finding in the early postoperative period.

IVC and Hepatic Veins

The normal hepatic vein Doppler waveform in a transplant liver is triphasic as a result of pressure variations in the right cardiac chambers during the cardiac cycle.

Biliary Anastomosis

The intrahepatic biliary tree should appear normal, and the extrahepatic ducts should be of normal caliber. T-tubes are rarely used in clinical practice, but if a T-tube is in place, the extrahepatic biliary ducts may appear thick walled. A small amount of free fluid in the perihepatic space is not unusual in the early postoperative period which usually resolves in 7–10 days (Caiado et al. 2007; Crossin et al. 2003) although may persist for considerably longer.

6.6.4.2 CT Appearances

Hepatic Artery Anastomosis

The hepatic artery is reconstructed with a “fish-mouth” anastomosis. The donor’s coeliac axis is anastomosed with the recipient artery either at the bifurcation of the hepatic artery or at the branch point of the gastroduodenal and proper hepatic arteries. In cases of small diameter recipient hepatic arteries, donor iliac artery interposition grafts are often directly anastomosed to the infrarenal or less commonly the supracoeliac aorta.

Portal Vein Anastomosis

This is typically an end-to-end type between the two portal veins. A venous jump graft from the donor portal vein or iliac vein may be used in cases of venous thrombosis or previous surgery. A sizeable hilar varix may be used. As a last resort in case of extensive thrombosis, arterialization of the portal vein (i.e., creation of anastomoses between both the portal vein and hepatic artery of the donor and arterial vessels of the recipient) may be used.

IVC Anastomosis

With recent developments, the retrohepatic IVC of the recipient is preserved, thereby maintaining uninterrupted blood flow during the operation. An anastomosis is created between the donor and recipient IVC in an end-to-side or side-to-side configuration. Piggyback techniques involve anastomosing the donor IVC and a common stump of the three hepatic veins (Fig. 6.43b). Other methods involve resection of the recipient retrohepatic IVC and forming an end-to-end anastomosis between the donor and recipient IVC.

Biliary Anastomosis

The gallbladder is removed, and the recipient common hepatic duct and the donor common bile duct are anastomosed. Preservation of the sphincter of Oddi is a major advantage using this technique. Historically, a T-tube was left in place for 3 months to provide access for cholangiography. This is now rarely use in modern practice. In cases where the recipient common bile duct is too small or diseased, a biliary-enteric anastomosis is fashioned using a Roux loop (Quiroga et al. 2001).

6.6.5 Postoperative Complications

The common early complications include vascular (overall incidence 9%), biliary complications, fluid collections, and graft rejection.

6.6.5.1 Graft Rejection

Graft rejection is the most common complication following OLT and occurs in 50% of patients. It is diagnosed mainly by clinical and biochemical features and requires histological confirmation from liver biopsy. Imaging plays no role in the diagnosis of rejection.

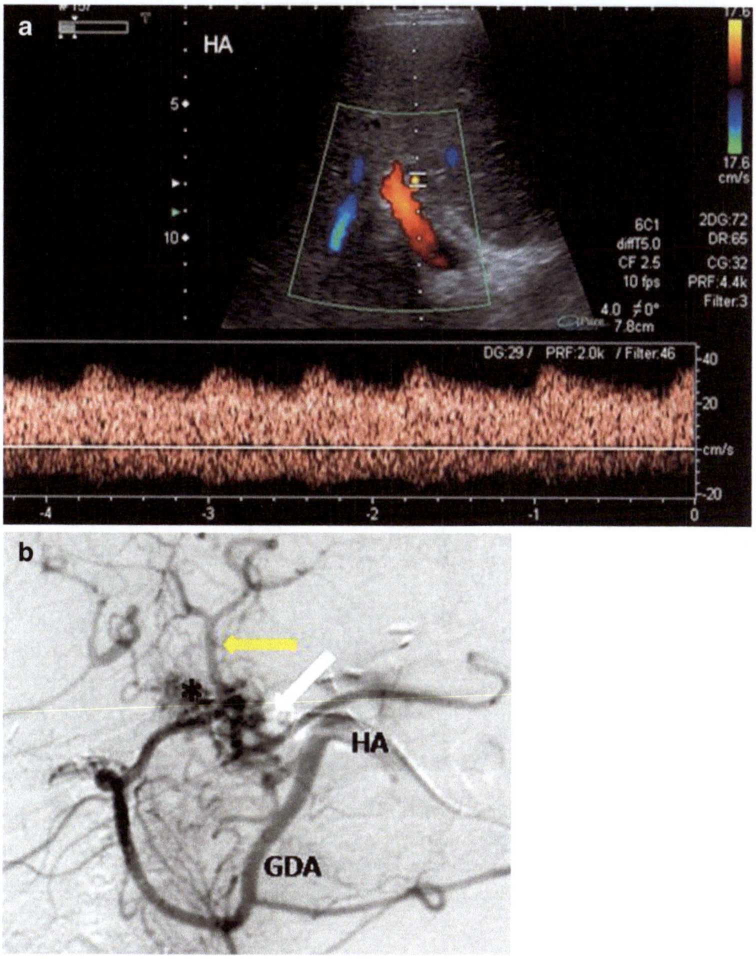

Fig. 6.46 Hepatic artery occlusion with formation of collaterals post liver transplant. The patient presented with recurrent cholangitis and deteriorating liver function tests. (**a**) Hepatic arterial waveform on Doppler ultrasound shows a delay in the systolic upstroke with a high end-diastolic flow ("parvus tardus" waveform), suspicious of hepatic artery stenosis. (**b**) Digital subtraction angiographic (DSA) views demonstrating a short segment occlusion of the hepatic artery (*HA*) between the gastroduodenal artery (*GDA*) and the donor hepatic artery (*white arrow*) proximal to its bifurcation. Multiple small collateral vessels (*) are noted in the vicinity, and the hepatic artery reforms distally (*yellow arrow*) just proximal to its bifurcation into the right and left branches. Splenic artery (SA)

6.6.5.2 Vascular Complications

Hepatic Arterial Complications

These include thrombosis and stenosis and have an incidence of 6–11% (Brancatelli et al. 2002). Early and prompt diagnosis is crucial because early intervention such as arterial reconstruction, thrombectomy, or angioplasty may allow graft salvage (Fig. 6.46). Absence of collateral vessels in the transplant as opposed to normal liver makes it vulnerable to liver infarction as a result of hepatic artery thrombosis or rarely portal vein occlusion (Fig. 6.47). In addition, donor bile ducts are particularly vulnerable as these are entirely supplied by the hepatic artery and reduced flow can result in bile duct ischemia and necrosis (see Sect. 6.6.5.3.1) (Nghiem et al. 1996). The development of a nonanastomotic biliary stricture or parenchymal liver abscess should prompt an assessment of the hepatic artery as both conditions are associated with arterial thrombosis.

Hepatic Artery Thrombosis

Doppler ultrasound is the primary imaging modality used in the immediate postoperative period. Absence of flow in the proper or intrahepatic artery at color or pulsed Doppler will establish the diagnosis. Contrast-enhanced multidetector CT (standard and angiographic protocols with vascular reconstruction) allows evaluation of vascular structures and the liver parenchyma. Gadolinium-enhanced MR (with three-dimensional spoiled gradient echo sequences) is another noninvasive method to assess the liver parenchyma and vessels. Abrupt cutoff of arterial flow is the criteria used to diagnose hepatic artery thrombosis on CT or MRI.

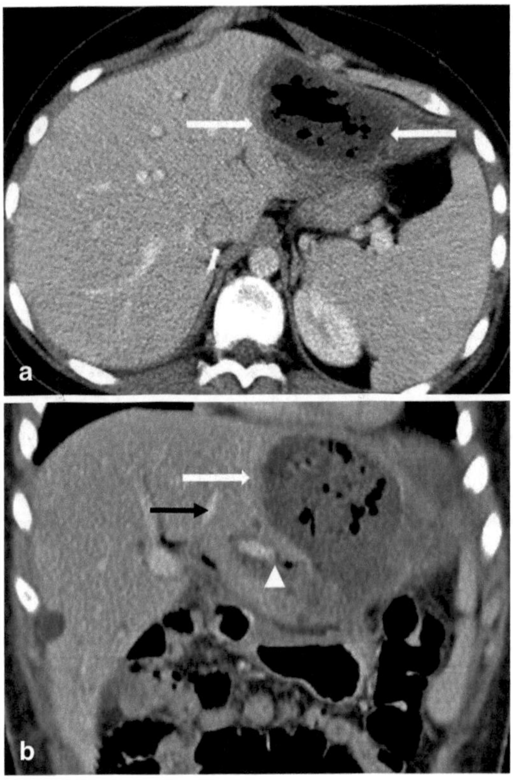

Fig. 6.47 (**a**, **b**) Posttransplant liver. The lateral branch of the left portal vein is occluded (*arrowhead*) resulting in segmental necrosis of the transplant liver (*white arrows*). The medial segmental branch of the left portal vein is patent (*black arrow*)

Hepatic Artery Stenosis

Hepatic artery stenosis usually occurs within 3 months following OLT at the site of anastomosis. Doppler ultrasound demonstrates an increased peak systolic velocity (>200 cm/s) at the anastomotic site or turbulent poststenotic flow. Intrahepatic waveforms may show a "tardus parvus" pattern depicted by a prolonged acceleration time of >0.08 s and a resistive index of <0.5. This can be confirmed by cross-sectional modalities or angiography. False-negative results can occur if there are extensive collaterals or with low-grade narrowing.

Hepatic Artery Pseudoaneurysm

This is uncommon. It usually occurs at the site of anastomosis and can cause hemobilia, hemoperitoneum, or gastrointestinal bleeding. On Doppler ultrasound, it appears as a color-filled cystic structure with turbulent flow. It is identified on contrast-enhanced CT or MR as an enhancing expansile structure. Other potential complications of a pseudoaneurysm include fistulation into the biliary tree or portal vein.

Liver Ischemia or Infarction

Infarcted liver segments appear as a peripheral well-defined wedge-shaped area of low density on CT. They can liquefy or develop secondary infection and at a later stage may become calcified (Quiroga et al. 2001).

Arterioportal Fistula

This is a recognized complication following liver biopsy. On CT, early enhancement of peripheral portal vein branches or transient, peripheral wedge-shaped area of parenchymal enhancement in the arterial phase can be recognized. These shunts are not usually of clinical significance and tend to close spontaneously (Quiroga et al. 2001).

Portal Vein and IVC Stenosis/Thrombosis

These occur in less than 3% of transplants (Boraschi and Donati 2004) (Fig. 6.47). On grayscale ultrasound, echogenic thrombus or luminal narrowing can be visualized. Doppler examination shows focal color aliasing (greater than three- to fourfold increased velocity) at the stenosis relative to the prestenotic segment. Persistent monophasic waveform is a sensitive but not a specific finding of hepatic vein stenosis. Suprahepatic caval stenosis can manifest as Budd-Chiari syndrome, a feature of which is a mosaic perfusion pattern on CT or MRI. It should be appreciated that varices and splenomegaly persist after transplantation but the lower portal pressure considerably reduces the risk of variceal hemorrhage.

6.6.5.3 Biliary Complications

These usually occur within 3 months following OLT and have an incidence of 5–15%.

Biliary Strictures

Biliary strictures commonly result from a fibrotic reaction at the site of the biliary anastomosis,

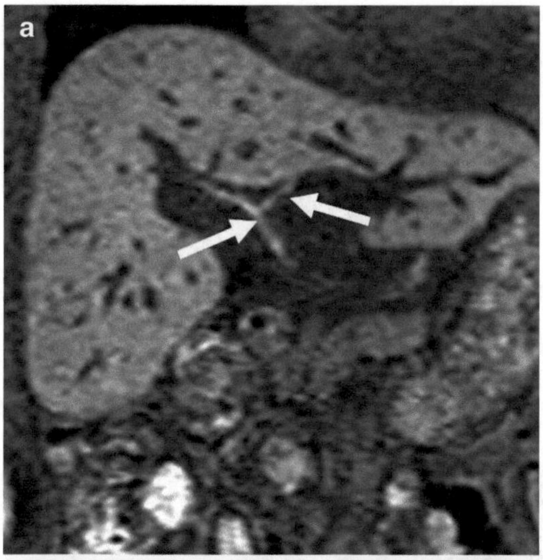

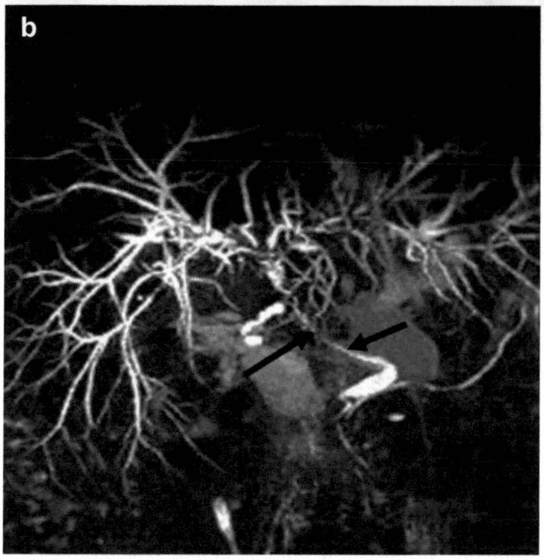

Fig. 6.48 Ischemic bile duct stricture post liver transplant for a neuroendocrine tumor. (**a**) Coronal GRE T1W fat-saturated image demonstrates a Y-shaped cast of biliary sludge (*white arrows*). (**b**) MRCP MIP image shows a long stricture involving the common hepatic and common bile duct (*black arrows*). There is dilatation of the intrahepatic biliary tree

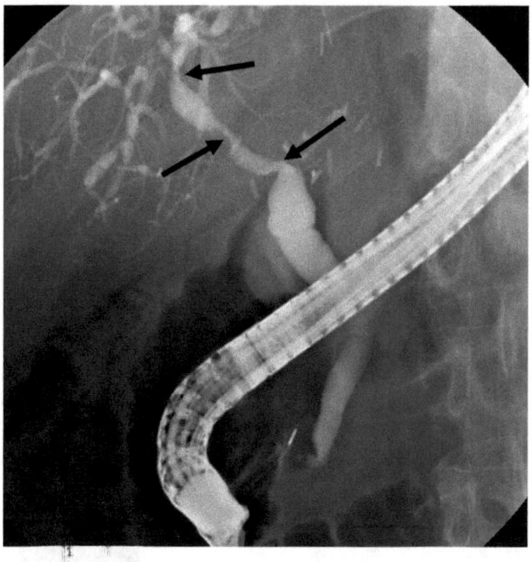

Fig. 6.49 Ischemic biliopathy. ERCP demonstrates multifocal predominantly extrahepatic biliary strictures (*arrows*) in a transplant patient with hepatic artery stenosis

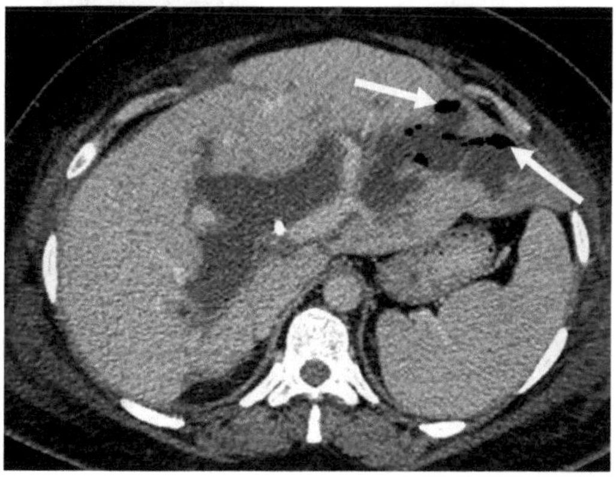

Fig. 6.50 Ischemic biliopathy. Axial CT in a post–orthotopic liver transplant patient with deteriorating LFTs. There is dilatation and necrosis of the intrahepatic biliary tree (bile lakes) secondary to hepatic artery thrombosis (confirmed with angiography). There is gas within the left lobe bile ducts (*arrows*)

clamp injuries causing focal stenoses adjacent to the anastomosis, or as a result of ischemic injury of the bile duct secondary to hepatic artery thrombosis or stenosis (less common) (Figs. 6.48 and 6.49). Ischemic biliopathy is increasing in frequency in units using non-heart-beating donors. Strictures at nonanastomotic sites may rarely be due to unrecognized pretransplant biliary diseases. Bile duct ischemia can also lead to bile duct necrosis leading to the formation of bile lakes which can become infected (Fig. 6.50). Ultrasound and MRCP are the principle means used to investigate biliary obstruction unless a T-tube has been left in situ. Management of bile duct strictures is generally conservative with ERCP (if no Roux loop present) or PTC and is discussed in Sects. 5.4.5 and 5.7.2.

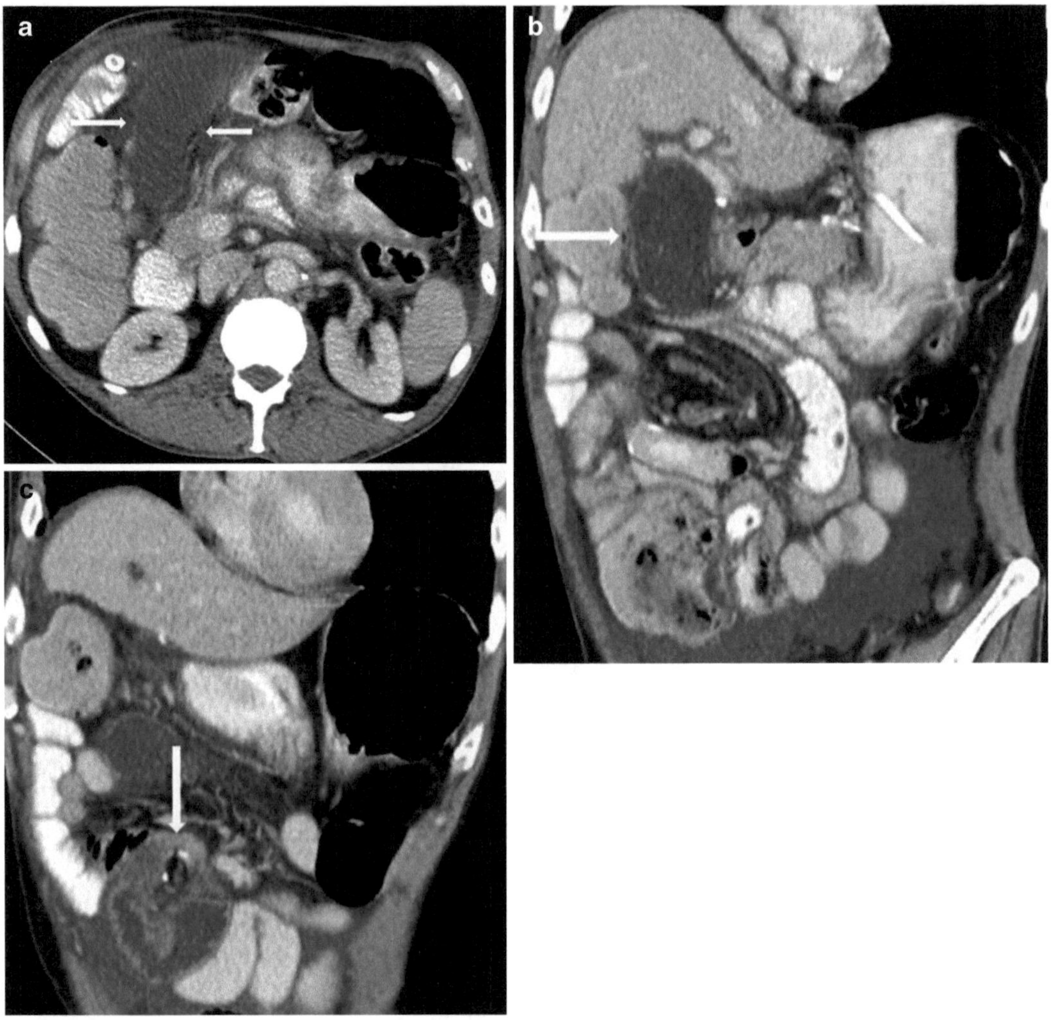

Fig. 6.51 Roux loop obstruction secondary to adhesions post-liver transplant. (**a**) Axial and (**b**) coronal reformatted CT images show a dilated Roux loop (*arrows*) in the right upper quadrant. (**c**) There is a caliber change and "kinking" of the distal Roux loop due to adhesions (*bottom arrow*). This was confirmed at laparotomy. Note that the Roux loop is "out of circuit" and therefore does not contain oral contrast unlike the rest of the small bowel

Bile Leak

Bile leaks may occur from the anastomosis, cystic duct stump, or other incompletely ligated ducts if a split graft is used. Bile will be seen on imaging as fluid in the perihepatic space or draining into the peritoneal cavity. In the immediate postoperative period, bile will be seen in the surgical drains, but if these have been removed, diagnostic aspiration using ultrasound may be required. Bile leaks are managed with percutaneous drainage and stenting via ERCP or PTC.

6.6.5.4 Fluid Collections

Fluid collections such as seromas and hematomas are usually found in the first few days after transplantation. They tend to occur near the vicinity of vascular or biliary anastomosis, and they usually resolve within few weeks. Hematomas appears high in density on CT and high signal on T1- and T2-weighted MR images which help to differentiate from other collections. It may not be possible to differentiate the exact nature of various collections on imaging. If there is clinical concern with regard to infection or a biliary leak, ultrasound-guided percutaneous aspiration is helpful. If a biloma is confirmed on aspiration, an ultrasound to assess patency of the hepatic artery and a cholangiogram to detect site of bile leak are required.

Right-sided pleural effusions are common.

6.6.5.5 Adrenal Hemorrhage

Ligation of right adrenal vein during removal of a portion of the inferior vena cava can result in right adrenal hemorrhage. This appears as high signal on T1- and T2-weighted MRI with a hypointense rim on T2 on MRI.

6.6.5.6 Small Bowel Ileus and Obstruction

Small bowel ileus is common in the immediate postoperative period and needs to be differentiated from mechanical small bowel obstruction. Obstruction can be due to adhesions from prior surgery or peritoneal thickening resulting from recurrent episodes of bacterial peritonitis (which is of increased incidence in decompensated cirrhotics with ascites). Roux-en-Y small bowel loops may become obstructed either at the anastomosis or due to internal hernias (Fig. 6.51). Patients with a history of PSC secondary to Crohn's disease and prior resections are particularly at risk of complex small bowel obstruction.

6.6.5.7 Late Complications

Almost all conditions that lead to the initial liver failure may recur in the graft. Despite careful selection of patients for transplantation with HCC, recurrence occurs in approximately 10%. The most common site of recurrence of hepatocellular carcinoma is in the lung. This is followed by the liver allograft and then the regional or distant lymphatic system. Recurrence of hepatocellular carcinoma appears as an enhancing nodule on the arterial phase within the liver allograft on dynamic contrast-enhanced CT or MRI. Early detection of recurrence is important so that prompt treatment can be considered.

Patients with OLT are at increased risk of developing malignancies, partly due to immunosuppressive treatment. The commonest malignancy is posttransplant lymphoproliferative disease (PTLD). This is a B-cell lymphoma and

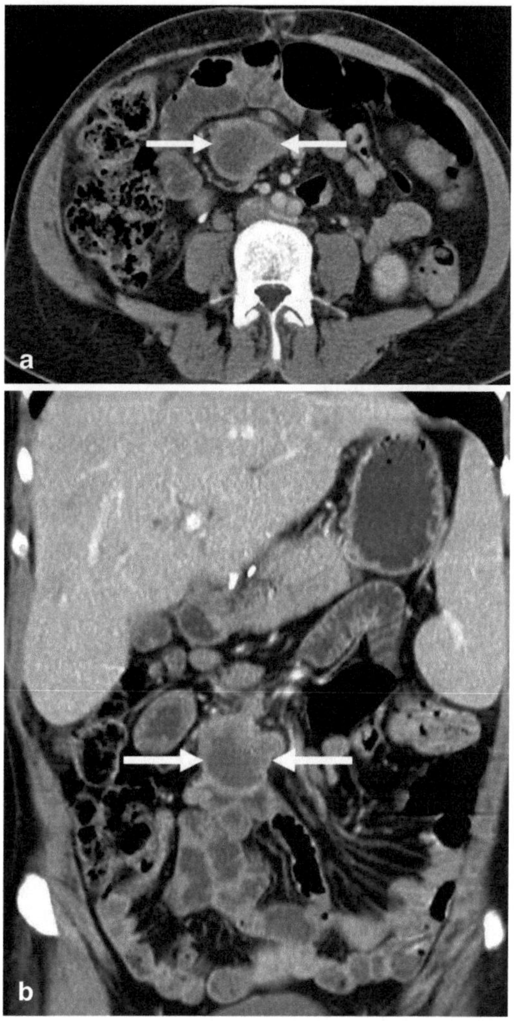

Fig. 6.52 Posttransplant lymphoproliferative disease. Portal venous phase CT in (**a**) axial and (**b**) coronal planes demonstrates a nodal mass (*arrows*) within the small bowel mesentery 2 years posttransplant for primary sclerosing cholangitis

occurs in up to 2% of patients. The manifestations of PTLD are similar to that of non-Hodgkin's lymphoma. It usually occurs 4–8 months following transplantation, but may occur years later, and is more common in patients receiving cyclosporine immunosuppressive therapy. The lymph nodes and gastrointestinal tract are the most common sites of involvement (Fig. 6.52). Imaging findings include adenopathy, localized bowel wall thickening or mass and liver lesions that are hypoechoic on ultrasound or hypodense on CT. When the liver is involved, it is more commonly diffusely infiltrated.

Skin cancer is another potential complication following liver transplant.

6.6.6 Teaching Points

- Knowledge of vascular and biliary anastomoses post-OLT with modifications of surgical technique is important for adequate postoperative assessment.
- Ultrasound is the most common modality used in the early postoperative period.
- Detection of arterial complications is crucial to maintain graft viability.
- Bile duct complications can be due to anastomotic site fibrosis or ischemia.
- The development of liver abscesses should prompt assessment of the hepatic artery.
- Persistence of varices and splenomegaly does not imply portal vein stenosis or graft dysfunction.
- Recurrence of hepatocellular carcinoma is most commonly seen in the lung followed by the liver.

References

Akahane M, Koga H, Kato N, Yamada H, Uozumi K, Tateishi R, Teratani T, Shiina S, Ohtomo K. Complications of percutaneous radiofrequency ablation for hepato-cellular carcinoma: imaging spectrum and management. Radiographics. 2005;25 Suppl 1:S57–68.

Bismuth H. Surgical anatomy and anatomical surgery of the liver. World J Surg. 1982;6(1):3–9.

Boraschi P, Donati F. Complications of orthotopic liver transplantation: imaging findings. Abdom Imaging. 2004;29(2):189–202.

Brancatelli G, Katyal S, Federle MP, Fontes P. Three-dimensional multislice helical computed tomography with the volume rendering technique in the detection of vascular complications after liver transplantation. Transplantation. 2002;73:237–42.

Brown DB, Geschwind JH, Soulen MC, Millward SF, Sacks D. Society of interventional radiology position statement on chemoembolization of hepatic malignancies. J Vasc Interv Radiol. 2006;17:217–23.

Caiado AH, Blasbalg R, Marcelino AS, da Cunha PM, Chammas MC, da Costa LC, Cerri GG, de Oliveira AC, Bacchella T, Machado MC. Complications of liver transplantation: multimodality imaging approach. Radiographics. 2007;27(5):1401–17.

Cammà C, Schepis F, Orlando A, Albanese M, Shahied L, Trevisani F, Andreone P, Craxì A, Cottone M. Transarterial chemoembolization for unresectable hepatocellular carcinoma: meta-analysis of randomized controlled trials. Radiology. 2002;224(1):47–54.

Catalano O, Singh A, Uppot R, et al. Vascular and biliary variants in the liver: implications for surgery. Radiographics. 2008;28:359–78.

Choi H, Loyer EM, DuBrow RA, Kaur H, David CL, Huang S, Curley S, Charnsangavej C. Radio-frequency ablation of liver tumors: assessment of therapeutic response and complications. Radiographics. 2001;21 Spec No:S41–54.

Couinaud C. Le foie. In: Etudes anatomiques et chirurgicales. Paris: Masson & Cie; 1957.

Couinaud C. Liver anatomy: portal (and suprahepatic) or biliary segmentation. Dig Surg. 1999;16(6):459–67.

Crossin JD, Muradali D, Wilson SR. US of liver transplants: normal and abnormal. Radiographics. 2003;23(5):1093–114.

Dromain C, de Baere T, Elias D, Kuoch V, Ducreux M, Boige V, Petrow P, Roche A, Sigal R. Hepatic tumors treated with percutaneous radio-frequency ablation: CT and MR imaging follow-up. Radiology. 2002;223(1):255–62.

Farid SG, Aldouri A, Morris-Stiff G, Khan AZ, Toogood GJ, Lodge JP, Prasad KR. Correlation between postoperative infective complications and long-term outcomes after hepatic resection for colorectal liver metastasis. Ann Surg. 2010;251:91–100.

Fong Y, Cohen AM, Fortner JG, Enker WE, Turnbull AD, Coit DG, Marrero AM, Prasad M, Blumgart LH, Brennan MF. Liver resection for colorectal metastases. J Clin Oncol. 1997;15:938–46.

Gates J, Hartnell GG, Stuart KE, Clouse ME. Chemoembolization of hepatic neoplasms: safety, complications, and when to worry. Radiographics. 1999;19(2):399–414.

Jarnagin WR, Gonen M, Fong Y, DeMatteo RP, Ben-Porat L, Little S, Corvera C, Weber S, Blumgart LH. Improvement in perioperative outcome after hepatic resection. Analysis of 1803 consecutive cases over the past decade. Ann Surg. 2002;236:397–407.

Katyal S, Oliver JH, Peterson MS, Chang PJ, Baron RL, Carr BI. Prognostic significance of arterial phase CT for prediction of response to transcatheter arterial chemoembolisation in unresectable hepatocellular carcinoma: a retrospective analysis. Am J Roentgenol. 2000;175(6):1665–72.

Kim W, Clark TW, Baum RA, Soulen MC. Risk factors for liver abscess formation after hepatic chemoembolization. J Vasc Interv Radiol. 2001;12:965–8.

Kokudo N, Makuuchi M. Current role of portal vein embolization/hepatic artery chemoembolization. Surg Clin North Am. 2004;84(2):643–57.

Letourneau JG, Steely JW, Crass JR, Goldberg ME, Grage T, Day DL. Upper abdomen: CT findings following partial hepatectomy. Radiology. 1988;166(1):139–41.

Liau KH, Blumgart LH, DeMatteo RP. Segment-oriented approach to liver resection. Surg Clin North Am. 2004;84(2):543–61.

Lim HK, Choi D, Lee WJ, Kim SH, Lee SJ, Jang HJ, Lee JH, Lim JH, Choo IW. Hepatocellular carcinoma treated with percutaneous radio-frequency ablation: evaluation with follow-up multiphase helical CT. Radiology. 2001;221(2):447–54.

Lim HS, Jeong YY, Kang HK, Kim JK, Park JG. Imaging features of hepatocellular carcinoma after transcatheter arterial chemoembolization and radiofrequency ablation. AJR Am J Roentgenol. 2006;187(4):W341–9.

Lo CM, Fan ST, Liu CL, Lai EC, Wong J. Biliary complications after hepatic resection: risk factors, management, and outcome. Arch Surg. 1998;133(2):156–61.

Lortat-Jacob JL, Robert HG, Henry L. Un cas d'hepatectomie droit reglee. Memoires de la Academie de Chirurgie. 1952;78:244–51.

Matsui O, Kadoya A, Yoshikama J, et al. Posterior aspect of segment 4: patterns of portal venule branching at helical CT during arterial portography. Radiology. 1997;205(1):159–62.

McGhana JP, Dodd 3rd GD. Radiofrequency ablation of the liver: current status. AJR Am J Roentgenol. 2001;176(1):3–16.

Nagorney DM, van Heerden JA, Ilstrup DM, Adson MA. Primary hepatic malignancy: surgical management and determinants of survival. Surgery. 1989;106: 740–8.

Nghiem HV. Imaging of hepatic transplantation. Radiol Clin North Am. 1998;36:429–43.

Nghiem HV, Tran K, Winter 3rd TC, Schmiedl UP, Althaus SJ, Patel NH, Freeny PC. Imaging of complications in liver transplantation. Radiographics. 1996;16(4):825–40.

Nishimine K, Uchida H, Matsuo N, Sakaguchi H, Hirohashi S, Nishimura Y, Guo Q, Ohishi H, Nagano N, Yoshioka T, et al. Segmental transarterial chemoembolization with Lipiodol mixed with anticancer drugs for nonresectable hepatocellular carcinoma: follow-up CT and therapeutic results. Cancer Chemother Pharmacol. 1994;33(Suppl):S60–8.

Overman MJ, Maru DM, Charnsangavej C, Loyer EM, Wang H, Pathak P, Eng C, Hoff PM, Vauthey JN, Wolff RA, Kopetz S. Oxaliplatin-mediated increase in spleen size as a biomarker for the development of hepatic sinusoidal injury. J Clin Oncol. 2010;28 (15):2549–55.

Pol B, Campan P, Hardwigsen J, Botti G, Pons J, Le Treut YP. Morbidity of major hepatic resections: a 100 case prospective study. Eur J Surg. 1999;165:446–53.

Quiroga S, Sebastià MC, Margarit C, Castells L, Boyé R, Alvarez-Castells A. Complications of orthotopic liver transplantation: spectrum of findings with helical CT. Radiographics. 2001;21(5):1085–102.

Rhim H, Dodd 3rd GD, Chintapalli KN, Wood BJ, Dupuy DE, Hvizda JL, Sewell PE, Goldberg SN. Radiofrequency thermal ablation of abdominal tumors: lessons learned from complications. Radiographics. 2004;24(1):41–52.

Robinson PJA, Ward J. Chapter 12: MRI of liver tumours after treatment. In: MRI of the liver. A practical guide. New York: Taylor and Francis Group; 2006. p. 328–56.

Rutkauskas S, Gedrimas V, Pundzius J, Barauskas G, Basevicius A. Clinical and anatomical basis for the classification of the structural parts of the liver. Medicina (Kaunas). 2006;42:98–106.

Seamen DS. Adult living donor liver transplantation: current status. J Clin Gastroenterol. 2001;33:97–106.

Simmonds PC, Primrose JN, Colquitt JL, Garden OJ, Poston GJ, Rees M. Surgical resection of hepatic metastases from colorectal cancer: a systematic review of published studies. Br J Cancer. 2006;94(7):982–99.

Starzl TE, Marchioro TL, Vonkaulla KN, Hermann G, Brittain RS, Waddell WR. Homotransplantation of the liver in humans. Surg Gynecol Obstet. 1963;117: 659–76.

Wah TM, Arellano RS, Gervais DA, Saltalamacchia CA, Martino J, Halpern EF, Maher M, Mueller PR. Image-guided percutaneous radiofrequency ablation and incidence of post–radiofrequency ablation syndrome: prospective survey. Radiology. 2005;237(3):1097–102.

Yamada R, Sato M, Kawabata M, Nakatsuka H, Nakamura K, Takashima S. Hepatic artery embolization in 120 patients with unresectable hepatoma. Radiology. 1983;148(2):397–401.

The Small Bowel

7

James C. Lenton, Adeshina S. Fawole,
John Brittenden, and Damian J.M. Tolan

Contents

7.1 **Introduction** ... 228

7.2 **The Small Bowel in the Postoperative Period** ... 228
7.2.1 Ileus and Small Bowel Obstruction (SBO) ... 228
7.2.2 CT in the Assessment of Dilated Small Bowel ... 229
7.2.3 Causes of Mechanical SBO in the Postoperative Patient ... 232

7.3 **Small Bowel Operations** ... 233
7.3.1 Roux-en-Y Enteroenterostomy ... 233
7.3.2 Small Bowel Resection ... 234
7.3.3 Common Modifications ... 234
7.3.4 Postoperative Complications ... 234
7.3.5 Teaching Points ... 241

7.4 **Feeding Jejunostomy** ... 241
7.4.1 Surgical Technique ... 241
7.4.2 Postoperative Complications ... 241

7.5 **Postoperative Abdominal Hernias** ... 242
7.5.1 Hernia Repair ... 242
7.5.2 Surgical Technique ... 243
7.5.3 Postoperative Imaging ... 243
7.5.4 Postoperative Complications ... 244
7.5.5 Incisional Hernia ... 244
7.5.6 Richter's Hernia ... 244
7.5.7 Postoperative Internal Hernias ... 245
7.5.8 Complications of Hernias ... 246
7.5.9 Teaching Points ... 246

7.6 **Ileal Pouch-Anal Anastomoses (IPAA or Ileal Anal Pouch)** ... 246
7.6.1 Clinical Indication ... 247
7.6.2 Surgical Technique and Postoperative Anatomy ... 247
7.6.3 Normal Postoperative Imaging ... 248

7.7 **Postoperative Complications** ... 249
7.7.1 Small Bowel Obstruction (SBO) ... 249
7.7.2 Pouch-Related Sepsis ... 250
7.7.3 Pouchitis ... 250
7.7.4 Anastomotic Stricture ... 250
7.7.5 Anastomotic Leak ... 250
7.7.6 Pelvic Infection and Abscess ... 251
7.7.7 Fistulas ... 252
7.7.8 Pouch Outlet Obstruction ... 252
7.7.9 Teaching Points ... 252

References ... 253

J.C. Lenton, MBChB, MRCS(Ed), FRCR
Department of Radiology,
Mid Yorkshire Hospitals NHS Trust,
Wakefield, UK

A.S. Fawole, MBBS, MD, FRCS
Department of Surgery,
Mid Yorkshire Hospitals NHS Trust,
Wakefield, UK

J. Brittenden, MBChB, MRCP, FRCR
Department of Radiology,
Mid Yorkshire Hospitals NHS Trust,
Wakefield, UK

D.J.M. Tolan, MBChB, MRCP, FRCR (✉)
Department of Clinical Radiology,
Leeds Teaching Hospitals NHS Trust,
Lincoln Wing, St James's University Hospital,
LS9 7JT, Leeds, UK
e-mail: damian.tolan@leedsth.ns.uk

J. Brittenden, D.J.M. Tolan (eds.), *Radiology of the Post Surgical Abdomen*,
DOI 10.1007/978-1-4471-2775-8_7, © Springer-Verlag London 2012

7.1 Introduction

Anatomically, the small intestine comprises the duodenum, jejunum, and ileum and is of variable length (average of 4–6 m). Clinically, the term small intestine usually excludes the duodenum which is covered in Chap. 3. The jejunum refers to the proximal half of the small intestine commencing at the duodenojejunal junction, although there is no clear anatomical distinction between the jejunum and ileum. The jejunum and ileum lie in the free edge of the mesentery. The small bowel mesentery extends from the duodenojejunal junction at the level of the second lumbar vertebra passing diagonally downward to the right sacroiliac joint. The root of the small bowel mesentery measures approximately 15 cm and is situated on the posterior abdominal wall. It contains vessels, lymphatics, and autonomic nerves.

The jejunum has a thicker wall and a wider diameter than the ileum. The mesenteric vessels form only one or two arcades in the jejunum with long narrow arteries leading from these to the jejunal wall. In the ileum, there are usually 3–5 arcades with shorter terminal arteries leading to the bowel wall.

7.2 The Small Bowel in the Postoperative Period

The small bowel is frequently affected by postoperative insult. The most common clinical scenario involves patients who are slow to recover normal bowel function. The main clinical conundrum is in the differentiation between ileus and high-grade small bowel obstruction (SBO). In this setting, imaging has an important role to guide management. Many patients with mechanical SBO in the postoperative period are often successfully managed conservatively with nasogastric decompression and fluid resuscitation. Patients with signs suggestive of closed loop or strangulating obstruction from any cause require emergency surgery, but again imaging can first suggest this diagnosis, especially in difficult to assess patients, such as those on ITU or the morbidly obese.

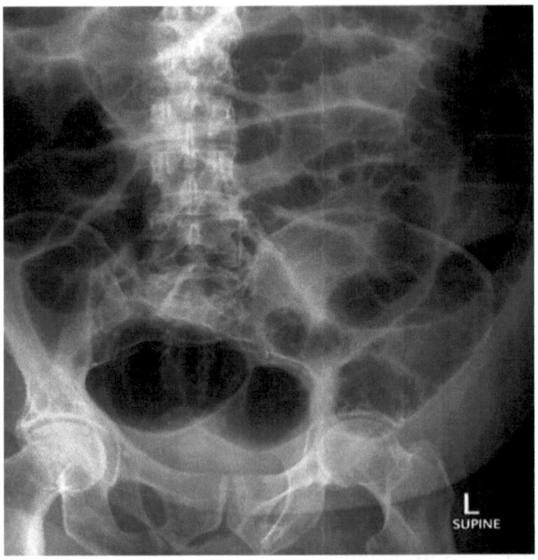

Fig. 7.1 Postoperative ileus. Supine abdominal film demonstrating multiple dilated loops of small and large bowel of varying caliber

7.2.1 Ileus and Small Bowel Obstruction (SBO)

Many patients undergoing abdominal surgery will experience small bowel ileus due to manipulation of the small bowel, even when it has not been directly involved in the surgical procedure. Differentiating between paralytic ileus (Fig. 7.1), incomplete (low grade) and complete (high grade) small bowel obstruction can be difficult. The plain abdominal radiograph is often the initial imaging modality in postoperative patients with symptoms of bowel obstruction. Studies comparing surgical correlation and the accuracy of abdominal radiographs have demonstrated sensitivities and specificities of only 50–60%. Serial films are helpful because with increasing obstruction less gas is seen within the colon (Fig. 7.2). Potential pitfalls in interpretation include the absence of gas-filled loops of small bowel due to fluid within the bowel lumen (Fig. 7.3) and small bowel dilatation due to large

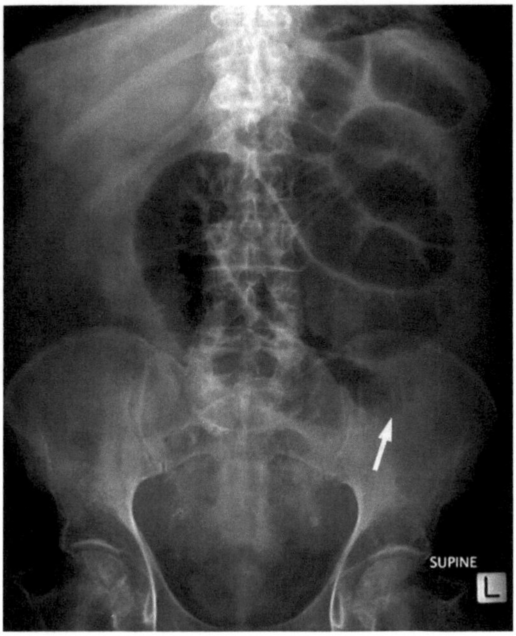

Fig. 7.2 Mechanical SBO. Supine abdominal film showing significantly dilated loops of proximal small bowel with abrupt cutoff (*arrow*) and no distal bowel gas

bowel obstruction in the presence of an incompetent ileocecal valve. Furthermore, the site and cause of small bowel dilatation cannot be accurately determined on plain abdominal X-rays and other important conditions producing dilatation such as ischemia/infarction or intra-abdominal collections cannot be evaluated.

Some centers advocate the use of a modified water-soluble follow-through study when the diagnosis of SBO is clinically and radiologically equivocal. One hundred milliliters of a hyperosmolar oral water-soluble contrast agent (e.g., Gastrografin) is administered, and an abdominal radiograph is taken at 4 h. Failure of oral contrast to reach the colon within 4 h is defined as abnormal since in ileus contrast will normally pass into the colon, whereas in high-grade obstruction, it will not (Fig. 7.4). Some authors advocate its use as a predictive test in patients with obstructive symptoms who can be managed conservatively since where contrast fails to reach the colon surgery is usually required (Abbas et al. 2007) (Fig. 7.5).

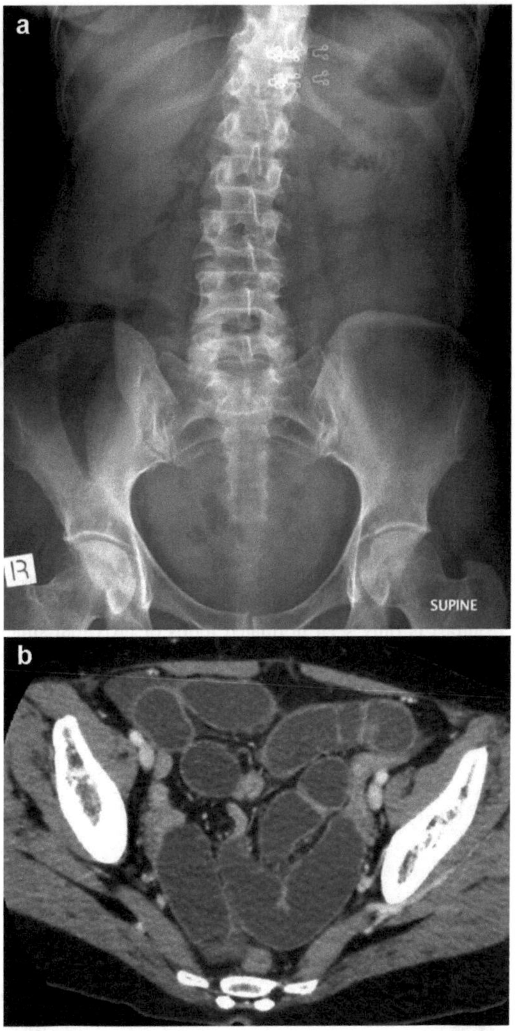

Fig. 7.3 (**a**,**b**) Mechanical SBO but normal supine abdominal film. There is an absence of bowel gas due to multiple dilated fluid-filled loops seen on a subsequent CT scan

7.2.2 CT in the Assessment of Dilated Small Bowel

CT is now routinely used in the assessment of patients with suspected SBO. CT can detect the precise location of SBO with high sensitivity and specificity (Frager et al. 1994). CT can be performed rapidly, is readily available, and provides a global evaluation of the gastrointestinal tract and abdomen.

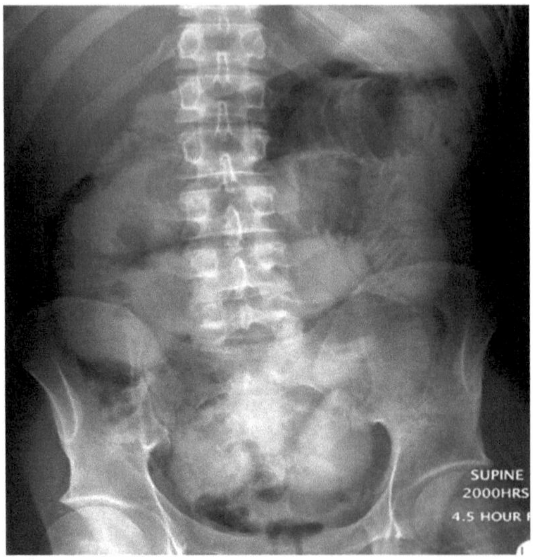

Fig. 7.4 Complete SBO. Water-soluble contrast follow-through taken 4.5 h after administration of contrast. Contrast is only seen in dilated loops of proximal small bowel with none in the right colon. Note the generalized poor density of the contrast due to its dilution in the retained fluid within the bowel lumen

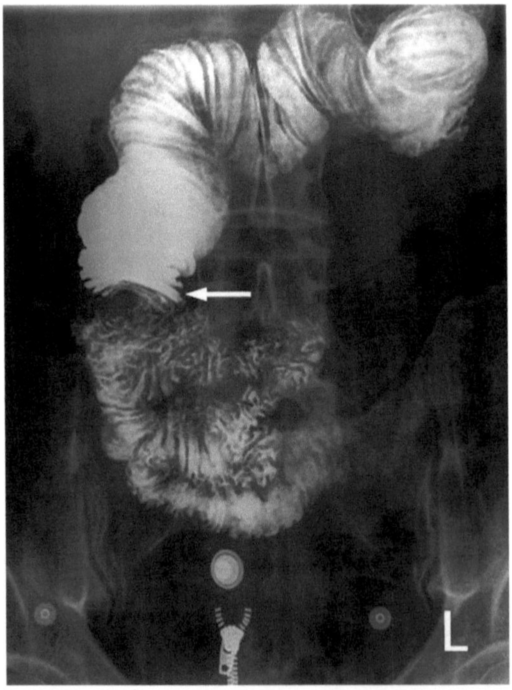

Fig. 7.5 Partial SBO with contrast examination demonstrating dilated proximal loops of small bowel with an abrupt transition point (*arrow*) and collapsed distal loops

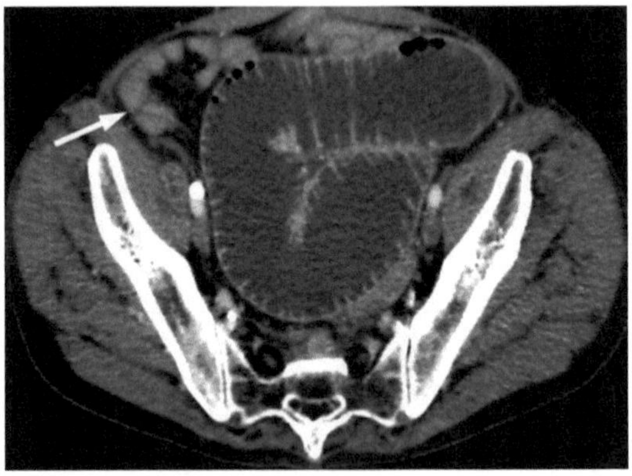

Fig. 7.6 Mechanical SBO. Contrast-enhanced CT showing significantly dilated loops of proximal small bowel and collapsed distal loops (*arrow*)

7.2.2.1 CT Technique

If the abdominal radiograph shows definite or likely SBO, oral contrast is not required for the CT examination, as fluid in dilated small bowel loops provides inherent contrast. Oral contrast is also unlikely to reach the point of obstruction by the time of the CT examination. It is also diluted by fluid proximal to the site of obstruction, and the additional oral fluid load may precipitate or exacerbate vomiting that may in turn increase the risk of aspiration. In patients with equivocal clinical and plain film findings, positive contrast can be useful particularly where patients have complex postoperative anatomy and poor intrinsic contrast (e.g., gross soft tissue edema or those where intravenous contrast is contraindicated).

7.2.2.2 CT Image Analysis

Small bowel dilatation is defined as a diameter exceeding 2.5–3 cm but this does not differentiate obstruction from paralytic ileus alone.

CT findings in SBO include:

- Abrupt transition point between dilated and collapsed distal small bowel
- Collapsed distal small and large bowel (Fig. 7.6)
- Gas and particulate matter seen within the lumen proximal to the obstruction (small bowel feces sign) (Catarina et al. 2009)

In SBO, the presence of small bowel feces alone should be interpreted with caution as this finding may be present in normal individuals, particularly if enteric feeding tubes have been used or in cystic

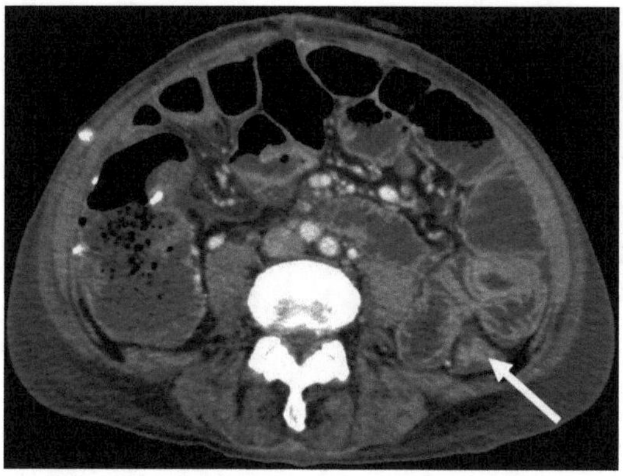

Fig. 7.7 Ileus. Contrast-enhanced CT showing generalized dilatation of the small and large bowel. No transition point was found in the examination. Note the descending colon is collapsed (*arrow*) due to compression and dependency which should not be mistaken for obstruction

fibrosis patients. If a point of obstruction is identified on CT, the relative length of collapsed and dilated small bowel is assessed in order to ascertain the level of obstruction. In SBO, dilated bowel loops may move from their normal position because of distension and twisting of the mesentery. This may lead to inaccuracy in defining the point of obstruction if normal anatomical landmarks are used in isolation. The presence of dilated small bowel without a transition point and normal caliber colon suggests either ileus or incomplete SBO (Fig. 7.7).

7.2.2.3 Closed Loop Obstruction and Ischemia

Closed loop obstruction occurs when a loop of bowel is obstructed at two adjacent points along its length at both ends. The most common causes affecting the small bowel are band adhesions (at the base of the mesentery) or herniation of a loop of small bowel through a mesenteric defect. The latter is a particular risk in patients undergoing laparoscopic surgery, where the mesenteric defects produced during bowel resection are not usually repaired. Closed loop obstruction is not always suspected clinically, but where a radiological diagnosis is made, urgent surgical intervention is required. This is because of the risks of developing ischemia resulting from either arterial occlusion (rotation of the mesentery) or venous infarction (increased intraluminal pressure impeding venous return).

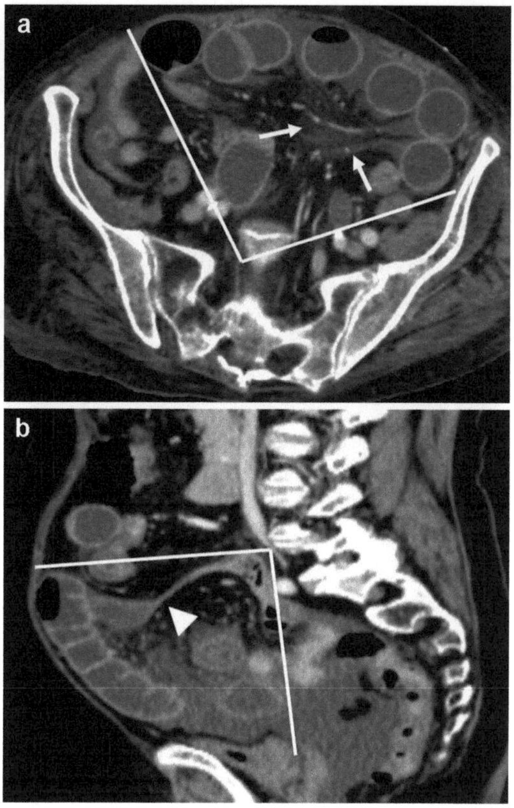

Fig. 7.8 (**a**,**b**) Closed loop small bowel obstruction. Contrast-enhanced CT shows SBO in a sectoral distribution. There is edema in the mesentery (*arrows*) with thickening and increased enhancement of the small bowel wall. The transition point (*arrowhead*) is smooth and tapered suggestive of a volvulus or adhesional band

CT findings in closed loop obstruction depend on the orientation of the closed loop within the abdomen and include (Silva et al. 2009) (Figs. 7.8 and 7.9):

- Radiating loops of dilated small bowel with the proximal and distal ends of the obstructed loop in close proximity
- Prominent mesenteric vessels converging toward the point of torsion
- U- or C-shaped dilated small bowel loop (depending on the orientation of the obstructed loop)
- Beak sign – due to torsion of the bowel loop
- Whirl sign – due to rotation of the small bowel and vessels around the point of obstruction
- Bowel wall thickening and increased enhancement

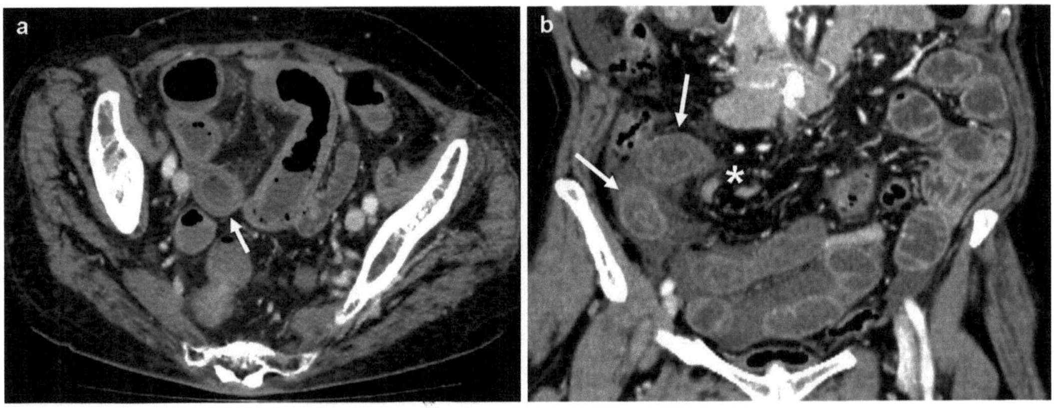

Fig. 7.9 (**a**,**b**) Closed loop small bowel obstruction. Contrast-enhanced CT in patient with mechanical SBO showing several loops of grossly thickened poorly enhancing ischemic bowel (*arrows*). The mesenteric vessels are twisting round each other indicating volvulus (*asterisk*). Emergency surgery is indicated

As obstruction progresses, CT features of ischemic bowel may be present (Sandrasegaran and Maglinte 2005):

- Bowel wall thickening
- Reduced bowel wall enhancement (arterial infarction)
- Increased bowel wall enhancement (venous infarction)
- Edema within the small bowel mesentery
- Ascites (simple and hemorrhagic)
- Pneumatosis intestinalis
- Gas within the superior mesenteric/portal veins or liver
- Perforation

All radiologists interpreting abdominal CT should be highly vigilant for these signs in patients with small bowel dilatation. Although some of the findings can be subtle, misdiagnosis can have catastrophic consequences for the patient.

7.2.3 Causes of Mechanical SBO in the Postoperative Patient

Adhesions are the most common cause of mechanical SBO in the postoperative period. Other causes include abdominal wall and internal hernias (Sect. 7.5.7), recurrent malignancy (serosal deposits), and rarely intussusception (Sect. 7.2.3.3).

7.2.3.1 Adhesions

Adhesions can cause chronic abdominal pain and small bowel obstruction. Imaging features of SBO on CT include:

- An abrupt transition point but no demonstrable obstructing lesion or cause
- Sharply angulated bowel loops with "twisting" of the adjacent mesentery
- Close approximation of the small bowel to the anterior abdominal wall

Adhesions are classified as visceral (extending between small bowel loops or to adjacent organs) or parietal (connecting the bowel to the anterior peritoneal surface).Visceral adhesions are more commonly associated with SBO and parietal with chronic abdominal pain (Maglinte et al. 2007). A range of modalities including CT enterography, CT enteroclysis and fluoroscopy can be employed to investigate symptomatic patients with a history of previous abdominal surgery. While some authors advocate a role for CT enteroclysis in the obstructed patient to allow decompression and assessment of the degree of obstruction (Maglinte et al. 2007), this has not been widely adopted.

7.2.3.2 Postoperative Hernias

Postoperative hernias are classified as either internal or external. Internal hernias are either naturally occurring (e.g., foramen of Winslow into the lesser sac or at the duodenojejunal flexure) or surgically created defects in the mesentery. External hernias can occur through surgical peritoneal defects in the abdominal wall created during laparoscopic surgery or stoma sites. Internal herniation of small bowel is associated with a high risk of strangulation and requires prompt surgical intervention. The management of external hernias is defined by other factors including the size of the hernia neck, the presence of visceral contents, and patient symptomatology.

7.2.3.3 Intussusception

It is most likely that physiological intussusception will be encountered as an observation during interpretation of a postoperative CT scan. This is typically seen in the proximal jejunum and is characterized as a short intussusception (<3 cm) without any identifiable pathological lead point. Intussusception is a very rare cause of small bowel obstruction in postoperative patients. Causative factors include increased peristalsis of bowel that has been extensively handled and the presence of potential "lead points" such as feeding tubes and sutures. CT will demonstrate the mesenteric fat and vessels of the intussusceptum within the distal intussuscipiens. Proximal small bowel obstruction may be present.

7.3 Small Bowel Operations

Operations on the small bowel involve either resection for disease or resection of a segment of small bowel for use as a conduit elsewhere (e.g., urinary conduits). Any patient undergoing small bowel surgery may develop the complications described in Sect. 7.2. In this section, we will describe the most common surgical procedures involving the small bowel and the specific complications related to each surgical intervention. Small bowel anastomoses are also used in the following surgical procedures and will be discussed in the relevant chapters:

- Biliary drainage procedure – hepatico- or choledochojejunostomy (Sect. 5.6)
- Bariatric Roux-en-Y gastric bypass – gastrojejunostomy (Sect. 3.5.3.1)
- Whipple procedure – pancreaticojejunostomy, gastrojejunostomy, and hepaticojejunostomy (Sect. 4.2)
- Pancreatic procedures in chronic pancreatitis (e.g., Frey, Beger, and Puestow procedure) – pancreaticojejunostomy (Sect. 4.4)
- Liver transplantation (occasionally) – hepaticojejunostomy (Sect. 6.6)
- Jejunal free flap – pharyngeal reconstruction (Sect. 2.3)
- Jejunal interposition – following total esophagectomy (Sect. 2.3)
- Urological operations – urinary conduit (Sect. 9.2)

7.3.1 Roux-en-Y Enteroenterostomy

This is a commonly performed small bowel operation and has many indications. It derives its name from the Swiss surgeon, César Roux, who first described it and the Y-shaped configuration of the small bowel following anastomosis. This is created by joining the end of a proximal limb of small bowel to the side of a more distal loop of small bowel. Roux loops are discussed in more detail in Chaps. 3, 4, 5, and 6.

7.3.1.1 Indications

- Gastric bypass for obesity surgery – The Roux loop is used in bariatric surgery to create a malabsorptive limb.
- Gastrectomy – This can be used to prevent bile reflux into the stomach or esophagus after a partial or total gastrectomy.
- Hepaticojejunostomy and choledochojejunostomy.

7.3.1.2 Postoperative Complications

These are similar to other small bowel operations described above but also specifically internal herniation especially through Petersen's space. This is the space behind the mesentery of the Roux loop and the colonic mesentery created during gastric bypass operations. Incidence of Petersen's internal hernia can be as high as 6% and this is a frequently missed radiological diagnosis (Bauman and Pirrello 2009). It is characterized by small bowel loops protruding to the anterior abdominal wall in the left upper abdomen and shift of superior mesenteric vessels to the left, while transmesocolic internal hernias produce clustered small bowel loops in the left upper quadrant through the mesocolic defect (Kawkabani Marchini et al. 2011) (Fig. 3.61 Chap 3).

7.3.2 Small Bowel Resection

This is a commonly performed surgical procedure.

7.3.2.1 Clinical Indications

- Small bowel obstruction (adhesions, hernias)
- Strictures (Crohn's disease, radiation induced, tuberculosis, malignancy)
- Benign small bowel tumors (lipoma, GIST, adenoma, hamartoma)
- Malignant small bowel tumors (carcinoid, lymphoma, adenocarcinoma)
- Traumatic injury (penetrating or blunt)
- Iatrogenic
- Ischemic bowel

7.3.2.2 Surgical Technique and Postoperative Anatomy

Operative summary – small bowel resection:

- This can be performed as an open operation or via a laparoscopic approach
- Mesentery divided
- Segment of small bowel resected
- Free ends anastomosed to restore continuity (end-to-end, end-to-side, or side-to-side)
- The anastomosis is hand sewn or stapled (the staple line is easy to identify on CT)

7.3.3 Common Modifications

7.3.3.1 Small Bowel Bypass

In cases where small bowel is stuck to unresectable intra-abdominal malignancy, en bloc resection may not be possible. Therefore, it may be more appropriate to bypass the diseased segment. In a small bowel bypass procedure, a loop of small bowel proximal to the diseased segment is placed side by side with a distal loop and an anastomosis is created.

7.3.3.2 Stricturoplasty/Strictureplasty

Stricturoplasty is used to treat benign small bowel strictures without having to resect small bowel. This is particularly useful in patients with Crohn's disease who may have multiple strictures. This technique preserves bowel length and prevents multiple resections and the associated risk of short gut syndrome. A longitudinal incision along the stricture extending into healthy small bowel is made (enterotomy). The narrowed segment is widened perpendicular to the stricture using either a hand-sewn or stapled technique (Fig. 7.10). One of the effects of the procedure is to sometimes create saccular dilatation of the treated small bowel loops. As a "new" abnormality on a postoperative small bowel evaluation, it is important not to confuse this finding with pseudosacculation arising from chronic Crohn's disease or dilatation from subacute obstruction. In this setting, a clear understanding of whether resection or stricturoplasty was performed is very important since imaging is usually requested in response to new symptoms and an incorrect diagnosis of ongoing obstruction may precipitate unnecessary further surgery.

7.3.4 Postoperative Complications

Patients requiring assessment for suspected complications in the early postoperative period are often investigated with CT, ideally following oral and IV contrast. Patients that develop delayed complications such as anastomotic stenosis or disease recurrence (tumor, adhesion, or inflammatory bowel disease) may be investigated with a combination of small bowel contrast studies or CT and MRI.

7.3.4.1 Anastomotic Leak

Anastomotic leaks involving the small bowel usually result from staple gun failure or ischemia at the anastomosis (Sandrasegaran et al. 2004). CT is the modality of choice for detecting leaks from an enteroenteric anastomosis. Leaks can be

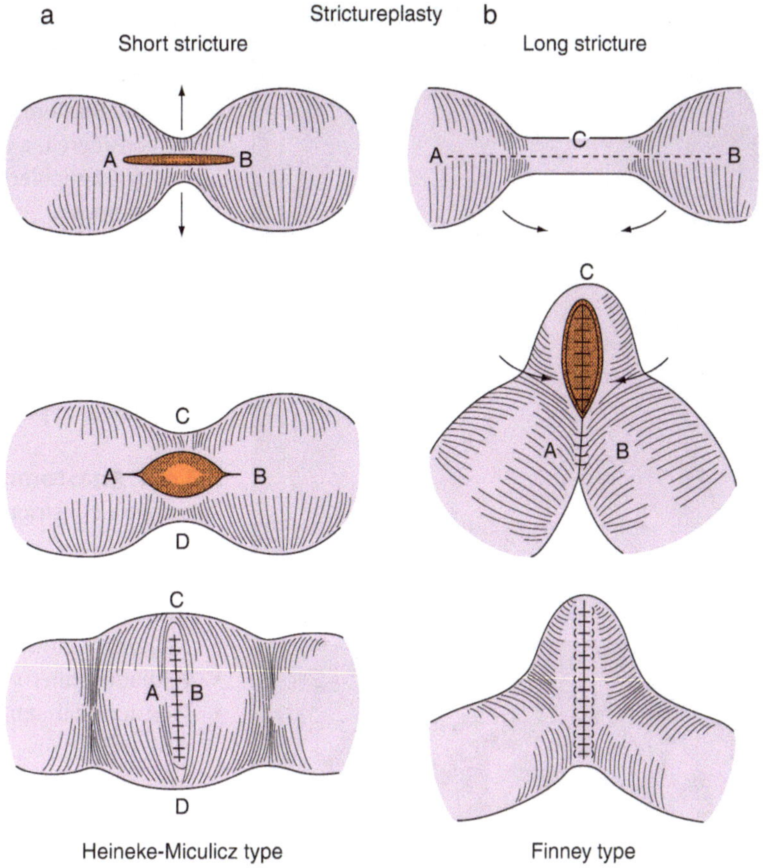

Fig. 7.10 (**a**,**b**) Strictureplasty procedures in the management of small bowel Crohn's strictures

made more conspicuous by the addition of higher than normal strength oral iodinated contrast (e.g., 8% vs. 2–4%). The diagnosis is suggested by excessive free intraperitoneal fluid and gas or focal collections of fluid and gas around the anastomosis. Free spill of oral contrast is characteristic. Patients with gastroenterostomies are usually initially investigated with upper GI contrast studies, providing they are able to tolerate the procedure, but CT can have an important supplementary role and may detect a subtle leak of contrast not appreciated on the contrast swallow. It should be remembered that contrast may be administered where appropriate via a nasogastric tube.

7.3.4.2 Abscess

Abscess formation may be secondary to a small anastomotic leak or a fluid collection/hematoma that becomes infected. Ultrasound can be extremely useful both in diagnosis and treatment but has a limited role in the diagnosis of deeper intra-abdominal sepsis. CT is far more sensitive and will often allow percutaneous drainage at the same sitting. Collections are classically of fluid density with an enhancing rim and may contain gas.

7.3.4.3 Blind Pouch Syndrome

A blind pouch is an enlarged aperistaltic loop of small bowel (Fig. 7.11), usually complicating a side-to-side small bowel anastomosis. The direction of bowel peristalsis causes ongoing filling of the pouch (Sandrasegaran et al. 2004). An incorrectly performed end-to-side anastomosis can result in a similar complication, i.e., if the end of the distal bowel is anastomosed to the side of the proximal bowel, peristalsis will propel the bowel contents into the blind end of the proximal limb (Lappas 2003). Blind pouches are often asymptomatic but present as a late complication months or years after initial surgery

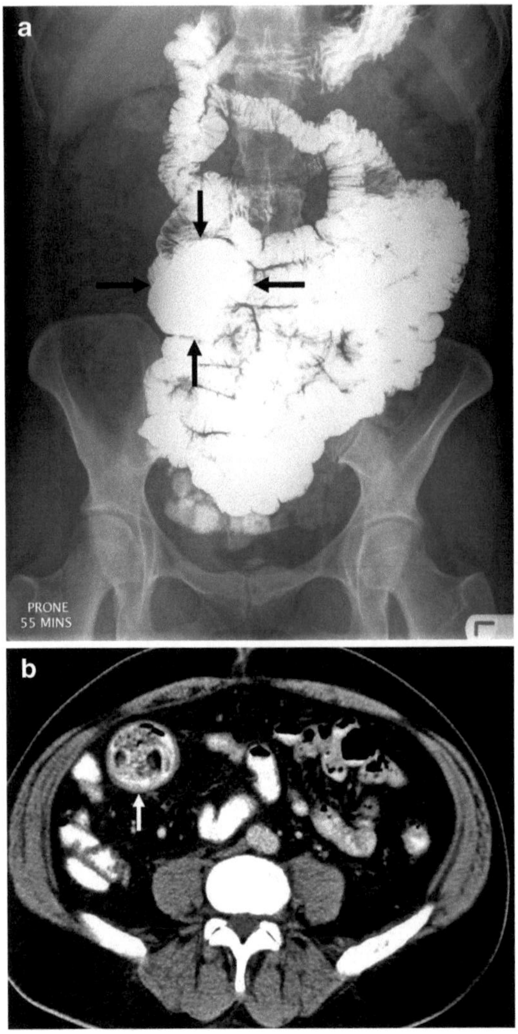

Fig. 7.11 (**a**,**b**) Blind pouch syndrome. (**a**) Barium follow examination shows a solitary dilated section of small bowel with no evidence of obstruction (*arrows*). (**b**) Contrast-enhanced CT on the same patient shows that the dilated segment corresponds to a blind pouch following previous side-to-end small bowel anastomosis (*arrow*)

complicated by gastrointestinal bleeding due to mucosal ulceration, malabsorption (due to bacterial overgrowth), or perforation.

A blind pouch will be positioned adjacent to a surgical staple line. The redundant loop may be of variable length and caliber. The appearances on postoperative imaging are characteristic and should not be mistaken for a diverticulum or perienteric abscess. Use of CT with positive oral contrast or small bowel barium studies with either compression or enteroclysis may assist where there is distorted small bowel anatomy (e.g., adhesions or multiple previous small bowel resections and anastomoses). Where blind pouch is being considered, a dynamic evaluation with fluoroscopy (particularly with enteroclysis if a distal anastomosis) can confirm the preferential filling of the blind loop and assess the degree of associated dilatation. It can be very difficult to appreciate the small bowel filling and anatomy during a standard small bowel meal where the patient drinks contrast with plain films obtained intermittently at preset time intervals.

7.3.4.4 Anastomotic Stricture

Anastomotic strictures occur due to the following:

- Postoperative fibrosis (typically quite short)
- Recurrent Crohn's disease
- Malignant infiltration
- Radiation enteropathy
- Nonsteriodal anti-inflammatory drug-induced strictures

SBO with a transition point at the anastomosis suggests the diagnosis (Fig. 7.12), but it is often not possible to differentiate from other conditions such as band adhesions. In patients who have undergone surgery for malignancy, previous imaging should also be carefully reviewed and compared to look for evidence of tumor recurrence at the anastomosis. This is particularly important where barium studies are being performed since extraenteric evaluation is not possible and extrinsic malignant disease may not be appreciated (or may have been misinterpreted as part of a bowel loop on prior cross sectional imaging).

7.3.4.5 Disease Recurrence

Patients who have undergone small bowel resection for benign or malignant disease may develop SBO due to recurrence of the original pathology such as carcinoma or Crohn's disease. Serosal deposits from more distant primary tumors (Fig. 7.13) may lead to SBO (ovary, breast, colon, stomach, and pancreas). CT is insensitive at detecting low-volume peritoneal and serosal disease. This diagnosis should be suspected in

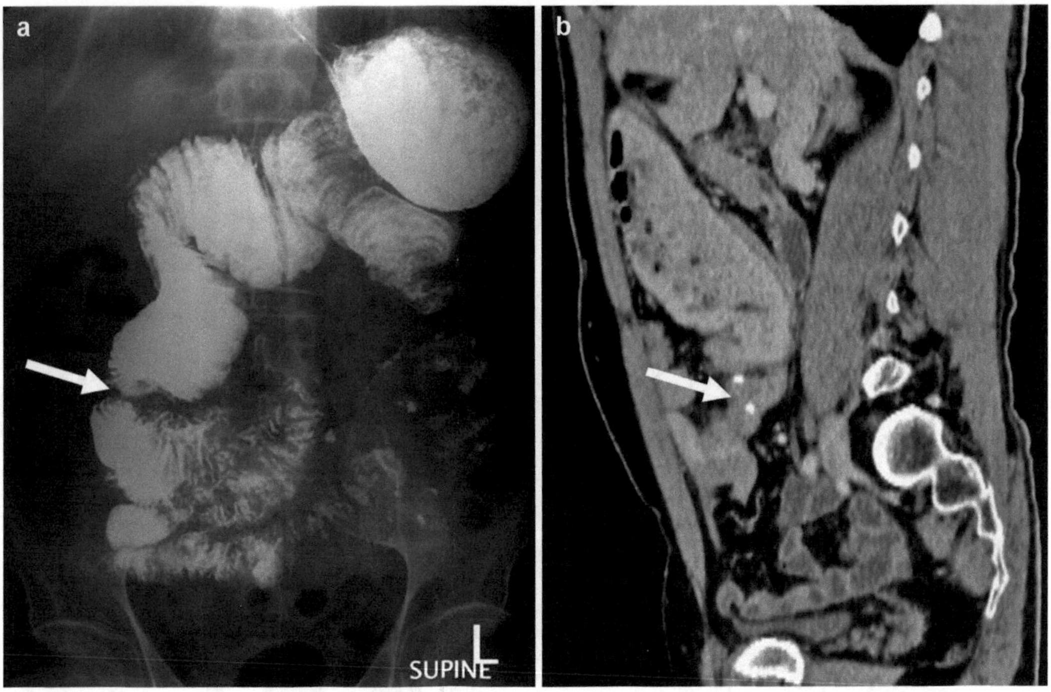

Fig. 7.12 (**a**,**b**) Anastomotic stricture in a patient 18 months following partial gastrectomy and Roux loop construction with symptoms of subacute obstruction. Barium follow through shows dilation of the proximal small bowel from a short stricture (*arrow*). (**b**) Sagittal CT in the same patient shows stricture at the distal Roux loop anastomosis – note staple line (*arrow*). Resection confirmed a benign stricture

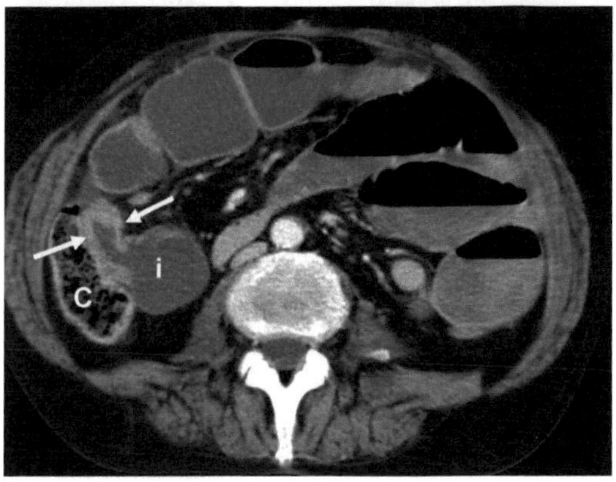

Fig. 7.13 Serosal recurrence in patient with prior Billroth 2 gastrectomy for cancer. Axial CT shows annular stricture (*arrows*) in the mid ileum (*i*) adjacent to ascending colon (*C*) but distal to the small bowel anastomosis (*not shown*)

patients with symptoms suggestive of recurrent disease or unexplained rising tumor markers. The earliest signs can be nonspecific, particularly in the early postoperative period, but specific features to observe include persistent free fluid, peritoneal nodules, and omental thickening. It should be remembered that surgical examination of the peritoneum is most sensitive in detection of small peritoneal metastatic deposits. Where there is doubt regarding the diagnosis, options include serial imaging, PET CT (but this can be misleading and false positive can occur in the early postoperative period), or image-guided/laparoscopic biopsy. This patient group may have multiple sites of obstruction contributing to their symptoms and consequently surgery for palliation has variable success.

7.3.4.6 Radiation Enteropathy

The small bowel is particularly sensitive to radiation toxicity. Radiotherapy fields are specifically chosen to minimize risk of inadvertent damage to the small bowel, and bladder filling and laxatives are sometimes also used to mitigate against this. However, radical radiotherapy with intent to cure for the treatment of pelvic malignancies

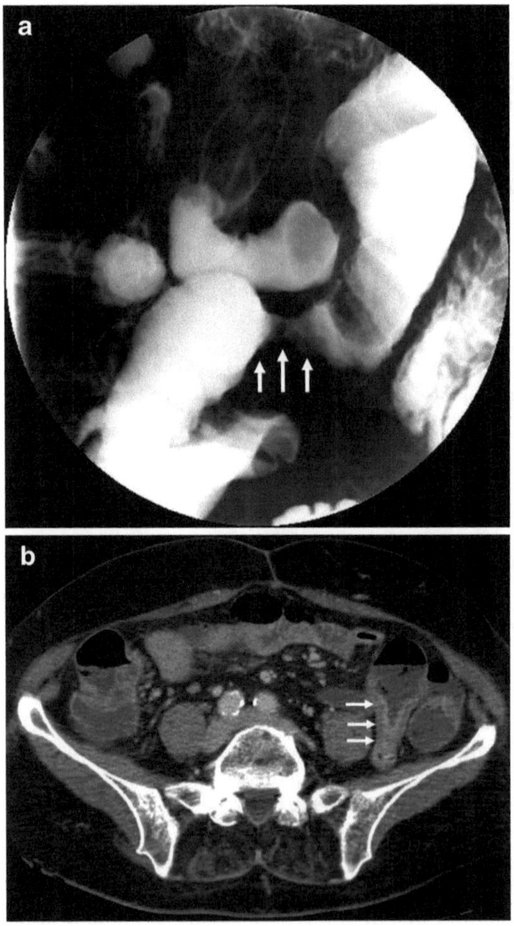

Fig. 7.14 (**a**,**b**) Radiation enteropathy. Elderly female 10 years following radiotherapy for endometrial cancer with intermittent abdominal colic. (**a**) Short-tapered stricture with irregular ulcerated mucosa at barium enteroclysis (*arrows*). (**b**) CT on later admission with small bowel obstruction confirms focal wall thickening (*arrows*) and proximal dilatation from radiation-induced stricture, later resected

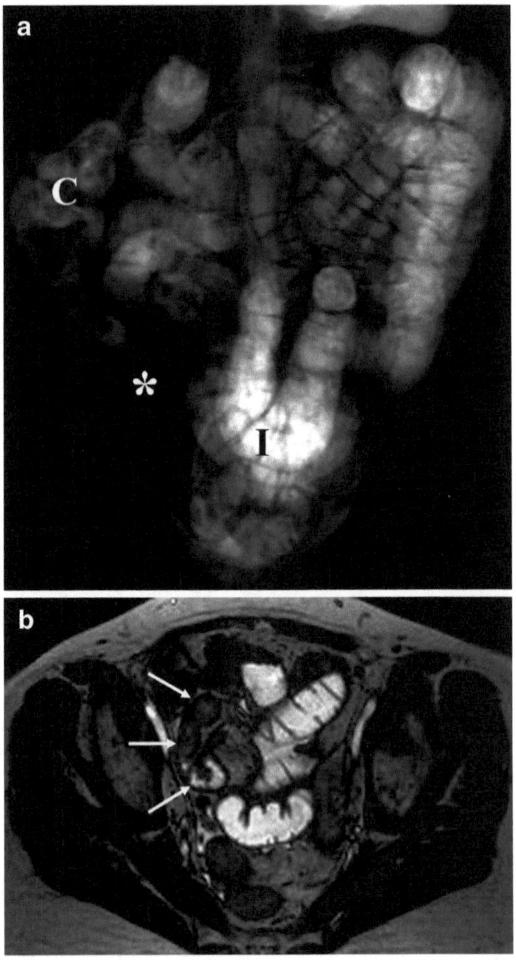

Fig. 7.15 (**a**,**b**) Radiation enteropathy. MR enteroclysis in a patient following chemoradiotherapy for cervical carcinoma with recurrent abdominal pain. Initial thick slab T2 shows nonfilling of bowel in the right iliac fossa (*) despite filling of ileum (*I*) and colon (*C*). Axial FISP shows persistent collapse of a 5-cm segment of ileum resulting from radiation-induced stricture (*arrows*) requiring resection

(e.g., cervical and prostate carcinoma) may catch pelvic bowel loops within the radiation field. Toxicity is increased with concurrent chemotherapy. A further risk factor is previous abdominal surgery where the presence of adhesions may tether the small bowel within the pelvis. The ileum is the most common site affected due to its predilection to a pelvic position (Addley et al. 2010) (Figs. 7.14 and 7.15). The effects of radiotherapy typically manifest at least 6–12 months after treatment resulting in endarteritis obliterans producing a vasculitic effect on the bowel. The resultant initial mural and mucosal inflammation proceeds to fibrosis and stricture formation. Patients may present with obstructive symptoms or failure to thrive secondary to malabsorption, particularly where a long segment of small bowel is affected.

The diagnosis can be very difficult to make without an accompanying history but may be suggested by disease conforming to a clearly demarcated radiation field also affecting adjacent organs (e.g., bladder or rectum) (Fig. 7.16). The specific imaging findings are difficult to differentiate from Crohn's disease with formation of deep ulcers, fistulas to skin or adjacent

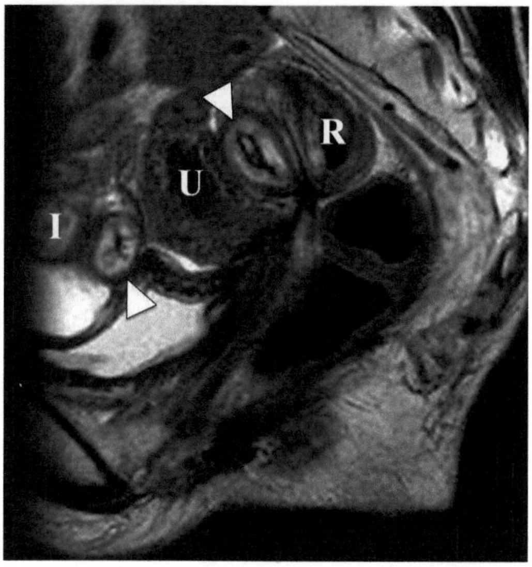

Fig. 7.16 Radiation enteropathy. Patient with abdominal pain and diarrhea 9 months after completion of chemoradiotherapy for cervical cancer. Uterus (*U*). Sagittal T2 HASTE MRI sequence shows wall thickening and high-signal submucosal edema (*arrowheads*) within pelvic ileal loops (*I*) and the upper third of the rectum (*R*). This is within the radiation field indicating radiation enterocolitis

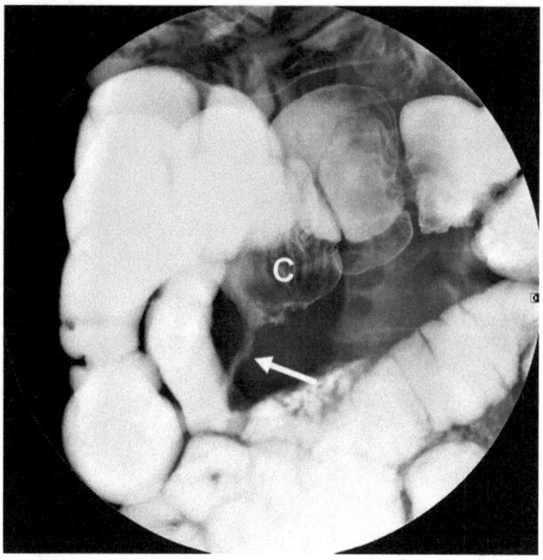

Fig. 7.17 Recurrent Crohn's disease on barium follow through supplemented with pneumocolon 12 months following ileocolic resection. The neoterminal ileum is strictured (*arrow*) with diffuse ulceration. Colon (*C*)

organs and transmural thickening. Despite these difficulties, radiologists are often the first to suggest the diagnosis.

7.3.4.7 Complications Specific to Surgery for Crohn's Disease

Postoperative patients with Crohn's disease represent a challenging group for radiologists to investigate, as the clinical picture overlaps with non-Crohn's disease-related complications. Traditionally, barium follow through examinations have been the mainstay for assessment of small bowel for recurrent Crohn's disease (Fig. 7.17). However, more recently, enterography and enteroclysis using CT or MRI have been used because of their ability to identify disease activity by detecting wall thickening and hyperenhancement while using multiplanar assessment to overcome problems with overlapping loops. An additional advantage is the detection of extraluminal complications including fistula formation and abscess as well as other markers of disease activity such as increased vascularity of the vasa recta, enhancing lymphadenopathy and fibrofatty proliferation of the mesentery (Tolan et al. 2010).

MRI allows assessment of the bowel without radiation, which is an important consideration in this patient group that often undergoes repeated high-dose radiation imaging with CT. In addition to multisequence assessment to determine the presence of inflammatory edema and enhancement pattern, it allows potential for functional assessment of strictures utilizing cine imaging (Fig. 7.18). However, 24-h access to MRI is often limited, which is relevant in the acute setting, whereas CT is more widely available and allows more rapid image acquisition and higher image resolution for multiplanar reformation with similar results with respect to detecting Crohn's disease-related strictures (Schreyer et al. 2010).

Fistulas may form between adjacent loops of large or small bowel, the urogenital organs, or the skin. They may reflect progression of the disease process or the sequelae of anastomotic leakage. Small bowel contrast studies can demonstrate the tract (Fig. 7.19a). combined with fistulography (via direct contrast injection down the tract). On CT, the tract may be seen outlined by oral contrast material or, more often, a soft tissue density tract can be identified

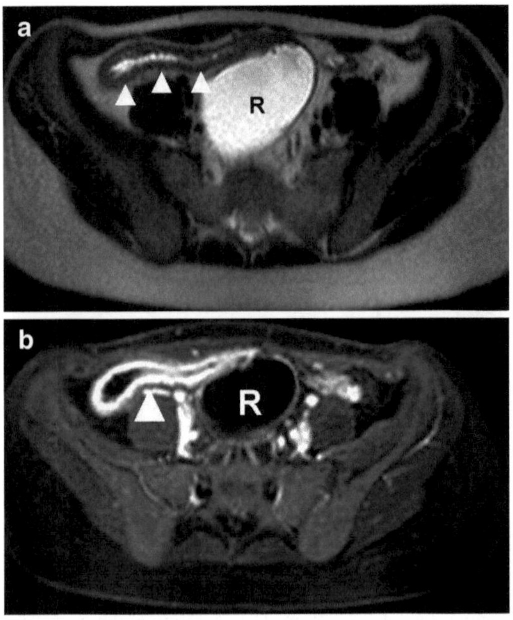

Fig. 7.18 (**a**,**b**) MR confirming recurrent Crohn's disease at the ileorectal anastomosis following subtotal colectomy. (**a**) Axial T2-weighted sequence shows wall and fold thickening (*arrowheads*). (**b**) Axial T1 fat-saturated post gadolinium demonstrates diffuse enhancement (*arrowhead*) indicating active disease with rectal sparing (*R*)

between adjacent structures, which may or may not contain gas (Fig. 7.19b). MRI may also detect fistulas because of its superior contrast resolution seen as either a high-signal tract on T2-weighted sequences or an enhancing linear structure on post gadolinium fat-saturated T1-weighted sequences.

7.3.4.8 Short Gut Syndrome

Short gut syndrome is due to inadequate residual small bowel following resection of a significant proportion (approximately two thirds). It can also occur following a small bowel bypass procedure. The symptoms of short gut syndrome are due to malabsorption (Lappas 2003) with diarrhea, abdominal pain, and steatorrhea along with associated vitamin and trace element deficiencies. The creation of a gastroileostomy or jejunoileal bypass may be intentional, during bariatric surgery, or accidental. Bariatric surgery of this type is no longer performed due to excessive protein and calorie malabsorption (Scheirey et al. 2006).

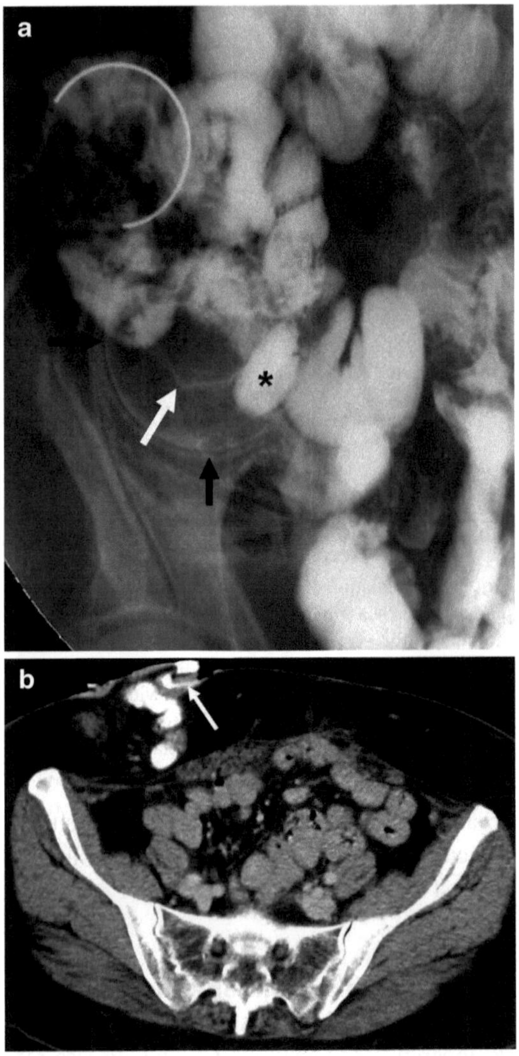

Fig. 7.19 (**a**,**b**) Recurrent peristomal fistulating Crohn's disease after panproctocolectomy and end ileostomy with pain around the stoma. Follow through examination demonstrates a small linear fistula (*white arrow*) tract near the stoma site (*asterisk*) (*black arrows* denotes stoma bag). (**b**) Fistula location confirmed on CT (*arrow*)

The diagnosis is usually apparent on follow-through barium studies in patients with an appropriate surgical history. In patients with a jejunal bypass, CT may show multiple unopacified loops of mid small bowel with oral contrast within the proximal small bowel and right colon only (Sandrasegaran and Maglinte 2005). These appearances may also be seen in patients with small bowel fistulas in active Crohn's disease. In a process called intestinal adaptation, physiological changes to the remaining small bowel occur to increase its absorptive capacity (resulting in dilatation and fold hypertrophy to increase absorptive area). It should be remembered that dilatation in patients with short gut is not necessarily a result of obstruction. Treatment options include parenteral nutrition and small bowel transplantation.

7.3.5 Teaching Points

- Small bowel operations include primary resection for pathology or use for conduits in other operations.
- Adhesions are the most common cause of SBO.
- Distinguishing small bowel ileus from obstruction can be difficult.

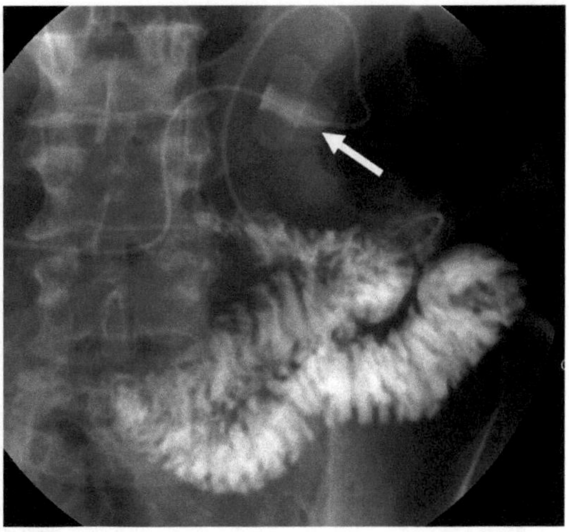

Fig. 7.20 Feeding jejunostomy. Normal tubogram with contrast filling the proximal jejunum with no leak. Fixation device to the anterior abdominal wall (*arrow*)

7.4 Feeding Jejunostomy

This refers to the placement of a tube into the jejunum to allow direct enteral feeding. It is indicated in patients with gastroduodenal obstruction or if there is contraindication to gastrostomy placement, e.g., intrathoracic stomach or gastric malignancy.

7.4.1 Surgical Technique

Operative summary – feeding jejunostomy:

- Feeding tube inserted through the skin and abdominal wall.
- Tube then inserted through jejunal wall into bowel lumen and then secured to the anterior abdominal wall.
- This can be performed via a percutaneous, open, or laparoscopic approach.

7.4.2 Postoperative Complications

Complications associated with feeding jejunostomy placement include leakage, malpositioning, enterogastric reflux, coiling, kinking, and rarely intussusception (Lappas 2003). General complications such as small bowel ileus or abscess formation may occur but are rare. Fluoroscopic retrograde infusion of water-soluble contrast is usually performed. With a correctly sited jejunostomy, the infused contrast outlines the proximal jejunum with rapid distal drainage. No extraluminal contrast should be seen (Fig. 7.20).

7.4.2.1 Tube Site Infection and Leak

Jejunostomy tube site infection is a clinical diagnosis characterized by erythema and pain around the tube site. Occasionally, ultrasound is utilized to diagnose and treat an associated superficial collection. Tube site leakage occurs when small bowel contents or feed leaks around the jejunostomy tube either into the peritoneal cavity or along the tract site. A contrast study through the jejunostomy tube will demonstrate the leak (Fig. 7.21). CT is less commonly performed but may be requested in the unwell patient with peritonitis. Excessive free intra-abdominal fluid and gas are the clues to the diagnosis, which can be confirmed by on-table injection of oral contrast into the jejunostomy tube.

7.4.2.2 Tube Occlusion

Radiology is rarely helpful in confirming tube occlusion, as contrast injection is not usually

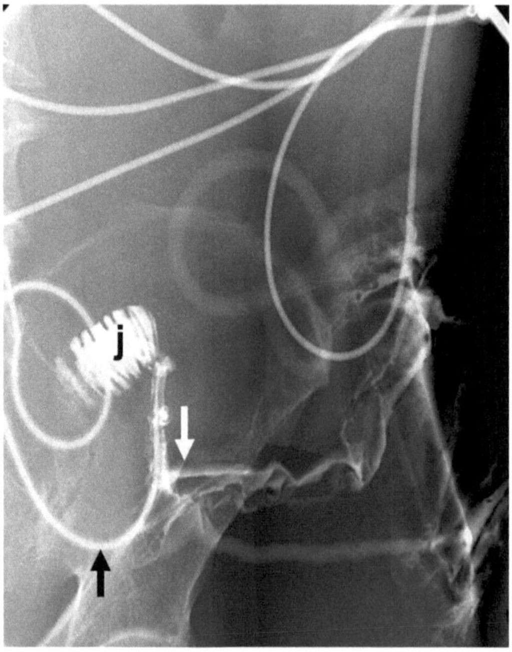

Fig. 7.21 Feeding jejunostomy leak. Tubogram shows leaking around the contrast-filled tube (*black arrow*), which is within the jejunum (*j*), retrogradely onto the skin surface (*white arrow*)

possible. When attempting a tube flush, it is important to use a small-volume syringe since this allows a higher injection pressure to be generated. Occasionally, an attempted passage of a wire may dislodge the object causing the blockage, which is typically congealed feed resulting from inadequate flushing after enteral nutrition infusion.

7.4.2.3 Tube Displacement

The tube may become completely displaced from the bowel lumen. A tubogram will outline small bowel loops with no contrast seen within the bowel lumen if inadequate time has passed for a fistula tract to form (typically at least 2–3 weeks is required for a tract to form). Where contrast is seen filling bowel loops, but the catheter is not within the lumen, it may be possible to manipulate the tube using a wire back into an intraluminal position. In some situations, it may be necessary to exchange the tube (particularly where it has a subcutaneous cuff as a retention device that has proven inadequate) for a small retention balloon catheter. Where possible, a dedicated feeding tube should be used, as urinary catheters may quickly degrade once enteral feeding is commenced.

7.5 Postoperative Abdominal Hernias

A hernia is a protrusion of viscera, omentum, or fat through the wall of the cavity in which it is normally contained. A detailed discussion of the most common anatomical hernias is beyond the scope of this chapter. The most common hernias in the postoperative setting are laparoscopic port site and incisional hernias (see Sect. 1.7). This section will discuss hernias occurring in the postoperative patient and general complications of hernia repair.

7.5.1 Hernia Repair

Small hernia defects can be repaired with sutures but most postoperative hernias require repair using a mesh. This significantly reduces the risk of recurrence but involves implantation of a foreign body, which increases the risk of infection, seroma, and hematoma formation. There are three positions for mesh placement: onlay, sublay, and inlay (Fig. 7.22).

7.5.1.1 Onlay Mesh

The hernia defect is identified and the sac is reduced into the abdominal cavity. The defect is usually sutured closed and a mesh is placed overlying the anterior rectus sheath. The mesh is then secured in place with sutures or staples.

7.5.1.2 Sublay (Underlay) Mesh

The hernia defect is again visualized and the sac reduced. In this technique, a space is created using a combination of blunt and sharp dissection in the extraperitoneal space. A mesh is then placed in this space and anchored with sutures or staples. Care needs to be taken to ensure that the underlying

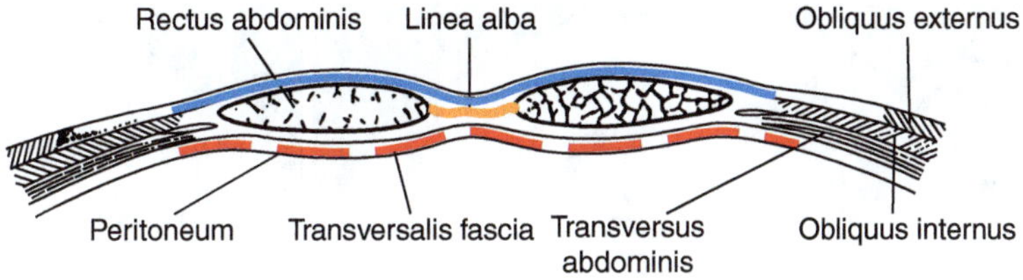

Fig. 7.22 Mesh placement. Illustration showing onlay (*blue line*), sublay (*red dotted line*), and inlay (*orange line*) placement of mesh during hernia repair

peritoneum is not breached as this can lead to herniation of a loop of bowel from the abdominal cavity into the extraperitoneal space resulting to bowel obstruction. Another technique of sublay mesh placement is a retrorectus placement, which places the mesh in the space between the rectus muscle and the posterior aponeurosis of the rectus sheath. This is only possible above the arcuate line (the midpoint between the umbilicus and the pubic bone) since there is no posterior abdominal wall muscle aponeurosis below this point.

7.5.1.3 Inlay Mesh

This technique is not often used as it has a high recurrence rate. In this procedure, the mesh is sutured to the edges of the hernia defect after reduction of the sac.

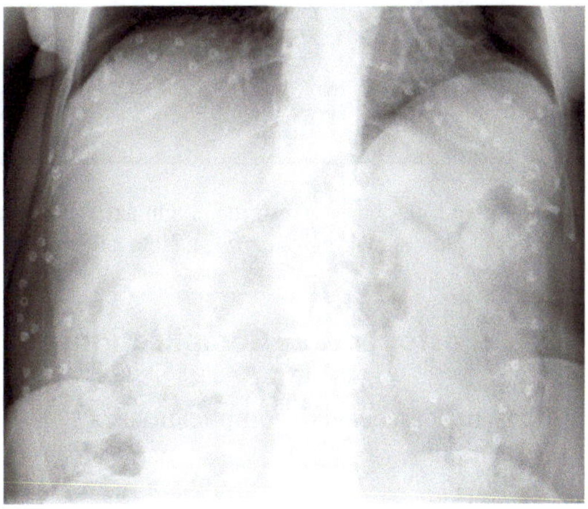

Fig. 7.23 Abdominal X-ray following extensive abdominal wall hernia repair with a multitude of clips outlining the boundaries of the mesh

7.5.2 Surgical Technique

Hernias are repaired by an open or laparoscopic approach. The laparoscopic technique for the repair of ventral/incisional hernias usually involves an intraperitoneal onlay mesh (IPOM) placement. This requires the use of specially engineered meshes that discourage bowel from sticking to the mesh material, and these can be placed directly on the peritoneal surface and secured in place usually with staples or absorbable tacks. These meshes are relatively expensive and usually only used in the laparoscopic approach to ventral hernia repair where it is difficult to create an extraperitoneal space with laparoscopic instruments.

It is, however, relatively easy to create an extraperitoneal space in the groin and thus avoid contact of mesh and bowel. There are two methods of creating an extraperitoneal space in the groin during hernia repair: totally extraperitoneal (TEP) and transabdominal preperitoneal (TAPP). In the TEP technique, the peritoneal cavity is not entered and all the dissection is performed within the extraperitoneal space. The laparoscope is inserted into the peritoneal cavity during the TAPP technique and then an incision is made in the peritoneum to access the extraperitoneal space. Following mesh insertion, the peritoneum is closed with sutures or staples.

7.5.3 Postoperative Imaging

The clips used to secure the mesh to the abdominal wall are often easily identified on plain radiographs which show the extent of the repair (Fig. 7.23). The mesh may be seen as a thin line on CT (Aguirre et al. 2005) and MRI (Fig. 7.24) but is often difficult to appreciate, particularly when there is no accompanying history to indicate its presence.

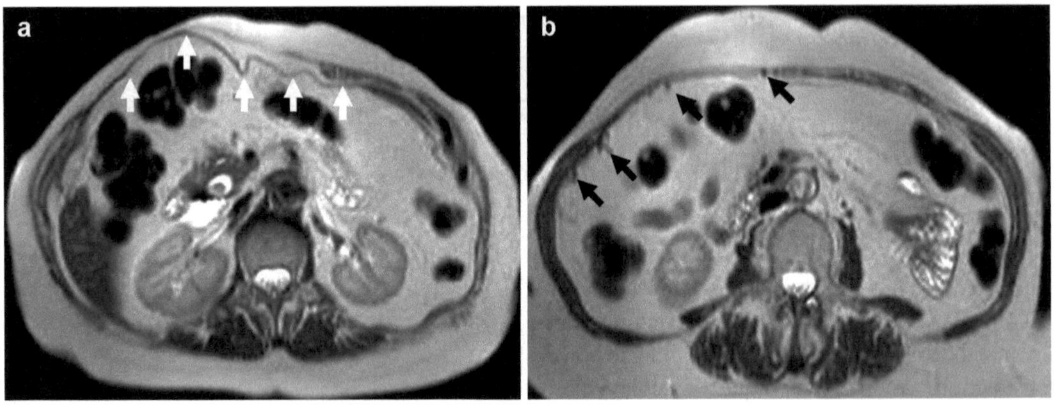

Fig. 7.24 (**a**,**b**) Extensive mesh repair. On axial T2-weighted MRI, the mesh is a thin low-signal line (*white arrows*) and clips are low signal (*black arrows*). Note gallstone in the CBD

7.5.4 Postoperative Complications

Meshes and associated complications are also discussed in Sect. 1.4.2.2.

7.5.4.1 Bleeding

Bleeding following hernia repair may lead to hematoma or seroma formation around the mesh. This may be identified and drained either with ultrasound or with CT if the hematoma becomes infected but usually spontaneously resorbs over time.

7.5.4.2 Mesh Infection

This may arise de novo or within a hematoma related to the repair. Imaging may be normal or show a collection surrounding the mesh. The presence of gas within a collection or adjacent to the mesh is highly suggestive of infection.

7.5.4.3 Testicular Atrophy

The testicular vessels may be damaged during inguinal hernia repair. The atrophic testis will be smaller with reduced flow on ultrasound examination.

7.5.5 Incisional Hernia

This is one of the most common long-term complications following any abdominal operation and occurs following small abdominal incisions. It is important to appreciate the most common incision sites during abdominal surgery in order to be aware of potential sites of herniation.

Common abdominal wall incisions are illustrated in Fig. 7.25:

A. Midline (linea alba) incision
B. Paramedian (rectus) incision
C. Subcostal incision
D. Roof-top incision
E. McBurney's incision
F. Grid iron (right side) and Pfannenstiel's (lower abdominal)
G. Thoracoabdominal (lateral)
H. Extended midline for thoracic access
I. Paramedian (rectus) incision with muscle splitting
J. Pararectus incision
K. "Hockey stick" (thoracoabdominal) incision

7.5.6 Richter's Hernia

In a Richter's hernia, the antimesenteric border of the bowel wall herniates through a fascial defect. Although intestinal obstruction does not occur, the involved segment of bowel wall may strangulate and perforate. These are often hard to identify on imaging but knowledge of and scrutiny of the port sites on postoperative CT is essential.

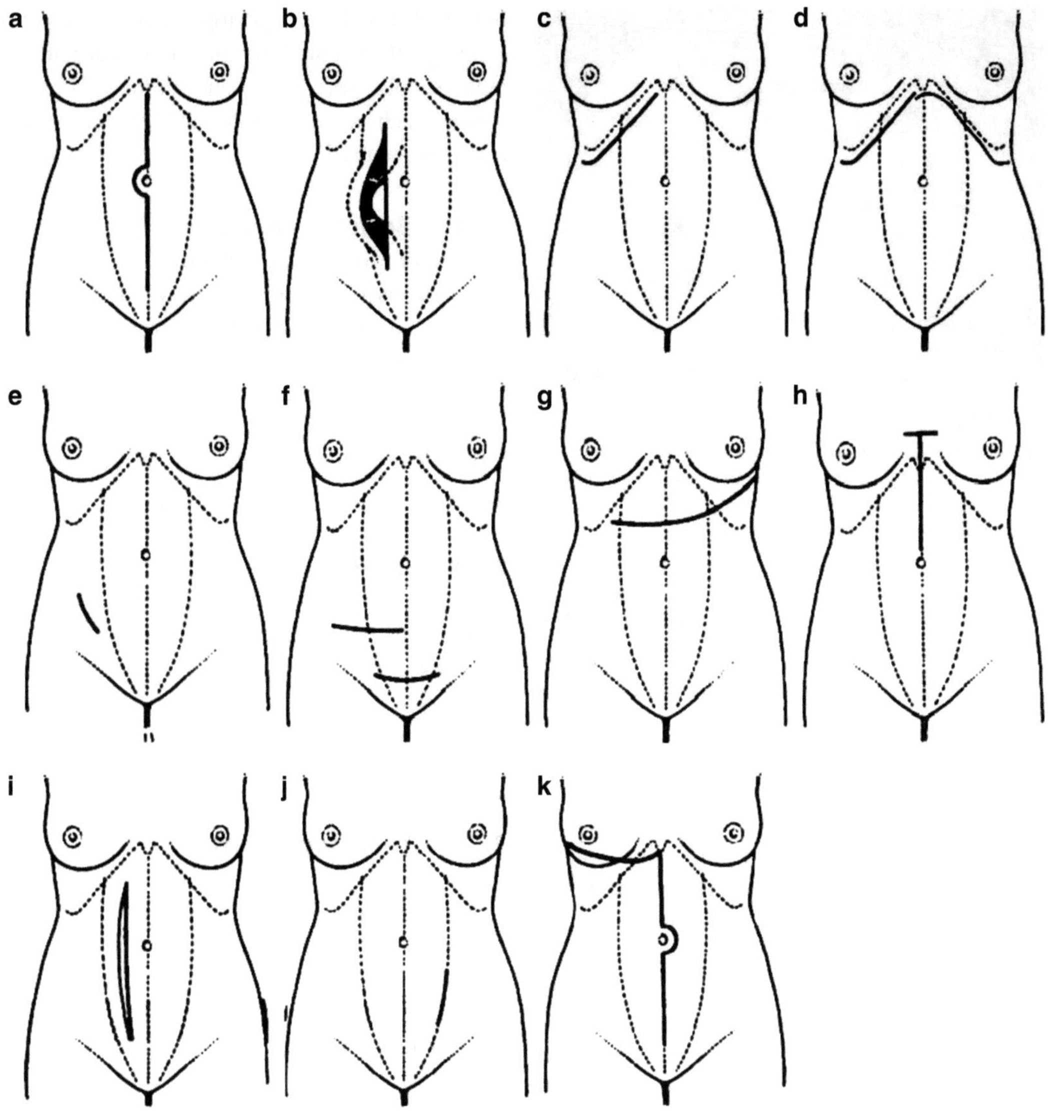

Fig. 7.25 Common abdominal surgical incisions. (**a**) Midline (linea alba) incision, (**b**) paramedian (rectus) incision, (**c**) subcostal incision, (**d**) roof top incision, (**e**) McBurney incision, (**f**) grid iron (right side) and Pfannenstiel (lower abdominal), (**g**) thoracoabdominal (lateral), (**h**) extended mid line for thoracic access, (**i**) paramedian (rectus) incision with muscle splitting, (**j**) pararectus incision and (**k**) "Hockey stick" (thoracoabdominal) incision (*see text*)

7.5.7 Postoperative Internal Hernias

The small bowel may herniate through any defect in the mesentery, such as that created in the transverse mesocolon during the formation of a Roux loop. Following colonic resection, the mesenteric defect is closed, but if this fails, there is potential for small bowel herniation.

The CT appearances are of a closed loop obstruction (Sect. 7.2.2.3).

Specific signs related to a defect in the transverse mesocolon include:

- Loops of dilated small bowel anterior to the stomach
- Downward displacement of the transverse mesocolon

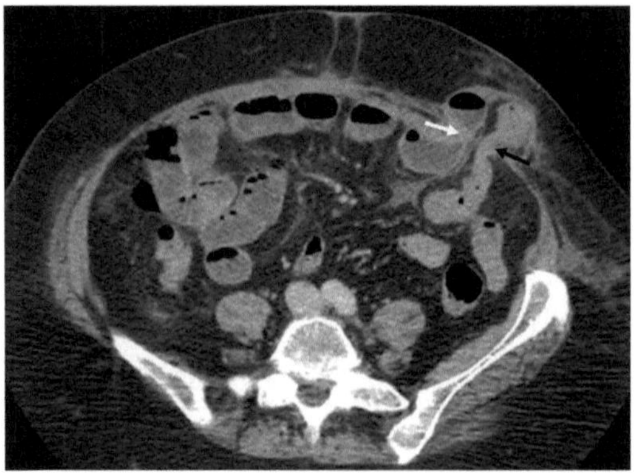

Fig. 7.26 SBO due to a small parastomal incisional hernia. Axial CT shows SBO with a transition point as the afferent ileal loop passes through the anterior abdominal wall (*white arrow*) just inferior to an end colostomy. The efferent ileal loop is collapsed (*black arrow*)

- Mesenteric vascular abnormities in the region of the stomach and transverse mesocolon (Sandrasegaran et al. 2004)

It is very important to recognize the difference between a "typical" postoperative bowel obstruction caused by adhesions and an internal hernia. The main distinguishing feature on CT is the abnormal, unusual clustering of bowel loops, resulting from them passing through the narrow mesenteric defect, which forms the neck, and the secondary mass effect of these obstructed bowel loops on adjacent viscera (such as colon, vessels, or omentum). In adhesive obstruction, the bowel is generally dilated down to the point of obstruction and does not tend to produce localized mass effect on structures. While classification of the precise type of internal hernia is less important, the diagnosis of closed loop obstruction has an important bearing on the management of the patient since these are taken for surgical reduction and repair, whereas adhesive obstruction is commonly treated conservatively in the first instance. Therefore, be vigilant of an obstructed postoperative small bowel and ask the question: "Could this be an internal hernia?"

7.5.8 Complications of Hernias

7.5.8.1 Bowel Obstruction

Hernias are one of the most common causes of small bowel obstruction after adhesions (Fig. 7.26). Before diagnosing adhesional small bowel obstruction on postoperative CT, careful scrutiny of potential hernia sites, particularly laparoscopic port sites, and clinically occult regions such as the obturator and femoral hernial canals is required.

7.5.8.2 Bowel Strangulation

This refers to ischemia of bowel or other tissue such as omentum that may have become trapped in the hernia defect resulting in a compromised blood supply. This can be difficult to diagnose with confidence on imaging, and the features are generally those of a closed loop obstruction which has already been discussed.

7.5.8.3 Incarceration

This term is often also used to refer to strangulated or obstructed hernias, but strictly speaking, this describes a hernia where the contents are irreducible. The diagnosis is made on clinical examination rather than with imaging.

7.5.9 Teaching Points

- Hernias are a common cause of SBO in the postoperative patient.
- Careful scrutiny of previous incision, port sites, and hernial orifices should be made in patients with SBO.
- Internal hernias produce closed loop obstruction and should be considered in any small bowel obstruction with unusual features.

7.6 Ileal Pouch-Anal Anastomoses (IPAA or Ileal Anal Pouch)

Ileal pouch-anal anastomosis is an ileal reservoir or pouch constructed following panproctocolectomy and anastomosed to the anus.

Advantages include:

- Avoidance of a permanent stoma
- Preservation of the sphincters and maintenance of continence
- Removal of diseased rectal mucosa and risk of developing recurrent colitis or carcinoma

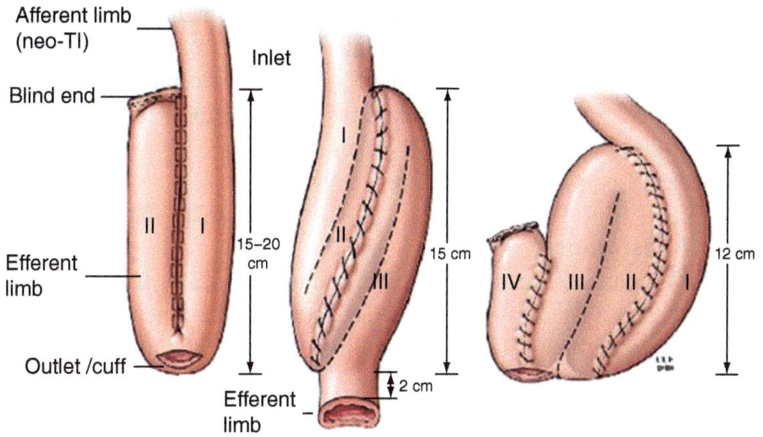

Fig. 7.27 Types of ileal-anal pouch (J, S, and W)

7.6.1 Clinical Indication

Patients with chronic ulcerative colitis and familial polyposis coli (increased risk of developing colorectal carcinoma).

7.6.2 Surgical Technique and Postoperative Anatomy

Ileal pouch-anal anastomosis (IPAA) can be performed in a number of stages:

- 1 stage
  - (i) Total abdominal colectomy and creation of an ileal reservoir without defunctioning ileostomy.
- 2 stage
  - (i) Total abdominal colectomy and creation of an ileal reservoir with defunctioning ileostomy.
  - (ii) Reversal of the loop ileostomy 2–3 months later. Pouch integrity is usually checked with a retrograde pouch study in combination with E.U.A. at the time of closure and, in some units, pouchoscopy.
- 3 stage
  - (i) Subtotal abdominal colectomy (sparing rectum) is often formed in the acute setting such as fulminant colitis, perforation, or toxic dilatation due to the high morbidity and mortality from acute proctectomy. This is also performed in patients on high doses of steroids or immunosuppression, which increase the risks of pouch complications following colectomy. It is also sometimes performed to conserve fertility in females.
  - (ii) Proctectomy and creation of an ileal reservoir with defunctioning ileostomy.
  - (iii) Reversal of the loop ileostomy commonly 2–3 months later.

7.6.2.1 Pouch Construct

There are a number of different ways in which pouches are formed. The principles are to create a pouch of reasonable volume while accepting that each suture line runs risks of complications. The number of times the small bowel is "looped" has given rise to the J, S, and W formations (Fig. 7.27).

- The S-pouch is uncommonly used because of functional problems which often requires the need to self-catheterize.
- There are theoretical advantages of a W-pouch with regard to volume, but this has not been found to confer significant advantage over the J-pouch in practice.
- The most common pouch operation forms a J-pouch which is the easiest and quickest to construct. This is formed by folding two 15–25 cm limbs of the terminal ileum with a linear stapler and anastomosing it to the anus with a side-to-end anastomosis.

- S- and W-pouches have end-to-end anastomoses, are globular, and have an efferent limb. This produces a short length of small bowel joining the pouch to the anus. In a J-pouch construct, the pouch is directly anastomosed to the anus. The S-, W-, and J-pouches all have afferent limbs.

7.6.2.2 Anastomosis

- IPAA is accomplished either through a double-stapled or a hand-sewn method. The latter takes longer and is technically more difficult and cannot be visualized radiologically.

7.6.2.3 Alternative Surgical Procedures

- Total proctocolectomy with end ileostomy – patients have a permanent ileostomy.
- Kock pouch (continent ileostomy) stoma – requires regular reservoir catheterization but avoids the requirement to wear a stoma bag. It has a valve mechanism on the inside to preserve continence.

7.6.2.4 Background

IPAA is indicated for patients with chronic ulcerative colitis of the colon and in familial adenomatous polyposis (FAP).

Contraindications include:

- Presence of mesenteric desmoid tumor which may form in patients with FAP and Gardner's syndrome and can interfere with pouch construct and function.
- Patients with Crohn's disease because of the high risk of recurrent disease in the small bowel and perineum. Some centers advocate IPAA for Crohn's colitis with concomitant prophylactic infliximab treatment, but this is experimental.

Occasionally, preoperative differentiation between Crohn's disease and UC is not possible. IPAA may be performed in indeterminate colitis although it is associated with a higher failure rate and perineal complications postoperatively. Ileorectal anastomosis in FAP is associated with a risk of developing carcinoma in the rectal mucosa and requires surveillance for rectal polyps. This is a good alternative in young people who usually have relative rectal sparing although proctectomy is usual required within 10–15 years. Mucosectomy removes the residual rectal epithelium as a cuff of anorectal mucosa. This is at risk of developing carcinoma in FAP or "cuffitis" in ulcerative colitis. This operation is infrequently performed because of poor functional results.

7.6.3 Normal Postoperative Imaging

7.6.3.1 GI Contrast Studies

Assessment of the pouch is usually performed at 2–3 months with a 14 F or larger Foley balloon catheter (Alfisher et al. 1997). Patients usually undergo digital and proctoscopic examination prior to the contrast study. The retrograde pouch examination may be performed with either water-soluble contrast or barium although barium studies are usually avoided because of the small risk of barium peritonitis if a leak is present.

It is important to ensure that control films in two orthogonal planes are performed prior to contrast administration so that staple lines are not misinterpreted as subtle leaks. After this, lateral, AP, and oblique views of the pouch are performed to view the pouch-anal anastomosis (Fig. 7.28) and to detect clinically occult leaks.

The J-pouch has two raphes or ridges corresponding to the anastomosis and has an appendage posteriorly called the J-pouch appendage, which is due to a small amount of closed reflected ileum not incorporated into the reservoir. The length of the J-pouch appendage can vary but should not be mistaken for a leak (Fig. 7.29). The S-pouch is more globular, has a greater volume, and occupies a higher position in the pelvis.

Pouch volume increases with time and the average volume is approximately 400 ml. There is a marked variation in the degree of emptying. As the ileum adapts as a neorectum, it develops indentations similar to normal rectal valves. However, in a typical postoperative study, this remodeling will not have occurred and a more typical ileal pattern of folds will be observed. It is also usual for contrast within the defunctioned pouch to trigger active peristalsis in the pouch and the efferent defunctioned limb of ileum downstream from the ileostomy, and contrast will usually flow proximally to fill the ileostomy stoma bag that is normally positioned in the right iliac fossa.

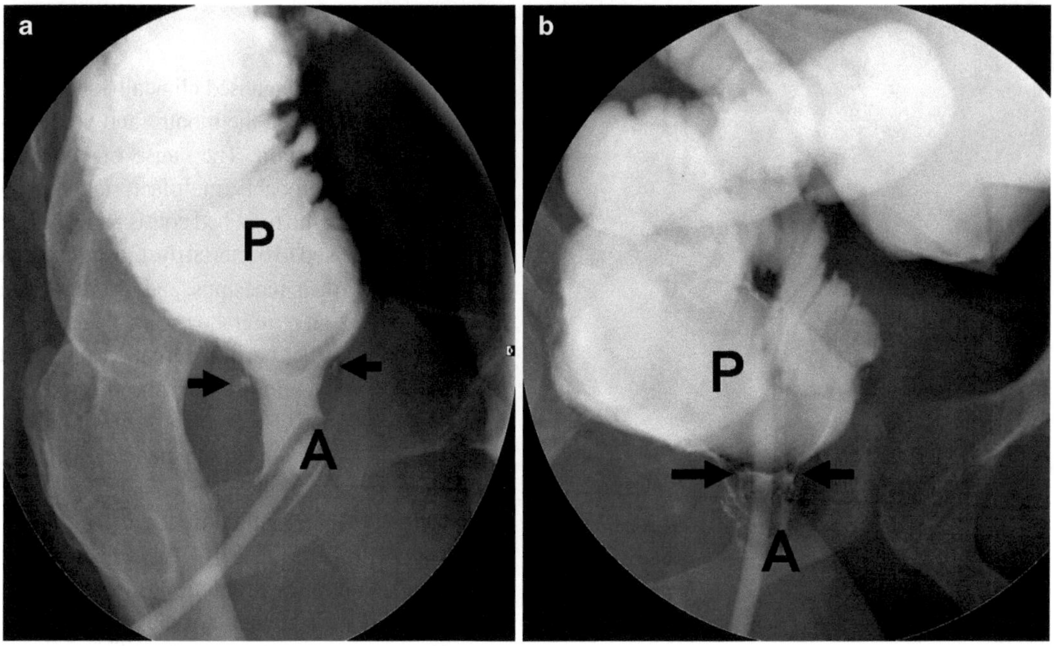

Fig. 7.28 (**a**,**b**) Two examples of normal pouch-anal anastomosis. Gastrografin studies following pouch construct post total colectomy for ulcerative colitis. Pouch (*P*), anus (*A*), staple line (*arrows*). Note the longer redundant blind loop in (**b**)

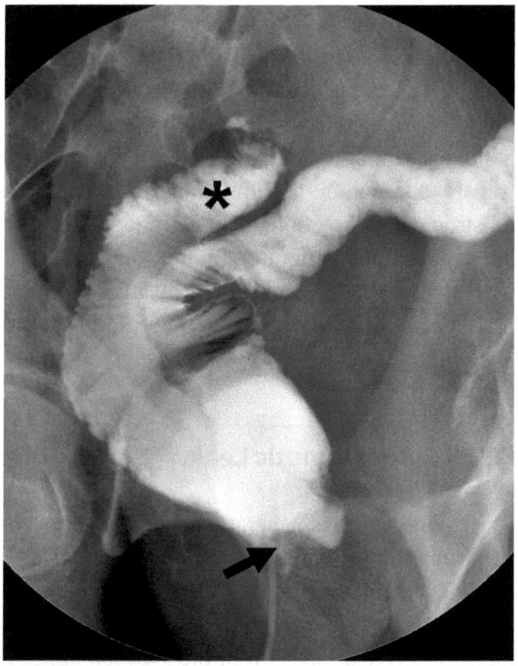

Fig. 7.29 J Pouch. Normal gastrografin enema prior to ileostomy closure shows the pouch-anal anastomosis (*arrow*) and long J-pouch appendage (*asterisk*)

7.6.3.2 CT

CT is indicated when a pelvic abscess is suspected. It can be performed with positive oral contrast alone (Fig. 7.30) or with oral and rectal contrast; the latter is administered via a flexible Foley catheter. The presence of a gas or fluid collection should be evaluated along with its relationship to the wall of the pouch, and an appraisal of whether image-guided intervention may be appropriate to deal with the sepsis (Broder et al. 2010).

7.7 Postoperative Complications

7.7.1 Small Bowel Obstruction (SBO)

SBO is the most common recognized complication following IPAA pouch formation. It can occur either before or after loop ileostomy closure. The most common site of obstruction is at the ileostomy closure site or the small bowel distal to it, i.e., adjacent to the pouch. Obstruction is due to adhesions, stricture, or small bowel volvulus

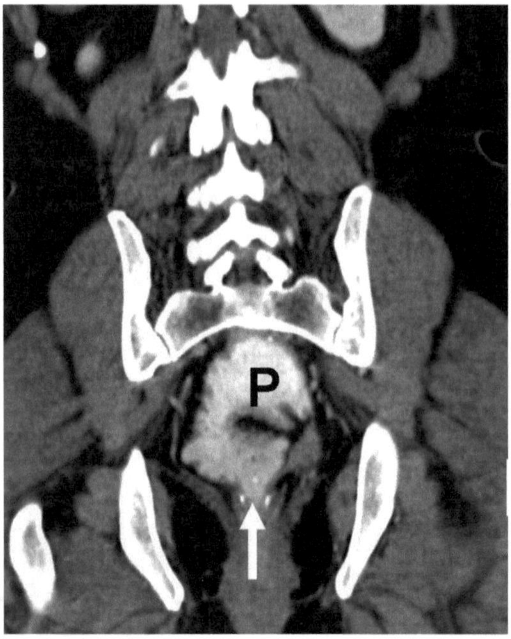

Fig. 7.30 Coronal CT of a J-pouch (*P*). Pouch-anal anastomosis indicated (*arrow*)

(caused by inadvertent torsion to the pouch prior to surgical anastomosis).

7.7.2 Pouch-Related Sepsis

In the first few weeks of the postoperative period, effluent can build up within a defunctioned pouch due to secretions or overflow from the loop ileostomy. Patients present nonspecifically unwell with low-grade pyrexia and occasionally raised inflammatory markers. Cross-sectional imaging is often requested to assess for a delayed presentation of anastomotic leak. Imaging will show a dilated fluid-filled pouch (which should not occur as the patient has been defunctioned with a proximal loop ileostomy). CT may also show wall thickening and mural enhancement. Interestingly, patients do not have an urge to empty the pouch. Management involves draining the pouch with a Foley catheter, which usually yields foul-smelling bowel contents (and sometimes pus) with a rapid improvement of patient symptoms.

7.7.3 Pouchitis

Pouchitis is usually diagnosed clinically and endoscopically and occurs in the months and years following pouch formation. The cause of pouchitis is unclear and is probably multifactorial. It only occurs in patients who have had colitis and not FAP and, in part, is related to bacterial dysbiosis. Patients present with diarrhea, tenesmus, and bleeding. The imaging findings on retrograde contrast studies are generally nonspecific, but inflammation may lead to loss of the normal fold pattern in the affected segment. Pelvic MR and CT can exclude pelvic collections while also demonstrating pouch dilatation, wall thickening, mucosal enhancement (Fig. 7.31), peripouch stranding, or fluid and reactive lymphadenopathy (Broder et al. 2010). Treatment is principally with antibiotics, probiotics, or novel agents (e.g., bile salt sequestrants, arsenic suppositories, etc.). However, intractable pouchitis may require pouch excision and end ileostomy.

7.7.4 Anastomotic Stricture

This occurs at the ileoanal anastomosis and is usually diagnosed during digital examination. It can be a consequence of a postoperative leak and may be treated with dilatation. Occasionally, patients with pouchitis present with unexplained sepsis due to an accumulation of pus in an obstructed defunctioned pouch secondary to an anastomotic stricture. In this situation, CT will demonstrate a fluid-filled distended pouch. Patients will rapidly respond to digital rectal decompression.

7.7.5 Anastomotic Leak

Postoperative leaks generally occur at the pouch-anal anastomosis and are referred to as anastomotic separation (Fig. 7.32). Less commonly, leakage occurs from the pouch staple line (Marcello et al. 1993) and rarely from the J-pouch appendage (Fig. 7.33). Most leaks are small and can be managed conservatively providing there are no signs of sepsis. Management options include delay

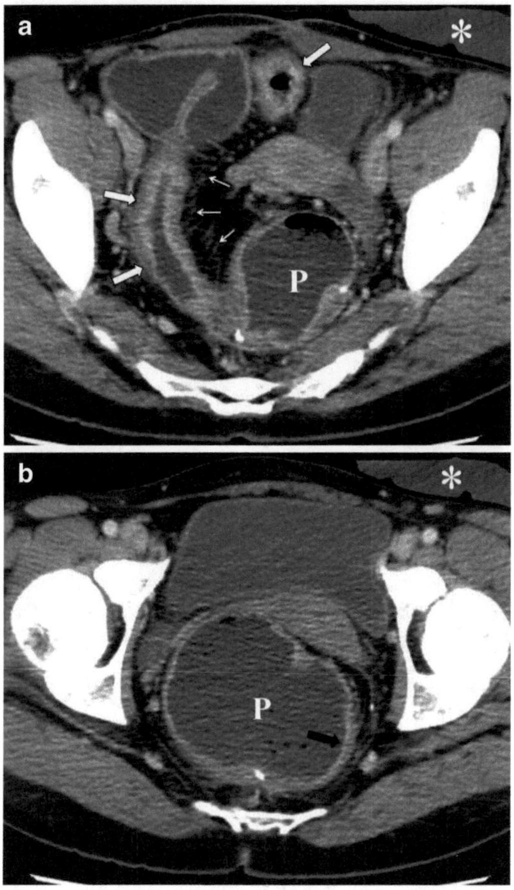

Fig. 7.31 CT to assess abdominal pain and diarrhea 2 years following ileoanal J-pouch (*P*) formation after colectomy for ulcerative colitis – patient remains defunctioned with loop ileostomy. Stoma bag (*). (**a**) The ileum is thickened with marked mucosal enhancement (*thick white arrows*) and injected vasa recta (*thin arrows*). (**b**) The pouch wall is thickened and distended (despite diversion) with mucosal hyperenhancement (*black arrow*) indicating severe pouchitis

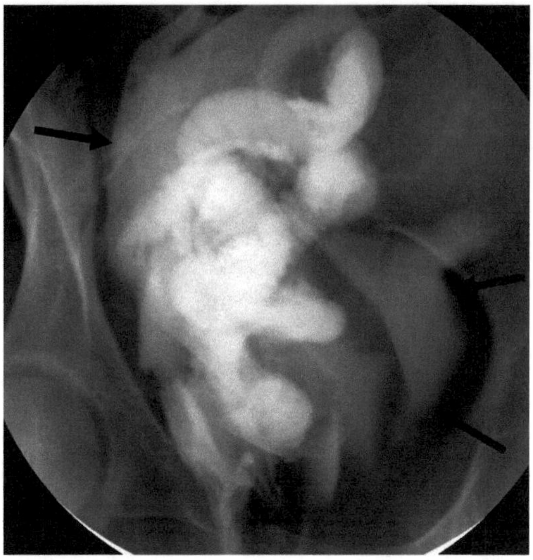

Fig. 7.32 Gross anastomotic breakdown 1 week after pouch formation. Despite some contrast filling the distal ileum, there is free leakage of contrast into the peritoneum (*arrows*)

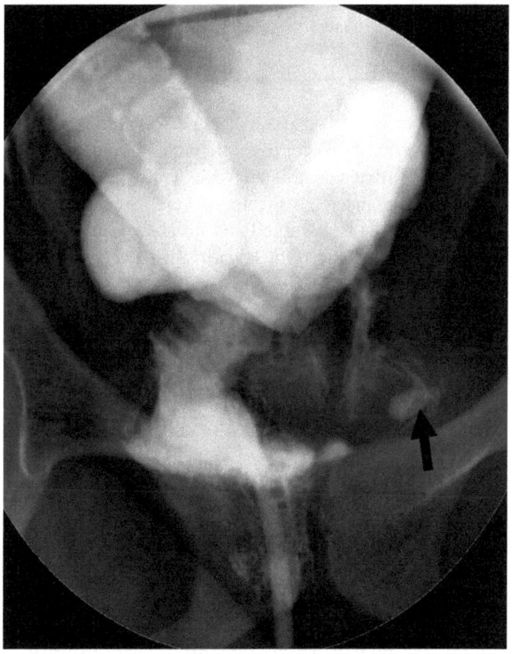

Fig. 7.33 Pouchogram demonstrates a small leak from the blind end of the J-pouch (*arrow*)

of ileostomy closure, fecal diversion if the ileostomy has already been reversed, surgical repair of the defect (Fig. 7.34), and drainage of associated collections (Fig. 7.35). Sizeable collections can be drained via the transgluteal route in order to minimize disruption to the pouch-anal anastomosis.

7.7.6 Pelvic Infection and Abscess

Most cases of pelvic infection occur prior to ileostomy closure and are associated with either pelvic contamination during surgery or pouch leakage. Clinical presentation includes sepsis, postoperative ileus, and pouch discharge. Treatment is with antibiotics, CT-guided drainage, and delay of ileostomy closure (Broder et al. 2010).

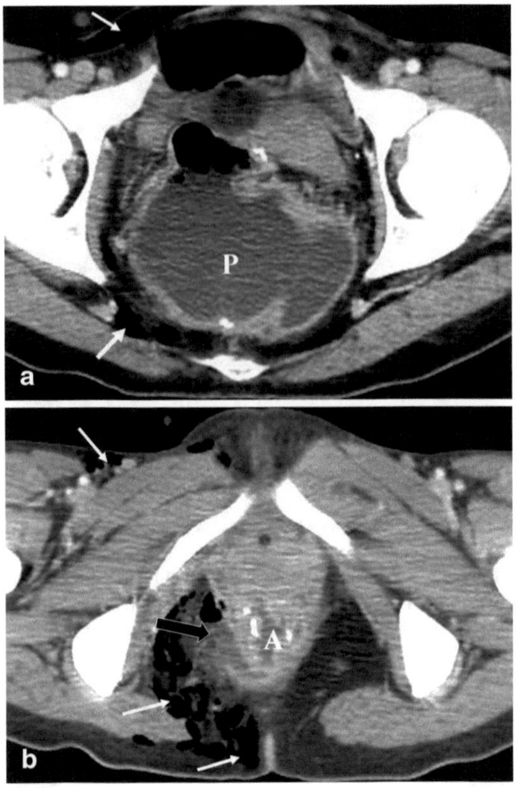

Fig. 7.34 (**a**,**b**) Perianal pain after period of diarrhea following reversal of ileostomy for ileoanal pouch. (**a**) Pouch (*P*) is fluid filled and dilated with wall thickening and increased enhancement from severe pouchitis. (**b**) Anastomosis (*A*) is disrupted and an abscess has formed rupturing through the right levator ani (*black arrow*). A gas-forming infection (*white arrows*) is producing surgical emphysema in the ischioanal fossa and subcutaneous tissues. Extensive debridement and resection of pouch followed

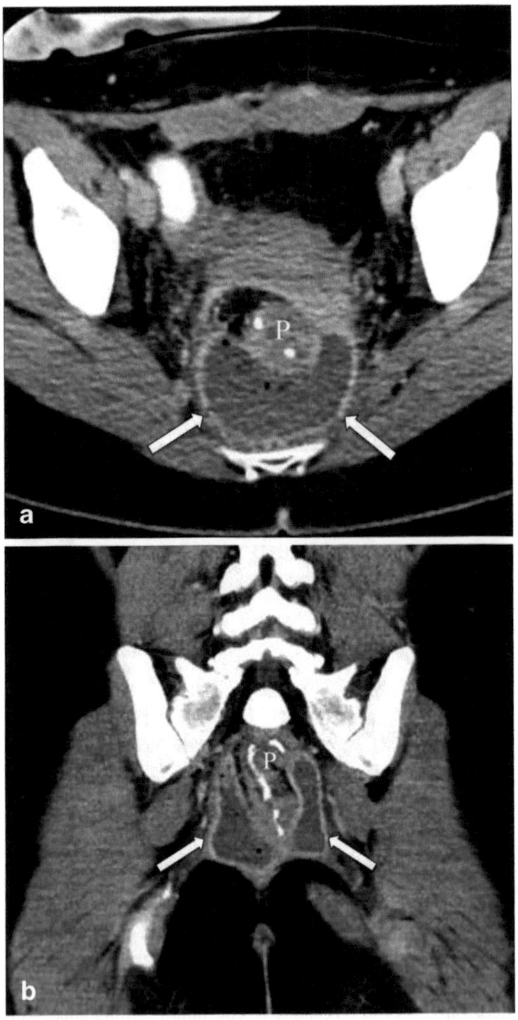

Fig. 7.35 (**a**,**b**) Postoperative sepsis after pouch formation. (**a**) Axial and (**b**) coronal CT shows a rim enhancing abscess (*arrows*) wrapping around the pouch (*P*) requiring transgluteal drainage (*not shown*)

7.7.7 Fistulas

Fistulas can occur between the pouch and anus, bladder, or vagina. This may occur where the pouch has been formed for indeterminate colitis which has later declared itself as Crohn's disease. During contrast studies, it is important to assess the patient in a lateral or prone position as most fistulas are to anterior structures. Management options include delay of ileostomy closure or, if this has already been performed, proximal fecal diversion. Ultimately, pouch excision may be required.

7.7.8 Pouch Outlet Obstruction

This occurs in patients with an S-pouch and is due to the weight of the superiorly placed pouch compressing the long efferent segment. Surgical revision with shortening of the efferent limb is usually performed.

7.7.9 Teaching Points

- IPAA is a reservoir formed from ileum which is anastomosed to the anal canal.

- Clinical indications include ulcerative colitis and familial polyposis coli.
- Sphincter function is preserved. The colon is removed, the chosen pouch formed, and the potential sequelae of pelvic sepsis is mitigated (fecal diversion) with a loop ileostomy which is typically reversed 2–3 months later.
- Retrograde contrast evaluation of the pouch is routinely performed prior to ileostomy closure.
- Most complications are managed conservatively.
- Knowledge of the type of pouch construct is essential for image interpretation.

Acknowledgments We would like to thank Mr. Chris Macklin (Consultant Surgeon, Mid Yorks NHS Trust) for his help with the pouch section of this chapter.

References

Abbas S, Bissett IP, Parry BR. Oral water soluble contrast for the management of adhesive small bowel obstruction. Cochrane Database Syst Rev. 2007;CD004651.

Addley HC, Vargas HA, Moyle PL, Crawford R, Sala E. Pelvic imaging following chemotherapy and radiation therapy for gynecologic malignancies. Radiographics. 2010;30:1843–56.

Aguirre DA, Santosa AC, Casola G, Sirlin CB. Abdominal wall hernias: imaging features, complications, and diagnostic pitfalls at multi-detector row CT. Radiographics. 2005;25:1501–20.

Alfisher MM, Scholz FJ, Roberts Counihan T. Radiology of ileal pouch-anal anastomosis: normal findings, examination pitfalls and complications. Radiographics. 1997;17:81–98.

Bauman R, Pirrello J. Internal hernia at Petersen's space after laparoscopic Roux-en-Y gastric bypass: 6.2% incidence without closure – a single surgeon series of 1047 cases. Surg Obes Relat Dis. 2009;5:565–70.

Broder JC, Tkacz JN, Anderson SW, Soto JA, Gupta A. Ileal pouch-anal anastomosis surgery: imaging and intervention for post-operative complications. Radiographics. 2010;30:221–33.

Catarina A, Pimenta M, Guimardes LS. Small bowel obstruction: what to look for. Radiographics. 2009;29: 423–9.

Frager D, Medwid SW, Baer JW, Mollinelli B, Friedman M. CT of small-bowel obstruction: value in establishing the diagnosis and determining the degree and cause. AJR Am J Roentgenol. 1994;162:37–41.

Kawkabani Marchini A, Denys A, Paroz A, et al. The four different types of internal hernia occurring after laparoscopic Roux-en-Y gastric bypass performed for morbid obesity: are there any multidetector computed tomography (MDCT) features permitting their distinction. Obes Surg. 2011;21(4):506–16.

Lappas J. Imaging of the post surgical small bowel. Radiol Clin North Am. 2003;41:305–26.

Maglinte D, Sandrasegaran K, Lappas J, Chiorean M. CT enteroclysis. Radiology. 2007;245:661–71.

Marcello PW, Roberts PL, Schoetz Jr DJ, Coller JA, Murray JJ, Veidenheimer MC. Long-term results of the ileoanal pouch procedure. Arch Surg. 1993;128(5): 500–4.

Sandrasegaran K, Maglinte D. Imaging of small bowel related complications following major abdominal surgery. Eur J Radiol. 2005;53:374–86.

Sandrasegaran K, Maglinte D, Lappas J, Howard T. Small bowel complications of major gastrointestinal tract surgery. Am J Roentgenol. 2004;185:671–8.

Scheirey C, Scholz F, Shah P, Brams D, Wong B, Pedrosa M. Radiology of the laparoscopic Roux-en-Y gastric bypass procedure. Conceptualization and precise interpretation of the results. Radiographics. 2006;26: 1355–71.

Schreyer AG, Hoffstetter P, Daneschnejad M, et al. Comparison of conventional abdominal CT with MR-enterography in patients with active Crohn's disease and acute abdominal pain. Acad Radiol. 2010;17: 352–7.

Silva AC, Pimenta M, Guimarães LS. Small bowel obstruction: what to look for. Radiographics. 2009;29: 423–39.

Tolan DJ, Greenhalgh R, Zealley IA, Halligan S, Taylor SA. MR enterographic manifestations of small bowel Crohn's disease. Radiographics. 2010;30:367–84.

The Colon

8

Chris Macklin, John Brittenden, David Jayne, and Damian J.M. Tolan

Contents

8.1 Introduction 256

8.2 Colon Resections 256
8.2.1 Clinical Indications 256
8.2.2 Surgical Technique and Postoperative Anatomy 256
8.2.3 Normal Postoperative Imaging 260
8.2.4 Postoperative Complications 261
8.2.5 Teaching Points 268

8.3 Anastomosis 268
8.3.1 Nomenclature 268
8.3.2 Anastomosis Construct 269

8.4 Stomas 269
8.4.1 Ileostomy 270
8.4.2 Colostomy 271
8.4.3 Stoma Complications 271

8.5 Recurrent Rectal Cancer and Pelvic Exenteration 272
8.5.1 Imaging of Recurrent Rectal Cancer 272
8.5.2 Complications of Pelvic Exenteration 275
8.5.3 Teaching Points 276

8.6 Image-Guided Colonic Intervention 276
8.6.1 Colonic Stenting 276
8.6.2 Cecostomy 278
8.6.3 Sigmoidopexy 278

8.7 Surgery for Fistula-in-Ano 279
8.7.1 Background 279
8.7.2 Parks Classification System for Fistula-in-Ano 280
8.7.3 Surgical Techniques for Fistula-in-Ano 280
8.7.4 Postoperative Imaging 281
8.7.5 Postoperative Complications 282
8.7.6 Teaching Points 282

8.8 Surgery for the Pelvic Floor and Defecatory Disorders 282
8.8.1 Clinical Indication 282
8.8.2 Summary of Management for Pelvic Floor Disorders 283
8.8.3 Surgery for Slow Transit Constipation 284
8.8.4 Surgery for Obstructed Defecation: Technique and Postoperative Anatomy 284
8.8.5 Surgery for Full-Thickness Rectal Prolapse: Techniques and Postoperative Anatomy 285
8.8.6 Surgery for Incontinence 286
8.8.7 Postoperative Complications 287
8.8.8 Normal Postoperative Imaging 288
8.8.9 Pitfalls in Postoperative Pelvic Floor Radiological Assessment 289
8.8.10 Teaching Points 291

References 292

C. Macklin, BMedSci, BM, BS, FRCS (Gen Surg), DM
Department of Surgery, Mid Yorkshire Hospitals NHS Trust, Wakefield, UK

J. Brittenden, MBChB, MRCP, FRCR (✉)
Department of Radiology, Mid Yorkshire Hospitals NHS Trust, Wakefield, UK
e-mail: john.brittenden@midyorks.nhs.uk

D. Jayne, BSc, MB, BCh, MD, FRCS
Department of Surgery, St James's University Hospital, Leeds Teaching Hospitals NHS Trust, Leeds, UK

D.J.M. Tolan, MBChB, MRCP, FRCR
Department of Clinical Radiology, Leeds Teaching Hospitals NHS Trust, Lincoln Wing, St James's University Hospital, LS9 7JT, Leeds, UK

J. Brittenden, D.J.M. Tolan (eds.), *Radiology of the Post Surgical Abdomen*, DOI 10.1007/978-1-4471-2775-8_8, © Springer-Verlag London 2012

8.1 Introduction

Historically, the role of the early coloproctologist was to treat the multitude of anorectal conditions with which mankind suffers. The ancient Egyptians as early as 1,700 BC recorded descriptions for treating many diseases with such concoctions as honey and sweet beer enemas. The Greeks however were more "surgical," and Hippocrates wrote famously on the surgical approach to hemorrhoids and fistulas. The transition from simple proctology to abdominal surgery occurred with the diagnosis of appendicitis in Edward VII, immediately prior to his coronation in 1902. The Royal surgeon Frederick Treves drained the appendiceal abscess successfully, and the move to abdominal surgery was made.

There have been numerous technological advancements to aid the modern colorectal surgeon in the treatment of colorectal diseases. Advances in anesthesia, antisepsis, blood transfusion, and surgical instruments have lead to improved surgical outcomes and postoperative survival. Simple instruments and suture materials have been replaced with advanced surgical staplers, modern energy sources (e.g., harmonic scalpel), and laparoscopic techniques, and even robotics have made colorectal surgery one of the most exciting and pioneering specialties. It is now possible to remove the whole colorectum through an incision 3–4 cm in diameter, insert an artificial bowel sphincter, or restore continence with stimulation of the sacral nerves.

Advancements in imaging have been crucial to the preoperative planning and postoperative assessment of colorectal patients, particularly those with colorectal cancer. Colorectal cancer is the third most common malignancy in the UK, and in 2007, there were 38,608 new recorded cases (Cancer Research UK). Cross-sectional imaging determines the preoperative management of rectal cancer with neoadjuvant chemoradiotherapy commonplace prior to surgery and, currently, within the auspices of the FOxTROT trial, is potentially going to have a similar role in colonic cancer. Other emerging modalities such as CT colonography and endoluminal ultrasound are becoming commonplace in the diagnosis of colorectal pathology.

8.2 Colon Resections (Fig. 8.1)

8.2.1 Clinical Indications

For benign and malignant disease involving the colon:

- Carcinoma of the colon
- Diverticular disease
- Inflammatory bowel disease
- Intestinal polyposis

8.2.2 Surgical Technique and Postoperative Anatomy

8.2.2.1 Right Hemicolectomy (RHC) (Fig. 8.1a)

- Resection of the terminal ileum, cecum, and ascending colon. Ligation of the ileocolic and right colic arteries and formation of an ileotransverse colon anastomosis.
- Extended right hemicolectomy involves resection of the above along with the proximal transverse colon (Fig. 8.1a). Occasionally, the resection extends to and includes the splenic flexure with division of the middle colic artery.

8.2.2.2 Transverse Colectomy (Fig. 8.1b)

- The middle colic artery is ligated, and the ascending and descending colon are anastomosed. This is less commonly performed with surgeons favoring an extended right or extended left hemicolectomy.

Fig. 8.1 Illustrations of colonic resections. (**a**) Right hemicolectomy and extended right hemicolectomy. (**b**) Transverse colectomy. (**c**) Left hemicolectomy. (**d**) Sigmoid colectomy. (**e**) Hartmann's procedure. (**f**) Anterior resection – *dotted lines* (distal limit of resection margin). Extra levator APER – *solid line* (performed when there is invasion of the external sphincter). Cylindrical APER (*dashed lines*). (**g**) Total colectomy with (A) ileorectal anastomosis (*arrow*) and (B) end ileostomy

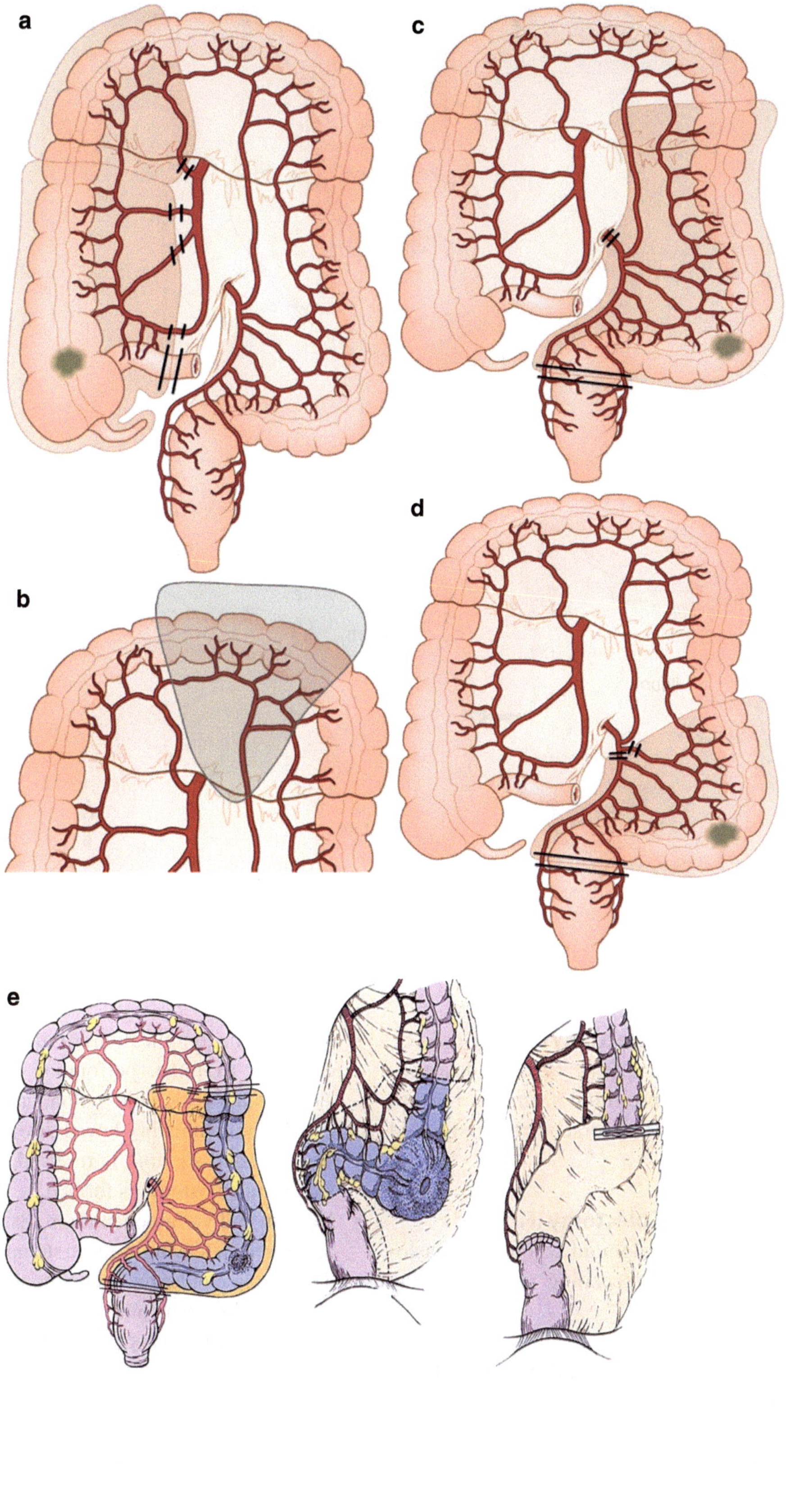
a
b
c
d
e

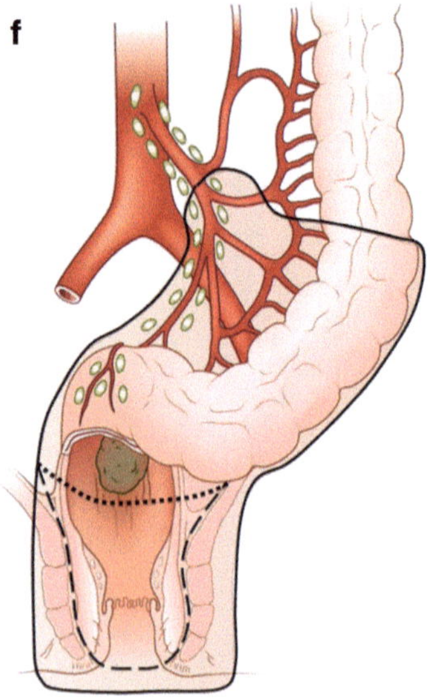

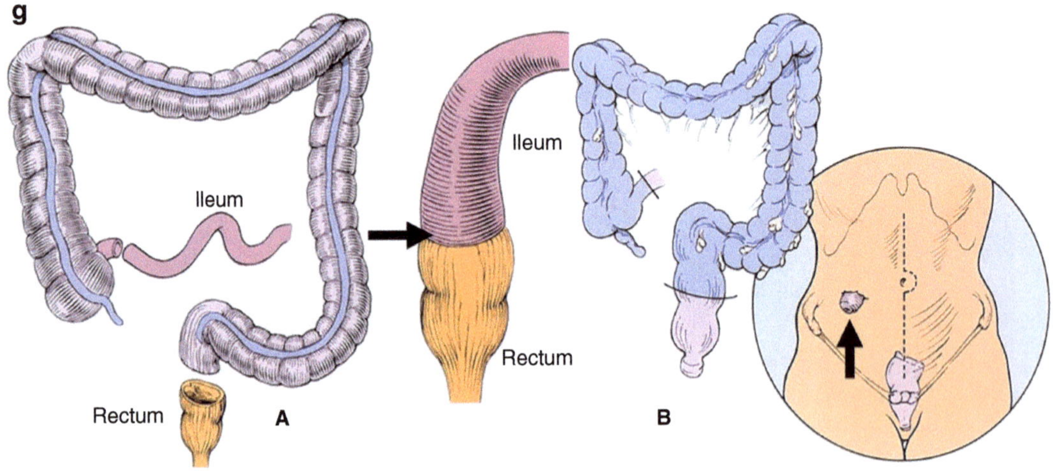

Fig. 8.1 (continued)

8.2.2.3 Left Hemicolectomy (LHC) (Fig. 8.1c)

- Resection of the splenic flexure, descending colon, and proximal sigmoid. Formation of a transverse colon-sigmoid anastomosis.

8.2.2.4 Sigmoid Colectomy (Fig. 8.1d)

- Resection of the sigmoid colon and anastomosis of the descending colon to the rectum.

8.2.2.5 Hartmann's Procedure (Fig. 8.1e)

- Performed when a primary colonic anastomosis is considered unsafe following sigmoid resection.
- Indicated in complications of diverticular disease, for example, perforation or stricture, carcinoma of sigmoid colon, and in some cases of inflammatory bowel disease.
- The diseased sigmoid is resected, and a left-sided end colostomy is formed.
- Rectum and variable length of distal sigmoid are closed off leaving a "rectal stump" (Fig. 8.2). The stump can be reattached to the proximal colon within 3–6 months of the primary surgery.
- A mucous fistula is occasionally formed. This is an end colostomy that communicates with the defunctioned colon that leads down to the anus. It discharges mucous only through the anterior abdominal wall.

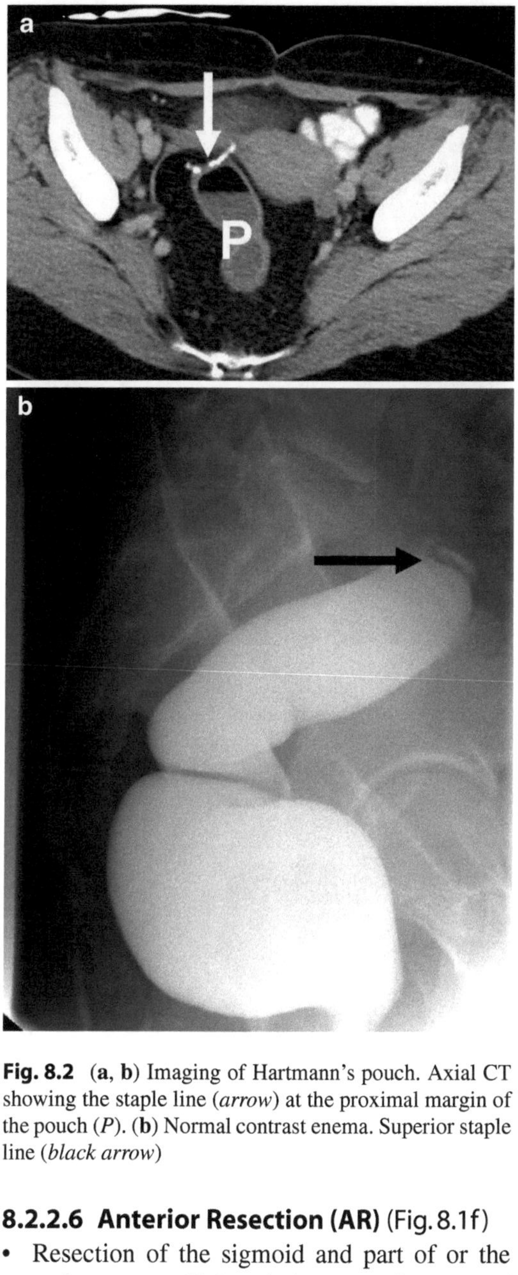

Fig. 8.2 (**a**, **b**) Imaging of Hartmann's pouch. Axial CT showing the staple line (*arrow*) at the proximal margin of the pouch (*P*). (**b**) Normal contrast enema. Superior staple line (*black arrow*)

8.2.2.6 Anterior Resection (AR) (Fig. 8.1f)

- Resection of the sigmoid and part of or the entire rectum. If the whole rectum is removed (low anterior resection), a coloanal anastomosis is used; otherwise, the anastomosis is colorectal. The sphincters are preserved. The consequences of an anastomotic leak (more common in low anastomoses) are mitigated against by diverting the fecal stream into a temporary defunctioning stoma, that is, a right-sided loop ileostomy or a transverse loop colostomy. This is often reversed after at least 6–8 weeks following surgery. A contrast enema is commonly performed prior to stoma reversal to exclude a postoperative leak or stenosis at the anastomosis.

8.2.2.7 Abdominoperineal Excision of Rectum (APER) (Fig. 8.1f)

- APER involves resection of the anus, rectum, and a portion of the distal sigmoid colon through incisions made in the abdomen and perineum. It is indicated for malignancy of the lower third of the rectum or anal canal and for salvage of anal cancer that fails to respond to chemoradiotherapy. The residual sigmoid colon forms the left-sided colostomy.

8.2.2.8 Total Colectomy (TC) (Fig. 8.1g)

- Resection of the entire colon; the rectum is preserved and is anastomosed to the terminal ileum (A). Fecal continence is preserved, although increased frequency of defecation is common. If performed for colonic polyposis, regular follow-up surveillance of the rectum is required. If an ileorectal anastomosis is not performed, an end ileostomy is fashioned in the right iliac fossa (B).
- Ileorectal anastomosis is performed following total colectomy in patients with familial adenomatous polyposis (FAP), multiple synchronous colonic polyps, or cancers and uncommonly for chronic ulcerative colitis. Ileorectal anastomosis in FAP is associated with a risk of developing carcinoma and requires surveillance for rectal polyps but is a good alternative in young people who have relative rectal sparing. However, proctectomy is usually required within 10–15 years.

8.2.2.9 Proctocolectomy (PC)

- Resection of the rectum and colon with formation of a permanent ileostomy in the right iliac fossa. To avoid an ileostomy, an ileoanal anastomosis is sometimes performed after establishment of an ileal anal pouch which gives rise to the term "restorative proctocolectomy."

8.2.2.10 Subtotal Colectomy (STC)

- Resection of the colon proximal to the distal sigmoid colon with an ileosigmoid anastomosis.

8.2.2.11 Types of Anastomosis

An ileocolic or colocolic anastomosis may be constructed using an end-to-end, end-to-side, or side-to-side anastomosis. The type will depend on surgeon preference and the diameters of the bowel involved. The end to end is the most physiological (although there do not appear to be functional differences in anastomotic construct) but requires similar bowel diameters. If different, an end-to-side anastomosis may be performed. A side-to-side anastomosis is least likely to leak but may lead to the formation of a blind pouch. Colonic anastomoses are also discussed in Sect. 8.3.

8.2.3 Normal Postoperative Imaging

8.2.3.1 Lower GI Contrast Studies

The routine use of lower GI contrast studies to assess the postoperative colon varies according to local practice. Some surgeons will request a water-soluble contrast enema to assess the anastomosis prior to reversal of the defunctioning stoma. Barium is contraindicated in the early post surgical period because of the risks of barium peritonitis if there is a leak. A Foley catheter is preferable to reduce the risk of anastomotic dehiscence and should be used without inflating the balloon. The use of a rigid rectal tube is relatively contraindicated, particularly in low anastomoses (Fig. 8.3).

A control spot film will demonstrate a ring of staples at the level of the anastomosis (if a staple gun has been used). Anastomotic leaks are most often posterior in location, and it is important to obtain good AP, lateral, and oblique views. Some leaks are only identified during emptying, and the anastomosis should be screened at the end of the procedure. It is important not to misinterpret a side-to-end anastomosis as a postoperative leak.

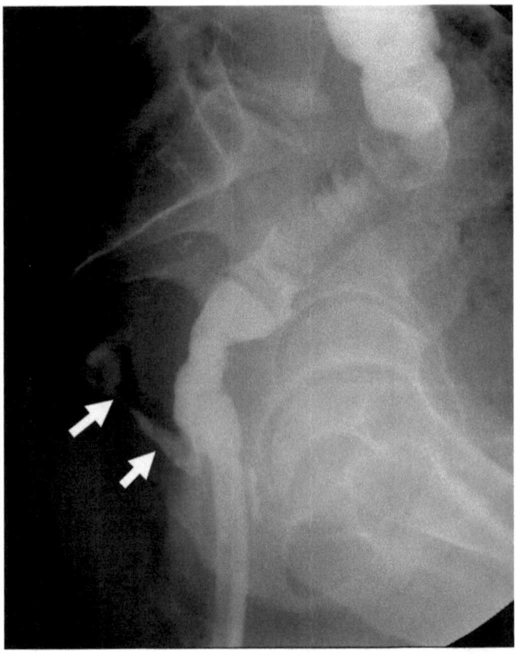

Fig. 8.3 Water-soluble contrast enema post anterior resection for a midrectal cancer. There is a posterior leak (*arrows*). A rigid tube has been used for the study, which should be generally avoided due to the risk of inadvertent perforation

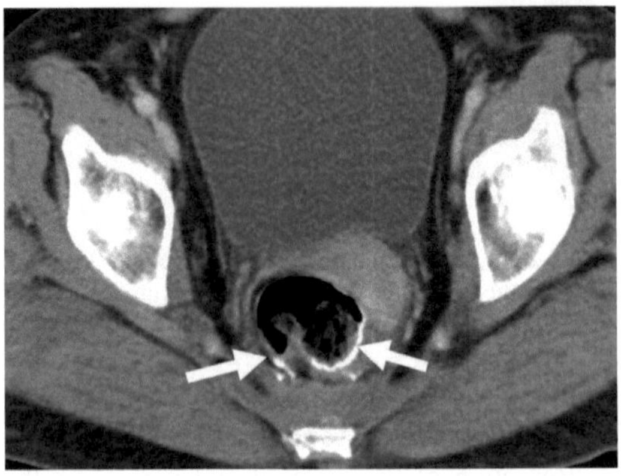

Fig. 8.4 Normal CT appearances of an intact staple line (*arrows*) post anterior resection. There is thickening of the presacral space due to postoperative fibrosis

8.2.3.2 CT

CT is not usually performed in the early postoperative period unless there are suspected complications such as an anastomotic leak, fistula, abscess, or bowel obstruction (Zissin and Gayer 2003). CT can be performed with rectal contrast injected via a Foley catheter to assess the integrity of distal colonic anastomoses. In the assessment of more proximal colonic anastomoses (RHC), the authors advocate using higher than usual strength of oral contrast, for example, 20 ml of Omnipaque 300 mg/ml in 250 ml of water (8% strength; see Sect. 1.2). Widening of the CT windows is used to detect any leaks. The anastomotic staple line should be in continuity (Fig. 8.4). CT findings of anastomotic leaks vary from subtle

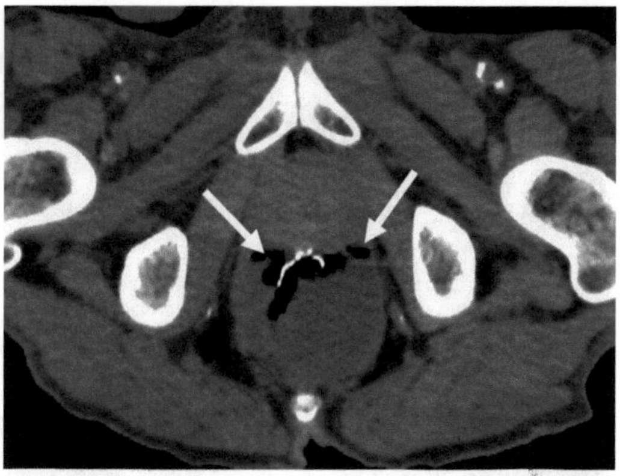

Fig. 8.5 Anastomotic breakdown post anterior resection. CT demonstrates disruption of the staple line with air outside the anastomosis (*arrows*)

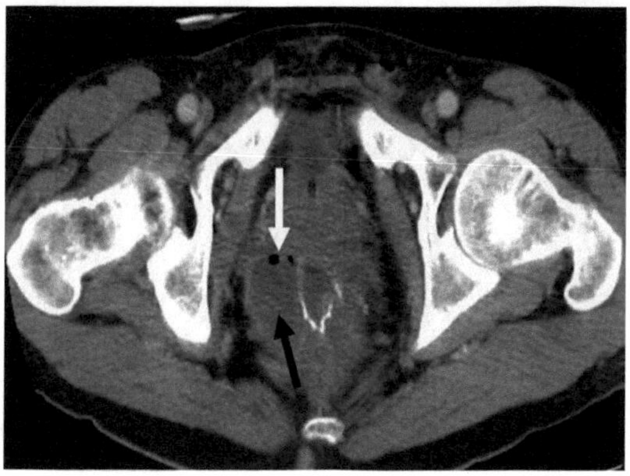

Fig. 8.6 Small leak post anterior resection. CT shows extraluminal gas (*white arrow*) and a small collection (*black arrow*). The staple line appears intact

disruption of the staple line to complete dehiscence. Supporting features include the presence of intramural or pericolonic gas and fluid collections (Figs. 8.5, 8.6, 8.7, 8.8). The presacral space is widened postoperatively, and fluid is often seen in this location. An enhancing fluid collection should alert the radiologist to the presence of a collection. If the patient is at increased risk of local recurrence or if there has been neoadjuvant radiotherapy or a postoperative collection, the CT appearances of the pelvis can be difficult to interpret. Therefore, an early scan at 3 months will serve as a useful baseline for future comparison. The timing and frequency of follow-up CT varies between institutions, but the highest risk of recurrence or metastasis is in the first 2–3 years

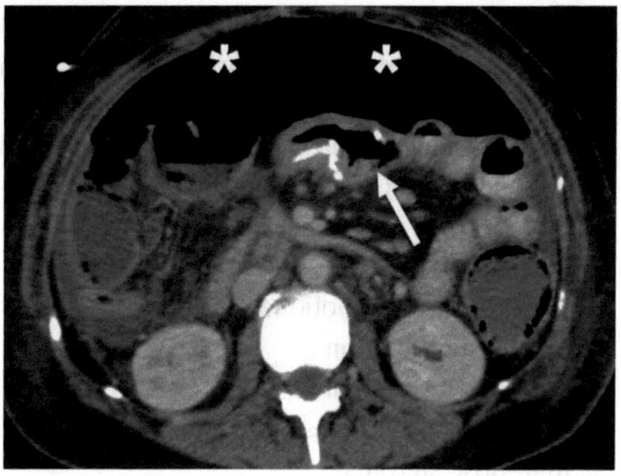

Fig. 8.7 Anastomotic breakdown post extended right hemicolectomy. There is disruption to the staple line (*arrow*) and gross pneumoperitoneum (*asterisks*)

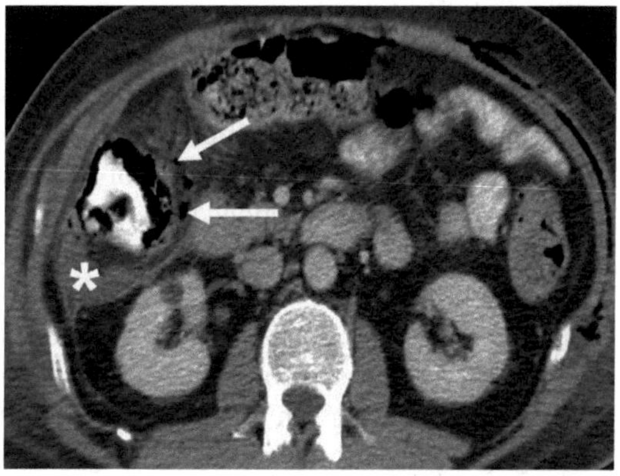

Fig. 8.8 Anastomotic leak 10 days post right hemicolectomy. CT demonstrates extramural air (*arrows*) and a small collection (*asterisk*). Although extramural air can be seen in the immediate postoperative period, it is usually pathological a week or more following surgery

following diagnosis. It would be reasonable to ensure a minimum annual imaging follow-up CT of the thorax, abdomen, and pelvis for at least this time period since localized recurrence and metastases can be successfully resected with curative intent.

8.2.4 Postoperative Complications

8.2.4.1 Anastomotic Leak and Abscess

This is the most common major complication of colonic surgery occurring in 5–10% of patients, usually within 2 weeks of surgery (Scardapane et al. 2005). Postoperative anastomotic leaks that require surgical intervention are associated with significant morbidity such as poor colonic function, permanent stomas, incisional hernia, and open abdomens. Contributing factors to anastomotic leaks are:

- Ischemia
- Excessive anastomotic tension
- Stapler malfunction
- Poor nutritional status
- Immunosuppression – chemotherapy and high-dose steroids
- Preoperative radiotherapy
- Sepsis

Incidence is independent of suture type, for example, hand-sewn or staples. The risk of a postoperative leak increases the nearer the anastomosis is to the anal verge, that is, a low anterior resection versus high anterior resection. It is important to appreciate the difference between a contained or free leak and knowledge of whether the patient has been defunctioned.

Leaks from low anastomoses, for example, low or ultralow anterior resections, are generally contained within the pelvis and can be drained transrectally by the surgeon (either digitally or endoscopically using an Endosponge drain) or image guided via a transrectal, transvaginal, or transgluteal route (Fig. 8.9).

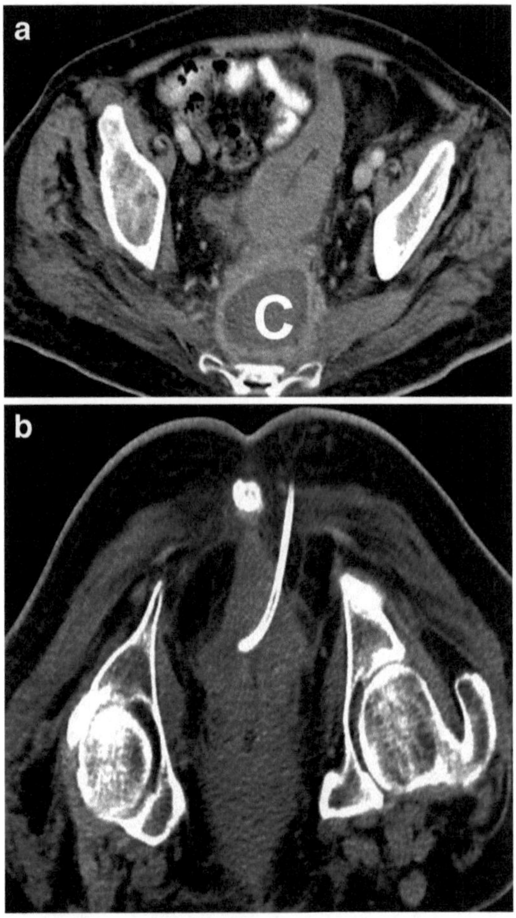

Fig. 8.9 (**a**) Presacral collection post APER (*C*). (**b**) Placement of a 10-Fr drainage catheter via a transgluteal approach using CT guidance

Leaks from a high anterior resection or a more proximal colonic anastomosis are associated with free spillage into the intraperitoneal space and therefore are associated with much higher morbidity. This is compounded if the fecal stream has not been diverted from the anastomosis with either a temporary loop ileostomy or loop colostomy (Fig. 8.10).

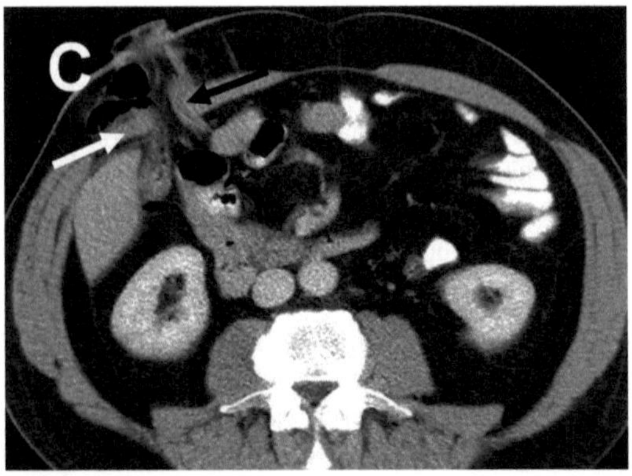

Fig. 8.10 Axial CT demonstrating a defunctioning transverse loop colostomy (*C*). Afferent limb (*white arrow*) and efferent limb (*black arrow*)

Contrast studies will show extraluminal extravasation, collections, or peritoneal spill. Most anastomotic leaks in the pelvis occur posteriorly. Signs of dehiscence on CT include discontinuity of the staple line, gas within or adjacent to the bowel wall, pneumoperitoneum, or free fluid. In rectal anastomotic leaks, the double rectum sign has been described. This is attributable to the anterior rectum coupled with a posterior fluid collection which may or may not enhance (Fig. 8.11).

It is important to recognize that surgical devices placed at the time of surgery can mimic collections.

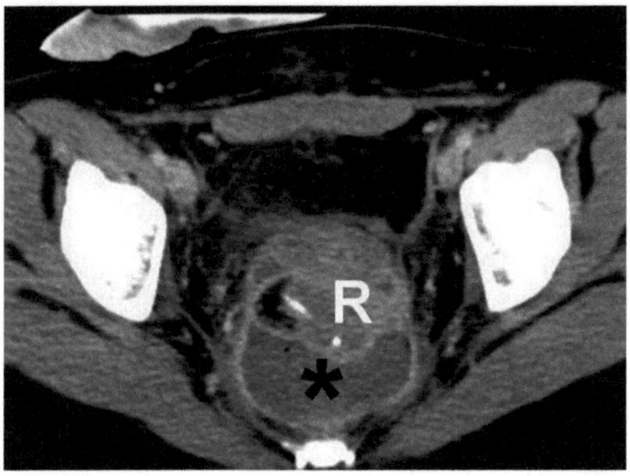

Fig. 8.11 Double rectum sign on CT following a leak post anterior resection with the rectum (*R*) anterior to the rim enhancing collection (*asterisk*)

Surgicel or oxidized regenerated cellulose, (Ethicon, Livingston, UK) is a bioabsorbable hemostasis agent which can trap air and be mistaken for an abscess within the surgical bed. Some surgical drains contain a balloon which can be misinterpreted as a fluid collection. Surgically placed corrugated drains are typically of soft tissue attenuation but have parallel areas of air density within the substance of the drain, producing a characteristic appearance (Fig. 8.12).

Surgical management of anastomotic failure is dependent on the site of the anastomosis and on local surgical practice. If a distal leak is small, it may spontaneously heal particularly as the fecal stream is diverted through a proximal stoma. Any associated collections are drained to improve the chances of healing, and a contrast enema is performed a few months later to ascertain whether the anastomosis is intact. Significant distal leaks are generally treated conservatively as refashioning the anastomosis is technically difficult and rarely successful. The radiologist, where possible, should assist in draining any associated pelvic collections where an image-guided route allows access, to prevent unnecessary surgery and prolonged hospital stay.

Small proximal leaks, for example, following right hemicolectomy, are managed with bowel rest and total parenteral nutrition with any associated collections drained under imaging guidance. The surgeon will then cautiously rechallenge the bowel at a later date. Significant leaks with intraperitoneal spillage of bowel contents require immediate surgery and intra-abdominal washout. The anastomosis is repaired but is temporarily protected by fashioning an upstream ileostomy.

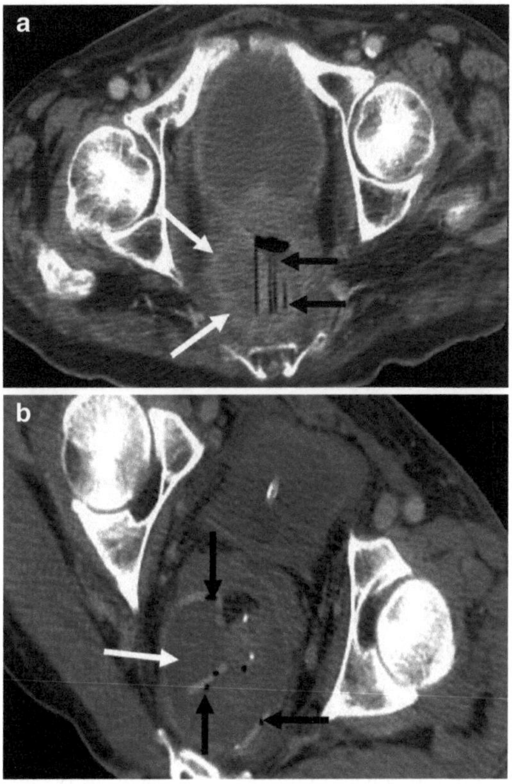

Fig. 8.12 (**a**, **b**) Examples of intraoperatively placed pelvic corrugated surgical drains in two patients. CT demonstrated collections (*white arrows*). Note that the drains are typically soft tissue attenuation and often contain air which follows the parallel lines of the corrugation (*black arrows*)

Transgluteal Drainage of Deep Pelvic Collections

Transgluteal drainage under CT guidance is an important specialist technique required in the management of a select group of patients where transrectal and transabdominal access to the collection is either not possible or inappropriate (e.g., recent ileorectal pouch or low anterior resection). The essential components of the technique are not dissimilar to other drainages in terms of preparation (see Sect. 1.10). Although this technique is associated with less morbidity than a repeat surgical procedure, it is important that the patient is made aware of postprocedure discomfort and the possibility of contamination of the gluteal muscle compartment via the drain tract. It is a matter of personal preference whether positive oral and/or intravenous contrast is administered to opacify pelvic organs and vessels – it can be particularly useful in the early postoperative period where normal fat planes are obliterated by edema/fluid overload. Patients require prone positioning and must be able to lie still during the procedure. In some cases, this will require the addition of sedation or even general anesthetic which adds to the complexity and planning of the procedure. It is critical that there is no movement between the initial planning scans and needle placement to prevent misregistration. A long cannula is used for access, and during needle advancement, deep infiltration with local anesthetic is performed. The needle tip should be aimed with a skin position that is as far lateral as reasonable (to prevent the patient lying on the catheter in a weight-bearing position that may precipitate formation of a pressure ulcer) while aiming to penetrate the pelvic sidewall as posteromedially as possible (to avoid injury to the neurovascular structure exiting the sciatic notch). When the needle is successfully inserted, then a Seldinger technique is used with wire placement and dilatation of the tract to accept a catheter of 8–10 Fr diameter. The collection should be aspirated to dryness and left on free drainage with a recommendation to remove it in 48–72 h for patient compliance and to minimize the risk of sinus formation.

8.2.4.2 Fistula

Fistulae result from anastomotic leaks and can communicate with the skin (Fig. 8.13) or genitourinary tract, particularly the vagina. The latter occurs when the vagina has been included within the stapled anastomosis or when a leak communicates through the vaginal cuff in patients with previous hysterectomy. Fistulae can also communicate with the presacral space and form chronic collections. Imaging with CT, pelvic MRI (Fig. 8.14), and contrast studies (Fig. 8.15) can evaluate complex fistulation. Management involves bowel rest and parenteral nutrition

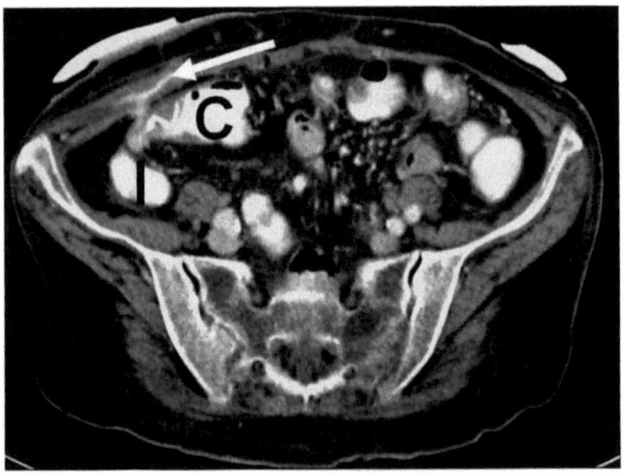

Fig. 8.13 Enterocutaneous fistula post right hemicolectomy. CT demonstrates a tract (*arrow*) originating at the ileocolonic anastomosis staple line and penetrating the anterior abdominal wall which is filling a drainage bag on the skin surface with contrast. Ileum (*I*) and colon (*C*)

8.2.4.3 Ileus and Obstruction

This is described in detail in Sect. 7.2.1.

8.2.4.4 Anastomotic Stricture

This may result from a postoperative leak or ischemia to the anastomosis and occurs within 2–12 months following surgery but is an infrequent complication. Patients present with increasing constipation but may be asymptomatic if they have been defunctioned with a proximal diverting stoma. Anastomotic strictures are often detected on a routine contrast enema study performed prior to closure of the stoma (Fig. 8.16). CT is less sensitive at detecting anastomotic strictures particularly if there is a diverting stoma as the colon between the stoma and the stricture is generally decompressed. Patients with an anastomotic stricture that is in intestinal continuity are at particular risk of obstruction and perforation. The colon above the stricture will be dilated (Fig. 8.17). Anastomotic strictures can be treated successfully with serial balloon dilatation (Fig. 8.18) but often require surgical revision.

8.2.4.5 Local Tumor Recurrence

The local recurrence rate for patients who undergo potentially curative surgery for colorectal cancer varies between 3% and 30%. This depends on factors including:

- The pathological stage of the primary tumor (T staging and the degree of differentiation)

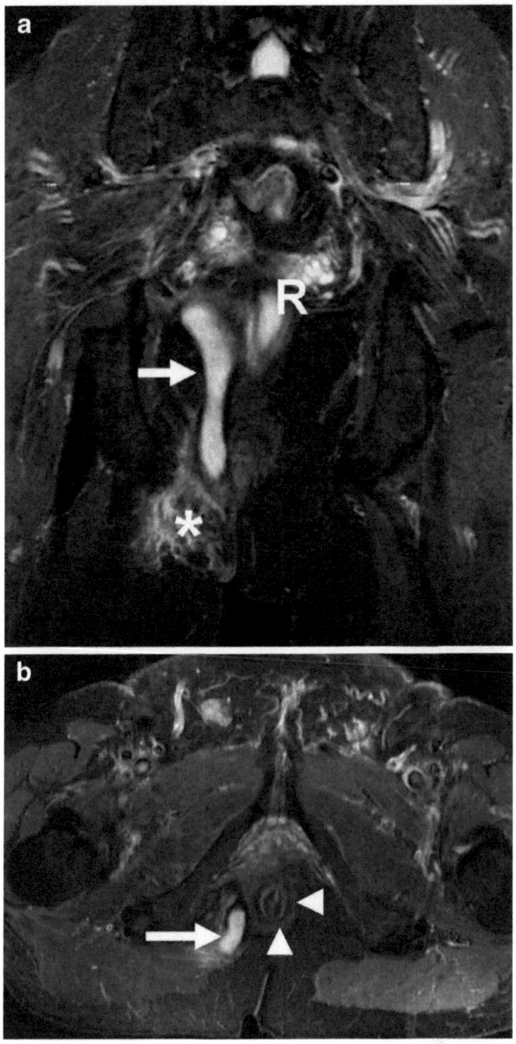

Fig. 8.14 Fistula post anastomotic leak following anterior resection. (**a**) Axial and (**b**) coronal STIR MRI shows a right extrasphincteric fistula (*arrow*) traversing the levator plate originating at the anorectal anastomosis (*R*). Note marked induration of the ischioanal fat adjacent to the fistula (*asterisk*). The external opening is lateral to the external sphincter (*arrowheads*) at 8 o'clock

- Presence of lymphovascular invasion
- Involvement of the circumferential resection margin
- Tumors in the lower third of the rectum
- Colonic tumors which have caused obstruction or perforation
- Whether preoperative neoadjuvant treatment was given for rectal cancer

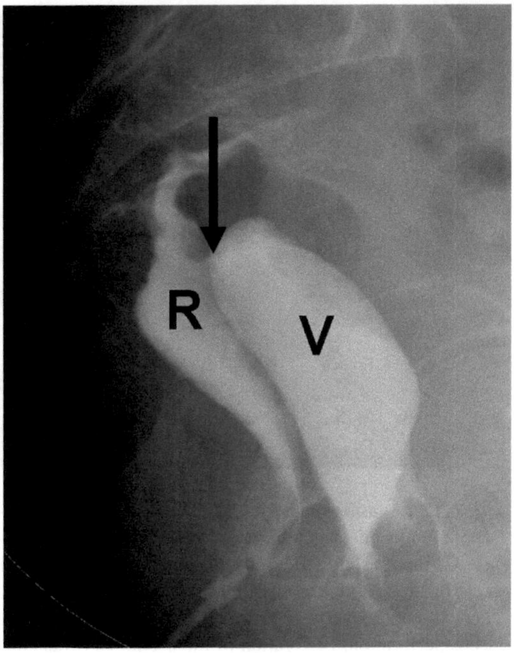

Fig 8.15 Rectovaginal fistula (*arrow*) complicating an anastomotic leak post anterior resection. Rectum (*R*) and vagina (*V*)

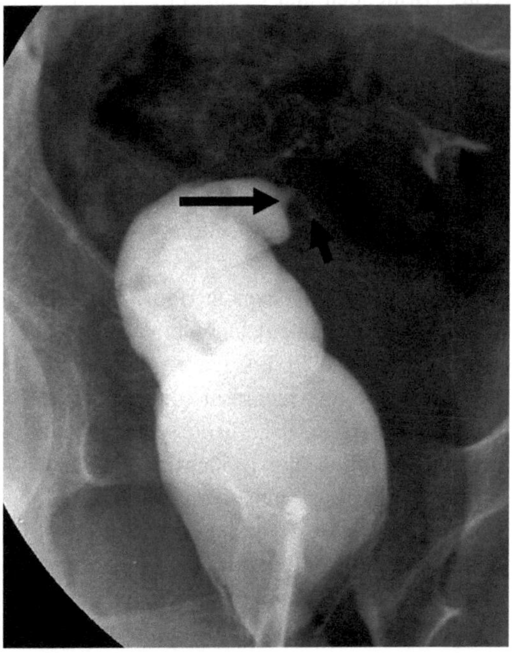

Fig. 8.16 Tight anastomotic stricture post anterior resection. Water-soluble contrast enema at 3 months prior to defunctioning loop ileostomy closure shows severe stenosis (*long arrow*) at the staple line (*short arrow*). Minimal contrast passes into the sigmoid colon proximally (*arrowheads*)

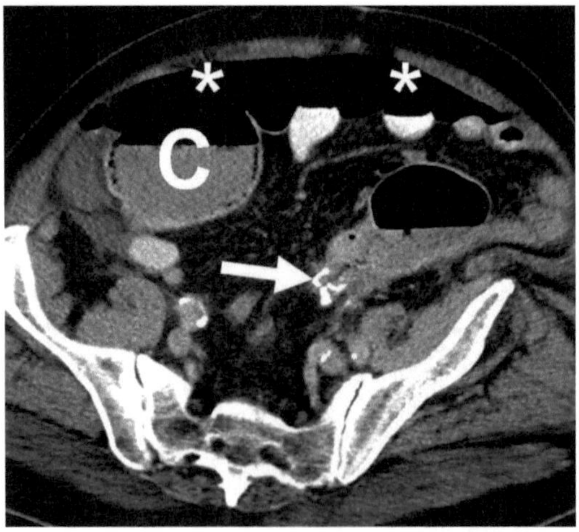

Fig. 8.17 Anastomotic stricture. Acute colonic obstruction 9 months post sigmoid colectomy for diverticular disease. CT demonstrates a closed loop large bowel obstruction due to stricture at the anastomotic staple line (*arrow*). There is pneumoperitoneum (*asterisk*) indicating hollow viscus perforation. Perforation of the cecum (*C*) was confirmed at surgery due to benign anastomotic stricture

Malignancy recurs in 80% of cases within 2 years (Brittenden and Chalmers 2007). Without treatment, the 5-year survival rate is less than 5%. Recurrence can be classified as local or systemic:

1. Local:
   - Anastomotic – due to seeding during surgery
   - Nodal – spread to locoregional lymph nodes
   - Pelvic viscera and sidewall – highest risk after incomplete resection
2. Systemic:
   - Spread to liver, omentum (Fig. 8.19) and peritoneum (Fig. 8.20), lungs, brain, and bones

CT, MRI, and PET CT are complementary in assessing for recurrent disease. Locally recurrent disease usually originates outside the bowel lumen and is identified as an exophytic enlarging mass on cross-sectional imaging (Figs. 8.21 and 8.22). CT can also demonstrate distant metastases which may preclude surgical resection or pelvic exenteration. Radiological evaluation of the post surgical pelvis can be complex because of the difficulties distinguishing between residual fibrosis and detecting foci of recurrent disease. This is compounded by postoperative complications and neoadjuvant/adjuvant treatments which add to the extent of the fibrosis and interpretive

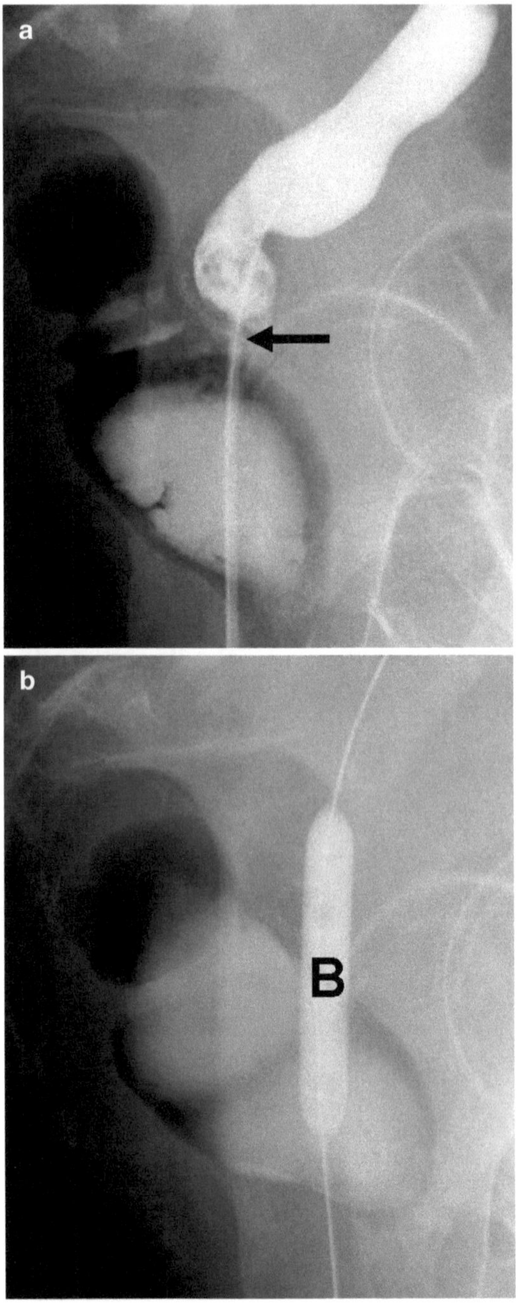

Fig. 8.18 (**a**, **b**) Balloon dilatation of an anastomotic stricture at the site of an end-to-side sigmoid to rectal anastomosis following sigmoid colectomy for diverticular disease. A sheath and a stiff wire have been placed beyond the tight stricture (*arrow*) with combined endoscopic/fluoroscopic guidance. Angioplasty balloon (*B*)

difficulty (Fig. 8.23). Detecting foci of recurrent disease can be difficult. Serial imaging can assist, but PET CT is increasingly being used in

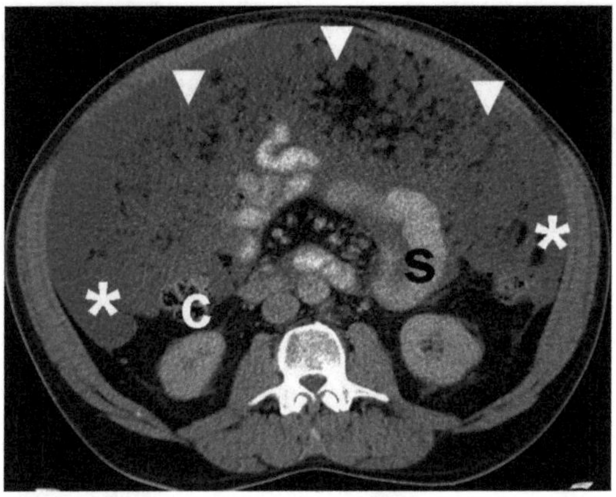

Fig. 8.19 CT of extensive omental infiltration (*arrowheads*) and ascites (*asterisk*) in a patient 1 year postresection for a T4 right colonic tumor. Small bowel is opacified with positive oral contrast (*S*), and residual colon (*C*) is demonstrated

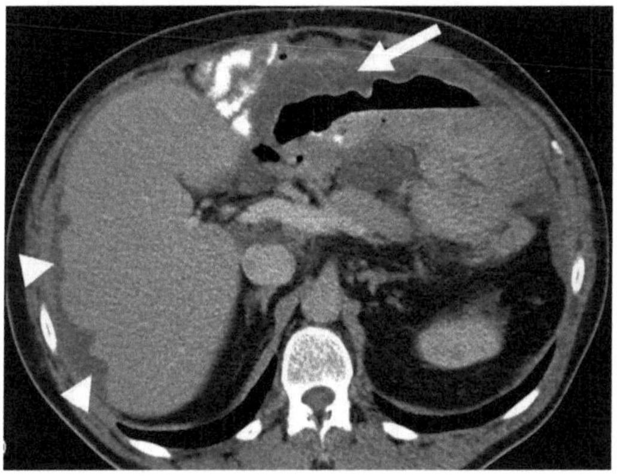

Fig. 8.20 CT demonstrating peritoneal tumor recurrence producing characteristic scalloping of the right lobe of the liver indicating subcapsular infiltration (*arrowheads*) along with invasion of the lesser omentum compressing the stomach (*arrow*)

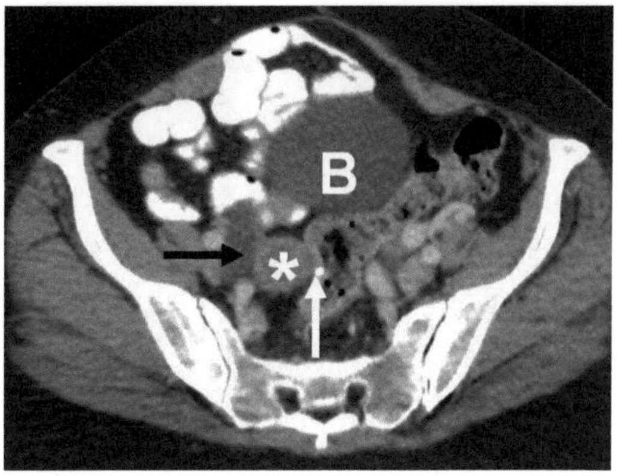

Fig. 8.21 Extraluminal recurrence. CT in a patient 2 years post high anterior resection with an elevated CEA. There is an extraluminal soft tissue mass (*asterisk*) causing right ureteric dilatation (*black arrow*). Bladder (*B*) and anastomotic staple line (*white arrow*)

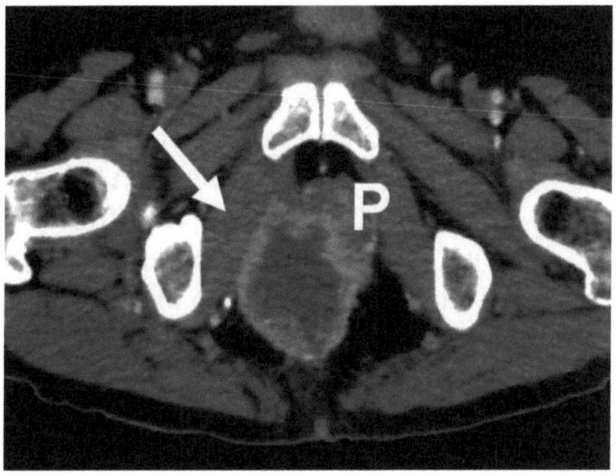

Fig. 8.22 Recurrent rectal cancer post APER. Tumor invades the prostate anteriorly (*P*) and the right obturator internus muscle (*arrow*). Note characteristic irregular rim enhancement often seen in large-volume local pelvic recurrence that may be mistaken for abscess

high-risk patients with equivocal imaging and elevated tumor markers. Recurrent rectal cancer is discussed in Sect. 8.5.

8.2.4.6 Complications Specific to the Site of Surgery

Right Colon Resection

Duodenal injury, anastomotic failure and bleeding.

Transverse Colon Resection

Inadequate mobilization of both cut ends, resulting in tension on the suture line and anastomotic leak.

Left Colon Resection

Injury to the spleen and left ureter. Mobilization of the splenic flexure is performed in patients undergoing a low anterior resection in order to bring the colon into the pelvis and ensure a tension-free anastomosis. It is also performed in sigmoid colectomies when the sigmoid colon is short or if there is concern regarding blood supply to the left colon. Mobilization changes on CT manifest as inflammatory changes within the surgical bed in the left upper quadrant and should not be misinterpreted for acute pancreatitis (Fig. 8.24).

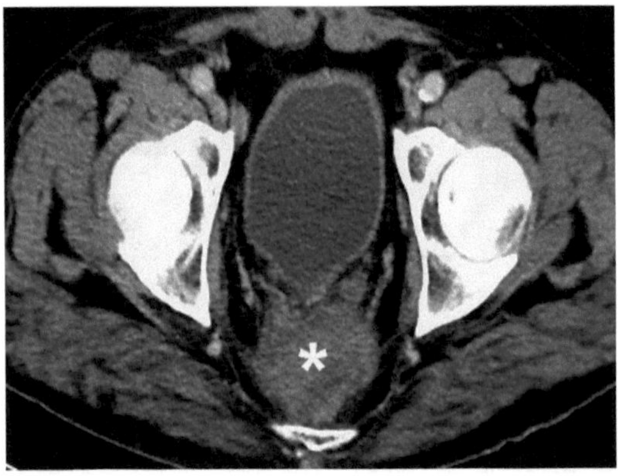

Fig. 8.23 CT 6 months following a postoperative leak shows an ill-defined presacral mass (*asterisk*). This remained stable on follow-up imaging consistent with postoperative fibrosis within the pelvis. This can be very difficult to differentiate from local recurrence without additional imaging or follow-up

Ischemia of the splenic flexure can also occur in left-sided colonic resections. This is due to ligation of the inferior mesenteric artery close to its origin and a subsequent "steal effect" via the arcade of Riolan. Blood is diverted from the SMA territory supplying the splenic flexure (branch of middle colic artery) to the anastomosis distally. The splenic flexure may appear thick walled on CT secondary to ischemia (Fig. 8.25).

8.2.5 Teaching Points

- Radiological assessment of the postoperative colon requires knowledge of the type of resection and anastomosis used.
- Most complications occur early within the postoperative period.
- CT (+/− rectal contrast) and fluoroscopy are most commonly used to investigate suspected complications.

8.3 Anastomosis

A surgical anastomosis is the connection of two hollow structures to restore continuity or provide an anatomical bypass.

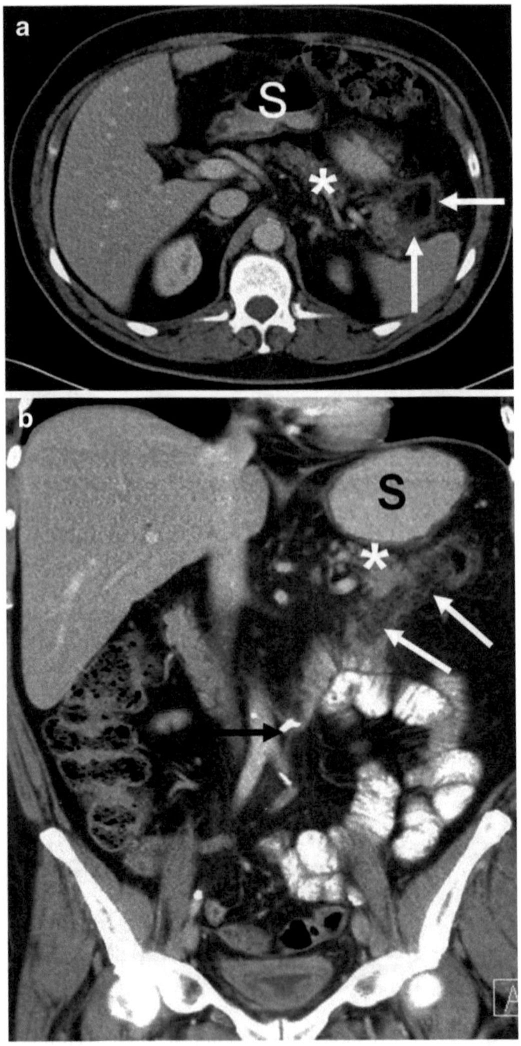

Fig. 8.24 Surgical bed changes post left hemicolectomy. (**a**) Axial and (**b**) coronal CT show inflammatory changes (*white arrows*) adjacent to the spleen, tail of pancreas (*asterisk*), and stomach (*S*). The inferior mesenteric artery has been clipped (*black arrow*). While this appearance can mimic acute pancreatitis, there is usually no associated history and is often seen following mobilization of the splenic flexure colon for sigmoid colectomy

8.3.1 Nomenclature

The naming of a type of anastomosis normally begins with the proximal part and then names the distal part. In colorectal surgery, this gives rise to the familiar anatomical terms ileocolic, colorectal, coloanal, and pouch-anal anastomoses. Similarly, the naming of an anastomosis can describe its structure according to whether the

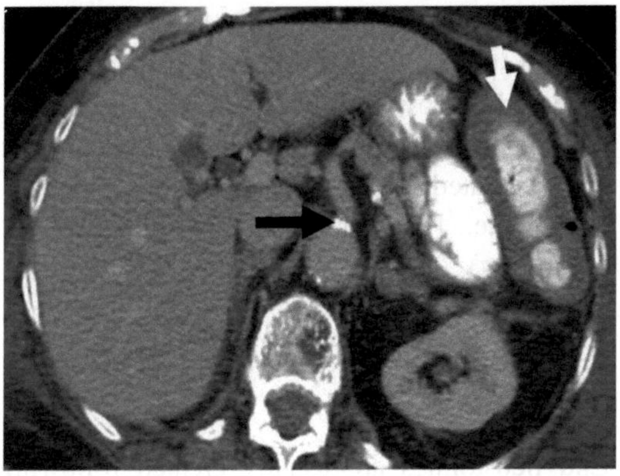

Fig. 8.25 Ischemia of the splenic flexure post–right hemicolectomy. CT demonstrates concentric thickening of the splenic flexure (*white arrow*) with calcified atheroma at the coeliac artery origin (*black arrow*)

side or end of the bowel is used, for example, end-to-end, side-to-end, end-to-side, or side-to-side anastomosis (less common in colonic surgery). It should be remembered that the name follows the same proximal/distal format so that a side-to-end colorectal anastomosis joins the side of the proximal colon to the end of the rectum, whereas an end-to-side ileocolic anastomosis joins the end of the ileum to the side of the colon (Keighley and Williams 2007). Examples of anastomoses used following anterior resection are illustrated as normal contrast studies in Figs. 8.26, 8.27, 8.28.

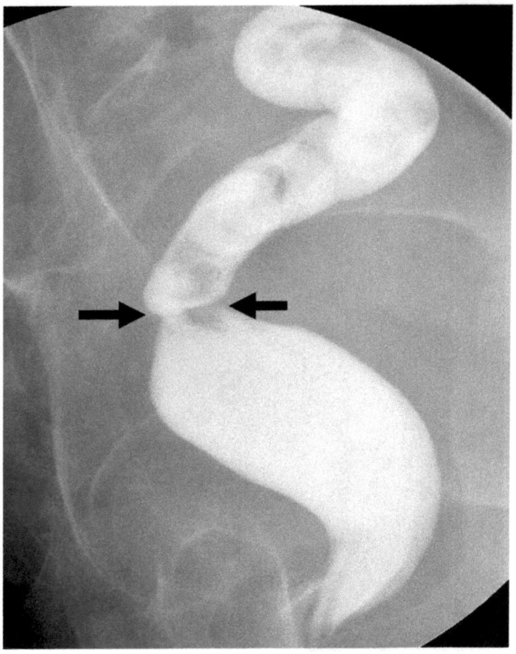

Fig. 8.26 End-to-end anastomosis. Water-soluble contrast study in a patient post–high anterior resection. Anastomotic staple line (*arrows*)

With the increasing use of laparoscopic surgery, vascular staplers are used to divide major blood vessels. These staples are similar to those used for bowel anastomosis but close more tightly to ensure hemostasis.

8.3.2 Anastomosis Construct

An anastomosis can be constructed in a number of ways. The two principal methods are hand-sewn and stapled (and combinations thereof). There are a number of additional novel methods such as the anastomosis ring, but these have not gained significant acceptance in the surgical fraternity at present.

Sutures are not visible on postoperative imaging, but staples can be seen and appear in either in a linear or circular configuration. Linear staplers can shed closed staples where there is no bowel between the jaws of the device. These staples should not be confused with anastomotic dehiscence. Occasionally, the staple line may be visible a reasonable distance from the anastomosis due to stapling of the adjacent mesentery.

8.4 Stomas

A stoma is an "opening" or "mouth" which in gastrointestinal surgery effectively means a surgical connection of the gastrointestinal tract to the skin. An estimated 100,000 people in the UK have a stoma, and about 65% of these stomas are permanent.

Stomas are described by their organ of origin, for example, gastrostomy, jejunostomy, ileostomy, or colostomy, and whether they use a loop or the end of the bowel. Stomas can also be described according to their intended function, that is, temporary or permanent, and "defunctioning" to indicate diversion of the fecal stream.

Loop stomas are described as having "afferent" and "efferent" limbs, leading "toward" and "away from" the stoma, respectively. Some surgeons

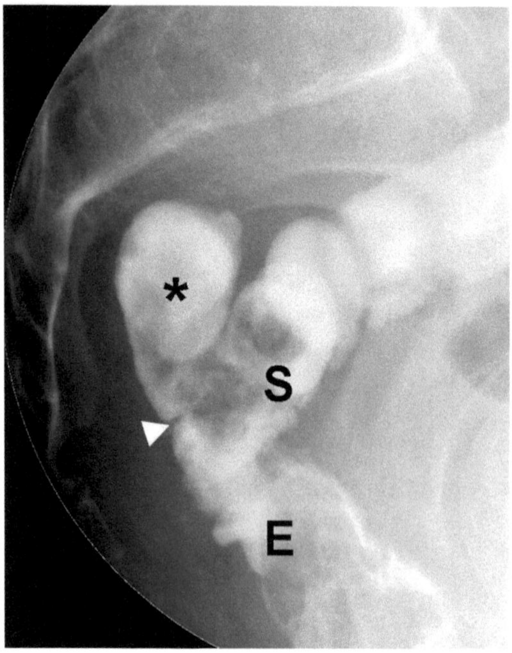

Fig. 8.27 Side-to-end anastomosis. The side of the proximal colon (*S*) has been anastomosed to the end (*E*) of the distal colon with staple line (*arrowhead*) and blind loop of the proximal colon (*asterisk*)

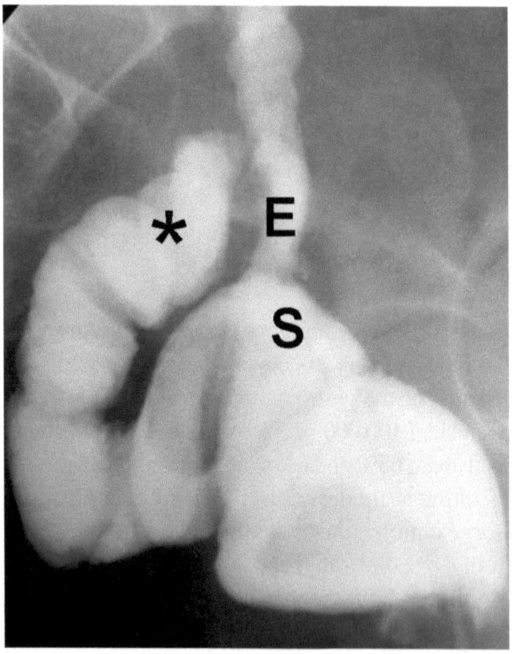

Fig. 8.28 End-to-side anastomosis. The end of the proximal colon (*E*) has been anastomosed to the side (*S*) of the midrectum with a long redundant end loop of the rectum (*asterisk*)

favor the placement of a rod to elevate the loop to prevent stomal retraction. The rod is typically left for 5–7 days postoperatively.

Stomas are commonly created surgically but can be created as a percutaneous endoscopic procedure (i.e., PEG for gastrostomy and PEC for colostomy).

8.4.1 Ileostomy

End ileostomies are usually created following subtotal colectomy for complicated inflammatory bowel disease or following emergency right hemicolectomy where anastomosis is inappropriate (e.g., right colon infarction in a sick patient).

A loop ileostomy is a favored option for defunctioning downstream bowel, for example, following low anterior resection to mitigate the consequences of an anastomotic leak.

Advantages of defunctioning loop ileostomy versus loop colostomy include:

- Easier to manage than a loop colostomy
- Less odor
- Fewer appliance changes
- Fewer problems with stoma management, for example, prolapse
- Low anterior resection – leave untouched upstream colon

Disadvantages include:

- Downstream obstruction with a competent ileocecal valve does not adequately decompress the colon.

Anatomically, loop ileostomies are most commonly created in the right iliac fossa.

Construction of an ileostomy is often at the time of laparotomy, although a trephine or laparoscopic defunctioning ileostomy may be performed as an initial procedure, for example, prior to long-course chemoradiotherapy in cases of advanced rectal cancer. On CT examinations, it is important not to confuse end ileostomies with an ileal conduit performed following cystectomy. Ileal conduits do not usually contain contrast on portal venous phase imaging (oral or intravenous), and the ureters are attached to the proximal end. Ileostomies may be positioned within the left iliac fossa if the patient already has an ileal conduit or if the stoma needs to be refashioned, for example, due to parastomal hernia.

8.4.2 Colostomy

End colostomies are created in the following scenarios (Fig. 8.29):

- When colonic continuity cannot be achieved, for example, where the sphincter complex is excised following abdominoperineal excision
- Left-sided colonic resection where an anastomosis is likely to fail, for example, Hartmann's procedure for acute diverticulitis
- Where the functional result is unlikely to be acceptable, for example, colonic resection in a patient with fecal incontinence

A loop colostomy is used to decompress an obstructed colon especially if there are concerns that the ileocecal valve is competent, and therefore, a loop ileostomy would be inadequate.

Advantages of defunctioning loop colostomy versus loop ileostomy for obstruction are:

- Can be performed under local anesthetic
- Decompresses the proximal colon

Disadvantages:

- Difficult bulky stomas
- Prone to prolapse

A temporary loop colostomy (either transverse or descending colon) is an acceptable alternative to temporarily divert the fecal stream proximal to an anastomosis, although this author favors a loop ileostomy. Complete fecal diversion is not always achieved with a degree of overspill almost inevitable.

A mucous fistula is effectively an end colostomy that communicates with the defunctioned colon that leads down to the anus. No feces passes into this part of bowel, and it tends to discharge a little mucous only.

End colostomies are commonly placed in the left iliac fossa, whereas loop colostomies are often located in the left iliac fossa or right upper quadrant depending on whether the left colon or transverse colon has been utilized (Keighley and Williams 2007).

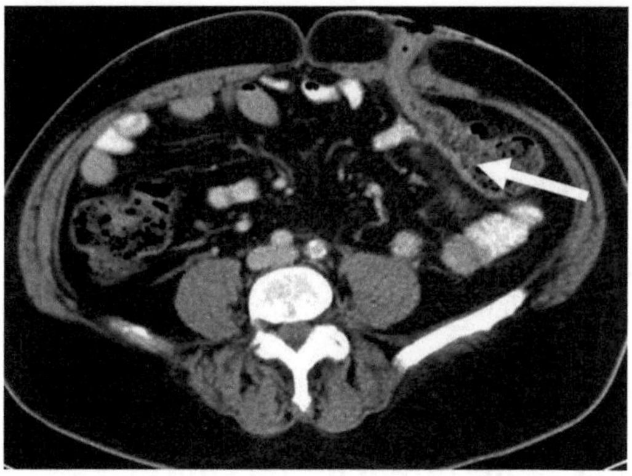

Fig. 8.29 Left-sided colostomy following Hartmann's procedure for acute diverticulitis. CT shows the left colon (*arrow*) and stomal orifice

8.4.3 Stoma Complications

8.4.3.1 Parastomal Hernia

The incidence of parastomal herniation may be as high 65% with many stomas ultimately forming parastomal hernias. Patients may be asymptomatic or develop minor symptoms such as a bulge or focal discomfort and in some cases life-threatening obstruction or strangulation. Repair can be local around the stoma, laparoscopic, or, at the time of laparotomy, with or without resiting of the stoma.

8.4.3.2 Prolapse

The incidence of prolapse for end colostomies and loop ileostomies is less than 5%, but transverse loop colostomies have a significantly higher incidence of up to 45%. This probably reflects not only the nature of loops as having a propensity to prolapse but also the circumstances in which the stoma was formed, that is, as an emergency in the presence of a dilated, edematous colon. Imaging seldom has a role in the management of these patients.

8.4.3.3 Stenosis and Retraction

Stomal stenosis or retraction occurs in up to 10% of patients. Stenosis can often be managed conservatively with dilatation but occasionally requires surgical reconstruction with either Z-plasty or resiting. Retraction may require refashioning of the stoma. These two complications can result from either tension at the time of surgery or relative ischemia of the colocutaneous anastomosis. Acute bowel obstruction is not usually seen as a complication compared with small bowel stomas. These complications are usually evaluated clinically with digital examination, but fluoroscopic examination can be helpful in excluding more proximal stenosis and defining the length of the stricture.

8.5 Recurrent Rectal Cancer and Pelvic Exenteration

Despite apparent curative resection of rectal carcinoma, local recurrence rates between 3% and 30% have been reported. 80% of cases occur within 2 years, with over half of these patients having disease confined to the pelvis.

Pelvic exenteration involves the evisceration of the organs of the pelvis. This may include some or all of the following: bladder, urethra, rectum, and anus and in the female the uterus and vagina. In cases with sacral involvement, then this may be performed in combination with partial sacrectomy.

The likelihood of recurrence depends on:

- The pathological stage of the primary tumor
- Involvement of the circumferential resection margin
- Tumors arising in the lower third of the rectum
- Tumors which have perforated or caused obstruction
- Quality of the initial surgery
- Use of neoadjuvant radiotherapy

Symptoms associated with recurrent rectal cancer are unpleasant, debilitating, and difficult to treat by nonsurgical means. Without treatment, the 5-year survival rate is less than 5%.

8.5.1 Imaging of Recurrent Rectal Cancer

Radiological evaluation of the post surgical pelvis is complex due to the problem of discriminating between residual fibrosis and recurrent tumor. This can be compounded by previous postoperative complications such as collections, hemorrhage, or leaks which add to the extent of fibrosis. Serial imaging with CT, MRI, PET CT, and measurement of tumor markers can be used to detect recurrence. The majority of anastomotic recurrences originate outside the bowel lumen and are often not accessible by endoscopic means. CT-guided biopsy may be required particularly where preoperative chemotherapy or radiotherapy are being considered (Fig. 8.30). The surgeon will also obtain additional information regarding tumor bulk and potential fixation with adjacent structures.

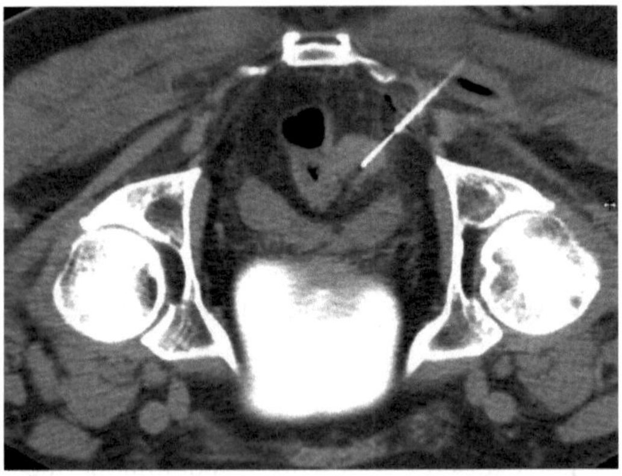

Fig. 8.30 Axial prone CT-guided transgluteal biopsy of new extraluminal soft tissue in a patient on surveillance following previous low anterior resection for rectal cancer with histology yielding adenocarcinoma, indicating recurrence

Demonstration of coexisting disease outside the pelvis is not an absolute contraindication to potential pelvic exenteration as resection and radiofrequency/microwave ablation can be performed to treat liver and lung metastases. However, the presence of disease outside the pelvis indicates another level of severity and therefore a poorer prognosis.

Contraindications to pelvic exenteration are:

- Sacral involvement above the S2/3 junction
- Tumor invasion of the pelvic sidewall
- Tumor traversing the greater sciatic foramen

The most favorable tumors for radical curative resection are central and invade the sacrum no higher than the S2/S3 disc space (Sagar and Pemberton 1996).

8.5.1.1 CT

Potential pitfalls in interpretation can be due to the presence of unopacified bowel loops and postoperative fibrosis. Indications of recurrent disease include lobulation or mass effect, increased enhancement (versus adjacent muscles), and a serial increase in size of the lesion. Malignancy can be confirmed with PET CT and/or biopsy. Biopsy is usually required in patients before undergoing neoadjuvant chemoradiotherapy prior to surgery (i.e., those who are radiotherapy naïve). Due to the position of most pelvic recurrences, a posterior transgluteal approach under CT guidance is often required for access since a large proportion of patients have high recurrences that are beyond the reach of transrectal ultrasound probes or have had APER and do not have access.

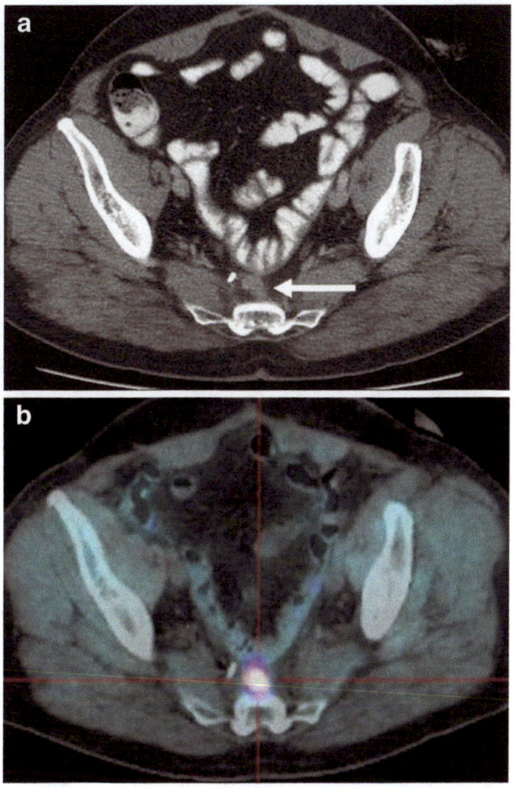

Fig. 8.31 Recurrent rectal cancer. (**a**) CT demonstrates a "nodule" within the presacral space (*arrow*), which is metabolically active on PET CT (**b**) confirming recurrence

8.5.1.2 PET CT

PET is very sensitive at detecting recurrence (Fig. 8.31). False-positive diagnoses can occur with persistent cavities following leaks and with normal physiological bowel uptake.

False-negative diagnoses can occur with mucinous tumors (Fig. 8.32), peritoneal disease, and with small liver metastases due to low-level FDG uptake and limited special resolution of PET scanner detectors (EVEN-SAPIR et al. 2004).

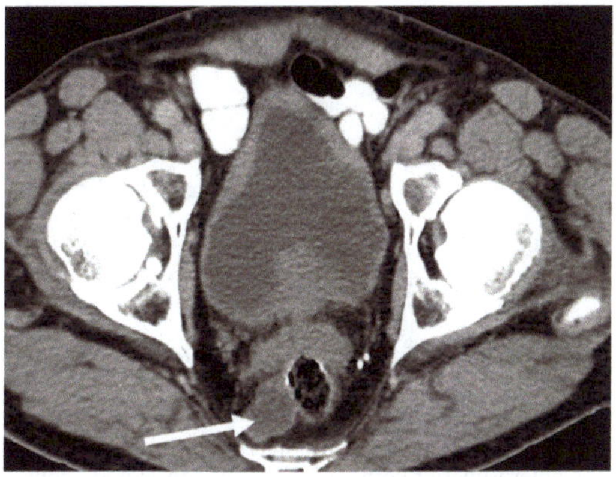

Fig. 8.32 Recurrent mucinous rectal cancer with extraluminal soft tissue (*arrow*) on CT. False-negative PET CT (*not shown*) with biopsy confirming tumor recurrence

8.5.1.3 MRI

MRI is an essential modality in the assessment of recurrent rectal cancer (Fig. 8.33). Its multiplanar abilities and use with contrast are important in distinguishing between recurrent tumor and postoperative fibrosis. A suggested MRI protocol includes (used in Leeds NHS Trust):

- T2W axial gradient echo sequences through the abdomen and pelvis to provide a general overview and to look for disease outside the pelvis
- T2W sagittal and axial sequences to provide anatomical detail
- T1W fat-saturated sequences pre- and post-contrast performed in all three planes to assess the relationship of tumor with the pelvic sidewall and anterior and posterior structures
- T2W fat-saturated or STIR sagittal and axial sequences of the pelvis to detect bone metastases (Fig. 8.34)

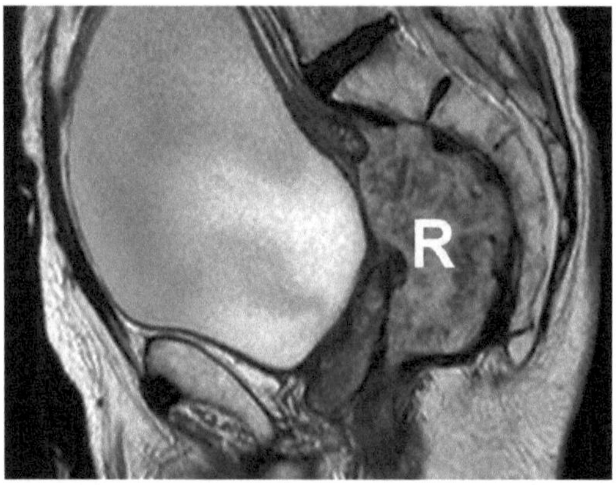

Fig. 8.33 Recurrent rectal cancer within the presacral space following previous APER. Sagittal T2W MRI shows a recurrent heterogeneous high-signal mass (*R*) secondary to mucinous tumor recurrence. There is contact with the sacrum at the S1/S2 level but no evidence of bone invasion

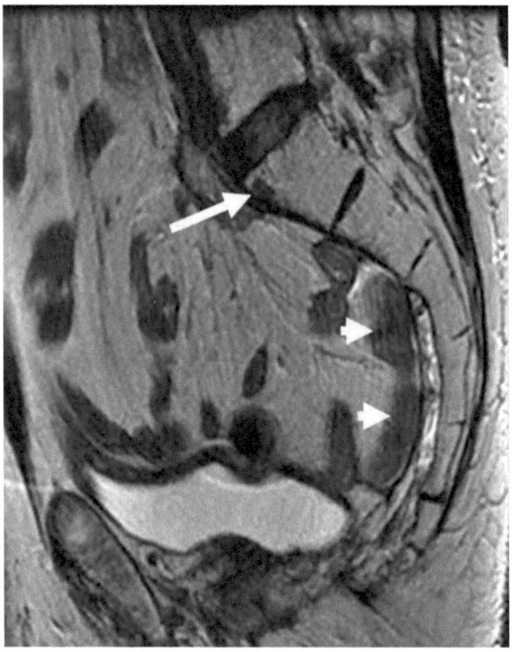

Fig. 8.34 Recurrent rectal cancer. Sagittal high-resolution T2W MRI demonstrates abnormal low signal within the anterosuperior corner of the S1 vertebral body consistent with malignant infiltration from recurrent rectal tumor (*large arrow*). Collapsed small bowel is present in the cavity at site of rectal excision (*small arrows*)

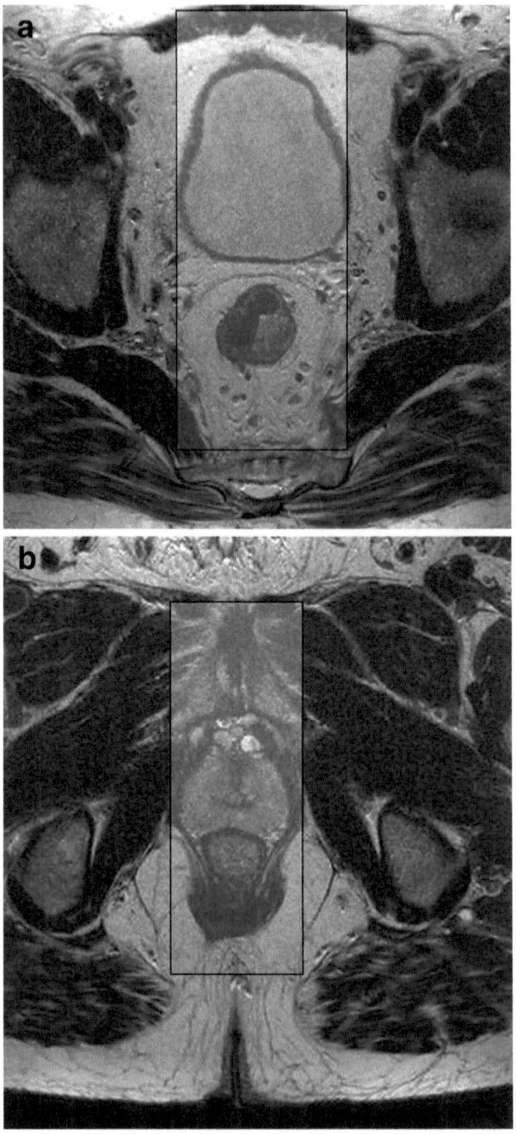

Fig. 8.35 (**a**, **b**) High-resolution axial T2W MRI pelvis demonstrating the anterior and posterior structures that are assessed when imaging recurrent rectal cancer in a male

Description of recurrence is recorded within the following compartments (MESSIOU et al. 2006):

- Anterior – structures threatened include the bladder and vagina, cervix, and uterus in women or prostate and seminal vesicles in men (Fig. 8.35).
- Lateral – involving the pelvic sidewall and greater sciatic foramen. Look for ureteric compromise (Fig. 8.36).
- Posterior – involving pelvic floor muscles, ischioanal fossa, presacral fascia, and the sacrum (Fig. 8.37).

MRI interpretation of recurrent rectal cancer is associated with numerous pitfalls. Tumor, granulation tissue, radiation-induced inflammatory changes, and hematoma can all display high signal on T2W images. Fibrosis is generally low signal on T2W sequences, but it is important to remember that fibrosis and recurrent tumor can coexist. The use of contrast is also not specific as enhancement can occur in both entities.

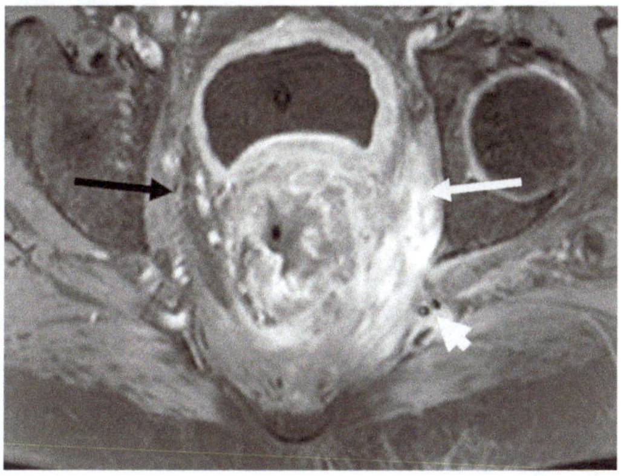

Fig. 8.36 Lateral recurrence. Axial T1 fat-sat MRI post-contrast shows recurrence extending to the left pelvic sidewall. There is abnormal enhancement involving left obturator internus (*long white arrow*) with encasement of the superior gluteal vessels (*short white arrow*). Right obturator internus indicated for comparison (*black arrow*)

Enhancement in recurrent disease includes a heterogeneous or rim pattern; the latter is not generally seen in fibrosis where there is usually only homogeneous low-level enhancement. Dynamic MRI is sometimes used which relies on the principle that recurrent tumor has both a greater blood supply than fibrosis and that the contrast peak occurs earlier. However, it is time-consuming and has not received widespread acceptance. In practice, MRI and PET CT are both complementary; MRI provides high-resolution anatomical detail required for preoperative planning, and PET CT allows supporting physiological evidence on the presence or absence of recurrence.

8.5.2 Complications of Pelvic Exenteration

The main complications following pelvic exenteration for recurrent rectal cancer include leak from the urinary conduit (Sect. 9.2.6.3), gastrointestinal/urinary fistula and obstruction, pelvic abscess, and hemorrhage. It is important to remember that such extensive resection often requires reconstruction of the soft tissues of the

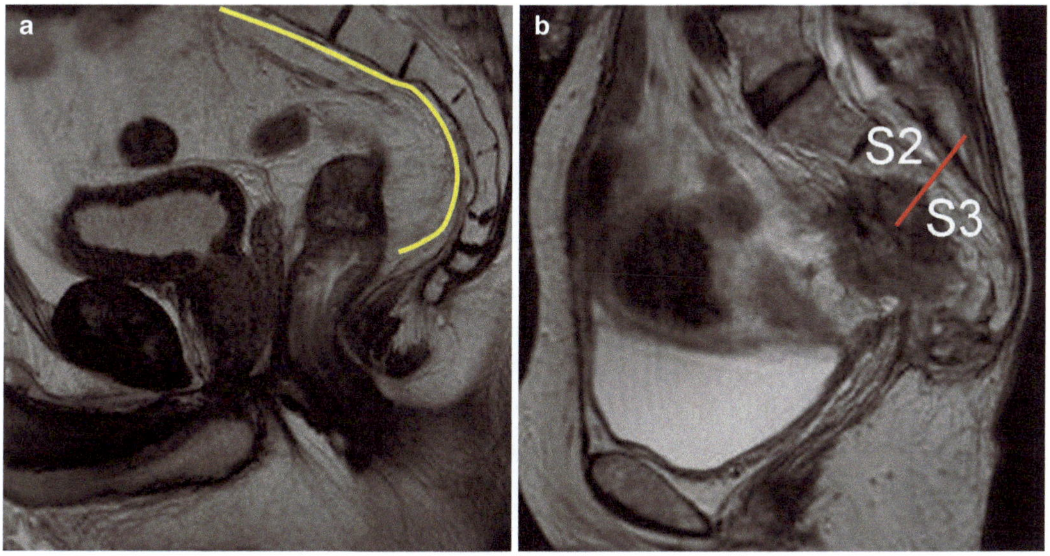

Fig. 8.37 Posterior compartment. Sagittal high-resolution T2W MRI demonstrates (**a**) the normal presacral fascia (*yellow line*) and sacral vertebrae. (**b**) Recurrence involving the S2 and S3 vertebrae. The *red line* demarcates the S2/S3 articulation. Tumor involvement above this boundary is generally a contraindication to pelvic exenteration

pelvis to fill the potential space created. Flap reconstructions are often mobilized by plastic surgeons in the form of the rectus abdominis or free flaps to fill the perineal defects. These are precious, and care needs to be taken during interventional procedures not to injure the vascular pedicle due to the risk of necrosis.

Five-year survival rates for pelvic exenteration in the literature are quoted between 20% and 30%.

8.5.3 Teaching Points

- Review all prior imaging.
- Triple assessment with CT, PET CT, and contrast-enhanced MRI is standard.
- MRI essential for assessment of resectability.
- Biopsy may be required for confirmation.
- MDT discussion is critical particularly to ascertain if neoadjuvant treatment is required before surgery.

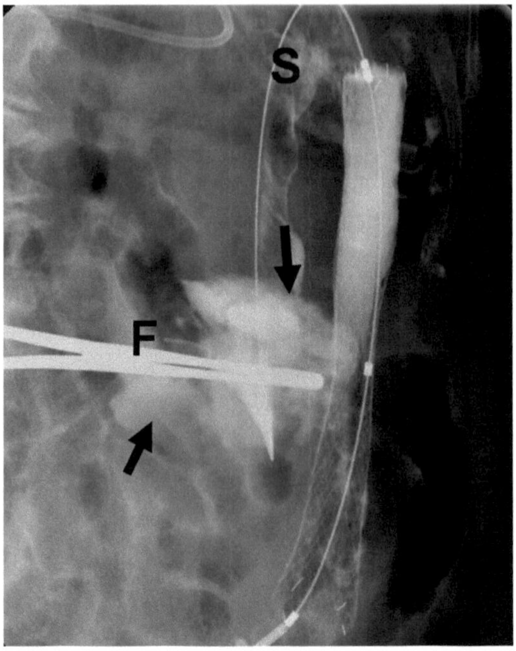

Fig. 8.38 Covered colonic stent placement for perforated diverticular disease in a 93-year-old patient too frail for surgery. Fluoroscopic image shows the stent within the descending colon and position relative to splenic flexure (*S*). Extravasated contrast (*arrows*) from the site of perforation, marked by position of forceps (*F*)

8.6 Image-Guided Colonic Intervention

8.6.1 Colonic Stenting

8.6.1.1 Clinical Indications

- Palliation in patients with obstructive symptoms due to inoperable colorectal cancer
- Bridge to surgery in patients with obstructing colorectal cancer
- Extrinsic compression due to pelvic malignancy (upper rectal strictures only as low rectal stents are associated with unacceptable tenesmus)
- Benign strictures and perforation (uncommon) (Fig. 8.38)
- Colovesical and colovaginal fistulas (covered stents)

8.6.1.2 Procedure Summary – Colonic Stenting (Fig. 8.39)

- Can be performed by a solo operator or as a combined procedure with or without endoscopic assistance.
- Malignant stricture traversed with guidewire using catheter or endoscope.
- Injection of iodinated contrast to delineate extent of the lesion.
- Deployment of uncovered expandable metal stent under fluoroscopic guidance.
- Lesions proximal to the splenic flexure are generally stented through the endoscope.

8.6.1.3 Contraindications

- Impending cecal perforation and suspected colonic ischemia

8.6.1.4 Background

The surgical treatment options for patients who present with obstruction from colorectal malignancy include resection with a primary anastomosis or a two-stage procedure involving resection and stoma formation (the stoma is reversed at a later date). Colonic stenting is increasingly being used as a method to alleviate intestinal obstruction, thus delaying surgery and the associated

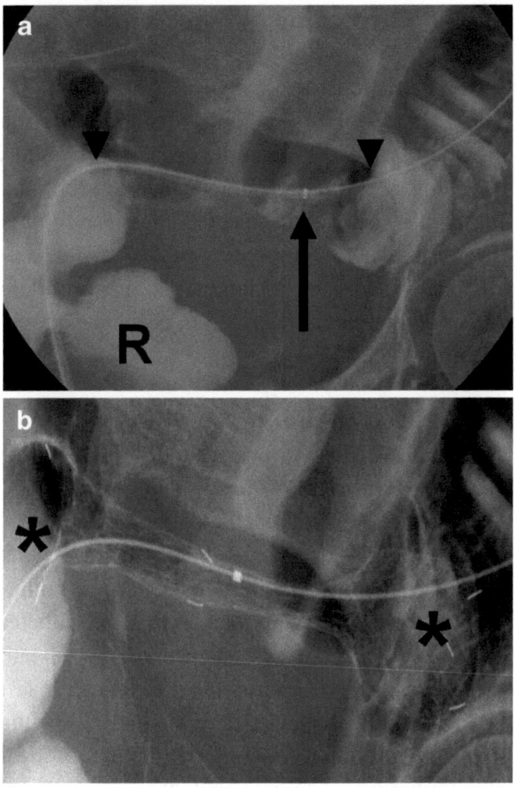

Fig. 8.39 (**a**, **b**) Uncovered colonic stent placement in the palliative management of rectosigmoid cancer. Stiff wire placed beyond the tumor by an endoscopist. Fluoroscopic delineation of the stricture (between *black arrowheads*) with iodinated contrast via a sheath (*long arrow*). Rectum (*R*). (**b**) Image taken after stent delivery. Note the flared ends of the stent (*asterisks*) indicate adequate coverage of the tumor

hazards of operating on acutely obstructed bowel (mortality following laparotomy for large bowel obstruction is 10–40%) (Mainar et al. 1999). The efficacy of stenting in acute colonic obstruction compared with surgical treatment is currently being studied in a UK multicenter randomized trial (ColoREctal Stent Trial – CREST). Primary resection without the requirement of a stoma is then performed at a later date (typically with an elective mortality of less than 5%). The intention of colonic stenting is to reduce perioperative morbidity, hospital stay, and stoma formation.

Colonic stents are manufactured to a range of lengths (40–140 mm) and diameters (18–32 mm) and may be covered or uncovered depending on the clinical indication. Stents can be deployed through the endoscope or over a guidewire alone. They usually have radiopaque markers at either end and sometimes in the center of the stent. In the opinion of the authors, a combined approach with expert endoscopy and radiology input allows the greatest chance for success.

8.6.1.5 Poststenting Imaging

Routine imaging is not mandatory, but an abdominal X-ray is sometimes performed within 12–24 h of stent placement. Accurately placed colonic stents will be narrowed in their central portion at the site of the stricture and opened at either end. Stents typically reach a maximum diameter after 24 h. A rapid increase in luminal diameter increases the risk of perforation, and for this reason, balloon dilatation should not be performed. Occasionally, overlapping stents are placed for long strictures. Successful deployment will result in decompression of dilated proximal colon and an improvement of symptoms. Contrast enemas may be performed where there is doubt regarding stent position and patency.

8.6.1.6 Poststenting Complications

The technical success rate in colonic stenting is typically 80–90%, but the clinical success rate is 10% lower. The most common complications are failure due to complete obstruction, bleeding, perforation, stent migration, and fracture (Khot et al. 2002).

8.6.1.7 Early Complications (Within 24 h)

Early complications include bleeding and perforation. Perforation rates are approximately 5%, caused by perforation from the guidewire or tumor rupture due to stent expansion. Similarly, bleeding occurs in 5% of patients and in most cases settles spontaneously within 24 h. Tenesmus, pain, and fecal incontinence can occur after lower rectal stent placement.

Failure of relief of colonic obstruction at 96 h should prompt reassessment to exclude stent migration or malposition.

8.6.1.8 Late Complications (>24 h)

Late complications include distal stent migration (Fig. 8.40), reobstruction due to tumor overgrowth, fecal impaction, stent fracture (Fig. 8.41),

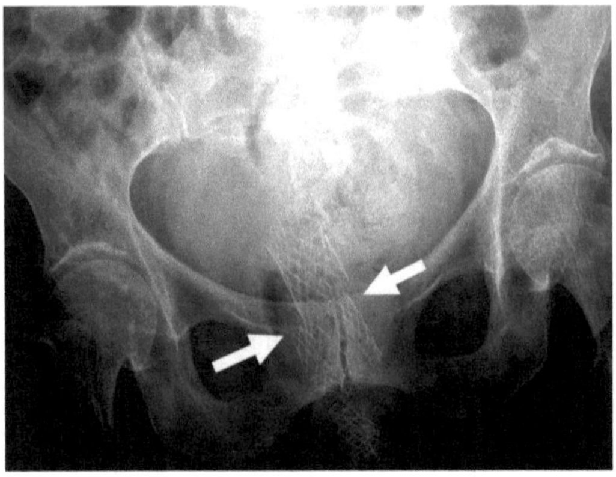

Fig. 8.40 Colonic stent migration and fracture. AXR 2 weeks following palliative stent placement for a midsigmoid tumor demonstrates the stent within the anorectum and discontinuity of the wire mesh, indicating fracture (*white arrows*)

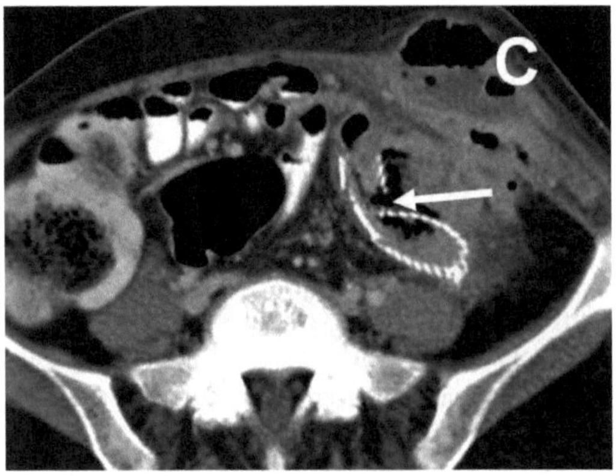

Fig. 8.41 Stent fracture. CT performed 1 month post emergency colonic stent placement for malignant large bowel obstruction. There is a fracture through the stent (*arrow*) with an enterocutaneous fistula and abdominal wall collection (*C*)

and erosion of the end of the stent through the colonic wall. This is a particular risk in patients who undergo stent placement followed by palliative or adjuvant chemotherapy; colonic wall changes associated with tumor regression as well as associated relative immunosuppression are probably the causative factors.

8.6.1.9 Teaching Points

- Colonic stents may be used as a palliative treatment or as a bridge to surgery in patients with malignant colonic obstruction.

8.6.2 Cecostomy

8.6.2.1 Indication

This is performed for colonic pseudoobstruction in patients where endoscopic decompression has been unsuccessful and surgery is in appropriate. It may also be used in selected cases for colonic irrigation, where colonoscopic assistance is usually required. This technique is inappropriate where there is concern for cecal ischemia/perforation.

8.6.2.2 Technique

The dilated cecum is located under fluoroscopic guidance. Up to four "pexy" sutures are positioned around the intended location of the percutaneous balloon catheter. A final puncture of the colon is performed to allow passage of a guidewire and dilation of the tract so that the catheter can be placed through a peel away sheath (Fig. 8.42). It is important that the catheter is left in situ for 4–6 weeks to allow maturation of the tract and minimize risk of free intraperitoneal contamination by colonic contents.

8.6.3 Sigmoidopexy

8.6.3.1 Indications

This is performed in cases of recurrent sigmoid volvulus in patients too frail for primary resection. It is contraindicated if there is clinical or endoscopic evidence of colonic ischemia or necrosis.

8.6.3.2 Technique

Sigmoidopexy may be carried out percutaneously or laparoscopically:

- Percutaneous – using a similar fixation technique to radiological insertion of gastrostomy (RIG) or cecostomy (see above). The sigmoid colon is decompressed and detorsed using a colonoscope, and the bowel is fixed to the anterior abdominal wall using two "pexy" sutures on either side of the apex of the sigmoid colon. This does not require placement of a percutaneous catheter.
- Laparoscopic sigmoidopexy – the sigmoid colon is extraperitonealized and fixed to the

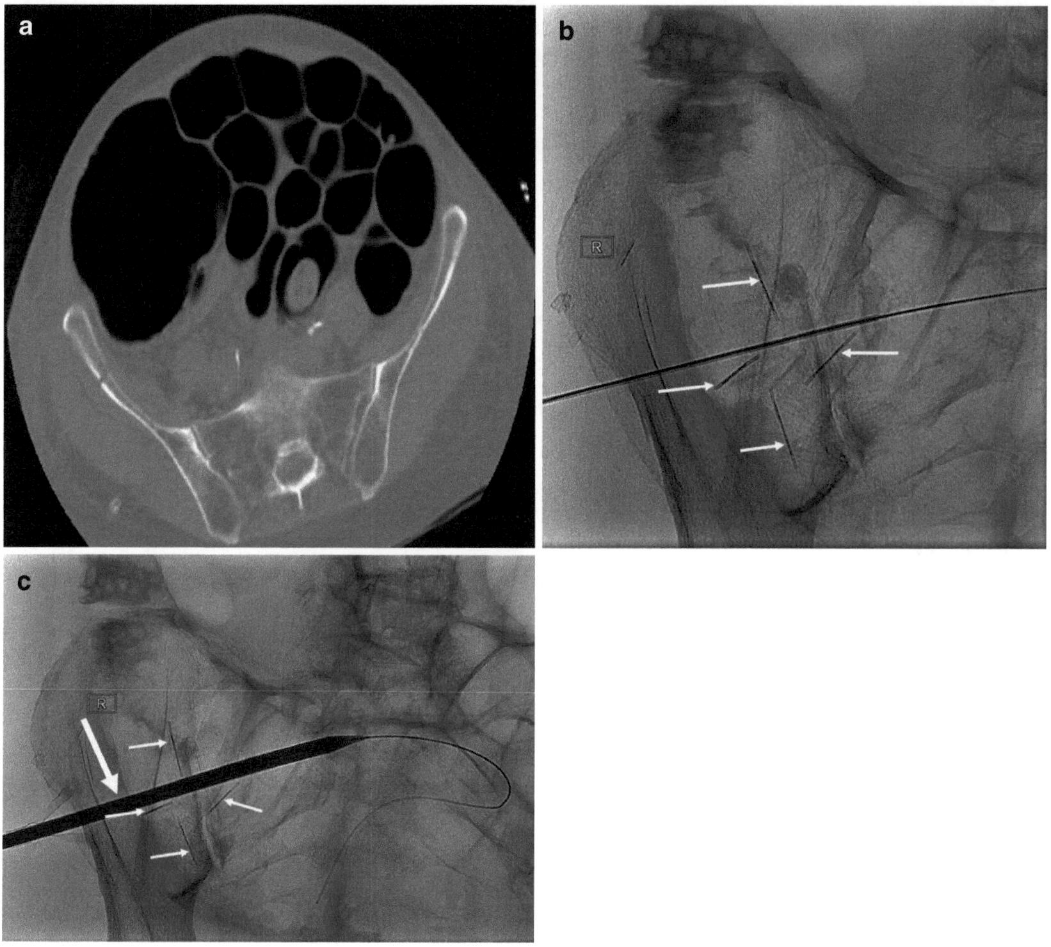

Fig. 8.42 Cecostomy. Postoperative global ileus in a patient on intensive care postsurgery for a C2 spine fracture requiring increased ventilatory support (due to abdominal distension). (**a**) CT confirms dilatation of the small bowel and colon. Endoscopic decompression of the colon was unsuccessful. (**b**) 4 pexy sutures (*white arrows*) were placed into the cecum under fluoroscopic guidance followed by (**c**) an 18.5-Fr peel away sheath (*large arrow*) to allow placement of a 14-Fr gastrostomy tube. The cecostomy was left in situ for 6 weeks to allow formation of a tract before it was eventually removed

anterior abdominal wall with sutures, thus preventing further volvulus.

- If sigmoidopexy is unsuccessful, sigmoid colectomy with end colostomy is performed.

8.7 Surgery for Fistula-in-Ano

8.7.1 Background

Anorectal sepsis is the most common colorectal emergency. Ninety percent of cases are due to cryptoglandular infection, that is, obstruction of the anal glands that lie in the intersphincteric space or anal ducts that traverse the internal anal sphincter (Morris et al. 2000). Subsequent spontaneous or surgical drainage may lead to a granulation tissue lined tract which causes recurrent symptoms. Other causes include inflammatory bowel disease (particularly Crohn's disease), malignancy, previous radiotherapy, unusual infections (e.g., actinomycosis, TB, and Chlamydia), and postoperative (e.g., stapled hemorrhoidopexy).

Up to 20% of anorectal abscesses will go on to produce a fistula-in-ano. A fistula is defined as an abnormal connection between two epithelialized surfaces which in the case of fistula-in-ano involves the anus/rectum and the perineal skin. Secondary tracts may radiate from the primary opening, leading to a complex fistula.

Knowledge of anatomy of the pelvic floor and sphincters is important to understand both the classification system of fistula-in-ano and the surgical techniques employed in their treatment.

8.7.2 Parks Classification System for Fistula-in-Ano

Fistulae-in-ano are described according to their primary tract and any abscess extensions in to the named anorectal spaces. Park's description of the four main fistula types remains useful (Parks et al. 1976):

- Intersphincteric – via the internal sphincter to the intersphincteric space communicating with the perineum. This accounts for 70% of anal fistulae.
- Transsphincteric – low origin via internal and external sphincters traversing the ischiorectal fossa and communicating with the perineum (25% of anal fistulae).
- Suprasphincteric – via the intersphincteric space extending superiorly above the puborectalis muscle into ischiorectal fossa and then to the perineum (5% of anal fistulae).
- Extrasphincteric – from the perianal skin through the levator ani muscles to the rectal wall completely outside the sphincter mechanism (1% of anal fistulae).

In addition, Goodsall's rule helps the surgeon and radiologist to anticipate the likely location of an internal opening. An external opening that lies in front of a line drawn transversely across the perineum through the anus will follow a radial tract. External openings behind this meridian follow a curved tract to open in the midline in the 6 o'clock position. Exceptions to this rule include Crohn's disease, external openings that lie distant from the anus (>3 cm), and abscesses that horseshoe around the anus.

Preoperative MRI has an important role in the evaluation of patients with complex disease, particularly those with one or more extensions, suspected supralevator and extrasphincteric fistulas, and patients with Crohn's disease; these groups will be most difficult to adequately characterize with surgical examination alone. MRI may be requested to evaluate disease distribution where a more complex disease distribution is suspected at initial examination under anesthetic in order to ensure that no sites of undrained sepsis are present before definitive fistula surgery. Where a seton has been placed, it appears as a central low signal point on axial sections traversing the high-signal edematous fistula tract (Halligan and Stoker 2006).

8.7.3 Surgical Techniques for Fistula-in-Ano

- Fistulotomy
- Core fistulectomy
- Seton placement
- Mucosal advancement flap (Williams 2009)

8.7.3.1 Fistulotomy

Fistulotomy is division of the tissue encircled in the fistulous tract to lay it open and allow healing by secondary intention:

- Indicated in most fistulae-in-ano (intersphincteric and low transsphincteric).
- Probe passed through internal and external openings and the tract is laid open with a scalpel or cauterization.
- At low levels in the anal canal, the internal and outer external sphincter fibers can be divided at right angles without affecting continence (not anteriorly in female patients).
- If the fistula extends higher into the sphincter mechanism, a seton should be placed.

8.7.3.2 Core Fistulectomy

Core fistulectomy is a formal excision of the fistulous tract without division of the muscle. Often, this is accomplished by delineating the tract at examination under anesthetic (EUA) with a probe and coring out the fistula following the probe up to and through the sphincter complex. The internal opening can then be closed (possibly combined with an advancement flap).

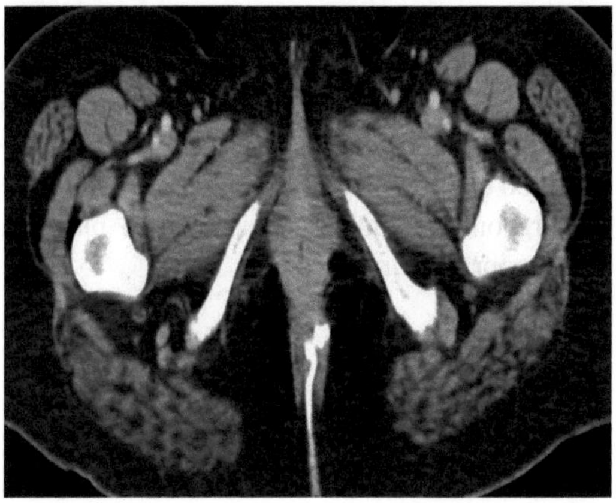

Fig. 8.43 Seton appearances on CT as a high-attenuation suture material traversing a low transsphincteric fistula

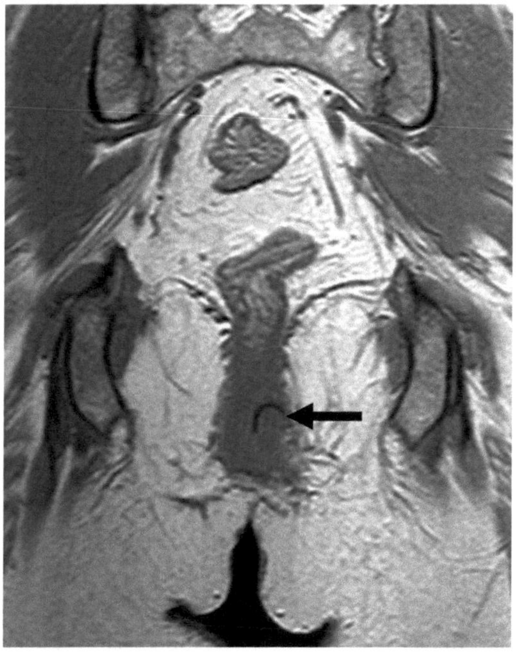

Fig. 8.44 Seton appearances on MRI. Coronal T1W MRI of the pelvis demonstrates a seton within the left anal canal (*arrow*)

8.7.3.3 Seton Placement

A seton is a foreign material that is placed in a fistula tract either to drain ongoing sepsis or to cut through the sphincter slowly to allow muscle fibrosis and scarring to help maintain the integrity of the sphincter mechanism (Figs. 8.43 and 8.44). Commonly used materials include nonabsorbable sutures or elastic (vascular sloops) bands. Cutting chemical setons are not widely used because of increased risks of incontinence:

- Indicated in high, complex, recurrent, or multiple fistulae.
- Can be placed in patients with poor preoperative sphincter pressures.
- Anterior fistula-in-ano in female patients.
- Setons promote fibrosis of the tract, slow transaction of the fistula, and provide visualization of the degree of sphincter muscle involvement.
- Setons comprise sutures, silastic, or rubber bands.
- Can be performed in conjunction with fistulotomy.

8.7.3.4 Advancement Flap

When traditional methods of fistulotomy and setons have failed or are inappropriate due to complex disease, then an advancement flap can be used. The tract can be curetted or excised as a core fistulectomy and the internal opening closed by raising a mucosal flap that is then sutured to cover the opening.

8.7.3.5 Novel Treatments: Fibrin Glue and Collagen Plugs

Recently, there has been considerable interest in the use of fibrin glue or collagen plugs to obliterate the fistulous tract. All ongoing sepsis needs eradicating (possibly by using a drainage seton) and the tract prepared with curettage. The tract is then either filled with fibrin glue or a collagen plug. Research continues to determine the most effective technique for dealing with this disease.

8.7.4 Postoperative Imaging

The role for imaging in recurrent fistula-in-ano is well established (Keighley and Williams 2007). MRI is superior to endoanal ultrasound in the evaluation of complex fistulas because of the limited beam penetration of ultrasound for evaluation of trans- and suprasphincteric fistulas and extensions and difficulties differentiating active fistulas from healed tracts. Therefore, ultrasound has a very limited role, reserved for patients with contraindication to MRI. Fluoroscopic fistulography is a historical footnote and is no longer practiced because of the lack of correlation of the position of the fistula track and extensions with the sphincter muscles.

MRI clearly defines the fistula classification, number and extent of fistulas, and extensions (which is particularly important in Crohn's disease) and the presence of abscesses and other unexpected complications that may account for nonhealing or recurrence (such as osteomyelitis). The majority of radiologists use either STIR or T2 sequences (with fat saturation) for MRI assessment using an axial and coronal plane inclined to the anal canal (Halligan and Stoker 2006). Gadolinium-enhanced T1 with fat saturation allows differentiation of fluid collection from soft tissue edema/granulation tissue. This is perhaps most useful in the evaluation of patients with Crohn's disease where anti-TNF immunomodulator therapy may be used rather than surgery, where the presence of an abscess is a contraindication to drug treatment without prior surgical drainage.

8.7.5 Postoperative Complications

8.7.5.1 Early Complications

- Urinary retention
- Bleeding

8.7.5.2 Late Complications

- Recurrence – up to 20% for low and simple fistulas and 40% for high and complex fistulas.
- Incontinence due to damage to the anal sphincters ranges from minor symptoms (such as involuntary passage of flatus) in up to 50% of cases to gross fecal incontinence in 3–5%.
- Anal stenosis secondary to fibrosis from the healing process is uncommon.

8.7.6 Teaching Points

- Anorectal abscesses and fistulae-in-ano form a continuum of disease and often coexist.
- Imaging in the acute presentation is often not necessary but may be appropriate for complex and recurrent disease to guide the surgeon at the time of surgery.
- Parks's classification and Goodsall's rule help to delineate fistulas.
- Good quality imaging and review between the surgeon and radiologist is vital to planning appropriate surgery.

8.8 Surgery for the Pelvic Floor and Defecatory Disorders

8.8.1 Clinical Indication

Pelvic floor dysfunction can present with symptoms related to the anterior compartment (bladder), middle compartment (vagina and uterus), posterior compartment (rectum), or any combination of these. This section will concentrate on the treatment of posterior compartment dysfunction, although it should be noted that in 30–40% of cases other compartments might be affected. As such, pelvic floor dysfunction should be treated within a multidisciplinary framework, including input from coloproctologists, urogynecologists, radiologists, physiologists, specialist nurses, and physiotherapists.

Posterior compartment dysfunction includes fecal incontinence, constipation/obstructed defecation, or rectal prolapse either alone or in combination.

It is estimated that some 10% of the adult population suffers from constipation, but this figure may represent the "tip of the iceberg." It is clinically useful to differentiate slow transit constipation (a failure to transport fecal content to the rectum) from obstructed defecation (a normal desire to defecate but an inability to satisfactorily evacuate the rectum). In a proportion of patients, slow transit constipation and obstructed defecation will coexist and may be further complicated by irritable bowel syndrome.

Between 1% and 10% of adults are affected by fecal incontinence with 0.5–1.0% experiencing regular fecal incontinence that severely affects quality of life. It is a source of social stigmatization and isolation. The majority of patients with constipation/obstructed defecation and fecal incontinence either self-medicate or are treated in the community. Referral to tertiary care usually denotes a significant impact on quality of life and a desire to undergo interventional therapy.

A careful history and physical examination is the cornerstone to diagnosis. Quantification should include assessment with a symptom specific scoring system. All patients should undergo endoscopic visualization of the left colon and rectum as a minimum. Further investigations include:

- Constipation: colonic transit studies (Figs. 8.45 and 8.46), defecating proctography (+/– dynamic MRI), anorectal physiology, and endoanal ultrasound
- Fecal incontinence: anorectal physiology and endoanal ultrasound (Stoker et al. 2001)

Based on the results of the above imaging/investigations, the disorder can be classified as an aid to preoperative decision making. The mainstay of treatment is conservative management in the first instance with escalation up the treatment algorithm as necessary.

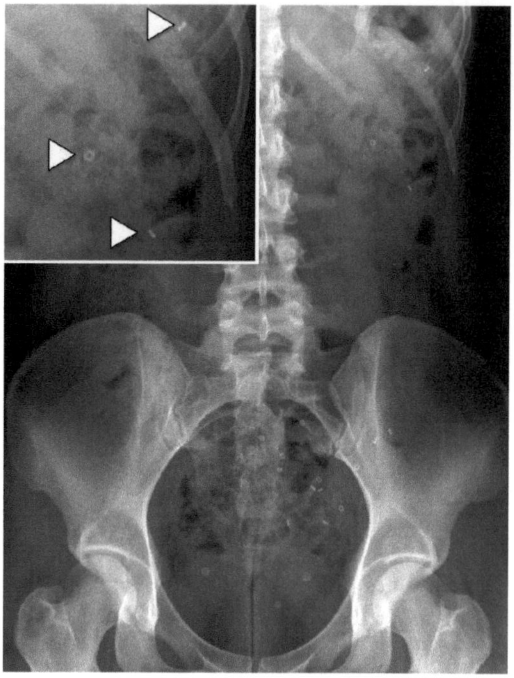

Fig. 8.45 Delayed colonic transit in a young female. Twenty-one out of thirty markers are retained within the colon (*arrowheads* – rings) on the abdominal radiograph performed 5 days after capsule ingestion

8.8.2 Summary of Management for Pelvic Floor Disorders

The following is an overview of possible management options:

8.8.2.1 Constipation

- Slow transit constipation: dietary modification, laxatives and enemas, irrigation techniques, sacral nerve stimulation, subtotal colectomy, and ileorectal anastomosis (rarely)
- Obstructed defecation: dietary modification, laxatives and enemas, biofeedback therapy, irrigation techniques, stapled transanal rectal resection (STARR), and laparoscopic ventral rectopexy

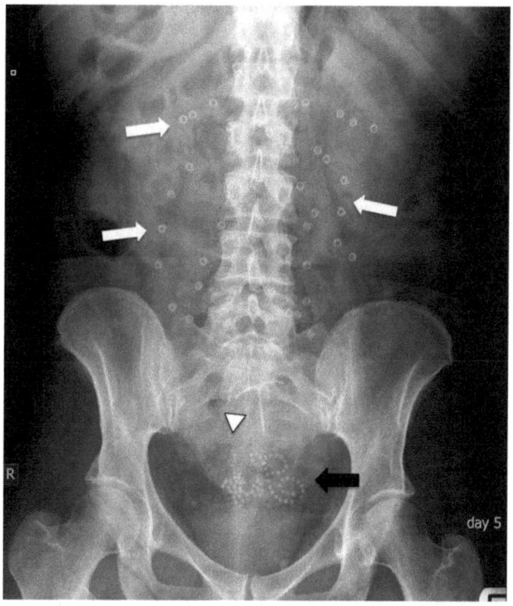

Fig. 8.46 Pitfalls in interpretation of colon transit studies. Normal transit study. Coils from previous mesh hernia repair (*white arrows*) and artifacts related to patient's underwear (*black arrow*) should not be mistaken for retained markers, and they do not conform to the normal path of colon. IUCD within the uterus (*arrow head*)

8.8.2.2 Fecal Incontinence

- Sphincter defect on endoanal ultrasound: constipating and bulking agents, irrigation techniques, anterior sphincter repair, sacral nerve modulation, and stoma formation

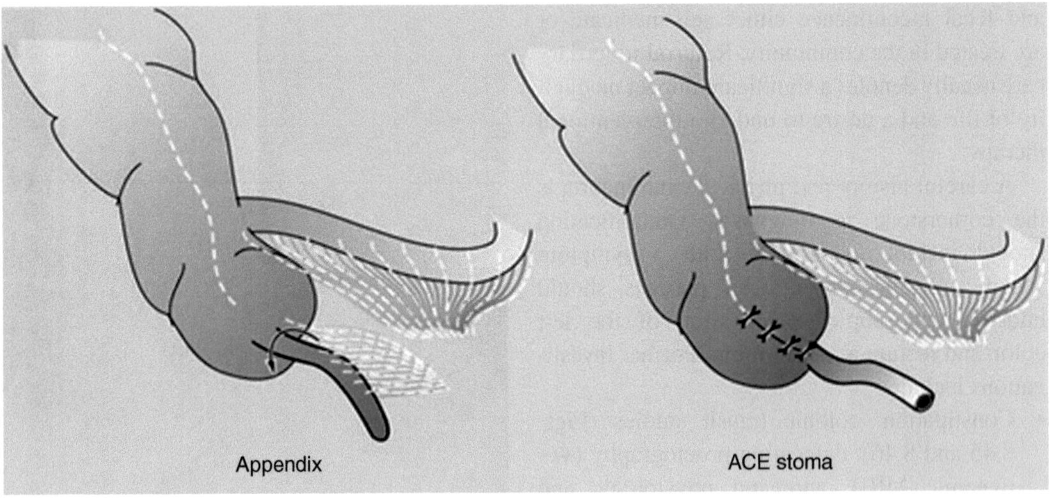

Fig. 8.47 ACE procedure. The appendix is used to make an antegrade colonic enema stoma

- No sphincter defect/weak sphincter on anorectal physiology: constipating and bulking agents, irrigation techniques, sacral nerve modulation, and stoma formation

8.8.2.3 Full-Thickness Rectal Prolapse

- Patient fit for abdominal surgery: laparoscopic rectopexy +/– sigmoid resection and laparoscopic ventral rectopexy
- Patient unfit for abdominal surgery: Delorme's procedure and perineal rectosigmoidectomy (Altemeier's procedure)

8.8.3 Surgery for Slow Transit Constipation

A proportion of patients that are refractory to oral laxatives for chronic constipation require antegrade colonic enema (ACE) to facilitate colonic emptying (Fig. 8.47). This is a minimally invasive option for patients who may otherwise be offered subtotal colectomy and ileorectal anastomosis. The operation involves creation of a stoma to the abdominal wall using the tunneled appendix (or ileum where the patient has undergone appendicectomy). This can then be intermittently catheterized to deliver a large-volume enema to empty the colon. In the immediate postoperative period, the appendix remains catheterized to maintain patency for up to 4 weeks.

8.8.4 Surgery for Obstructed Defecation: Technique and Postoperative Anatomy

8.8.4.1 Stapled Transanal Rectal Resection (STARR)

STARR corrects the mechanical obstruction to defecation (internal rectal prolapse/intussusception +/– rectocele) by achieving a transanal, full-thickness, circumferential resection of the distal rectum and associated anatomical defects (Fig. 8.48).

Two techniques are described based upon the stapling device employed. The PPH-STARR uses two firings of a circular stapler to produce separate anterior and posterior hemicircumferential resections. The Transtar procedure uses a curved stapler, specifically designed for STARR, to achieve a circumferential resection by means of multiple, sequential firings of the device. The end result of the two techniques is similar (Jayne and Stuto 2009).

8.8.4.2 Laparoscopic Ventral Rectopexy (Sacrocolporectopexy)

Laparoscopic ventral rectopexy corrects the mechanical obstruction to defecation (internal rectal prolapse +/– rectocele) by means of a mesh suspension of the posterior and middle pelvic compartments. Additionally, it closes the Pouch of Douglas and corrects any associated enterocele and supports the vaginal vault (Fig. 8.49).

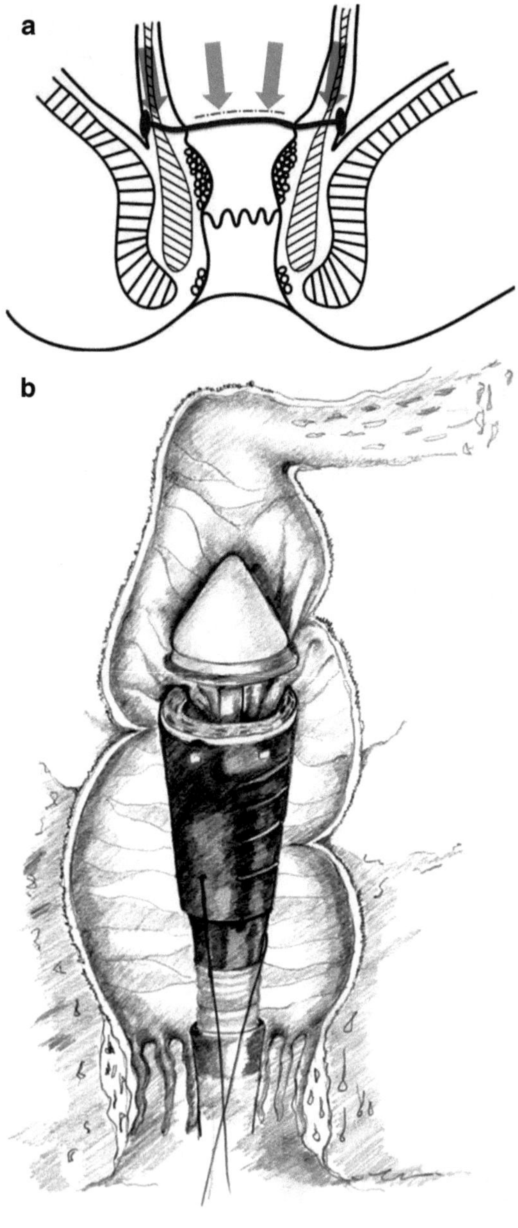

Fig. 8.48 (**a**, **b**) Stapled transanal resection of rectocele (STARR). A full-thickness resection of the bowel wall results in removal of the rectocele and shortening of the residual rectum (*arrows*) using a circumferential anastomosis (*continuous line*). (**b**) The full thickness of the bowel wall is pulled into the stapler for excision of rectocele

The right pararectal gutter is opened and the dissection extended over the anterior peritoneal reflection. Care is taken not to dissect in the posterior rectal plane to avoid rectal denervation. The rectovaginal septum is dissected as low as possible; a strip of mesh is inserted into the space created and sutured to the anterior rectal wall and posterior vaginal vault. The proximal end of the mesh is sutured to the fascia at the sacral promontory, resuspending the distal rectum and vaginal vault. The mesh is excluded from the pelvic cavity by reconstruction of the peritoneum (D'Hoore et al. 2008).

8.8.5 Surgery for Full-Thickness Rectal Prolapse: Techniques and Postoperative Anatomy

8.8.5.1 Perineal Procedures

Delorme's Procedure

A sleeve resection is performed of the prolapsing mucosa and submucosa, leaving the muscular rectal tube intact. The muscular tube is plicated in a longitudinal fashion to eradicate the prolapse and the foreshortened distal rectum returned to its anatomical position.

Perineal Rectosigmoidectomy (Altemeier's Procedure)

The outer bowel tube of the prolapsed rectum is incised within a few centimeters of the dentate line, entering the pelvic cavity proper from the transanal approach. Sequential division of the mesorectum (+/– mesosigmoid) allows delivery of the entire rectosigmoid transanally, which is resected and gastrointestinal continuity restored by either a stapled or hand-sewn anastomosis.

8.8.5.2 Abdominal Procedures

Laparoscopic Resectional Rectopexy

This combines posterior rectopexy with resection of the sigmoid colon and stapling of the colorectal anastomosis. It is used to treat full-thickness rectal prolapse associated with constipation. The procedure is associated with low rates of prolapse recurrence but with the added morbidity of an anastomosis.

Posterior rectopexy is performed by mobilization of the rectum in the total mesorectal excision (TME) planes with suture fixation at the level of the sacral promontory. When rectopexy is performed alone, without sigmoid resection, mesh placement is sometimes used to help secure the posterior fixation.

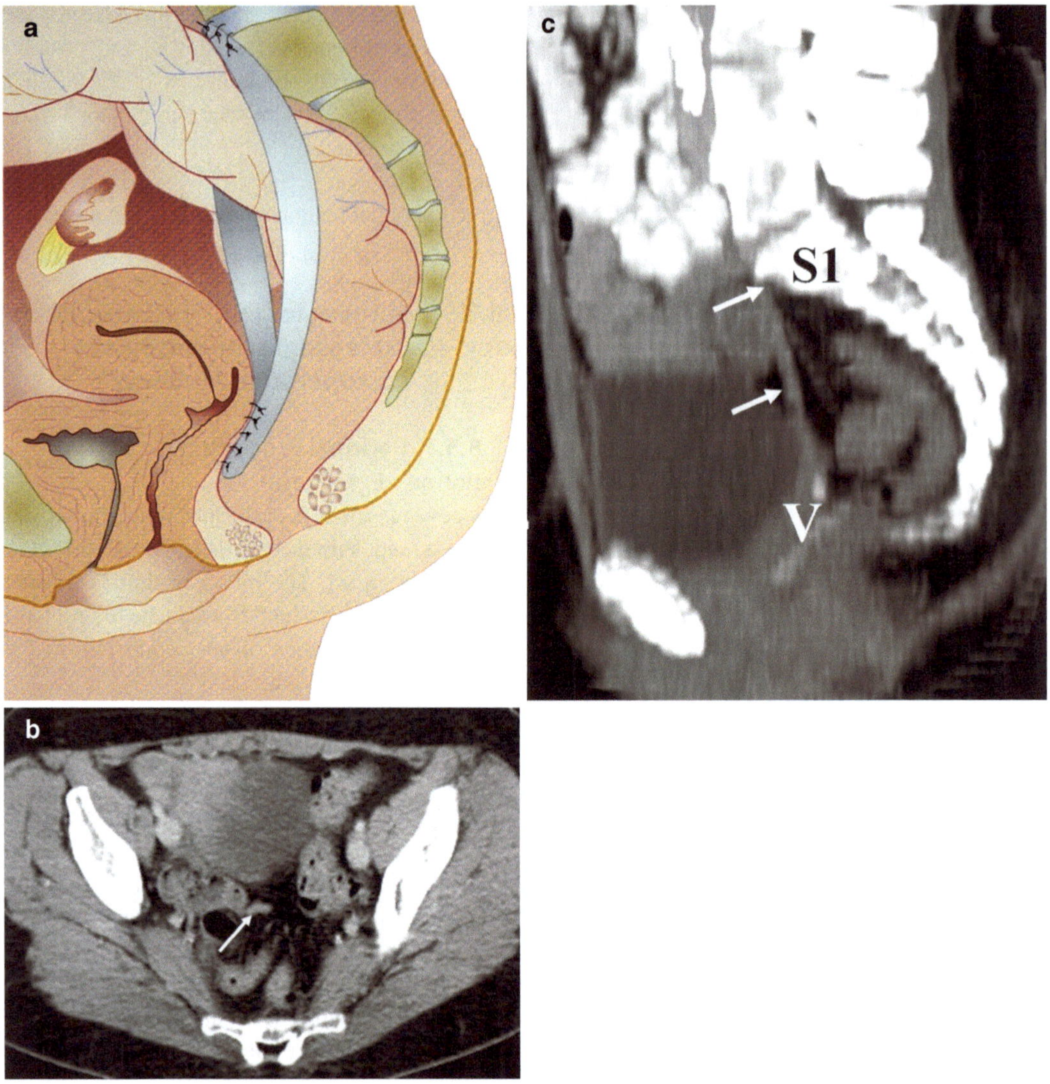

Fig. 8.49 (**a–c**) Laparoscopic ventral rectopexy (sacrocolporectopexy). (**a**) Surgical line drawing. (**b**, **c**) Ventral rectopexy mesh on CT. (**b**) The tape (*arrows*) is soft tissue attenuation and similar density to bowel loops. (**c**) It should be anchored between the sacral promontory and the vaginal vault (*V*) as seen on the sagittal thick MIP reconstruction

Laparoscopic ventral rectopexy (as described above) has been advocated as an alternative to posterior rectopexy with claimed benefits in terms of reduced postoperative constipation.

8.8.6 Surgery for Incontinence

8.8.6.1 Anterior Sphincteroplasty

Anterior sphincter defects are usually associated with obstetric trauma. Surgical management involves a transverse perineal incision (to access the perineum) with mobilization of the disrupted ends of the external anal sphincter (and internal sphincter if identifiable) which are then sutured together (usually in an overlapping repair).

8.8.6.2 Post-Anal Repair

This is rarely performed due to poor long-term outcomes. The procedure involves plication of the posterior levators in the post-anal space, resulting in a more pronounced anorectal angle.

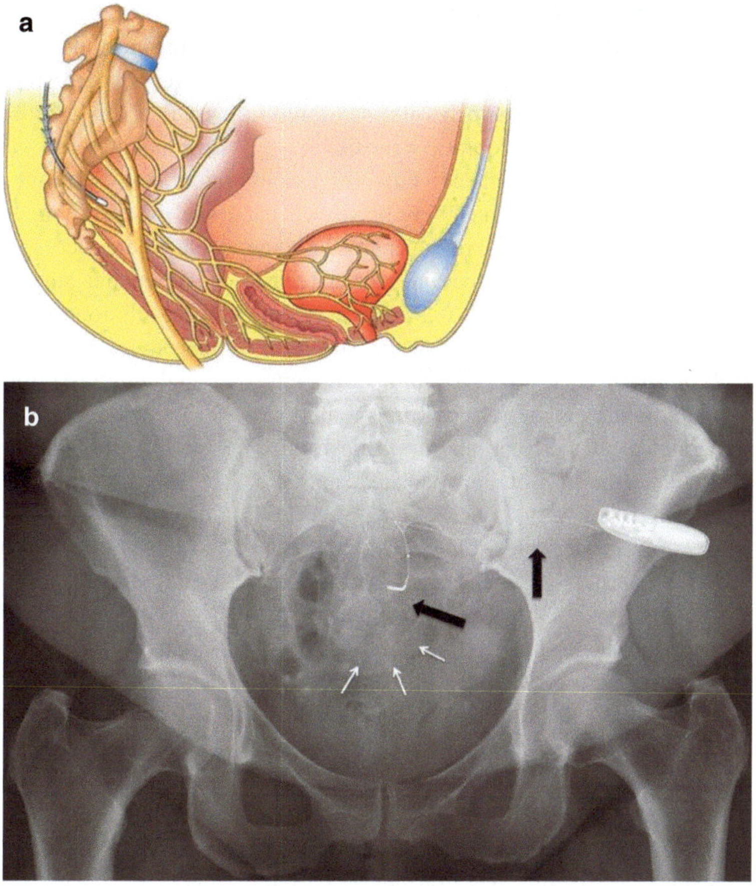

Fig. 8.50 (**a**) Line drawing of a sacral nerve stimulator InterStim (Medtronic, Minneapolis). (**b**) Normal plain film appearances of sacral nerve stimulator with wire positioned through the left S2 vertebral foramen (*black arrows*). Note metal suture line (*white arrows*) from previous subtotal colectomy and ileorectal anastomosis for slow transit

8.8.6.3 Sacral Nerve Modulation

Sacral nerve modulation is increasingly used as a first-line intervention for fecal incontinence. It is usually performed as a two-stage procedure: an initial "screening" temporary stimulation which, if successful in achieving greater than a 50% improvement in symptoms, can be followed by implantation of a permanent stimulator.

It is associated with low morbidity and can be performed as a day case procedure involving percutaneous placement of either the temporary or permanent electrode into the S3 (occasionally S4) sacral foramen (Fig. 8.50). Successful placement of the electrode and assessment of response are observed by a positive anal wink and toe flexion. Intraoperative fluoroscopic guidance is used to place the permanent electrode and may be helpful with difficult cases of temporary stimulator placement.

The temporary electrode is connected to an external battery pack, which is worn for the 2-week trial period. The permanent electrode is "barbed" to minimize migration. It is connected to the permanent battery, which is buried in the subcutaneous tissue of the buttock.

Sacral nerve stimulation is usually performed as a unilateral intervention, but occasionally, bilateral implants are placed.

8.8.7 Postoperative Complications

8.8.7.1 General Complications

- Complications of general anesthesia, including neuropraxia from poor patient positioning on operating table
- Complications of spinal anesthesia – urinary retention and spinal headache
- Pain-related complications – urinary retention and analgesic-induced constipation and impaction
- Wound infections (particularly perineal) resulting in failure of repair or mesh/implant infection

8.8.7.2 Specific Complications by Operation

- *ACE procedure* – intra-abdominal bleeding, visceral injury, port site hernia; anastomotic breakdown, and anastomotic stenosis
- *STARR* – defecatory urgency (20–30% usually temporary and resolving by 6–12 weeks, but occasionally protracted), postoperative bleeding (5%), staple line dehiscence with anorectal sepsis (4%), anastomotic stenosis (<1%), fecal incontinence (2%), and rectovaginal fistula (very rare)
- *Laparoscopic ventral rectopexy* – intra-abdominal bleeding, visceral injury, port site hernia, rectal perforation (rare), mesh infection, and mesh migration (isolated reports of up to 5% long term)
- *Delorme's procedure* – bleeding, rectal perforation, anastomotic dehiscence, perineal sepsis, constipation (up to 50%), incontinence, and recurrent prolapse (10–30%)
- *Perineal rectosigmoidectomy (Altemeier's)* – intra-abdominal bleeding, bladder injury, anastomotic leak, defecatory urgency, fecal incontinence (up to 50%, all grades), and recurrent prolapse (0–16%)
- *Laparoscopic resectional rectopexy* – intra-abdominal bleeding, visceral injury, port site hernia, anastomotic leak (<5%), constipation, fecal incontinence, and bladder and sexual dysfunction
- *Anterior sphincteroplasty* – bleeding, rectal perforation, rectovaginal fistula, wound infection, disruption of repair, pudendal nerve injury, and recurrent incontinence (50% at 5 years)
- *Sacral nerve modulation* – wound site infection, implant infection, lower limb paresthesia (inappropriate stimulation), electrode migration and electrode fracture (diagnosed by lateral pelvic X-ray), battery site pain and battery migration (permanent implant), and failure to improve symptoms (20–30%)

8.8.8 Normal Postoperative Imaging

The main role for radiology is in the assessment of surgical "failure" where patients' symptoms recur after one of the operations that have already been described. Imaging only has a limited role in the postoperative period. Unlike most rectal surgery where single contrast studies are often used to assess an anastomosis, stomas are infrequently formed following pelvic floor surgery because of the low incidence of leaks at the site of operation. Imaging therefore only has a role where there is unexpected delay in recovery giving rise to suspicion of leak or abscess. In this scenario, contrast-enhanced CT is probably the best modality for assessment (with or without rectal contrast) following the same principles described for evaluation of other rectal surgery that has already been described.

Fluoroscopic contrast examinations performed after surgery should show a more normal rectal outline without rectocele. The rectum may be circumferentially "pinched" or plicated at the site of rectocele repair with a more straightened rectal ampulla, whereas resectional rectopexy will anastomose sigmoid colon to the anal canal.

Fluoroscopy is used in the initial placement of sacral nerve stimulators. These have a similar appearance to other nerve stimulators (and single chamber pacemakers) with a box connected to a single wire, which enters one of the sacral foramina (S3 or S4). As this technology is new, many reporting radiologists are unaware of what these devices represent on plain radiographs. It is most important to ensure that there is no sign of wire fracture or displacement. Obviously, these patients are precluded from MRI assessment in the future as a result of their implant.

Endoanal ultrasound is a valuable tool in the assessment of adequacy of primary repair following sphincter trauma (Williams et al. 2001). In this setting, the critical assessment is the approximation of the external sphincter, since any accompanying internal sphincter defect is not repaired surgically. In obstetric injury, the tear is usually anterior, while iatrogenic injury, for example, following hemorrhoidectomy or lateral sphincterotomy for fissure in ano may occur in other positions. Scarring manifests as a hypoechoic defect in the striated heterogeneous external sphincter. A sonographic "good" repair will leave very little gap between the torn external sphincter fibers (Fig. 8.51). Where a wider

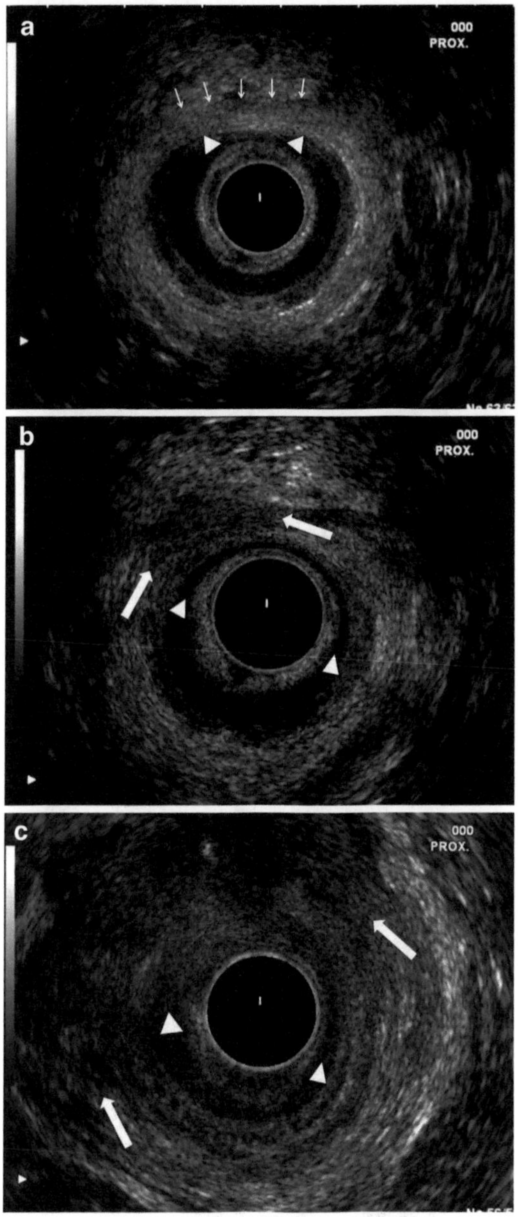

Fig. 8.51 (**a**–**c**) Three patients following anal sphincter repair after obstetric injury. (**a**) Excellent approximation of the external sphincter with complete overlap (*arrows*) – the internal sphincter defect is not repaired (*arrowheads*) and persists. (**b**) Reasonable repair with hypoechoic scarring bridging the gap between ends of the external sphincter (*arrows*) between 10 and 12 o'clock. The internal sphincter defect is larger in this case (*arrowheads*). (**c**) Poor result from primary repair. There is extensive deficiency of the internal sphincter and no approximation of the external sphincter with a large defect (*arrows*) extending from 8 to 2 o'clock (Images courtesy of Professor Stuart Taylor, University College Hospital, London, UK)

defect exists and there is accompanying incontinence with poor anal physiology, a secondary sphincter repair may be offered. It is important to note that a sphincter defect alone is not in itself an indication for surgery since a surprising number of patients maintain normal continence despite these injuries.

MRI has a role in patients developing late recurrent symptoms using MR proctography, as well as those who develop complications of sepsis such as collection or fistula. Where there is significant postoperative distortion, the addition of post–gadolinium-enhanced fat-saturated T1W sequences can help differentiate infected collection from simple fluid by assessing for increased rim enhancement. Fistulas may also show hyperenhancement which may improve conspicuity compared with sequences demonstrating "water/edema" such as T2 with fat saturation or STIR, where true pathology may be masked by postoperative changes.

8.8.9 Pitfalls in Postoperative Pelvic Floor Radiological Assessment

The following require careful consideration on postoperative imaging:

8.8.9.1 Postoperative Gas

It is important to remember that many of the operations should not involve transmural colonic resection (e.g., Delorme's) and that free gas should not be seen in any of the transperineal operations, with the exception of resectional rectopexy or perineal rectosigmoidopexy. In the setting of a localized transperineal operation, the main concern is creation of an inadvertent full-thickness defect in the rectum, leading to a localized leak, which should be contained within the mesorectal fascia. However, in patients undergoing the STARR procedure, there is potential for the transmural stapled resection to incorporate the peritoneal reflection where the rectovaginal septum is deficient (i.e., in the presence of peritoneocele) with potential for small bowel injury or intraperitoneal leak.

8.8.9.2 Surgical Materials

Stigmata of previous surgery may not be present such as an anastomotic staple line where a hand-sewn anastomosis has been created. In addition, the mesh used for ventral rectopexy repair may be difficult to appreciate on either MRI or CT and is invisible on fluoroscopy. However, as with hernia repairs using mesh, a mesh infection creates a loculated fluid collection around the "foreign body," making it visible where it would otherwise be hidden (since it is applied to the posterior wall of the vagina and anterior wall of the adjacent rectum and fixed to the presacral fascia superiorly). Mesh will appear on CT or MRI as a straight or wavy linear structure running from the sacral promontory into the rectovaginal septum.

8.8.9.3 Treatment Failure

The most common indication for postoperative evaluation is in patients in whom the first surgery has failed. In most cases, this is many months or years later. It is therefore important to be aware of the type of procedure performed and the interval since surgery and to employ a modality that allows evaluation for other pelvic findings than simply the one that was repaired (i.e., the anterior and middle compartment where an isolated rectocele repair has been performed in the past) (Siegmann et al. 2010). Local expertise in interpretation and access will determine which modality is chosen for suspected recurrent pelvic floor prolapse. MR proctography (Figs. 8.52, 8.53, 8.54) has benefits

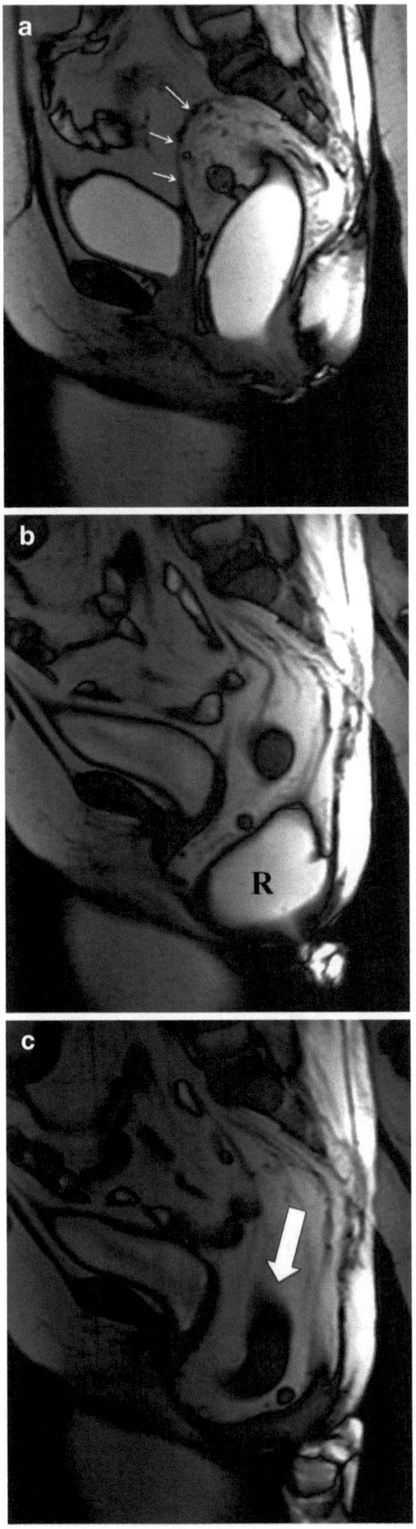

Fig. 8.52 (**a–c**) Sacrocolporectopexy performed 2 years previously with recurrent obstructive defecation (prior hysterectomy). (**a**) MR proctography FISP sequences during evacuation of contrast gel demonstrate the mesh (*arrows*) from previous repair which is anchored from vaginal vault to sacral promontory. (**b**) There is excessive perineal descent with formation of a rectocele (*R*). (**c**) Further emptying allows descent of a sigmoidocele (*large arrow*)

over fluoroscopic proctography, where evaluation of the anterior and middle compartments involves catheterization of the bladder and contrast injection into the vagina, which is quite intrusive for patients (Maglinte et al. 2011). MRI also allows evaluation of the levator ani muscles for signs of atrophy that may indicate pudendal neuropathy or muscular injury which may be an additional factor contributing to pelvic floor failure.

8.8.10 Teaching Points

- Clinical indications for pelvic floor surgery are incontinence, constipation, and prolapse.
- Postoperative imaging is usually reserved for patients with recurrent symptoms since complications are usually less common compared with surgery for rectal cancer.
- Knowledge of whether surgical mesh placement or rectal resection has been performed is important for accurate interpretation since these are not always readily apparent on imaging.
- Ultrasound has an important role for sphincter assessment in fecal incontinence and MR or fluoroscopic proctography for obstructive defecation.

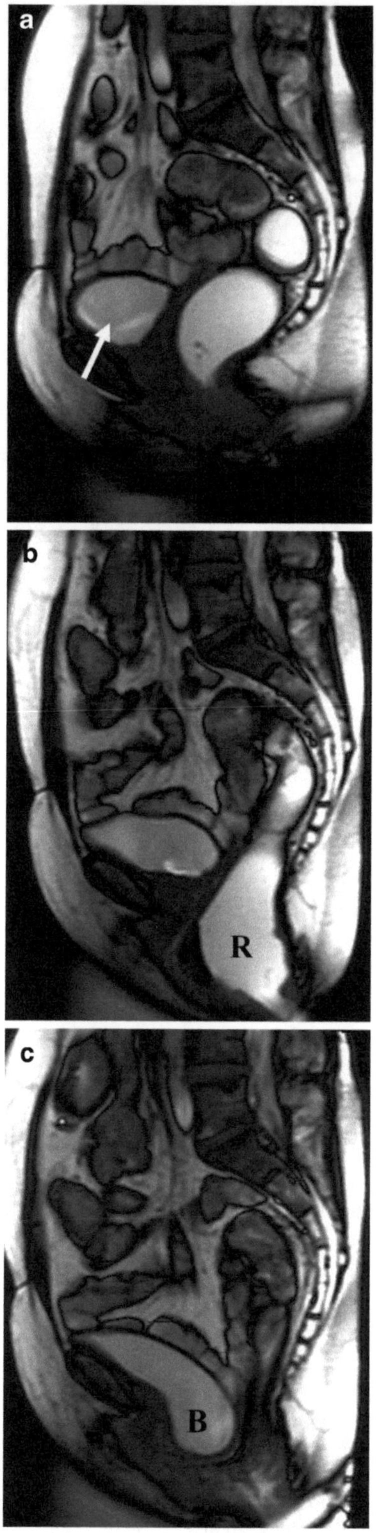

Fig. 8.53 (**a**–**c**) Previous sacrocolporectopexy and previous hysterectomy with new urinary and obstructive bowel symptoms. (**a**) Previous mesh cannot be identified with normal position of pelvic organs at rest (arrow denotes bladder). (**b**) Straining precipitates formation of a large rectocele (*arrow*) followed by (**c**) a large cystocele (*B*) implying failure of the previous repair. Rectum (*R*)

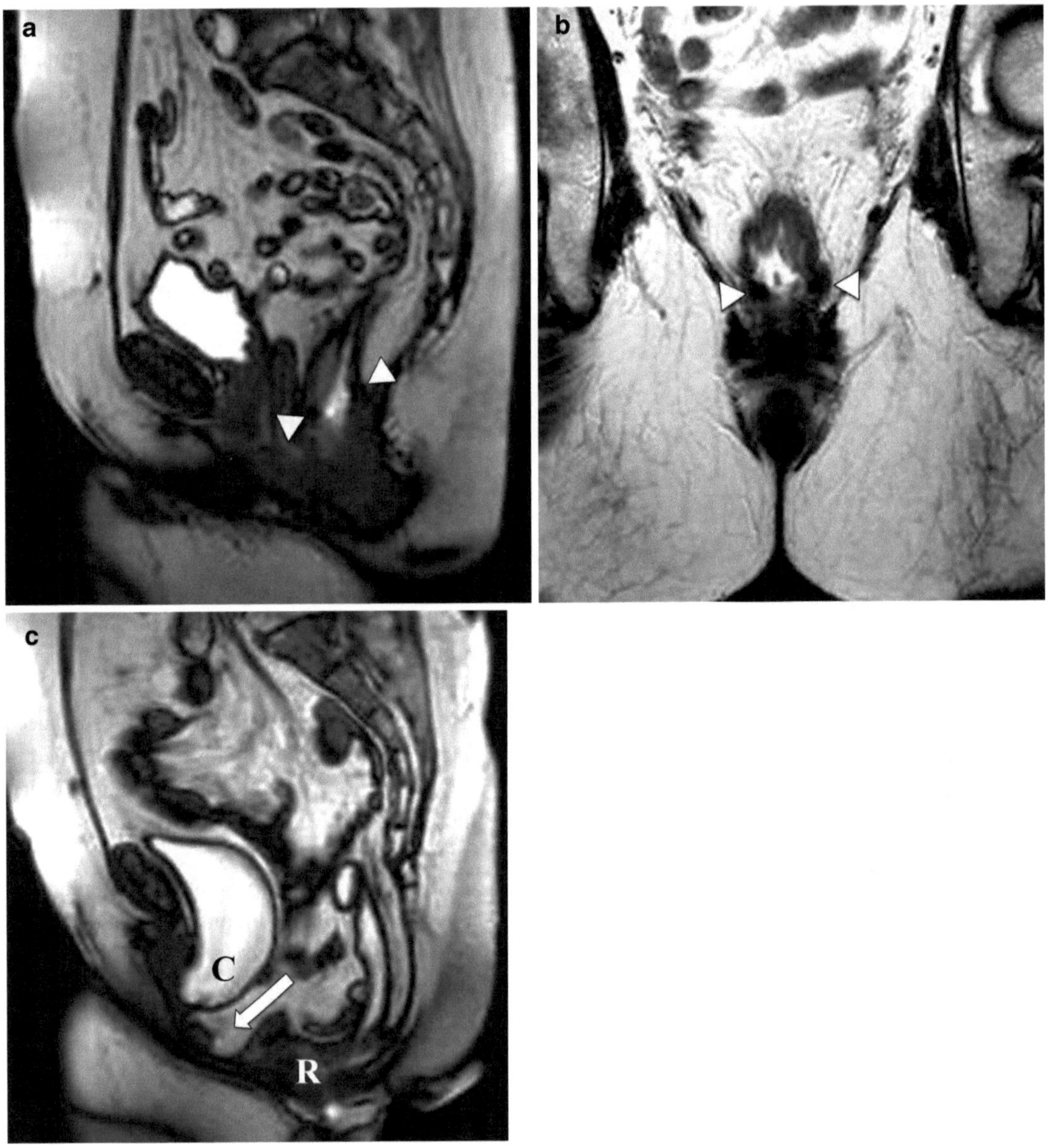

Fig. 8.54 (**a–c**) Recurrent obstructive symptoms following STARR procedure 6 months prior. (**a**) Susceptibility artifact on sagittal FISP (*arrowheads*). (**b**) Coronal HASTE indicates staple lines from previous surgery (*arrowheads*). (**c**) Evacuatory phase shows large cystocele (*C*), peritoneocele (*arrow*), and excessive perineal descent of rectum (*R*)

References

Brittenden J, Chalmers AG. Imaging of colorectal carcinoma. Radiol Update. 2007;6(2):55–67.

D'Hoore A, Vanbeckevoort D, Penninckx F. Clinical, physiological and radiological assessment of rectovaginal septum reinforcement with mesh for complex rectocele. Br J Surg. 2008;95(1):264–72.

Even-Sapir E, Parag Y, Lerma H. Detection of recurrence in patients with rectal cancer: PET/CT after abdominoperineal or anterior resection. Radiology. 2004;232:815–22.

Halligan S, Stoker J. State of the art: imaging of Fistula in Ano. Radiology. 2006;239:18–33.

Jayne D, Stuto A, editors. Transanal stapling techniques for anorectal prolapse. London: Springer; 2009.

Keighley M, Williams N. Surgery of the colon, rectum and anus. 1st ed. London: Elsevier; 2007.

Khot UP, Lang WA, Murali K, Parker MC. Systematic review of the efficacy and safety of colorectal stents. Br J Surg. 2002;89:1096–122.

Maglinte DD, Bartram CI, Hale DA, Park J, Kohli MD, Robb BW, et al. Functional imaging of the pelvic floor. Radiology. 2011;258:23–39.

Mainar A, De Gregorio A, Tejero E, Tobio R, Pinto I, Herrera M, Fernandez JA. Acute colorectal obstruction. Treatment with self-expandable metallic stents before scheduled surgery – results of a multicentre study. Radiology. 1999;210:65–9.

Messiou C, Chalmers AG, Boyle K. Surgery for recurrent rectal carcinoma. The role of magnetic resonant imaging. Clin Rad. 2006;61:250–8.

Morris J, Spencer J, Ambrose S. MR imaging classification of perianal fistulas and its implication in patient management. Radiographics. 2000;20:623–35.

Parks AG, Gordon PH, Hardcastle JD. A classification of fistula in ano. Br J Surg. 1976;63(1):1–12.

Sagar PM, Pemberton JH. Surgical management of locally recurrent rectal cancer. Br J Surg. 1996;83:293–304.

Scardapane A, Brindicini D, Fracella MR, Angelelli G. Post colon surgery complications: imaging findings. Eur J Radiol. 2005;53(3):397–409.

Siegmann KC, Reisenauer C, Speck S, et al. Dynamic magnetic resonance imaging for assessment of minimally invasive pelvic floor reconstruction with polypropylene implant. Eur J Radiol 2011;80(2): 182–7.

Stoker J, Halligan S, Bartram CI. Pelvic floor imaging. Radiology. 2001;218:621–41.

Williams R. Colorectal surgery. A companion to specialist surgical practice. 4th ed. London: Elsevier; 2009.

Williams AB, Bartram CI, Halligan S, et al. Anal sphincter damage after vaginal delivery using three-dimensional endosonography. Obstet Gynecol. 2001;97: 770–5.

Zissin R, Gayer G. Post operative anatomic and pathologic findings at CT following colonic resection. Semin US CT MR. 2003;25(3):222–38.

Genitourinary System

9

Christopher Wilkinson

Contents

9.1 Introduction 295

9.2 Urinary Diversion 295
9.2.1 Clinical Indication 295
9.2.2 Surgical Technique and Postoperative Anatomy 296
9.2.3 Normal Postoperative Imaging: Incontinent Conduit Diversion 298
9.2.4 Normal Postoperative Imaging: Continent Catheterizable Reservoir 302
9.2.5 Normal Postoperative Imaging: Orthotopic Neobladder 303
9.2.6 Postoperative Complications 304
9.2.7 Teaching Points 310

9.3 Ureteric Injury 310
9.3.1 Background 310
9.3.2 Contrast Studies 310
9.3.3 CT 311
9.3.4 Teaching Points 311

9.4 Bladder Injury 311
9.4.1 Background 311
9.4.2 Contrast Studies 312
9.4.3 CT 312
9.4.4 Teaching Points 314

9.5 Urethral Injury 314
9.5.1 Background 314
9.5.2 Contrast Studies 314
9.5.3 CT 315
9.5.4 Teaching Points 316

References 316

9.1 Introduction

A comprehensive overview of gynecological and urological surgical imaging is beyond the scope of this book. This chapter will focus on areas of genitourinary imaging applicable to abdominal and pelvic surgery in general, namely urinary diversions and iatrogenic injuries to the urinary tract. Urinary diversions can be encountered as part of gastrointestinal, urological, or gynecological procedures, particularly oncological surgery within these disciplines. Complications affecting genitourinary structures can arise secondary to any intra-abdominal or pelvic surgery, and therefore imaging features of ureteric and bladder injuries will also be discussed.

9.2 Urinary Diversion

9.2.1 Clinical Indication

To achieve urinary diversion following benign or malignant disease of the bladder:

- Bladder carcinoma (commonly transitional cell carcinoma) necessitating cystectomy

C. Wilkinson, BSc, MBChB, FRCR
Department of Radiology,
York NHS Trust, York, UK
e-mail: ctlwilkinson@hotmail.com

J. Brittenden, D.J.M. Tolan (eds.), *Radiology of the Post Surgical Abdomen*,
DOI 10.1007/978-1-4471-2775-8_9, © Springer-Verlag London 2012

- Exenteration secondary to rectal or cervical carcinoma
- Neuropathic bladder
- Radiotherapy-induced bladder injury
- Intractable urinary incontinence

9.2.2 Surgical Technique and Postoperative Anatomy

The three most common types of urinary diversions include the following:

- Incontinent conduit diversion
- Continent catheterizable reservoir
- Orthotopic neobladder

Common operative techniques for each type of urinary diversion are outlined in the following sections, but it is important to note that there can be wide local variations in the surgical methods used, even for the eponymous procedures.

9.2.2.1 Operative Summary: Incontinent Conduit Diversion

The most common procedure to achieve incontinent conduit diversion is ureteroileostomy (ileal conduit formation):

- A segment of ileum approximately 20 cm in length is divided and attached to its vascular pedicle (Fig. 9.1).
- Ileal continuity restored with end-to-end or end-to-side anastomosis (Fig. 9.2).
- Left ureter mobilized and brought through sigmoid mesentery.
- The proximal end of the ileal segment is sutured closed.
- The distal ureters are anastomosed to the proximal ileal segment. Ureteric stents are often placed.
- Distal end of ileal segment brought out through the anterior abdominal wall to form a stoma (Fig. 9.3).

9.2.2.2 Alternative Techniques

- Using the Bricker technique, the ureters are spatulated (i.e., incised longitudinally for a short section to allow greater circumference for anastomosis) and then anastomosed separately to the proximal end of the conduit (Fig. 9.4).

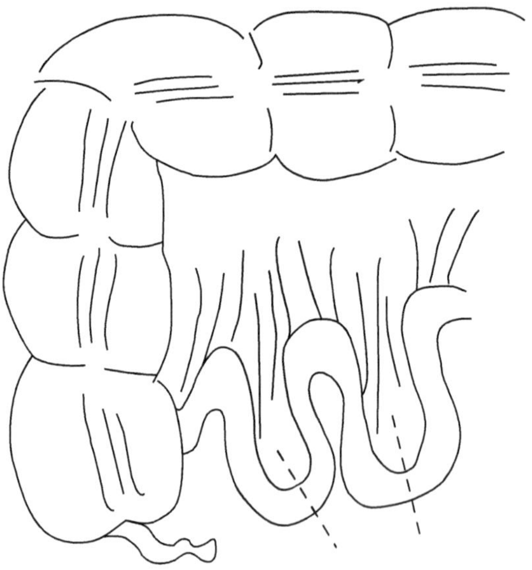

Fig. 9.1 Twenty-centimeter segment of ileum divided for ileal conduit

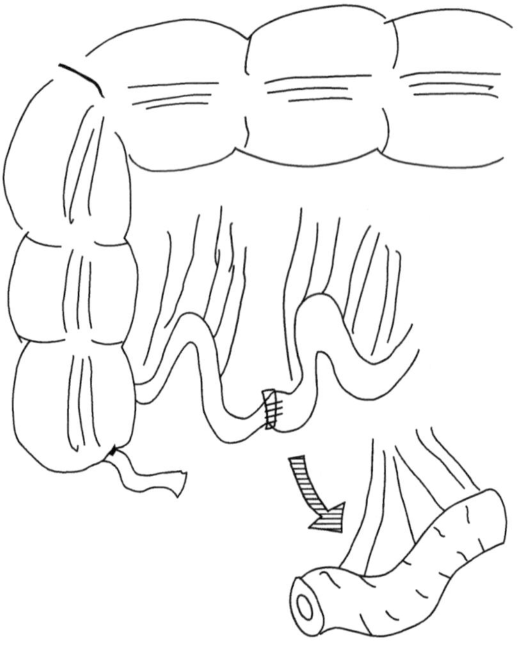

Fig. 9.2 Ileal continuity restored

- Using the Wallace technique, the ureters are spatulated and then sewn together before anastomosing as one to the proximal end of the conduit (Fig. 9.5).

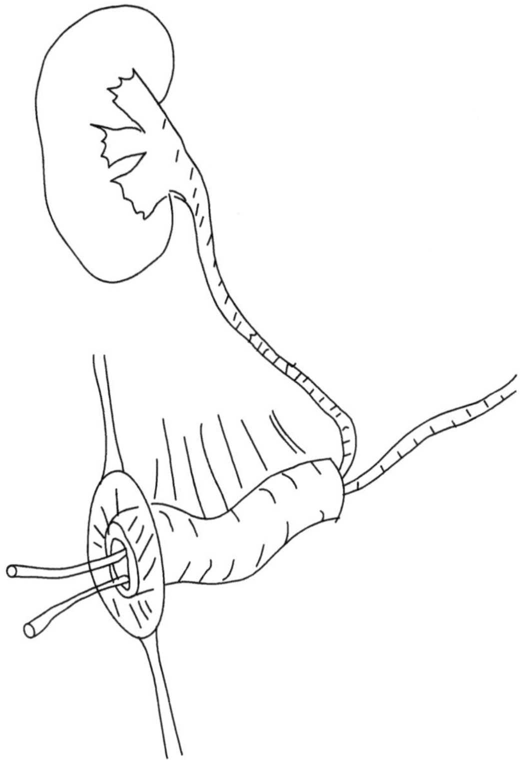

Fig. 9.3 Ileal conduit with ureteric stents

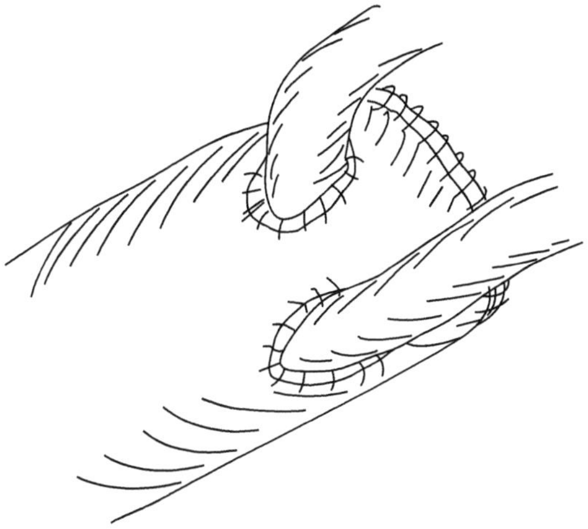

Fig. 9.4 Bricker technique of ureterointestinal anastomosis

9.2.2.3 Operative Summary: Continent Catheterizable Reservoir

A commonly utilized procedure to achieve continence via a catheterizable urinary reservoir (Indiana pouch):

- The cecum, ascending colon, and approximately 10 cm of terminal ileum are isolated (Fig. 9.6).
- Bowel continuity restored with an ileocolostomy (Fig. 9.7).
- The colonic segment is detubularized along its antimesenteric border, folded in on itself, and resutured to form a reservoir (a portion of the ileal segment can be used as a patch).
- The ureters are anastomosed separately into the posterior taeniae of the colonic segment, and ureteric stents placed.
- The terminal ileum is reduced in diameter by stapling the antimesenteric border to form a catheterizable stoma that is brought out through the anterior abdominal wall (Fig. 9.8). Commonly one or more cecostomy tubes and a stomal catheter are left in situ postoperatively.
- The intact ileocecal valve helps to maintain continence.

9.2.2.4 Alternative Techniques

- The Penn pouch uses the right colon and ileum to construct the reservoir, and utilizes the appendix as an appendicostomy for catheterization (Mitrofanoff principle).
- The Kock pouch uses a 70–80 cm length of small bowel to create the reservoir. This technique has a relatively high complication rate and is no longer commonly used.

9.2.2.5 Operative Summary: Orthotopic Neobladder

Orthotopic neobladder formation is commonly performed using the Studer technique:

- Long segment (up to 60 cm) of ileum is divided, and the distal 40 cm is detubularized on its antimesenteric border (Fig. 9.9).
- Ileal continuity restored with end-to-end or end-to-side anastomosis (Fig. 9.10).
- The distal 40 cm of the ileal segment is folded into a U shape, and the medial border sutured.
- The ureters are anastomosed to the proximal (isoperistaltic afferent) limb of the ileal segment using an end-to-side technique.
- The distal ileal segment is then folded and sutured to form a reservoir.
- A urethroenteric anastomosis is formed using the most dependent part of the reservoir (Fig. 9.11).
- A covering cystostomy tube is commonly left in situ.

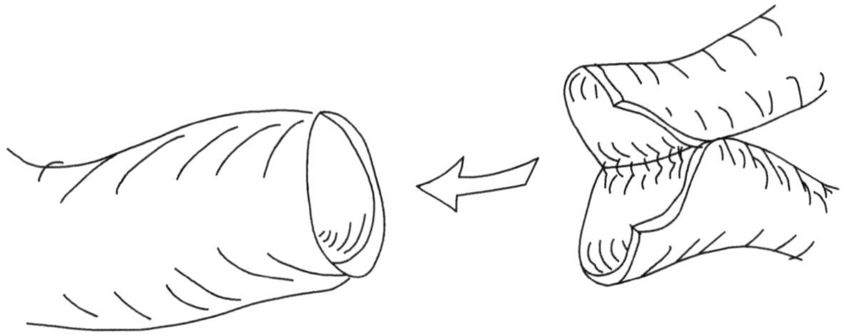

Fig. 9.5 Wallace technique of ureterointestinal anastomosis

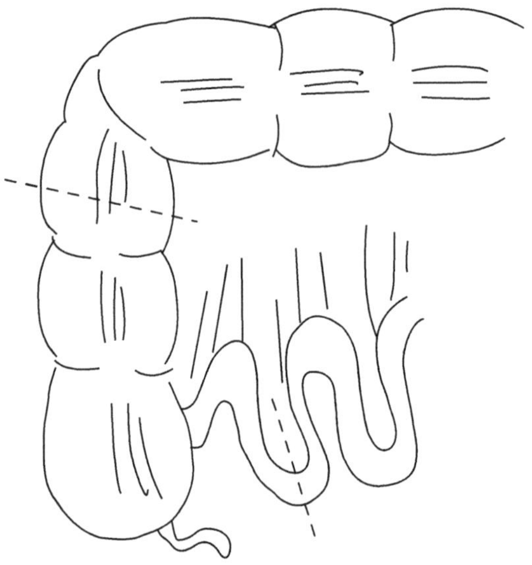

Fig. 9.6 Cecum, ascending colon, and terminal ileum divided for continent catheterizable reservoir formation

9.2.2.6 Alternative Techniques

- Hautmann neobladder uses a 60-cm segment of ileum sutured into a "W" configuration.

9.2.3 Normal Postoperative Imaging: Incontinent Conduit Diversion

9.2.3.1 Contrast Studies

A "loopogram" or "conduitogram" is performed by catheterizing the ileal conduit with a 14F Foley catheter or similar. The catheter balloon may be inflated to facilitate an adequate seal. Water-soluble contrast is injected and is seen to fill the conduit which is distensible and may demonstrate active peristalsis (Fig. 9.12).

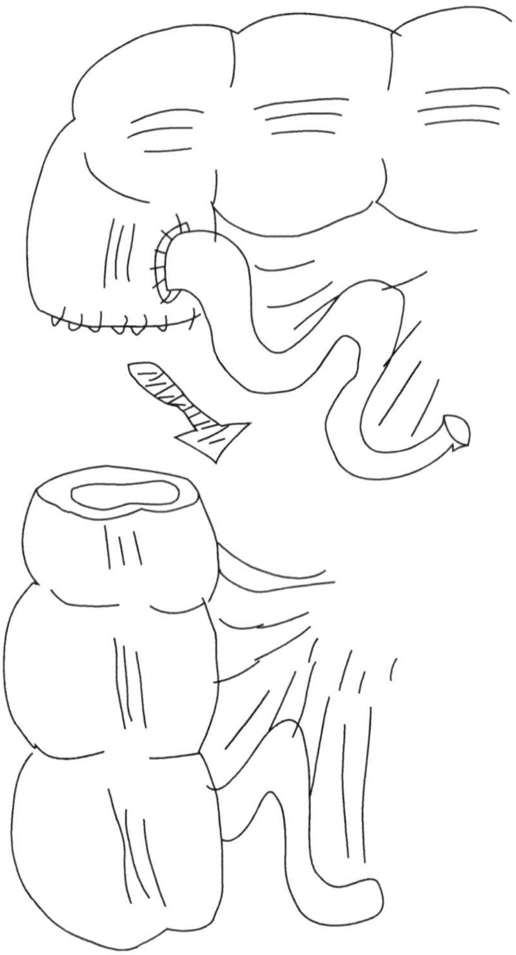

Fig. 9.7 Bowel continuity restored with ileocolostomy

Initially, the valvulae conniventes of the ileal segment will be visible (see Fig. 9.16), but with time these may disappear to produce a more smooth appearance to the conduit (compare with Fig. 9.12). Bilateral and equal reflux of contrast up both ureters and into the renal

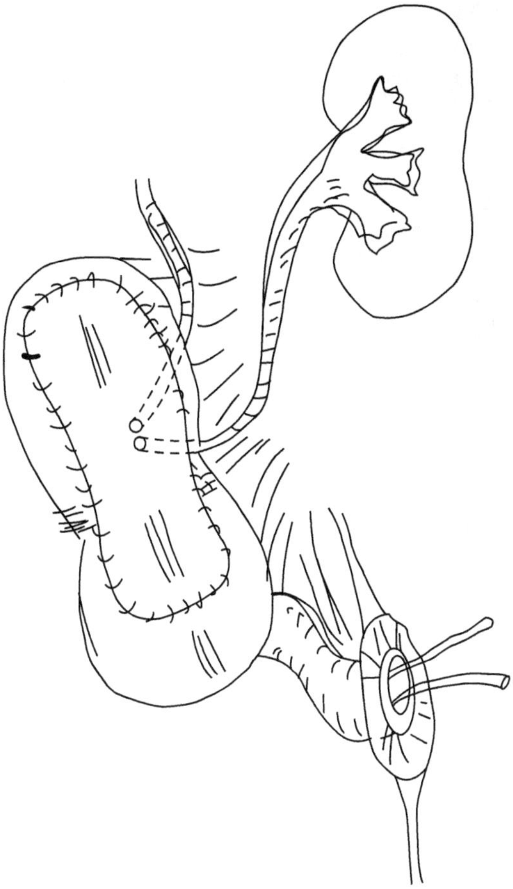

Fig. 9.8 Continent catheterizable reservoir with ureteric stents

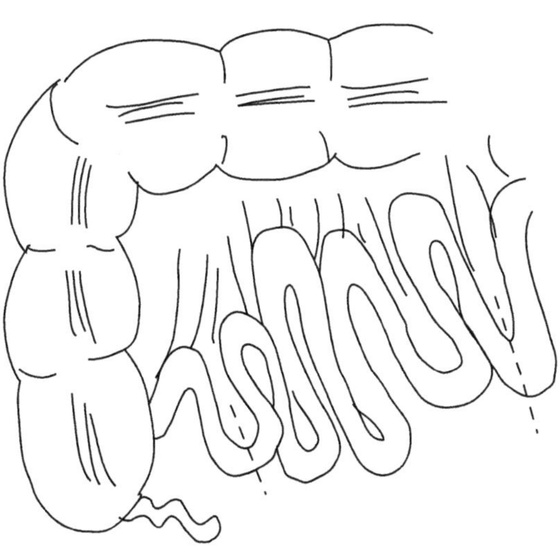

Fig. 9.9 Sixty-centimeter segment of ileum divided for neobladder formation

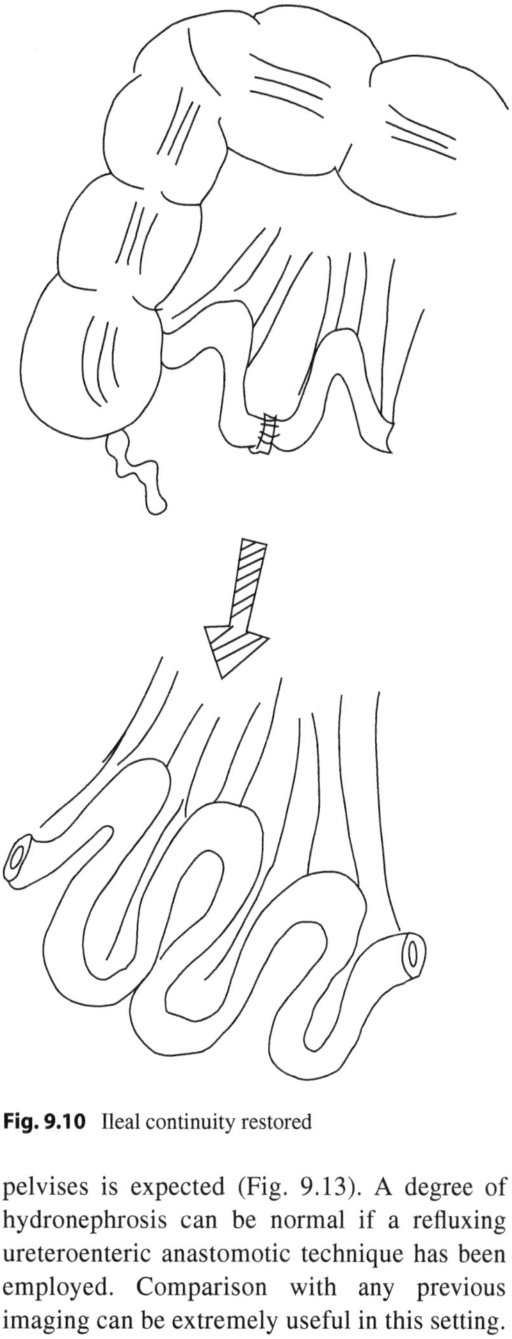

Fig. 9.10 Ileal continuity restored

pelvises is expected (Fig. 9.13). A degree of hydronephrosis can be normal if a refluxing ureteroenteric anastomotic technique has been employed. Comparison with any previous imaging can be extremely useful in this setting. Depending upon the surgical technique employed, the ureters either will be seen to arise separately from the conduit or, more frequently, will initially take a short common course before dividing. In either case, it is essential that the ureteroenteric anastomoses are adequately visualized, and this often requires the use of oblique fluoroscopic views.

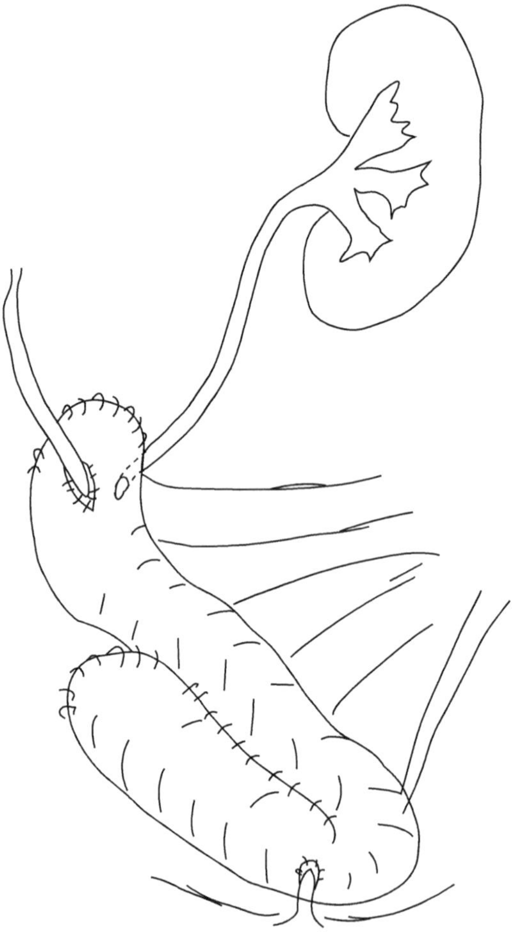

Fig. 9.11 Neobladder

If a long segment of ileum has been used to form the ileal conduit, it may be more difficult to generate sufficient pressure to cause adequate ureteric reflux (Fig. 9.14). In the immediate postoperative period, anastomotic edema may prevent reflux of contrast up one or both ureters. This should settle with time, and caution should be exercised in misdiagnosing genuine pathology or pathological obstruction.

Most surgeons will place bilateral ureteric stents during surgery that extend from the renal pelvis, down the ureter, through the conduit, and out through the stoma. If ureteric stents are present, it is possible to use these to deliver contrast into each renal pelvis separately, and then demonstrate antegrade filling of the conduit (Figs. 9.15, 9.16, and 9.17). The stents

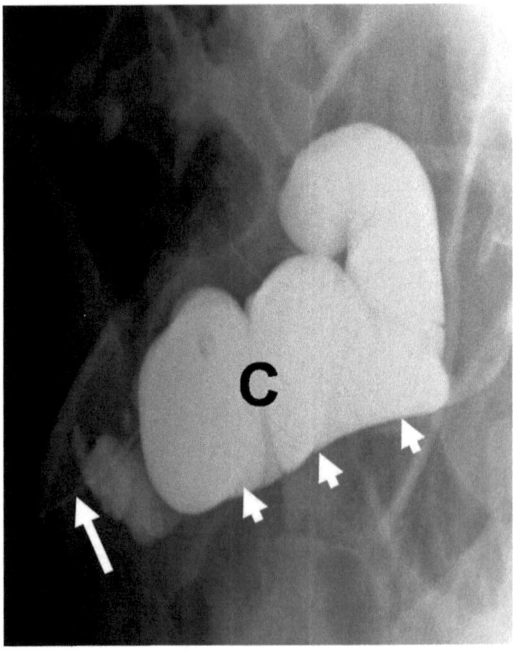

Fig. 9.12 Normal fluoroscopic appearances of an ileal conduit (*C*) filled via a Foley catheter (*arrow*) inserted into the stoma. Note the smooth outline to this 5-month-old conduit (*short arrows*)

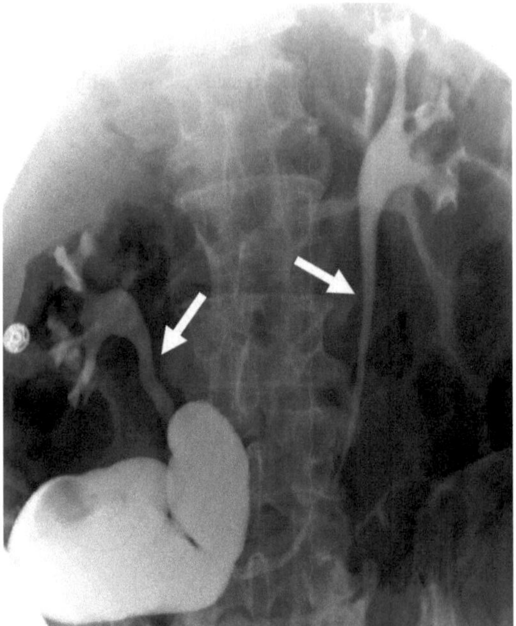

Fig. 9.13 Ileal conduitogram demonstrating normal and equal opacification of both ureters and pelvicalyceal systems (*arrows*)

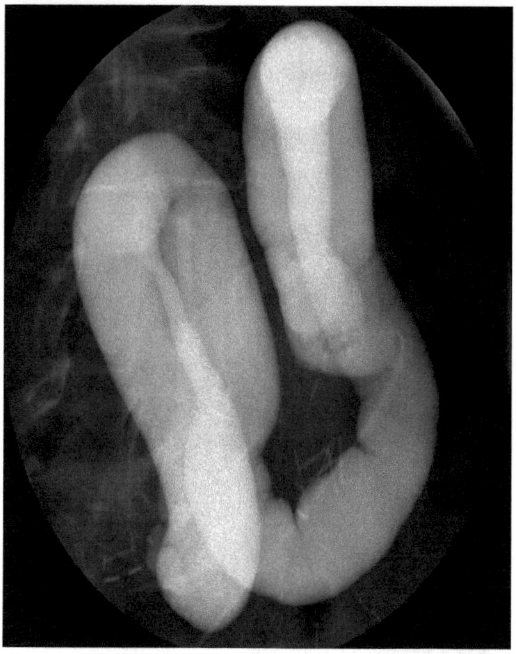

Fig. 9.14 Long-length ileal conduit opacified with contrast via a Foley catheter inserted into the stoma. Note that it has not been possible to opacify the ureters due to the long conduit

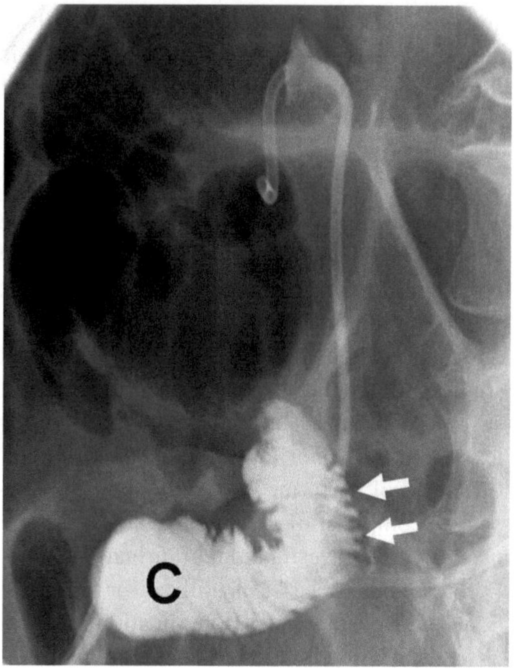

Fig. 9.16 The ileal conduit (*C*) has now been filled with contrast via the left ureteric stent. The right renal tract has yet to be opacified. Note in this recently fashioned conduit, the valvulae conniventes can be clearly seen (*arrows*)

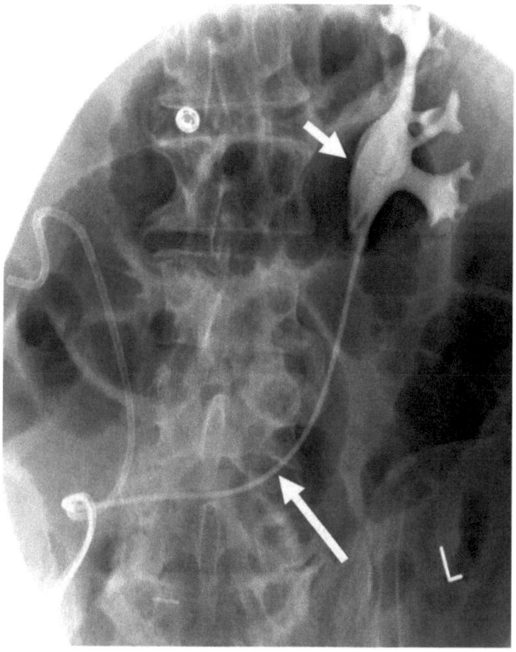

Fig. 9.15 In the early postoperative period, the conduit or reservoir can be filled via the ureteric stents. Here, contrast has been injected into the left ureteric stent (*long arrow*), opacifying the left pelvicalyceal system and the superior part of the left ureter (*short arrow*)

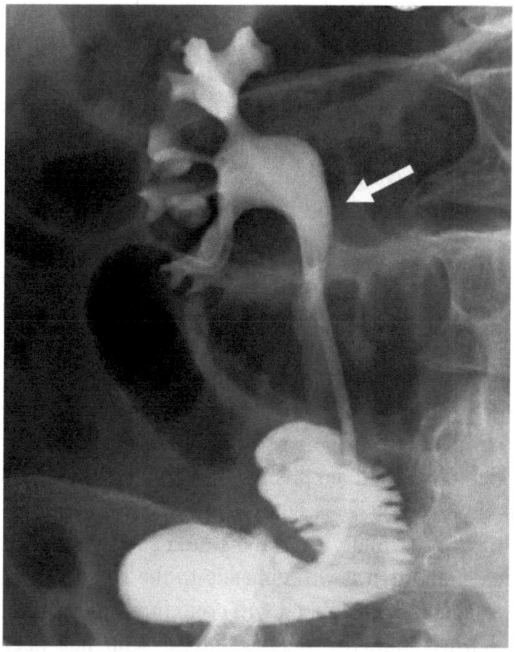

Fig. 9.17 Contrast is injected into the right ureteric stent, and the right pelvicalyceal system and right ureter are opacified (*arrow*)

are usually removed at around the seventh to tenth postoperative day. In some centers, it is routine to perform a loopogram prior to stent removal.

9.2.3.2 CT

CT is not routinely performed and will only be required in the immediate or early postoperative period if certain complications are suspected. While ureterointestinal leaks and urinary obstruction are better investigated with contrast studies, CT is the investigation of choice for suspected abscess, urinoma, and anastomotic leak from the donor bowel site. The particular CT protocol performed depends upon the suspected complication. Unenhanced CT can be used for the investigation of urinary calculi. Portal venous phase CT is utilized for the investigation of postoperative complications such as abscess or differentiation of ileus from mechanical gastrointestinal obstruction. Delayed phase CT can be useful to help confirm urinoma as extravasated contrast is seen to collect within the fluid cavity. A delay of a minimum of 10 min is necessary to opacify the ureters, and if the renal pelvis and ureters have not been opacified, a further scan with a longer delay may be necessary. This is often the case where abscesses or leaks are present due to stasis in the upper urinary tract. Three-phase multidetector CT urogram is being used increasingly in the investigation of postoperative complications in some centers as it allows simultaneous assessment of the continuity of the urinary tract as well as extraluminal complications (Catala et al. 2009). However, the radiation dose is not insignificant.

It is important to recognize that it can be very difficult to identify the ileal conduit as a separate structure from the rest of the small bowel, particularly where no positive oral contrast has been administered. It is helpful to trace the ileal segment proximally from the stoma site, where it is expected that it will enhance to the same degree as adjacent bowel and will contain urine of water density (unless a delayed phase scan has been performed).

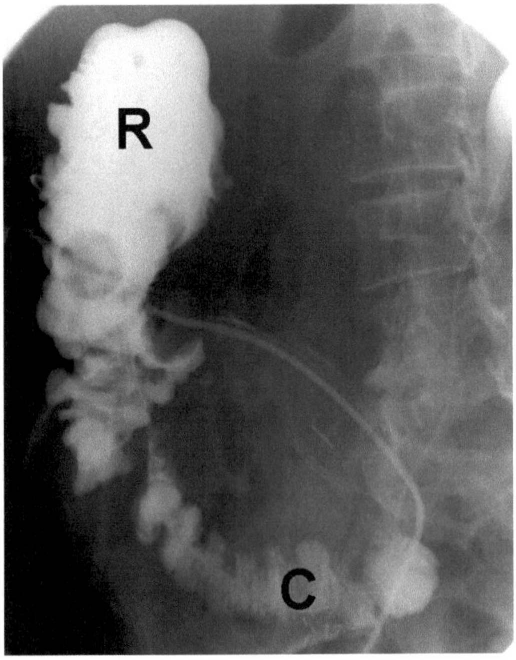

Fig. 9.18 Normal appearances of a continent catheterizable reservoir (*R*) formed using the right colon and distal ileum, opacified via a Foley catheter in the stoma. This patient also has an ileal conduit (*C*)

9.2.4 Normal Postoperative Imaging: Continent Catheterizable Reservoir

9.2.4.1 Contrast Studies

It is common to routinely image the continent catheterizable reservoir in the third to fourth postoperative week (Fig. 9.18). In the early postoperative period, the patient will have at least one cecostomy tube draining the reservoir and a Foley catheter placed through the stoma. The Foley catheter should be used to inject water-soluble contrast into the reservoir following clamping of the cecostomy tube. If the routine postoperative "pouchogram" shows no leak, then the surgeons will often remove the cecostomy and catheter. With an Indiana pouch, the ureters will be implanted in the posterior pouch wall. Initially, the pouch has a capacity of approximately 250 ml, but this increases to as much as 1 litre after a few months (Kenney et al. 1990). There should be only minimal residual fluid within the pouch following drainage.

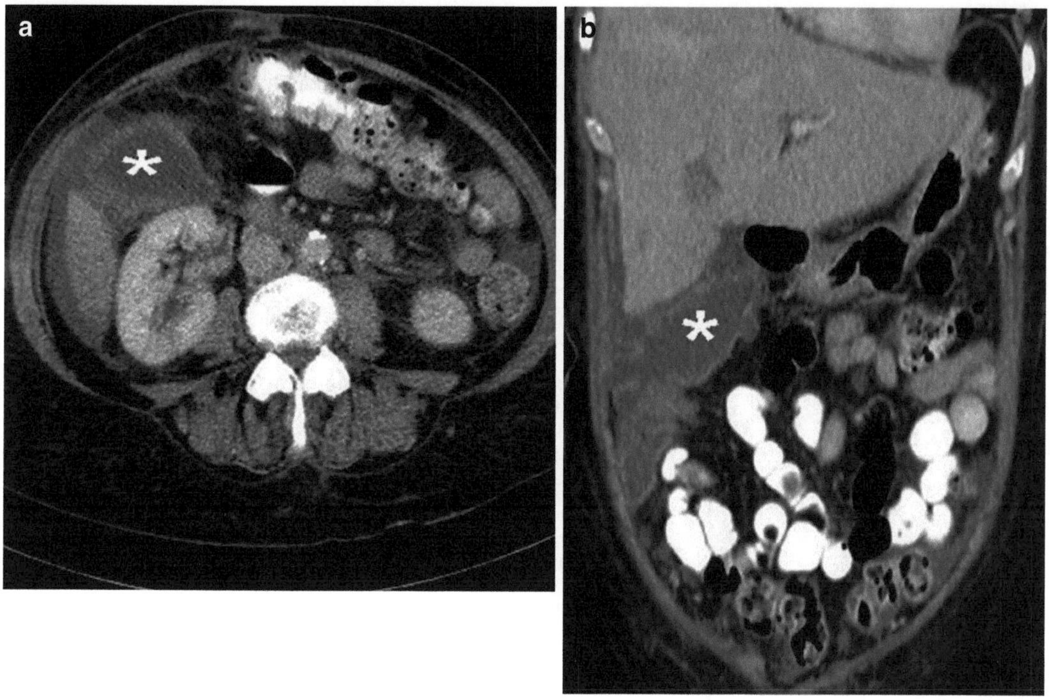

Fig. 9.19 (**a**, **b**) Normal axial (**a**) and coronal (**b**) CT appearances of a fluid-filled continent catheterizable reservoir (*asterisks*) formed from right colon and distal ileum

9.2.4.2 CT

As with other forms of urinary diversion, CT is usually only employed in the early postoperative patient if complications are suspected. In this early postoperative period, the reservoir will be empty if the drainage tubes are functioning correctly. Once the drains and stents are removed, the reservoir may be filled with fluid depending upon when it was last drained (Fig. 9.19). Normal mucous secretions may be seen within the reservoir as hypodense material, which is particularly apparent when the bladder is filled with contrast on delayed images following CT urography.

9.2.5 Normal Postoperative Imaging: Orthotopic Neobladder

9.2.5.1 Contrast Studies

The postoperative neobladder will be drained by both a urethral catheter and at least one cystostomy tube. Following water-soluble contrast administration, the neobladder usually forms a round or oval shape in the lower mid pelvis, and the afferent limb is most commonly seen in the right lower quadrant with valvulae conniventes clearly visualized. Both parts should be readily opacified with contrast (Figs. 9.20 and 9.21). As with all other types of urinary diversion, the ureteroenteric anastomosis in particular should be carefully scrutinized for leaks, although there is also risk of leak from the urethral reservoir anastomosis (see Fig. 9.20). At 6 months, a Studer pouch will have a capacity of approximately 600 ml (Heaney et al. 1999). Mild dilatation of both ureters and pelvicalyceal systems can be expected in the immediate postoperative period, but this is likely to settle or remain stable over time.

9.2.5.2 CT

As previously mentioned, CT is not routinely utilized in the early postoperative period. If performed, the fluid-filled pouch is seen centrally

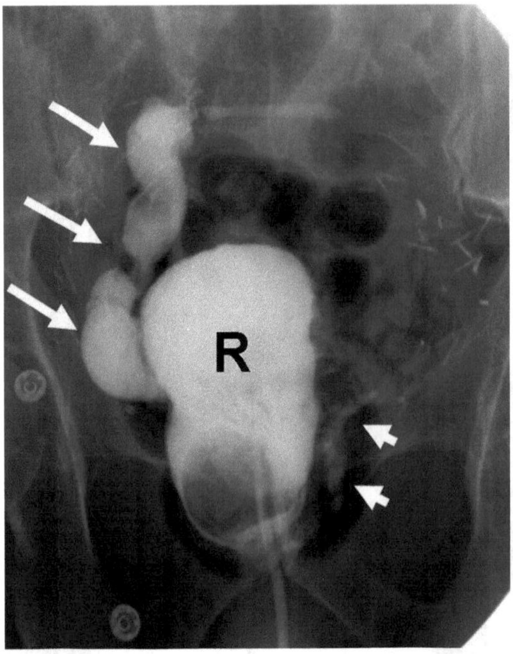

Fig. 9.20 Studer-type neobladder following radical cystectomy and lymph node dissection (surgical clips are seen bilaterally within the pelvis). Both the reservoir (*R*) and isoperistaltic limb (*long arrows*) are visible. The reservoir has been filled via a urethral Foley catheter. Note extraluminal contrast flowing from the most inferior part of the neobladder, indicating a urethral anastomotic leak (*short arrows*)

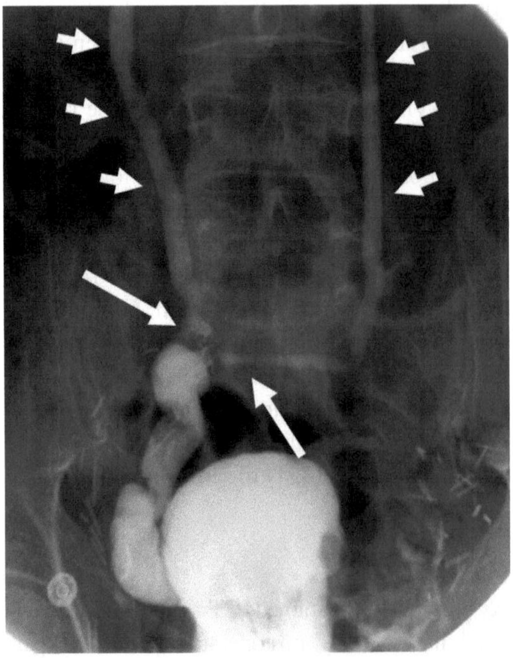

Fig. 9.21 Image of superior part of neobladder showing normal ureteric reflux (*short arrows*) and typical position of ureteric implantation into the isoperistaltic limb (*long arrows*)

within the pelvis with the tubular fluid-filled isoperistaltic afferent loop often in the right iliac fossa. The fluid volume of the neobladder will depend upon whether catheters are in situ and left on free drainage.

9.2.6 Postoperative Complications

While certain complications are more common following particular procedures (e.g., stone formation following ileal conduit), the complications are broadly similar, and the imaging findings will therefore be described collectively below.

Early complications (<30 days):

- Ileus
- Gastrointestinal anastomotic leak (from bowel donor site)
- Urinary leak
- Urinary infection (early or late)
- Hematoma
- Abscess
- Urinoma

Late complications (>30 days):

- Ureteric stricture (early or late)
- Calculus formation
- Fistulas
- Conduit stenosis
- Hernias
- Tumor recurrence

9.2.6.1 Ileus

Postoperative ileus is the most commonly encountered complication following cystectomy and urinary diversion and is found in approximately 20% of patients (Chang et al. 2002). CT may be useful to help differentiate between ileus and mechanical obstruction if normal bowel function is not resumed within the first 5 days postoperatively and clinical features are equivocal. The presence of uniformly dilated, fluid-filled bowel with the absence of a transition point favors ileus rather than mechanical obstruction, but this is described in more detail in Sect. 7.2.1.

9.2.6.2 Gastrointestinal Anastomotic Leak from Donor Bowel Site

In nearly all cases of urinary diversion, a part of the patient's own GI tract is utilized to form the urinary conduit or reservoir, therefore necessitating surgical anastomosis to restore continuity to the bowel. In any patient who is not making an appropriate postoperative recovery, it is important to bear in mind this anastomosis as a potential cause, particularly as it will not be visualized on screening studies performed to exclude urinary leaks. The gastrointestinal surgical anastomosis should be located and actively interrogated on any postoperative CT. The exact anastomotic technique differs between centers and for different procedures, but in our center, the gastrointestinal anastomoses are hand sewn. While in this particular setting it can be difficult to be sure exactly from where the leak is originating, excessive pneumoperitoneum or free fluid for the patient's postoperative status may be clues to the underling diagnosis. Where excessive gas is present, clinical correlation is always required before any intervention, and it is important not to confuse normal postoperative pneumoperitoneum for perforation. Use of positive oral contrast can be very helpful where there is doubt. In general, features of leak at this site are no different from those seen following surgery for non-urological indications, and are described in more detail in the small and large bowel chapters of this book (Chaps. 7 and 8) and will not be repeated here.

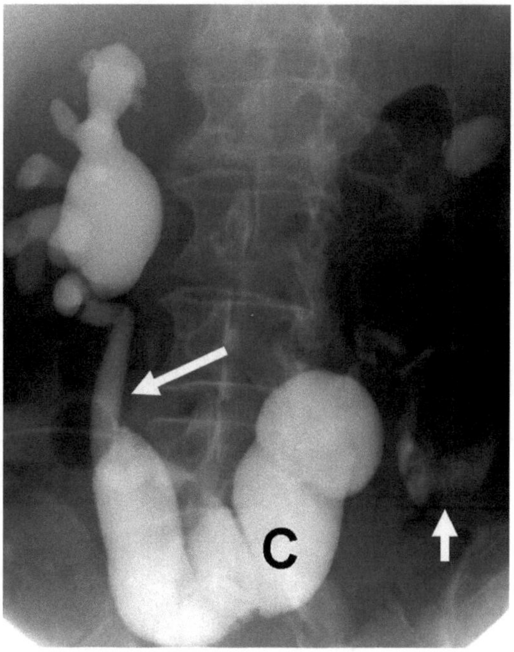

Fig. 9.22 Ileal conduit (*C*) opacified via Foley catheter. Smoothly outlined right ureter can be seen (*long arrow*). Leak demonstrated from the left distal ureter with extraluminal contrast in an irregular pattern not conforming to the normal shape of the ureter (*short arrow*)

9.2.6.3 Urinary Leak

Urinary leak occurs in approximately 4% of patients following urinary diversion (Catala et al. 2009). The most accurate way of determining the presence of a urinary leak is with contrast studies. Extravasation of contrast out with the normal shape of the conduit/reservoir and the ureters confirms urinary leak. This may manifest as anything from a small localized focus of extraluminal contrast which may be extremely subtle, to large leaks where contrast is seen to flow freely into the peritoneal cavity, outlining bowel loops and other structures.

The region of the ureteroenteric anastomosis should be particularly scrutinized for any contrast extravasation, as this is the most common site for leak (Fig. 9.22). However, urinary leaks may occur from the urinary reservoir itself (Fig. 9.23) or anywhere along the length of the ureters due to inadvertent injury following ureteric mobilization. Leaks will be readily demonstrated by instilling contrast into the conduit either via a Foley catheter in the stoma or via ureteric stents in the early postoperative period (Fig. 9.24).

CT is less accurate for determining the presence or absence of leak, but if this modality is utilized, delayed phase images can be useful especially in the absence of a discrete fluid collection. It is important not to simply dismiss free fluid as a normal postoperative finding, particularly when loculated fluid is present adjacent to the anastomosis. There should be a low threshold for performing additional delayed phase scans or suggesting a contrast study in this context. Where there is a urinary leak, contrast collects outside the urinary tract on delayed imaging. In addition, the presence of hydronephrosis does not necessarily equate to obstruction and is usually a normal postoperative finding. However, it may be asymmetric and more pronounced on the side where a ureteric leak is present. Most leaks can be treated

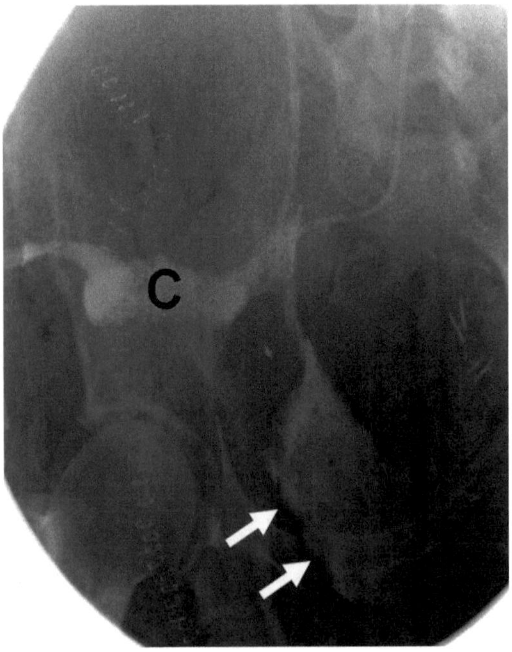

Fig. 9.23 Conduitogram demonstrating large leak (*arrows*) from the proximal part of the ileal conduit (*C*)

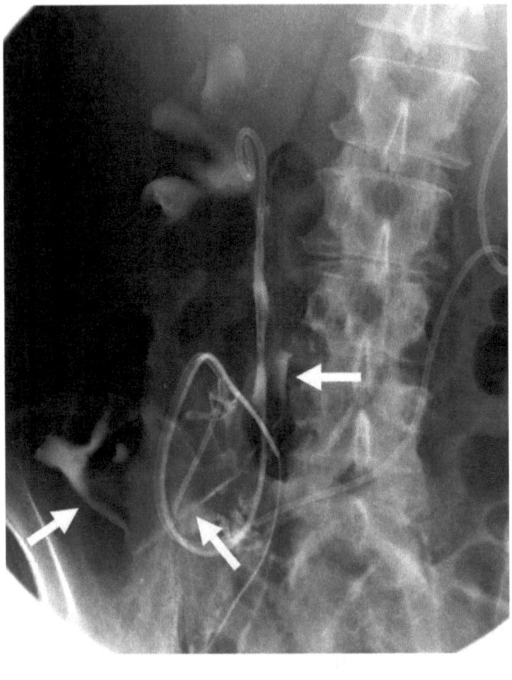

Fig. 9.24 Ileal conduit opacified via right ureteric stent. Extraluminal contrast can be seen flowing from the distal right ureter inferiorly into the right side of the pelvis (*arrows*). Such straight lines of contrast are rarely seen in normal anatomical locations

conservatively by leaving ureteric stents in situ, with further surgery rarely required.

9.2.6.4 Urinary Infection

Bacteriuria is extremely common following urinary diversion, but clinically apparent urinary tract infection is less so. Although usually a clinical diagnosis, imaging can be useful to exclude hydronephrosis, stones, and significant postvoiding urinary residuum in the reservoir.

9.2.6.5 Postoperative Collection

Commonly encountered postoperative fluid collections include urinoma, hematoma, and abscess. Urinomas are associated with urinary leaks in the early postoperative period and have already been described. It is important to note that urinoma is one of only a number of appearances that suggest urinary leak, and further imaging features are discussed elsewhere in this chapter. Delayed imaging on CT can be useful to differentiate urinoma from other fluid collections such as lymphoceles, as the former will typically fill with contrast. Urinomas often require image-guided percutaneous drainage due to the risk of infection.

Postoperative hematomas and abscesses often occur at the cystectomy site (Fig. 9.25), but the imaging features themselves are no different to postoperative hematomas and abscesses occurring secondary to any other abdominal or pelvic surgery. A hematoma is typically heterogeneous, hyperdense, and non-enhancing on CT and will not increasingly opacify on delayed phase imaging. Abscesses typically have an enhancing rim and may contain gas, but again do not opacify on delayed phase CT (Fig. 9.26). If typical features are not present, it can be very difficult to distinguish between infected and noninfected postoperative collections with imaging alone. In this situation, the clinical findings must be taken into account, with image-guided aspiration reserved for equivocal cases.

9.2.6.6 Ureteric Stricture

Strictures occurring in the early postoperative period may be due to surgical edema or due to improper surgical anastomotic technique. The former should recover quickly with time, whereas

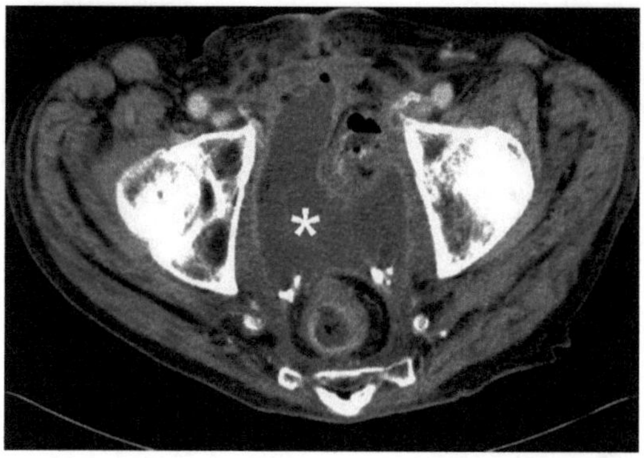

Fig. 9.25 Axial CT of a patient 6 days post cystectomy and ileal conduit. Well-defined, peripherally enhancing, gas-containing fluid collection consistent with abscess is seen in the cystectomy bed (*asterisk*)

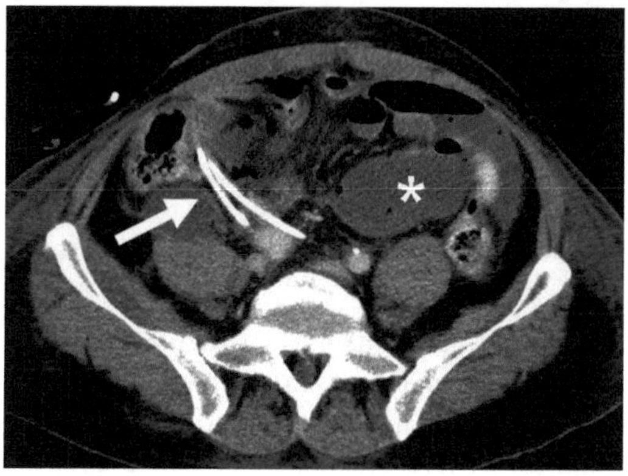

Fig. 9.26 Axial CT of a patient 5 days post cystectomy and ileal conduit demonstrates a well-defined fluid collection containing gas (*asterisk*). This did not opacify on delayed images (*not shown*) and subsequently proved to be an abscess. Both ureteric stents can be seen (*arrow*)

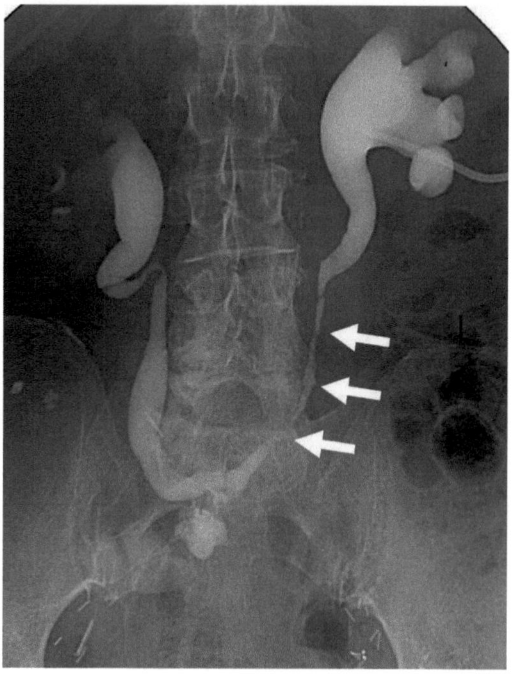

Fig. 9.27 Patient with ileal conduit. Left nephrostogram reveals a long, irregular left mid ureteric stricture (*arrows*) due to ischemia

the latter will persist and may require surgical treatment.

Causes of strictures occurring in the late postoperative period include tumor recurrence and ischemia (Fig. 9.27). The most common site of stricture is at the ureteroenteric anastomosis, and this is particularly true of the left ureter (Fig. 9.28). This has been attributed to ischemia secondary to damage of the left periureteric vessels as it is mobilized and taken across to the right side of the pelvis for anastomosis. Irregularly marginated strictures, an associated enhancing soft tissue mass, and evidence of recurrent disease elsewhere (such as with lymphadenopathy and distant metastases) are all features favoring a malignant cause, but it can be very difficult to differentiate benign from malignant causes of ureteric stricture whichever imaging modality is employed.

9.2.6.7 Calculus Formation

Calculus formation is more common following urinary diversion than in the general population, particularly after continent urinary reservoirs due to urinary stasis (Fig. 9.29). Stones may form as early as 4–5 months postoperatively, with a reported incidence of between 2.9% and 12.9% (Benson and Olsson 1999; Rowland and Kropp 1994; Terai et al. 1996). Urinary obstruction secondary to stone formation is a potentially serious complication, predominantly for patients with a single common ureteroenteric anastomosis. In these patients, bilateral hydronephrosis can result from a single obstructing calculus. Plain films, contrast studies, ultrasound, and unenhanced CT all have a role in the detection and follow-up of patients with calculi.

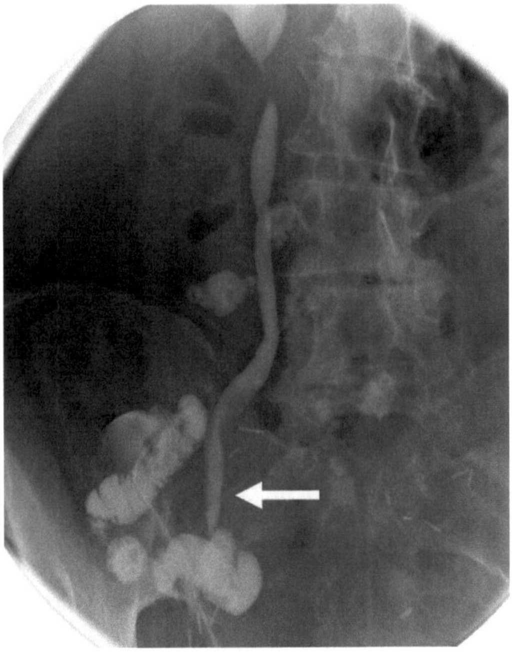

Fig. 9.28 Ileal conduitogram demonstrates normal reflux of contrast up the right ureter (*arrow*), but no contrast refluxes up the left ureter. This was due to a tight stricture at the left ureteroenteric anastomosis

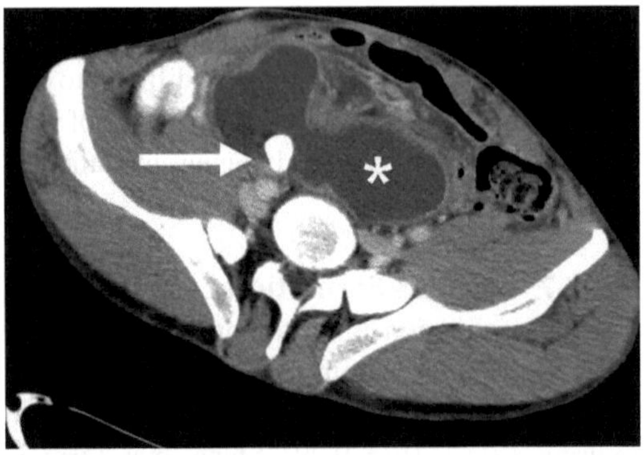

Fig. 9.29 Axial CT of a patient with a continent catheterizable reservoir (*asterisk*) with calculus demonstrated within the reservoir (*arrow*)

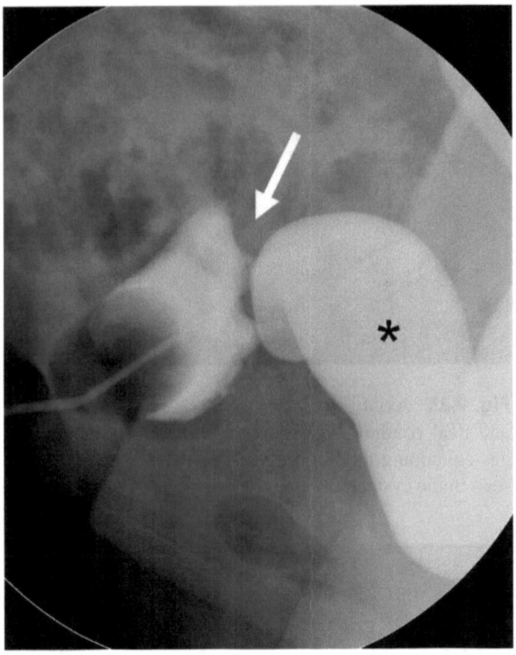

Fig. 9.30 Conduitogram via Foley catheter, demonstrating distal conduit stenosis (*arrow*). Contrast has flowed into the main part of the conduit, however (*asterisk*)

9.2.6.8 Fistulas

Fistulas occur in approximately 2% of patients following surgery for urinary diversion (Catala et al. 2009), and these include enteroconduit fistulas in patients with ileal conduits, enteropouch fistulas in patients with neobladders and continent catheterizable reservoirs, enterocutaneous fistulas from the gastrointestinal anastomosis, and enterovaginal fistulas (particularly following neobladder formation). Ureteroarterial and intestinoarterial fistulas have also been described but are very rare. Risk factors for fistula formation include radiotherapy and local tumor recurrence.

9.2.6.9 Conduit Stenosis

Conduit stenosis is a relatively rare complication of urinary diversion. It may occur within the main body of the ileal loop as a result of ischemia of the ileal segment, but is more common in close proximity to the stoma as it passes through the anterior abdominal wall musculature secondary to adhesions or parastomal herniation (Fig. 9.30). Conduit stenosis may also be caused by chronic inflammation and urinary tract infection. Stenosis may be mild and asymptomatic, or severe enough to cause bilateral hydronephrosis and warrant surgical revision. It is usually well demonstrated with contrast studies whereby a segment of the conduit is narrowed, with possible dilatation of the proximal ileal loop, ureters, and pelvicalyceal systems.

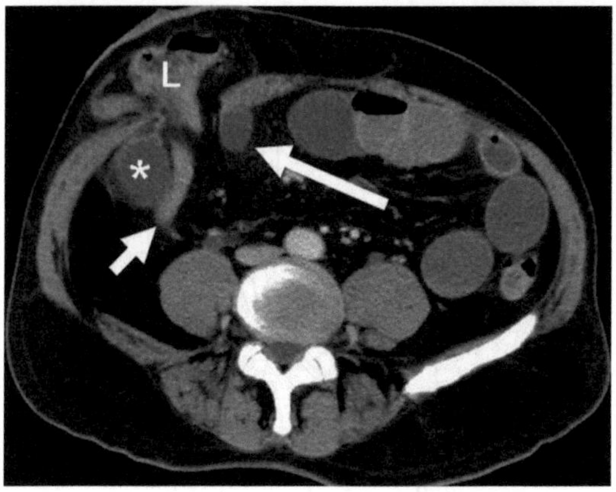

Fig. 9.31 Small-bowel obstruction caused by parastomal hernia. This patient had cystectomy and ileal conduit for TCC 4 years previously. Axial CT demonstrates a hernia containing unobstructed large bowel (*L*). A dilated loop of afferent small bowel can be seen entering the hernia (*long arrow*) with a collapsed efferent loop exiting (*short arrow*). The ileal conduit is also visible (*asterisk*)

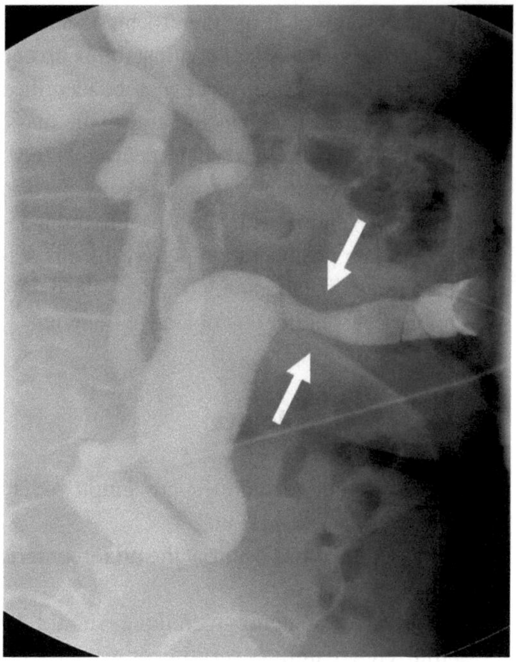

Fig. 9.32 Ileal conduitogram demonstrates mild conduit stenosis secondary to an abdominal wall hernia (*arrows*)

9.2.6.10 Hernias

Parastomal hernias are a relatively common late postoperative finding, occurring in up to 20% of patients (Catala et al. 2009). The consequences of parastomal herniation will depend upon the nature of the herniating bowel. If a loop of small or large bowel in normal gastrointestinal circuit is herniated, small or large bowel obstruction may result (Fig. 9.31). If the neck of the hernia is wide, there may be no resulting functional problem, but it may cause discomfort and a poorer cosmetic result. CT is the modality of choice to investigate for clinical complications arising secondary to parastomal hernias (usually bowel obstruction). The urinary reservoir or conduit itself may herniate into the parastomal space, and this is a recognized cause of urinary outflow obstruction (Fig. 9.32). Rarely the urinary conduit itself may herniate through other anatomical orifices such as the inguinal canal (Fig. 9.33). Contrast studies are the initial modality of choice to investigate complications thought to arise from urinary reservoir or conduit herniation.

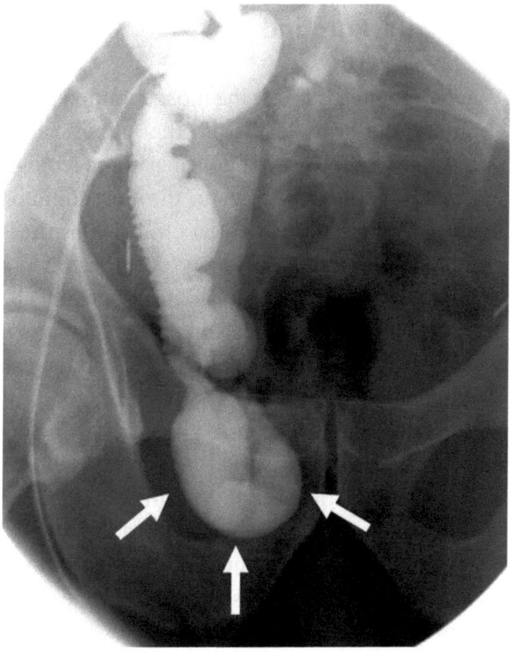

Fig. 9.33 This patient presented with bilateral hydronephrosis and raised creatinine 3 years following cystectomy and ileal conduit. Conduitogram demonstrates the conduit partially obstructed in a right inguinal hernia (*arrows*)

9.2.6.11 Tumor Recurrence

Tumor recurrence increases in frequency with more advanced primary tumor stage. Tumor recurrence may manifest on contrast studies as a ureteric stricture or, if present at the ureteroenteric anastomosis, with complete lack of contrast reflux up one ureter. On CT, tumor recurrence may be identified as a pelvic or ureteric enhancing soft tissue mass, with lymphadenopathy or distant metastases (e.g., liver or bone). Recurrence should be suspected in any patient presenting with new onset hydronephrosis in the late postoperative period. In this setting, increasing dilatation may be appreciated only with reference to earlier postoperative imaging.

9.2.7 Teaching Points

- Many different techniques are employed to achieve urinary diversion.
- Most complications occur at the ureteroenteric anastomosis.
- Postoperative imaging technique should be optimized to carefully scrutinize this site.

9.3 Ureteric Injury

9.3.1 Background

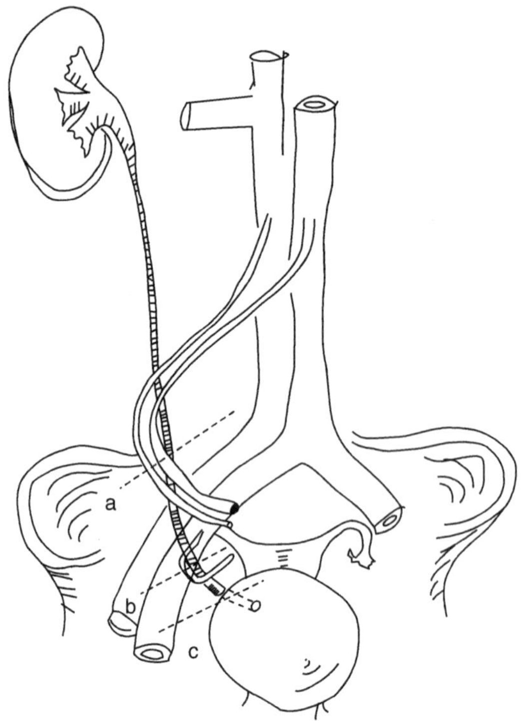

Fig. 9.34 Common sites of ureteric injury (*dashed lines*). *a* At the level of the pelvic brim, *b* along the pelvic sidewall, and *c* at the vesicoureteric junction

Whereas trauma is by far the most common cause of injury and urine leak from the kidney, iatrogenic injury following genitourinary, gynecological, or retroperitoneal surgery is the most common cause of ureteric leaks (Titton et al. 2003). Less commonly, ureteric injury may occur secondary to endourological procedures. The ureters may be subjected to full or partial thickness laceration, ischemia, crushing, or ligation. The ureter can theoretically be injured at any site along its abdominal or pelvic course, but the following sites are at risk (Fig. 9.34):

- At the level of the pelvic brim (base of the infundibulopelvic ligament) when ligating the gonadal vessels, particularly following abdominal hysterectomy or dissection of the mesorectum as part of total mesorectal excision for rectal carcinoma
- Along the pelvic sidewall when ligating the uterine vessels
- At the vesicoureteric junction during bladder/vaginal dissection

When the injury is not recognized intraoperatively and primarily repaired, the patient may present in the early or late postoperative period with a variety of symptoms and signs including pyrexia, sepsis, abdominal or loin pain, urinary obstruction, and fistulation. Unless the injury is severe, treatment is usually with antegrade or retrograde temporary urinary stent insertion, the choice depending upon local expertise and availability. Surgical repair is rarely required; it is reserved for when large defects are present or more conservative strategies have failed (that may necessitate formation of a urinary diversion). Small urinomas usually resolve spontaneously, but occasionally larger, persistent, or infected urinomas require percutaneous image-guided drainage. Rarely percutaneous aspiration is required to confirm the diagnosis of urinoma if other imaging has been equivocal.

9.3.2 Contrast Studies

Ureteric injury can be diagnosed on antegrade or retrograde pyelography, with extravasation of contrast. If a urinoma is present, contrast may collect

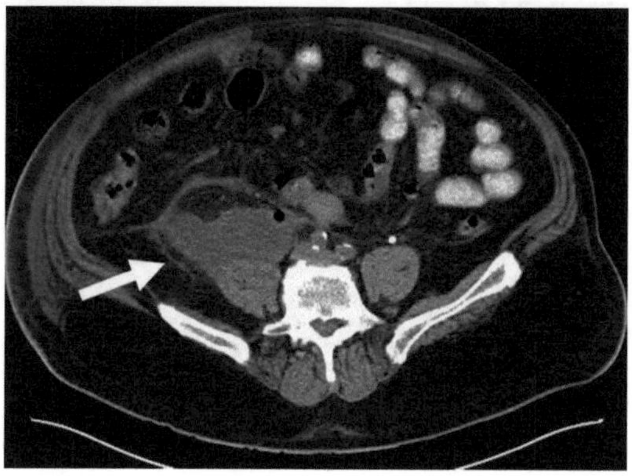

Fig. 9.35 CT demonstrating right retroperitoneal urinoma (*arrow*). The patient sustained a right ureteric injury during anterior resection for rectal carcinoma

in a well-defined extraluminal collection. An inadvertently ligated ureter will be opacified to a point of abrupt cutoff at the level of the ligation.

9.3.3 CT

The CT appearances of ureteric injury are highly variable. Ureteric laceration may produce a discrete well-defined urinoma (Fig. 9.35), a less well-defined fluid collection, or, less commonly, free urinary ascites. Sometimes the urinoma may not be adjacent to the site of laceration and can be seen at any site in the retroperitoneum or intraperitoneally. Normal fluid density (0–20 Hounsfield units) is seen initially on CT, and it may be impossible to distinguish urinoma from other types of collection and urinary ascites from other causes of free fluid unless delayed phase imaging is utilized (typically 10–20 min following intravenous contrast administration) (Fig. 9.36). A fluid-fluid level may be seen, with contrast settling in the dependent part of the collection. Fibrous and even rim-calcified chronic urinomas have been described, but often in the acute phase, no rim is present.

A ligated ureter results in hydronephrosis and hydroureter proximal to the level of the ligation, with a collapsed distal ureter.

9.3.4 Teaching Points

- The most common cause of ureteric injury is iatrogenic secondary to pelvic surgery.

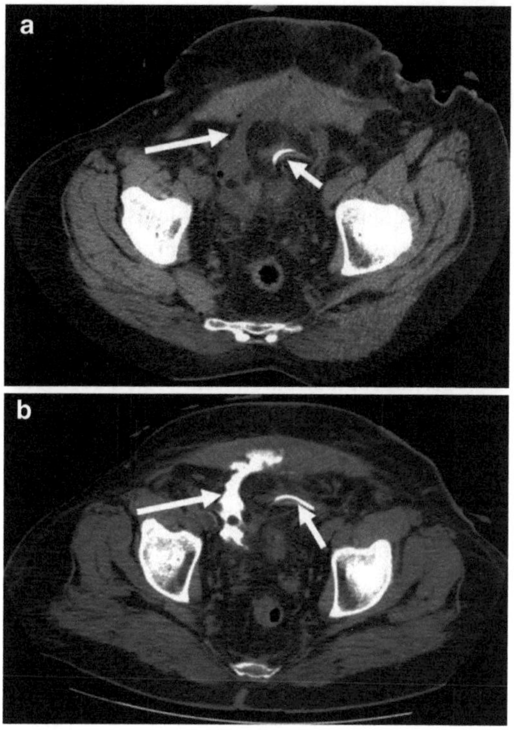

Fig. 9.36 Portal venous phase CT of a patient post anterior resection for bowel carcinoma, in whom ureteric leak was suspected. (**a**) Initial portal venous phase CT shows a fluid collection (*long arrow*) in the region of the right distal ureter. Left ureteric stent is also in situ (*short arrow*). (**b**) Delayed phase CT in the same patient shows leak of contrast into the collection (*long arrow*), confirming this to be a urinoma, left ureteric stent (*short arrow*)

- The appearances of a urine leak on CT are highly variable.
- Delayed phase CT urography can be extremely useful in diagnosis.

9.4 Bladder Injury

9.4.1 Background

The most common cause of bladder injury is blunt abdominal trauma, but iatrogenic injury following abdominal and pelvic surgery does occur. The majority of iatrogenic injuries occur secondary to gynecological surgery, with urological procedures (predominantly endourological) being the next most common (Dobrowolski et al. 2002), where the bladder is most often damaged while being mobilized from adjacent organs. Intraperitoneal leak is the most common type after iatrogenic injury, although extraperitoneal and combined types may be seen. Risk factors include pelvic inflammatory disease, endometriosis, and previous pelvic radiotherapy. Many bladder injuries constitute minor perforations, heal with conservative management, and never reach the attention of the radiologist. However, larger injuries may have significant consequences, and their imaging features should be readily appreciated, in particular, the differentiation between intraperitoneal and extraperitoneal leaks. Extraperitoneal leaks are often treated conservatively, whereas many intraperitoneal leaks are surgically repaired due to the risk of chemical peritonitis.

While discussing iatrogenic bladder injury, mention should be made of radiation damage. The bladder can be affected by both external beam radiotherapy and brachytherapy for the treatment of a wide variety of conditions, most commonly prostate carcinoma in men and cervical carcinoma in women. Radiation damage of the bladder has a spectrum of consequences ranging from asymptomatic nonvisible hematuria with no radiological manifestation through to bladder necrosis, fibrosis (rarely with mural calcification), and fistulation to surrounding organs. Occasionally, the first radiological presentation of radiation cystitis may be upper renal tract dilatation resulting from a low-volume, thick-walled bladder due to radiation fibrosis.

9.4.2 Contrast Studies

If inadvertent bladder injury is suspected during surgery, the patient is likely to have a urethral catheter in situ. This is used to slowly instill water-soluble contrast into the bladder, under the aid of gravity while intermittently screening. It is essential that the bladder is adequately distended to fully exclude small leaks and that oblique/lateral views and postdrainage films are taken to exclude posterior and posterolateral leaks. With intraperitoneal perforations, such as those involving the dome of the bladder, contrast will outline loops of bowel and may extend into the paracolic gutters (Fig. 9.37). Contrast may be confined to the perivesical space around the anterolateral bladder in extraperitoneal perforation (Fig. 9.38), where the base of the bladder has been injured. More extensive extravasation around the bladder may be seen (Fig. 9.39), sometimes extending as far as the thigh or scrotum. However, extraperitoneal leaks do not extend above the pelvis, and therefore any contrast material seen extending superiorly into the abdomen indicates intraperitoneal or a combined leak. These discriminating features apply equally to both fluoroscopic cystography and to CT cystography. A combination of intraperitoneal and extraperitoneal injury can occur, and with very small contained leaks, it can sometimes be difficult to accurately distinguish between the two.

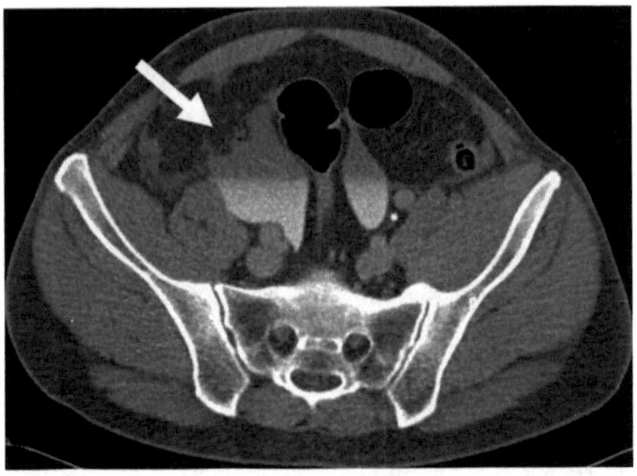

Fig. 9.37 Axial CT cystogram of a patient with intraperitoneal bladder leak following pelvic surgery. Fluid surrounds bowel loops and there is a fluid-fluid level with layering of extravasated contrast material (*arrow*)

9.4.3 CT

CT cystography has become the mainstay of detecting bladder injury in trauma but is not so readily used for suspected iatrogenic injury where fluoroscopic contrast studies remain the preferred modality in many centers. However, if the patient is clinically unwell or there is diagnostic uncertainty with general abdominal signs and symptoms, then CT may be preferred. On portal venous phase imaging, the only feature suggestive of bladder perforation may be the presence of free fluid with either extraperitoneal or intraperitoneal

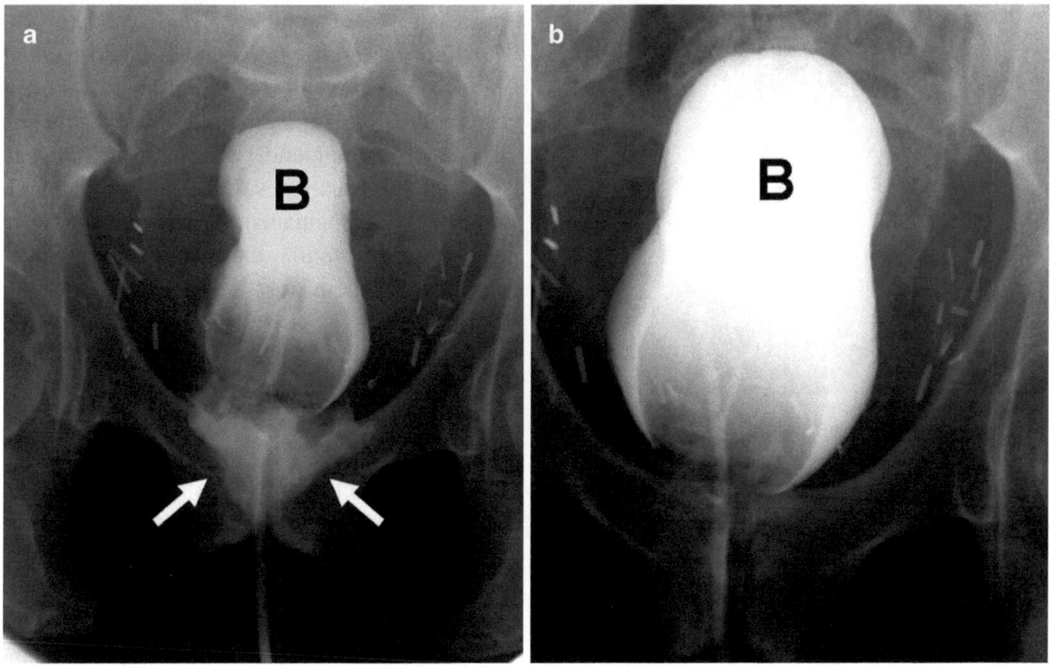

Fig. 9.38 Extraperitoneal bladder leak. (**a**) Cystogram via urethral Foley catheter, demonstrating extravasation of contrast into the perivesical space around the bladder base (*arrows*). Bladder (*B*). (**b**) Follow-up cystogram on the same patient shows the leak has healed. Note the smooth outline to the bladder (*B*) with no extravesical contrast

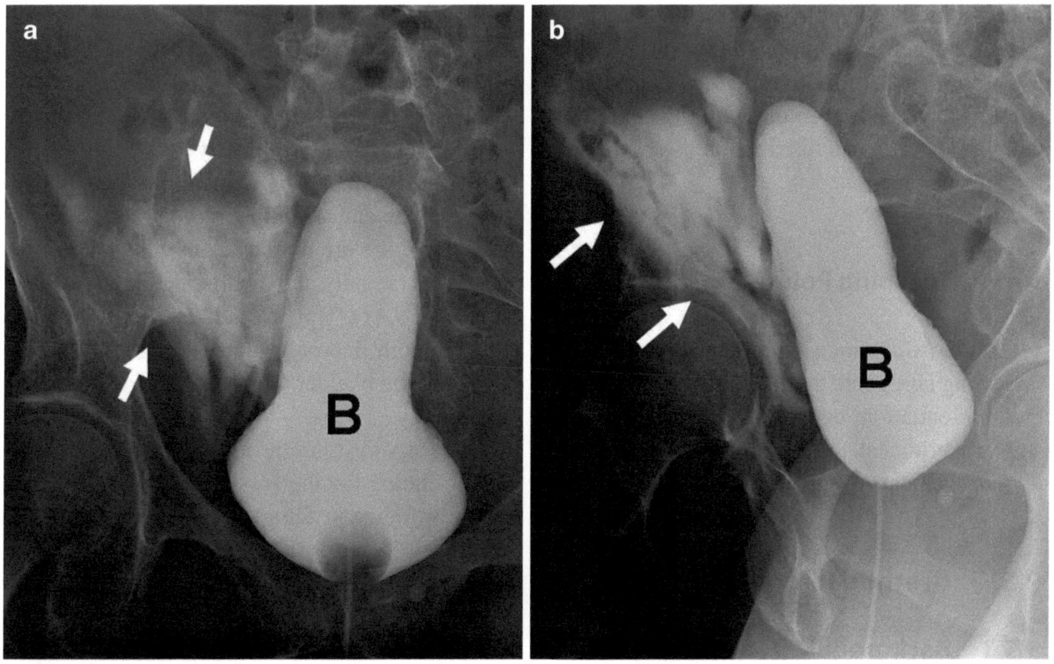

Fig. 9.39 (**a**) Cystogram demonstrating more extensive contrast extravasation into the perivesical space (*arrows*), indicating extraperitoneal leak. This patient had a full-thickness perforation following cystoscopic biopsy. (**b**) Cystogram oblique view of the same patient showing the anterior extent of contrast extravasation into the perivesical space (*arrows*). Bladder (*B*)

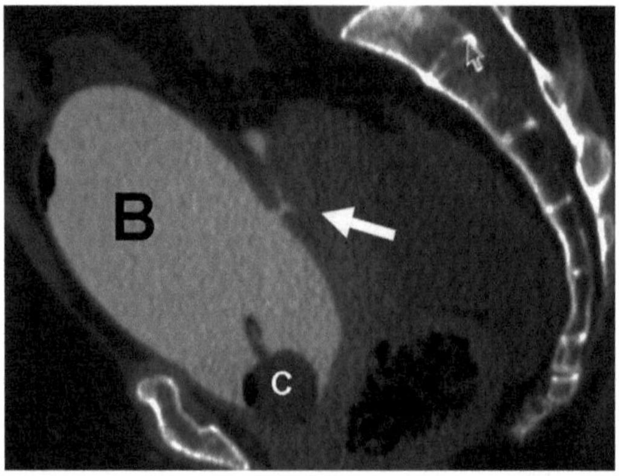

Fig. 9.40 Sagittal CT cystogram on a patient post transurethral resection of bladder tumor demonstrates leakage of contrast through a perforation in the posterior bladder wall (*arrow*). Bladder (*B*), catheter balloon (*C*)

distribution depending upon the site of injury. For confirmation of bladder perforation, a CT cystogram should be performed. This involves actively filling the bladder with approximately 200–400 ml of water-soluble contrast (4% strength is appropriate) via a urethral catheter, and then rescanning through the pelvis (Fig. 9.40). As with fluoroscopic cystography, it is essential to achieve adequate distension of the bladder to ensure small leaks are detected. Bladder leak is confirmed if contrast material is seen out with the confines of the bladder wall, in a distribution as described in the previous section.

9.4.4 Teaching Points

- The most common type of bladder leak following iatrogenic injury is intraperitoneal.
- Differentiation between intraperitoneal and extraperitoneal leaks is crucial to determine management.

9.5 Urethral Injury

9.5.1 Background

Iatrogenic urethral injury is rare, but can occur following surgery that involves deep pelvic resection when the normal pelvic anatomy has been disturbed such as with salvage surgery for recurrent rectal carcinoma. Transurethral procedures for resection of prostate or bladder tumor can also rarely result in urethral injury. Another cause of urethral injury in the surgical population is related to traumatic Foley catheter removal, although this usually results in only minor contusions that heal spontaneously without significant clinical manifestation. Iatrogenic urethral injury can involve both the anterior and posterior urethra.

9.5.2 Contrast Studies

Retrograde urethrography is the modality of choice for the investigation of suspected urethral injury in males. The patient lays supine, with the pelvis rotated to an approximately 30° oblique position (usually right posterior oblique) and the right leg flexed. A pediatric Foley catheter (commonly 8F) is placed with its tip approximately 2 cm into the urethra in the fossa navicularis (the catheter should be flushed with contrast prior to insertion to expel any air) and the balloon inflated slowly. In order to produce a good seal, the balloon may have to be inflated such that it is uncomfortable for the patient. Approximately 30 ml of contrast is injected slowly into the urethra via the catheter while intermittently screening (some centers advocate a single image following instillation of the entire volume of contrast). In a normal study, the urethra has a smooth contour that narrows gradually at the bulbomembranous junction (Fig. 9.41). The prostatic urethra is seen as a thin, smooth line of contrast, and reflux of contrast into the bladder may be visualized in a complete study.

Voiding cystourethrography is the modality of choice for the investigation of suspected urethral injury in females, and may be utilized in males if retrograde urethrography has not been conclusive and a posterior urethral injury is suspected. The bladder is filled with water-soluble contrast via either a urethral or suprapubic catheter, the patient actively voids usually in the upright position while screening, and spot images are obtained. The urethral catheter can be left in situ for the entire investigation. In a normal study, the bladder neck widens and the

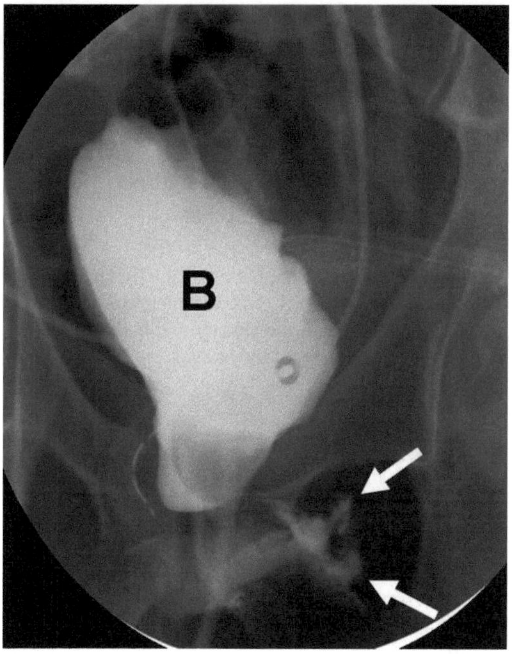

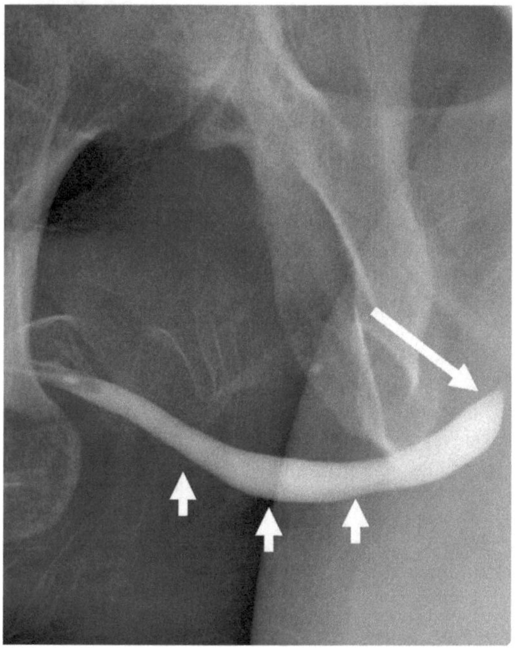

Fig. 9.41 Retrograde urethrogram showing the normal smooth contour of the urethra (*short arrows*) and gradual tapering at the bulbomembranous junction (*long arrow*)

Fig. 9.42 Cystogram of a patient with an upper prostatic urethral injury following abdominoperineal resection of recurrent rectal cancer. Extraluminal contrast can be seen in the extraperitoneal pelvic soft tissues (*arrows*). Bladder (*B*)

posterior urethra is distended more fully than in retrograde urethrography.

Whichever technique is employed, urethral rupture is diagnosed when extravasation of contrast is seen outside the normal confines of the urethra (Fig. 9.42). This may be locally confined within the periurethral tissues or, particularly with injuries near the bladder neck, may extend more diffusely into the extraperitoneal space.

9.5.3 CT

CT is not routinely used for postoperative imaging in suspected urethral injury in the postoperative patient. If CT has been performed, the urethral injury itself is unlikely to be visualized. There may be free extraperitoneal fluid present, especially if the patient has not been catheterized. If a catheter is in situ, a CT cystogram can be performed, with high-attenuation fluid seen in the extraperitoneal space in the pelvis if there is a urethral tear, although it can be difficult to distinguish this from a leak arising from a bladder base injury. Small-volume fluid focally within the urogenital diaphragm may point toward a urethral injury as the cause (Fig. 9.43). Often urethrography will be required to confirm urethral injury following nonspecific CT findings.

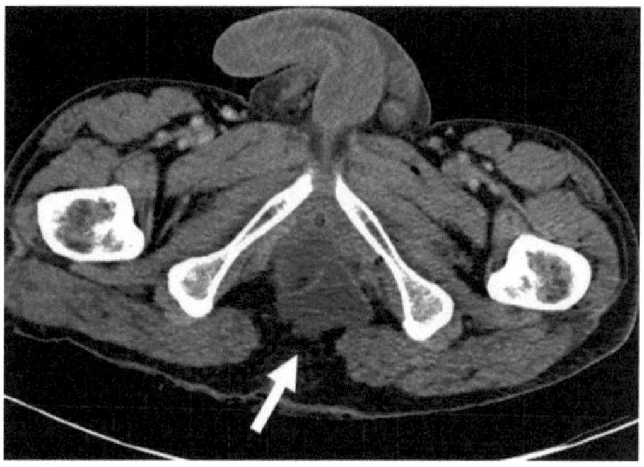

Fig. 9.43 Axial CT of a patient following radical resection of a locally advanced rectal carcinoma invading the prostate, requiring prostatectomy. CT performed for unexplained sepsis. Urethral anastomotic leak indicated by collection of fluid within the deep pelvic soft tissues posterior to the urethra (*arrow*). Confirmed on urethrogram (*not shown*)

9.5.4 Teaching Points

- Clinically significant urethral injury is a rare complication of pelvic surgery or transurethral procedures.
- Urethrography is usually required to confirm the diagnosis of urethral tear.

Acknowledgments I would like to thank Dr. Henry Irving (Consultant Radiologist, Leeds Teaching Hospitals NHS Trust) for his help with the chapter and his kind permission for the use of many of the images.

References

Benson MC, Olsson CA. Continent urinary diversions. Urol Clin North Am. 1999;26:125–47.

Catala V, Sola M, Samaniego J, et al. CT findings in urinary diversion after radical cystectomy: post surgical anatomy and complications. Radiographics. 2009;29: 461–76.

Chang SS, Cookson MS, Baumgartner RG, Wells N, Smith Jr JA. Analysis of early complications after radical cystectomy: results of a collaborative care pathway. J Urol. 2002;167:2012–6.

Dobrowolski ZF, Lipczynski W, Drewniak T, Jakubik P, Kusionowicz J. External and iatrogenic trauma of the urinary bladder: a survey in Poland. BJU Int. 2002;89: 755–6.

Heaney MD, Francis IR, Cohan RH, et al. Orthotopic neobladder reconstruction: findings on excretory urography and CT. Am J Roentgenol. 1999;172:1213–20.

Kenney PJ, Hamrick KM, Samuels LJ, Han SY, Bueschen AJ. Radiologic evaluation of continent urinary reservoirs. Radiographics. 1990;10:455–66.

Rowland RG, Kropp BP. Evolution of the Indiana continent reservoir. J Urol. 1994;152:2247–51.

Terai A, Ueda T, Kakehi Y, et al. Urinary calculi as a late complication of the Indiana continent urinary diversion: comparison with the Koch pouch procedure. J Urol. 1996;155:66–8.

Titton RL, Gervais DA, Hahn PF, et al. Urine leaks and urinomas: diagnosis and image-guided intervention. Radiographics. 2003;23:1133–47.

Index

A
Abdominal aortic aneurysm (AAA), 25
Abdominoperineal excision of rectum (APER), 17, 258, 259
Abnormal postoperative abdomen
  colonic pseudoobstruction, 15–16
  fluid collections and abscesses, 11–13
  generalized peritonitis, 11, 12
  large bowel obstruction, 16
  postoperative leaks, 13–14
  small bowel obstruction, 14–15
  spontaneous bacterial peritonitis, 13
Acalculous cholecystitis, 34
ACE. *See* Antegrade colonic enema (ACE)
Achalasia, 65–66
Acute ischemic colitis, 30
Acute pancreatitis, 136–137
Advancement flap, 281
Afferent loop obstruction/syndrome, 86
Alpha-fetoprotein (AFP), 202
Anastomosis
  construction, 269
  nomenclature, 268–270
Anastomotic leak, 182–183
  and abscess
    contributing factors, 261–262
    distal and proximal leaks, 263
    double rectum sign, 262–263
    loop colostomy and, 262
    surgical drains, 263
    transgluteal drainage, 263–264
  bypass and substitution, 61, 63, 64
  and duodenal stump leak
    comprehensive review
      importance, 85
    diagnostic pitfalls, 82, 83
    image-guided drainage, 85, 87
    successful management, 84
    total gastrectomy, 85, 86
  resection
    clinical features, 49
    complications and treatment, 52–53
    esophagogastric, 50–52
    mortality, 48–49
    pyloroplasty leak, 52
    upper GI contrast study, 49, 50
  small bowel
    operation, 234–235
    postoperative complications, 250–252
Anastomotic strictures
  biliary enteric anastomoses, 183, 184
  bypass and substitution, 65, 66
  colon resections, 264–266
  normal postoperative imaging, 86–88
  resection, 54–56
  small bowel
    operation, 236–237
    postoperative complications, 250
Angelchik antireflux prosthesis, 76
Antegrade colonic enema (ACE), 284
Anterior resection (AR), 258, 259
Anterior sphincteroplasty, 286
APER. *See* Abdominoperineal excision of rectum (APER)
AR. *See* Anterior resection (AR)
Arterioportal fistula, 220
Ascites, 198
Auxiliary liver transplantation, 216, 217

B
Bacteriuria, 306
Balloon dilatation, 55
Bariatric surgery. *See* Stomach and duodenum
Barium, 37–38, 142
Basal pulmonary atelectasis, 7–8
Beak sign, 231
Bedside suprapubic catheter placement, 17
Beger procedure, 132, 134
Belsey Mark IV repair, 76–77
Berne procedure, 133, 135
Bile duct injuries
  anatomy and common variants, 167, 168
  Bismuth's classification, 168, 169
  management, 168, 170
  Strasberg's classification, 167, 169
Bile leak, 197–198, 222
  causes, 170
  contrast-enhanced MRCP, 172, 173
  CT cholangiography, 172, 174
  HIDA, 171–172
  imaging, 170–172
  liver bilioma, 170, 171
  management, 174, 175

J. Brittenden, D.J.M. Tolan (eds.), *Radiology of the Post Surgical Abdomen*,
DOI 10.1007/978-1-4471-2775-8, © Springer-Verlag London 2012

Bile reflux gastritis, 89
Biliary anastomosis, 218
Biliary dilatation, 157
Biliary enteric anastomoses. *See* Biliary tree
Biliary obstruction
  biliary complications, 198
  cholecystectomy complications, 174, 176
  pancreas, 146–147
Biliary strictures, 174, 176, 220–221
Biliary tree
  background, 153–154
  cholecystectomy complications
    bile duct injuries, 167–170 (*see* Bile duct injuries)
    bile leak (*see* Bile leak)
    biliary obstruction, 174, 176
    biliary strictures, 174, 176
    cystic duct stump complications, 180
    dropped or spilled gallstones, 177–179
    laparoscopic, 180
    retained CBD stones, 176–178
    vascular injury, 179–180
  enteric anastomoses
    anastomotic leak, 182–183
    anastomotic strictures, 183, 184
    clinical indications, 181
    modifications, 181–182
    nonanastomotic strictures, 184
    stone formation, 184, 185
    surgical technique and postoperative anatomy, 181, 182
  laparoscopic cholecystectomy
    clinical indications, 154
    modifications, 154–156
    normal radiological appearances, 156–157
    surgical technique and postoperative anatomy, 154, 155
  Mirizzi's syndrome, 181
  MRCP interpretation tips and pitfalls
    bile duct air, 160–162, 164
    3D MRCP MIP image, 158, 159
    flow artifact, 159–160, 163
    pathology, 163, 167
    pseudocalculus, 160, 163
    single-shot FSE MRCP sequence, 157
    stents, clips, and drains, 162–163, 165, 166
    true FISP sequence, 158, 161
    vascular compression, 158–159, 162
Biliscopin, 174
Billroth II partial gastrectomy, 79, 80
Billroth I partial gastrectomy, 78, 80
Bismuth's classification, 168, 169
Bladder injury, 19, 26, 27
  background, 311–312
  contrast studies, 312, 313
  CT, 312, 314
Bladeless trocar technology, 25
Blind pouch syndrome, 235–236
Bowel strangulation, 246
Bricker technique, 296, 297
Budd-Chiari syndrome, 199–200, 220

C
Calculus formation, 307–308
Calot's triangle, 154
Caudatectomy, 191
CBD injury. *See* Common bile duct (CBD) injury
Cecostomy, 278, 279
Celiac artery stenosis, 146
Central pancreatectomy, 130–131
Chemical arteritis, 211
Chlorhexidine, 36
Cholecystectomy. *See* Biliary tree
Cholecystojejunal bypass, 182
Cholecystostomy, 155, 156
Choledochoduodenostomy, 181–182
Chronic kidney disease (CKD), 4
Chronic pancreatitis. *See* Pancreas
Chylothorax, 55
Closed loop obstruction and ischemia, 231–232
Clostridium difficile, 29
Collimation, 5
Collis gastroplasty, 77–78
Colon
  anastomosis
    construct, 269
    nomenclature, 268–270
  fistula-in-ano surgery
    background, 279–280
    Parks classification system, 280
    postoperative complications, 282
    postoperative imaging, 281–282
    surgical techniques, 280–281
  image-guided colonic intervention
    cecostomy, 278, 279
    colonic stenting (*see* Colonic stenting)
    sigmoidopexy, 278–279
  pelvic floor and defecatory disorders
    clinical indication, 282–283
    full-thickness rectal prolapse, 285–286
    incontinence surgery, 286–287
    laparoscopic ventral rectopexy, 284–286
    management, 283–284
    normal postoperative imaging, 288–289
    postoperative complications, 287–288
    postoperative gas, 289
    slow transit constipation surgery, 284
    STARR, 284, 285
    surgical materials, 290
    treatment failure, 290–292
  recurrent rectal cancer and pelvic exenteration
    complications, 275–276
    CT, 273
    factors, 272
    imaging of, 272
    MRI, 273–275
    PET CT, 273
  resection
    anastomosis types, 260
    anastomotic leak and abscess (*see* Anastomotic leak, and abscess)
    anastomotic stricture, 264–266
    APER, 258, 259

AR, 258, 259
clinical indications, 256
CT, 260–261
fistula, 264, 265
Hartmann's procedure, 257–259
LHC, 257, 258
local tumor recurrence (*see* Local tumor recurrence)
lower GI contrast studies, 260
PC, 259
RHC, 256, 257
sigmoid colectomy, 257, 258
STC, 259
surgery site complications, 267–269
TC, 258, 259
transverse colectomy, 256, 257
stomas
colostomy, 271
description, 269–270
ileostomy, 270–271
parastomal hernia, 271
prolapse, 271
stenosis and retraction, 271–272
technological advancements, 256
Colonic pseudoobstruction, 15–16
Colonic stenting
background, 276–277
clinical indications, 276
complications, 277–278
poststenting imaging, 277
procedure, 276, 277
Colon resections. *See* Colon
Colostomy, 271
Common bile duct (CBD) injury, 154
Computed tomography (CT). *See also* Small bowel
bladder injury, 312, 314
cholangiography, 172, 174
continent catheterizable reservoir, 303
IPAA, 249–250
normal postoperative anatomy (*see* Pancreas)
normal postoperative imaging, 46, 60–61
orthotopic neobladder, 303–304
protocol/technique optimization (*see* Postoperative abdomen)
ureteric injury, 311
urethral injury, 315
Conduit leak, 65
Conduit necrosis/ischemia and anastomotic leak, 61, 63, 64
Conduitogram, 298
Conduit stenosis, 308
Continent catheterizable reservoir
alternative techniques, 297
contrast studies, 302
CT, 303
procedure, 297–299
Contrast-enhanced MRCP, 172, 173
Contrast-induced nephropathy, 4
Core fistulectomy, 280
Couinaud's classification, 188
Crohn's disease, 239–240
CT. *See* Computed tomography (CT)
Cystic duct stump complications, 180
Cystic tumors, 128

D

Delorme's procedure, 285
Digital subtraction angiography (DSA), 144
Distal pancreatic operations, 131, 132
Dor fundoplication, 66, 67
DPPHR. *See* Duodenum-preserving pancreatic head resection (DPPHR)
DSA. *See* Digital subtraction angiography (DSA)
Dumping syndrome, 149
Duodenal obstruction and palliation, 122–124
Duodenal resection and surgery
duodenal obstruction and palliation
imaging, 123, 124
stent *vs.* surgery, 122–123
duodenal ulcer surgery
bleeding, 121
indications, 118–119
management, 120–121
perforated, 121
postoperative imaging and complications, 122, 123
PPTD and SD
clinical indications, 118
postoperative imaging and complications, 118, 120
technique, 118–120
uses, 117–118
Duodenum-preserving pancreatic head resection (DPPHR), 132, 135
Dysphagia, 67–69
Dysphagia and dysmotility, 73

E

Efferent loop obstruction
adhesive obstruction and distal anastomotic stricture, 107–109
internal hernia, 105–107
port site/incisional hernia, 107, 108
Endoscopic retrograde cholangiopancreatography (ERCP), 174
Endoscopy, 115
End-to-end anastomosis, 269
End-to-side anastomosis, 269, 270
Enteric complications, pancreas
delayed gastric emptying, 148
gastric outlet and afferent roux loop obstruction, 149
gastroenterostomy, 148–149
malabsorption, 149
ERCP. *See* Endoscopic retrograde cholangiopancreatography (ERCP)
Esophagotomy and leak, 66–67
Esophagus
bypass and substitution
anastomotic strictures and reflux, 65, 66
clinical indications, 58
conduit leak, 65

Esophagus (*cont.*)
conduit necrosis/ischemia and anastomotic leak, 61, 63, 64
conduit/substitute and position choice, 58–60
CT, 60–61
donor site complications, 65
upper GI contrast studies, 59, 61–63
general considerations, 41–42
Heller myotomy
clinical indications and surgical technique, 65–67
esophagotomy and leak, 66–67
postoperative dysphagia, 67–69
postoperative imaging, 66
reflux, 68
resection
anastomotic leak (*see* Anastomotic leak)
anastomotic stricture, 54–56
aspiration risk, 47
cardiovascular complications, 57
chylothorax, 55
clinical indications, 42
CT, 46
delayed emptying, 55, 57
hiatus and diaphragmatic hernias, 56–58
image-guided intervention role, 57–58
Ivor Lewis esophagectomy, 42–44
left thoracoabdominal approach, 44, 46
pulmonary and pleural complications, 47–49
three-stage esophagectomy, 43, 45
transhiatal esophagectomy, 44–46
tube necrosis/ischemia, 53–54
tube torsion, 54
upper GI contrast studies, 44–45
External hernias, 233
Extraperitoneal leak, 312
Extrasphincteric fistula, 280

F
Familial adenomatous polyposis (FAP), 248, 259
Fasciocutaneous flap necrosis, 63, 64
Fast spin-echo (FSE) sequences, 157
Fecal incontinence, 282–283
Feeding jejunostomy. *See* Small bowel
Fibrin glue and collagen plugs, 281
Fistula, 264, 265
Fistula-in-ano surgery. *See* Colon
Fistulas, 48, 252, 308
Fistulotomy, 280
Fluoroscopy, postoperative abdomen. *See* Postoperative abdomen
Frey procedure, 132, 133
FSE sequences. *See* Fast spin-echo (FSE) sequences
Full-thickness rectal prolapse, 285–286
Fundoplication
dehiscence, 76
principles and types, 72
Fundus-first cholecystectomy, 155

G
Gangrenous cholecystitis, 34
Gastric remnant malignancy, 89, 90
Gastric resections and surgery
additional operations, 91–92
afferent loop obstruction/syndrome, 86
anastomotic strictures, 86–88
Billroth II/polya partial gastrectomy, 79, 80
Billroth I partial gastrectomy, 78, 80
clinical indications, 78
efferent complications, 89–91
gastric remnant complications, 89, 90
gastroenterostomy, 80, 82
leak (*see* Anastomotic, and duodenal stump leak)
normal postoperative imaging, 82
parastomal ulceration, 89
subtotal gastrectomy with Roux loop reconstruction, 79
total gastrectomy, 80, 81
truncal vagotomy, 80
tumor recurrence, 91
wedge resection, 80
Gastroduodenal artery (GDA) stump, 144–146
Gastroesophageal reflux surgery. *See* Stomach and duodenum
Gastrointestinal anastomotic leak, 304–305
Gastrojejunostomy, 138–139
Gastroparesis, 89
GDA stump. *See* Gastroduodenal artery (GDA) stump
Generalized peritonitis, 11, 12
Genitourinary system
bladder injury
background, 311–312
contrast studies, 312, 313
CT, 312, 314
types, 296
ureteric injury
background, 310
contrast studies, 310–311
CT, 311
urethral injury
background, 314
contrast studies, 314–315
CT, 315
urinary diversion
alternative techniques, 296
calculus formation, 307–308
clinical indications, 295–296
complications, 304
conduit stenosis, 308
continent catheterizable reservoir (*see* Continent catheterizable reservoir)
fistulas, 308
gastrointestinal anastomotic leak, 304–305
hernias, 309
incontinent conduit diversion, 296–297
orthotopic neobladder, 297, 299, 300
postoperative collection, 306, 307
postoperative ileus, 304
tumor recurrence, 309–310
ureteric stricture, 306–308

urinary infection, 306
urinary leak, 305–306
Goodsall's rule, 280
Gossypiboma, 21
Graft ischemia, 53
Graft rejection, 218

H
Hartmann's procedure, 257–259
Hassan technique, 24
Hautmann neobladder, 298
HCC. *See* Hepatocellular carcinoma (HCC)
Heineke-Mikulicz pyloroplasty, 92, 93
Heller myotomy
clinical indications and surgical technique, 65–67
esophagotomy and leak, 66–67
postoperative dysphagia, 67–69
postoperative imaging, 66
reflux, 68
Hemostatic compounds, 9, 10
Heparin, 36
Hepatic artery anastomosis, 217, 218
Hepatic artery pseudoaneurysm, 220
Hepatic artery stenosis, 220
Hepatic artery thrombosis, 219
Hepaticojejunostomy (HJ), 181
Hepatic parenchymal atrophy, 211
Hepatocellular carcinoma (HCC), 188
Hernias, 309
Hiatus and diaphragmatic hernias, 56–58
Hiatus hernia repair
clinical indication, 77
postoperative complications and imaging, 78, 79
surgical technique, 77–78
HIDA, 171–172
Highly selective vagotomy, 91–92
HJ. *See* Hepaticojejunostomy (HJ)

I
Iatrogenic postoperative problems. *See* Postoperative abdomen
Ileal pouch-anal anastomoses (IPAA)
advantages, 246
background, 248
CT, 249–250
GI contrast studies, 248–249
pouch construct, 247–248
stages, 247
Ileostomy, 270–271
Image-guided colonic intervention
cecostomy, 278, 279
colonic stenting (*see* Colonic stenting)
sigmoidopexy, 278–279
Image guided drainage
access route, 34
causes, 34
coagulation status assessment, 35–36
consent, 35
modality choice, 34–35
technique, 36–37
Incarceration, 246
Incisional hernia, 107, 108, 244, 245
Incontinent conduit diversion
alternative techniques, 296–298
common procedure, 296, 297
contrast studies, 298–302
CT, 302
Infective colitis, 29
Inlay mesh, 243
Internal hernias, 105–107, 245–246
International Study Group of Pancreatic Surgery, 144
Intersphincteric fistula, 280
Intraoperative cholangiography (IOC), 155
Intraoperative injury, 18–19
Intraperitoneal leak, 311–312
Intraperitoneal onlay mesh (IPOM), 243
Intrathoracic wrap herniation, 74–76
Intravenous contrast, 3–5
IOC. *See* Intraoperative cholangiography (IOC)
IPAA. *See* Ileal pouch-anal anastomoses (IPAA)
Ischemic biliopathy, 221
Ivor Lewis esophagectomy, 42–44

J
J-pouch, 247–248

K
Kausch-Whipple procedure, 128–129
Knee jerk response, 13
Kock pouch, 248, 297

L
Laparoscopic adjustable gastric band (LAGB)
complications
erosion, 113
migration, 111–113
open, 113–114
port site infection, 115
tight, 110–112
tube and port related, 114–115
restrictive surgery, 93–94
Laparoscopic cholecystectomy. *See* Biliary tree
Laparoscopic/open bile duct exploration, 155, 156
Laparoscopic resectional rectopexy, 285–286
Laparoscopic surgery related complications. *See* Postoperative abdomen
Large bowel obstruction, 16
Left hemicolectomy (LHC), 257, 258
Left thoracoabdominal approach, 44, 46
Lewis-McKeown procedure, 43, 45
LHC. *See* Left hemicolectomy (LHC)
Lidocaine, 36

Linear staplers, 269
Liver
  anatomic resection, 187–188
  HCC, 188
  ischemia/infarction, 220
  normal anatomy
    Couinaud's classification, 188–189
    hepatic arterial supply, 189
    hepatic venous drainage, 190
  orthotopic liver transplantation
    background, 214
    biliary complications, 220–222
    fluid collections, 222–223
    graft rejection, 218
    late complications, 223–224
    modifications, 215–216
    normal postoperative imaging, 216–218
    small bowel ileus and obstruction, 222, 223
    surgical technique, 214–215
    vascular complications, 219–220
  resection and metastasectomy
    ascites, 198
    biliary complications, 197–198
    clinical indications, 190
    CT, 194–196
    modifications, 192–194
    MRI, 196
    recurrent disease imaging, 200–203
    sepsis, 197
    surgical technique and postoperative anatomy, 190–193
    vascular complications, 199–200
  RFA
    background, 202
    clinical indications, 204
    complications, 205–207
    features, 202–204
    imaging post-RFA, 205, 206
    modifications, 204, 205
    recurrent disease, 207–208
    technique, 204–205
  TACE
    advantages, 209
    clinical indications, 209
    complications, 211–212
    imaging post-TACE, 210–211
    recurrent malignancy post-TACE imaging, 212–214
    technique, 209–210
Living-donor liver transplantation, 215–216
Local tumor recurrence
  adjuvant treatments, 266–268
  classification, 266
  exophytic enlarging mass, 266–267
  factors, 264–265
Loopogram, 298
Loop stomas, 269
Luminal contrast, 2–4

M
Magenstrasse and Mill (M&M) procedure, 95, 96
Magnetic resonance cholangiopancreatography (MRCP), 33, 154. *See also* Biliary tree
Malabsorption, 149
Maximum intensity projection (MIP), 158
MDCT. *See* Multidetector CT (MDCT)
Mesenteric panniculitis, 8
Mesh-related erosion, 9–11
Mirizzi's syndrome, 181
M&M procedure. *See* Magenstrasse and Mill (M&M) procedure
Modified Lloyd-Davis position, 23
MRCP. *See* Magnetic resonance cholangiopancreatography (MRCP)
Multidetector CT (MDCT), 2
Myocutaneous flap necrosis, 63, 64

N
Necrotizing fasciitis, 28
Neuroendocrine tumors (NETS), 130
Neutral contrast, 3
Neutropenic enterocolitis, 32
Nissen fundoplication, 72
Nonanastomotic strictures, 184
Nonanatomic wedge resections, 193
Normal postoperative abdomen
  basal pulmonary atelectasis, 7–8
  free gas, 6–7
  smoke of battle, 6
  wet patient, 7

O
Obstructed defecation surgery
  laparoscopic ventral rectopexy, 284–286
  STARR, 284, 285
Ogilvie syndrome, 15
OLT. *See* Orthotopic liver transplantation (OLT)
Omental infarction, 19–20
Omnipaque, 260
Onlay mesh, 242
Oral contrast, 3
Orthotopic liver transplantation (OLT)
  background, 214
  biliary complications, 220–222
  fluid collections, 222–223
  graft rejection, 218
  late complications, 223–224
  modifications, 215–216
  normal postoperative imaging, 216–218
  small bowel ileus and obstruction, 222, 223
  surgical technique, 214–215
  vascular complications, 219–220
Orthotopic neobladder
  alternative techniques, 298
  contrast studies, 303, 304
  CT, 303–304
  procedure, 297, 299, 300
Oxaliplatin, 196

P

Pancreas
acute pancreatitis interventions, 136–137
chronic pancreatitis operations
Beger procedure, 132, 134
Berne procedure, 133, 135
complications imaging, 136
Frey procedure, 132, 133
Puestow procedure, 134
surgical outcomes, 135
surgical procedure, 131
distal pancreatic operations, 131, 132
duodenal, and ampullary tumor resections
central pancreatectomy, 130–131
Kausch-Whipple procedure, 128–129
NETS and RAMPS, 130
PPPD, 129–130
surgical modifications, 130
enteric complications
delayed gastric emptying, 148
gastric outlet and afferent roux loop obstruction, 149
gastroenterostomy, 148–149
malabsorption, 149
injury, 26, 27
normal postoperative anatomy, CT
fluid/fat stranding, 139
gastrojejunostomy, 138–139
hepaticojejunostomy, 138, 139
pancreatic atrophy, 142
pancreatic duct dilatation, 141
pancreaticojejunostomy, 137–138
peripancreatic inflammation, 141–142
perivascular cuffing, 139–140
pneumobilia, 140–141
pylorojejunostomy, 138
reactive lymphadenopathy, 140
resection margin, 141
pancreatic anastomotic leak, 142–143
postoperative upper GI contrast studies, 142
resections performed, 128
tumor recurrence, 149–151
vascular complications
abcess and acute pancreatitis, 147
biliary obstruction, 146–147
investigation, 144
radiological management, 144–147
Pancreas preserving total duodenectomy (PPTD)
clinical indications, 118
postoperative imaging and complications, 118, 120
technique, 118–120
uses, 117–118
Pancreatic atrophy, 142
Pancreatic duct dilatation, 141
Pancreaticoduodenectomy (PD), 128–129
Pancreaticojejunostomy, 137–138
Parastomal hernias, 271, 309
Parastomal ulceration, 89
Parietal adhesions, 232
Parks classification system, 280
PC. *See* Proctocolectomy (PC)
Pelvic exenteration and recurrent rectal cancer. *See* Colon
Pelvic floor and defecatory disorders. *See* Colon
Penn pouch, 297
Peptic ulcer disease
duodenal resection and surgery (*see* Duodenal resection and surgery)
gastric resection and surgery
additional operations, 91–92
afferent loop obstruction/ syndrome, 86
anastomotic strictures, 86–88
Billroth II/polya partial gastrectomy, 79, 80
Billroth I partial gastrectomy, 78, 80
clinical indications, 78
efferent complications, 89–91
gastric remnant complications, 89, 90
gastroenterostomy, 80, 82
leak (*see* Anastomotic leak, and duodenal stump leak)
normal postoperative imaging, 82
parastomal ulceration, 89
subtotal gastrectomy with Roux loop reconstruction, 79
total gastrectomy, 80, 81
truncal vagotomy, 80
tumor recurrence, 91
wedge resection, 80
Perineal rectosigmoidectomy, 285
Peripancreatic inflammation, 141–142
Perivascular cuffing, 139–140
Peroral image-guided gastrostomy (PIG), 117
Pigskin mesh, 10, 11
Plain film radiography, 48
Pleural effusions, 136–137
Pneumobilia, 140–141, 160–162, 164
Polya partial gastrectomy. *See* Billroth II partial gastrectomy
Portal vein anastomosis, 218
Portal vein thrombosis (PVT), 32
Port site hernia, 27, 28
Positive contrast, 3
Postablation syndrome, 207
Post-anal repair, 286
Postembolization syndrome, 211
Postoperative abdomen
abnormal
colonic pseudoobstruction, 15–16
fluid collections and abscesses, 11–13
generalized peritonitis, 11, 12
large bowel obstruction, 16
postoperative leaks, 13–14
small bowel obstruction, 14–15
spontaneous bacterial peritonitis, 13
assorted problems
acute cholecystitis, 32–34
acute colitis, 29–30
neutropenic enterocolitis, 32
PVT, 32
small bowel ischemia, 30–32
confusing findings
hemostatic compounds, 9, 10

Postoperative abdomen (*cont.*)
meshes, 9–11
preexisting pathology, 8
CT protocol/technique optimization
anatomical coverage, 5
factors, 2
intravenous contrast, 3–5
luminal contrast, 2–4
single-phase *vs.* multiphase acquisition, 5–6
slice thickness/collimation, 5
fluoroscopy and
contrast selection, 37–38
CT integration, 38
therapeutic effects, 38
iatrogenic postoperative problems
complications, 20–21
drain-related events, 16–18
hemorrhage, 19, 20
intraoperative injury, 18–19
omental infarction, 19–20
retained foreign material, 21–22
surgical material, 21
image-guided drainage
access route, 34
causes, 34
coagulation status assessment, 35–36
consent, 35
modality choice, 34–35
technique, 36–37
laparoscopic surgery related complications
general principles, 22–25
patterns, 25–27
port site hernia, 27, 28
retained tissues or objects, 27–28
wound, 28–29
normal
basal pulmonary atelectasis, 7–8
free gas, 6–7
smoke of battle, 6
wet patient, 7
ultrasound and, 38–39
Postoperative abdominal hernias. *See* Small bowel
Postoperative collection, 306, 307
Postoperative fluid/fat stranding, 139
Postoperative free gas, 6–7
Postoperative ileus, 304
Postoperative internal hernias, 245–246
Postoperative leaks, 13–14
Postpancreatectomy hemorrhage (PPH), 144
Posttransplant lymphoproliferative disease (PTLD), 223
Postvagotomy diarrhea, 91
Pouchitis, 250, 251
Pouch outlet obstruction, 252
Pouch-related sepsis, 250
PPH. *See* Postpancreatectomy hemorrhage (PPH)
PPPD. *See* Pylorus-preserving pancreaticoduodenectomy (PPPD)
PPTD. *See* Pancreas preserving total duodenectomy (PPTD)
Proctocolectomy (PC), 259
Pseudocalculus, 160
Pseudocysts, 136–137
PTLD. *See* Posttransplant lymphoproliferative disease (PTLD)
Puestow procedure, 134
PVT. *See* Portal vein thrombosis (PVT)
Pylorojejunostomy, 138
Pyloroplasty, 92, 93
Pylorus-preserving pancreaticoduodenectomy (PPPD), 129–130

R

Radiation enteropathy, 237–239
Radical antegrade modular pancreatosplenectomy surgery (RAMPS), 130
Radiofrequency ablation (RFA), 193
background, 202
clinical indications, 204
complications, 205–207
features, 202–204
imaging post-RFA, 205, 206
modifications, 204, 205
recurrent disease, 207–208
technique, 204–205
Radiological insertion of gastrostomy (RIG), 278
complications, 117
indications, 115
nonradiological techniques, 115, 116
PIG, 117
technique, 115–117
RAMPS. *See* Radical antegrade modular pancreatosplenectomy surgery (RAMPS)
Reactive lymphadenopathy, 140
Rectal contrast, 3, 4
Recurrent achalasia, 67–69
Recurrent rectal cancer and pelvic exenteration. *See* Colon
Reflux, 65, 66, 68
Restrictive surgery
LAGB, 93–94
sleeve gastrectomy, 93, 94
vertical banded gastroplasty, 93
Retrograde urethrography, 314
RFA. *See* Radiofrequency ablation (RFA)
RHC. *See* Right hemicolectomy (RHC)
Richter's hernia, 244
RIG. *See* Radiological insertion of gastrostomy (RIG)
Right hemicolectomy (RHC), 256, 257
Right posterior oblique (RPO) position, 99
Roux-en-Y enteroenterostomy, 233–234
Roux-en-Y gastric bypass (RYGB), 95–97
Roux-en-Y loop, 129
Roux loop obstruction, 149
RPO position. *See* Right posterior oblique (RPO) position
RYGB. *See* Roux-en-Y gastric bypass (RYGB)

S

Sacral nerve modulation, 287
Sacrocolporectopexy, 284–286
SD. *See* Segmental duodenectomy (SD)

Secondary achalasia, 73
Sedoanesthesia, 115
Segmental duodenectomy (SD)
  clinical indications, 118
  postoperative imaging and complications, 118, 120
  technique, 118–120
  uses, 117–118
Seldinger technique, 36
Selective internal radiation therapy (SIRT), 210
Serum creatinine, 4–5
Seton placement, 281
Short gut syndrome, 240–241
Side-to-end anastomosis, 269, 270
Sigmoid colectomy, 257, 258
Sigmoidopexy, 278–279
Single-port surgery (SILS), 23
SIRT. *See* Selective internal radiation therapy (SIRT)
Sleeve gastrectomy, 93, 94
Slow transit constipation surgery, 284
Small bowel
  anatomy, 228
  bypass, 234
  CT
    advantages, 229
    closed loop obstruction and ischemia, 231–232
    image analysis, 230–231
    technique, 230
  dilatation, 230
  feeding jejunostomy
    surgical technique, 241
    tube displacement, 242
    tube occulation, 241–242
    tube site infection and leak, 241, 242
  ileus and obstruction, 222, 223
  ileus and SBO, 228–230
  IPAA
    advantages, 246
    background, 248
    CT, 249–250
    GI contrast studies, 248–249
    pouch construct, 247–248
    stages, 247
  mechanical SBO causes
    adhesions, 232
    intussusception, 233
    postoperative hernias, 232–233
  operations
    abscess, 235
    anastomotic leaks, 234–235
    anastomotic stricture, 236–237
    blind pouch syndrome, 235–236
    common modifications, 234, 235
    Crohn's disease and, 239–240
    disease recurrence, 236–237
    radiation enteropathy, 237–239
    resection, 234
    Roux-en-Y enteroenterostomy, 233–234
    short gut syndrome, 240–241
    surgical procedures, 233
  postoperative abdominal hernias
    complications, 244, 246
    hernia repair, 242–243
    imaging, 243–244
    incisional hernia, 244, 245
    internal hernias, 245–246
    mesh placement, 242, 243
    Richter's hernia, 244
    surgical technique, 243
  postoperative complications
    anastomotic leak, 250–252
    anastomotic stricture, 250
    fistulas, 252
    pelvic infection and abscess, 251
    pouchitis, 250, 251
    pouch outlet obstruction, 252
    pouch-related sepsis, 250
    SBO, 249
  resection, 234
Small bowel obstruction (SBO), 14–15. *See* Small bowel
Smoke of battle, 6
Solid pancreatic tumors, 128
SonoVue, 205
Split liver transplantation, 215
Spontaneous bacterial peritonitis, 13
S-pouch, 247–248
Stapled transanal rectal resection (STARR), 284, 285
Steal effect, 268
Stenosis and retraction, 271–272
Stents, 58
Stomach and duodenum
  bariatric surgery
    anastomotic leaks, 100–103
    CT, 99–101
    duodenal switch with biliopancreatic diversion, 96–97
    efferent loop obstruction (*see* Efferent loop obstruction)
    fistula to excluded stomach, 102–104
    fluoroscopy, 97–100
    gastric channel and gastric outlet obstruction, 104–105
    gastric remnant and biliopancreatic limb obstruction, 109–110
    LAGB (*see* Laparoscopic adjustable gastric band (LAGB))
    M and M procedure, 95, 96
    morbid obesity, 92
    obese patients, 97
    restriction lack and weight gain, 110, 111
    RYGB, 95–97
    sleeve gastrectomy, 93, 94
    vertical banded gastroplasty, 93
  gastroesophageal reflux surgery
    clinical indications, 72
    dysphagia and dysmotility, 73
    fundoplication dehiscence, 76
    fundoplication principles and types, 72
    intrathoracic wrap herniation, 74–76

Stomach and duodenum (*cont.*)
normal postoperative imaging, 72–73
relevant historic antireflux procedures, 76–77
wrap migration/slipped wrap, 74
hiatus hernia repair
clinical indication, 77
postoperative complications and imaging, 78, 79
surgical technique, 77–78
peptic ulcer disease
duodenal resection and surgery (*see* Duodenal resection and surgery)
gastric resections and surgery (*see* Gastric resections and surgery)
RIG
complications, 117
indications, 115
nonradiological techniques, 115, 116
PIG, 117
technique, 115–117
Stomal stenosis, 148
Stomas. *See* Colon
Strasberg's classification, 167, 169
Stricturoplasty, 234, 235
Studer technique, 297
Sublay mesh, 242–243
Subtotal cholecystectomy, 155
Subtotal colectomy (STC), 259
Subtotal gastrectomy, 79
Supercharging, 61
Suprasphincteric fistula, 280
Surgicel, 263. *See also* Hemostatic compounds

T
TACE. *See* Transcatheter arterial chemoebolization (TACE)
TAPP technique. *See* Transabdominal preperitoneal (TAPP) technique
TC. *See* Total colectomy (TC)
TEP technique. *See* Totally extraperitoneal (TEP) technique
Testicular atrophy, 244
Textiloma, 21
Three-stage esophagectomy. *See* Lewis-McKeown procedure
TME. *See* Total mesorectal excision (TME)
Total colectomy (TC), 258, 259
Total gastrectomy, 80, 81
Totally extraperitoneal (TEP) technique, 243
Total mesorectal excision (TME), 285
Total pancreatectomy, 128
Transabdominal preperitoneal (TAPP) technique, 243
Transcatheter arterial chemoebolization (TACE), 193
advantages, 209
clinical indications, 209
complications, 211–212
imaging post-TACE, 210–211
recurrent malignancy post-TACE imaging, 212–214
technique, 209–210
Transhiatal esophagectomy, 44–46
Transsphincteric fistula, 280
Transverse colectomy, 256, 257
Truncal vagotomy, 80
Tube necrosis/ischemia, 53–54
Tube torsion, 54
Tumor recurrence, 149–151, 309–310
Tumor seeding, 207
T2W sequences, 273, 275
Typhlitis, 32

U
Ultrasound, postoperative abdomen, 38–39
Ureteric injury, 18
background, 310
contrast studies, 310–311
CT, 311
Ureteric stricture, 306–308
Ureteroileostomy, 296
Urethral injury
background, 314
contrast studies, 314–315
CT, 315
Urinary diversion. *See* Genitourinary system
Urinary infection, 306
Urinary leak, 305–306

V
Vascular complications
liver, 198–200
pancreas
abcess and acute pancreatitis, 147
biliary obstruction, 146–147
investigation, 144
radiological management, 144–147
post-RFA complications, 205–207
Vascular injury, 179–180
Vascular staplers, 269
Veress needle, 24
Vertical banded gastroplasty, 93
Visceral adhesions, 232
Voiding cystourethrography, 314

W
Wallace technique, 296, 297
Warfarin, 36
Wedge resection, 80
Whirl sign, 231
W-pouch, 247–248
Wrap migration/slipped wrap, 74

Y
Yttrium-90, 210

MIX
Papier aus verantwortungsvollen Quellen
Paper from responsible sources
FSC® C105338

If you have any concerns about our products,
you can contact us on
ProductSafety@springernature.com

In case Publisher is established outside the EU,
the EU authorized representative is:
Springer Nature Customer Service Center GmbH
Europaplatz 3, 69115 Heidelberg, Germany

Printed by Libri Plureos GmbH
in Hamburg, Germany